Doctor, Say What?

Doctor, Say What?

PART II

THE GUIDES

What Works and What Doesn't:
Step-by-Step Integrative Treatments for Over Ninety Medical Conditions

Larry Altshuler MD

ISBN: 1519269994
ISBN 13: 9781519269997

Contents

CHAPTER 1

Introduction to the Guides

By reading Part I of this book "*The Inside Scoop on Getting the Best Medical Care,*" you will have gained a significant amount of information on the three major medical approaches: preventive, conventional, and alternative. You will have learned in general what you may or may not expect from these medical approaches and what you need to know to avoid the negatives and obtain benefit from the positives. You will also have learned how nonmedical factors may influence the health care you receive and how to navigate the present health care system and future changes. You should now be empowered to take an active role in your health and health care!

The Guides provide potential options to help you control or even resolve specific medical conditions from which you may suffer. ***You need to realize, however, that this is just a guide***: This information will inform you of the many choices available to treat your condition and provide you suggestions on what treatments may help you the most from the preventive, alternative and conventional medical approaches. But ***you will then need to take this information to a practitioner who has expertise in that particular area.***

―――――⚭―――――

Disclaimer: *The recommendations made in the following pages are based on current research and expert opinion, both conventional and alternative. There is no way I can know everything about you: I don't know the results of your diagnostic tests, your physical examination, your other medical conditions, or what treatments you have already undergone. Remember, also, that all types of treatment may have side effects and complications, which I cannot predict. This book does not constitute a doctor-patient relationship for those reasons. This information and the recommendations should serve only as a basic road map to assist you and your practitioner in determining your best course of treatment. The author disclaims any liability arising directly or indirectly from the use of this book.*

―――――⚭―――――

A very important factor is to have faith. No matter how many medical conditions you have or how bad those conditions are, there may still be hope that you can control, help reverse, or maybe even resolve these diseases. A recent study evaluated disease and disability among centenarians and discovered that one-third had suffered from a disabling condition like COPD, diabetes, or dementia for over fifteen years yet had required only minimal or no assistance in their daily lives; you also may be able to achieve this goal and have a better of quality of life by following these guides.

Important Note:
Illness and Happiness: Can You Have Both?

We know that being ill can cause unhappiness, and in fact, research reveals that health influences happiness more than money. On the other hand, happiness can enhance health. So it behooves us to be happy, even when ill. Is that possible?

A study published in the *Journal of Happiness Studies* showed that it wasn't illness per se that determined happiness but rather how much an illness disrupts your daily functioning, that is, your quality of life (QOL).

In the following pages, I make recommendations to help you treat illnesses in the most cost-effective manner possible, but I realize that you may not be able to completely resolve your medical conditions. Even so, many of these recommendations will improve your quality of life, and that in itself is extremely important. If your quality of life is improved, you will be happier; and, in turn, your medical condition may also improve. Rather than a vicious cycle, it is a healing cycle.

CHAPTER 2

The Balancing Act: Getting the Most out of Your Treatment Choices

Your health is unique to you. Although the treatments suggested in the following pages work for many people, they don't work for everyone, and some initial steps may not work as well as later steps. You and your medical provider may need to appraise various methods to find the combination that provides the results you are seeking.

The evolution of health has gone from "hands-on" care to high-tech care. There certainly are advantages to our wonderful technology, but there are also some significant disadvantages. In many cases, returning to a more hands-on, alternative approach may be more effective for you as well as less expensive; but in other cases, the high-tech approaches may be your best bet.

There are several kinds of information provided in the *Guides*.

- ■ *What You Need to Know* will relate aspects of the condition that are important to understand so that you will be better able to determine your best course of treatment. Certain aspects of the condition (such as symptoms, causes, or testing) may not be described in depth as there are numerous resources available with this information. Treatment of the condition is the primary focus.

- ■ *Treatments for the Condition* will summarize the therapies used by the three major medical approaches for that particular condition and relate important facts that you may need to know about those therapies. *Preventive* treatments are not only intended to prevent the condition but also to prevent *worsening* of the condition and *improving* the condition if you already are afflicted with it. For *conventional* treatments, there may be categories that include several options (such as different medications that all can be beneficial for that condition) but I cannot suggest the best one for *you* as that can depend on many factors, including your age, gender, and other medical conditions you may have:

you will need to consult with your doctor. The same is true for some *alternative* therapies such as herbs and supplements: some may work better for you than others, and you will need to consult a naturopath or herbalist.

- ***Important Notes, Warnings, Cautions and Helpful Hints*** will be given to provide additional, relevant information that you need to know about specific therapies.
- ***Your Empowered Patient Action Plan for the Condition*** gives you general step-by-step guides for treating the condition and reasons why certain steps are suggested before others. Again, however, each of you is different, so the order of these steps may vary depending on other physical, psychological, and environmental factors that may affect you.
- ***Expected Outcome*** will describe what you may expect from these treatments.

Finding Qualified Practitioners

Again, *The Guides* only provide you with information regarding treatment options that may help your condition(s). The details of how to use these therapies most appropriately should be provided by a practitioner qualified in that medical approach. So, although you can use many alternative methods on your own, I recommend that you at least begin by seeing a qualified practitioner of that method. This is especially important with alternative therapies that require different types of diagnostics than conventional medicine, such as Chinese medicine. For many alternative practices, a knowledgeable, trained practitioner is able to help you determine the best approach within that method or may be necessary to provide that particular treatment.

With conventional medicine, it is certainly important for you to consult a physician(s) to determine the treatment that is best for your individual needs as many conventional treatments require a doctor's prescription, referral, or authorization. In addition, you may have other conditions or be undergoing other treatments that can interfere with each other, causing potential harm. It would be most helpful to find a physician who is at least open to helping you explore all methods for your particular condition(s). In general, for non-emergency medical problems, it may be best to start with a primary care physician (PCP) but if you are not improving, being evaluated by a specialist may be necessary.

By using the recommendations in chapter 2, you can empower yourself to find a practitioner who can work well with you and find the treatments that are best for you. You will also know how to evaluate all your options and choose the best one(s) for your health and well-being.

Determining Appropriate Treatments

In the following guides, I have discussed numerous treatments options and provided general step-by-step suggestions regarding which ones you may want to begin with. There are several general aspects that I use to determine my recommendations.

- First, conventional and alternative treatments may be equally effective in treating many conditions. When this is the case, the most cost-effective treatments with the least potential for side effects/harm will be recommended first.
- Also, treatments that involve invasive methods or surgery are usually recommended as a last resort for most conditions, unless they are clearly the best solution for resolving that condition.
- When a specific type of treatment contains several options that may be effective (for example: medications for blood pressure or supplements for heart disease), I delineate differences among them when possible but when not plausible, you will need to consult with a practitioner of that method to determine which one is the best for you
- Dosages for conventional medications are not listed in the guides since they must be determined and prescribed by your doctor.
- The dosages most commonly suggested by research findings and alternative practitioners will be provided when recommending alternative products. Understand, however, that such dosages can vary depending on the form of the product and the manufacturing process (see chapter 4 for further details). For Chinese herbs, you should consult with a practitioner certified in Chinese herbal therapy, especially with complex conditions.
- There are alternative devices, treatments and nutritional supplements as well as some conventional treatments recommended that you may be unfamiliar with. These have been discussed fully in chapters two to four in Part I and you should refer to those chapters before using these methods or refer to the Appendix for referral sources and to obtain more information on these methods from trained and certified practitioners.

To Your Optimal Health

Whatever your health condition and treatment options, I hope that this guide will help you find and use the most beneficial balance of preventive, alternative, and conventional methods for your personal and particular needs and conditions. My goal is to help you understand all your options, help you stay as healthy as possible, and enjoy an excellent quality of life.

CHAPTER 3

The Conditions

Allergic Rhinitis

What You Need to Know

Allergic rhinitis is one of the most common chronic diseases in the United States. Although you might think of allergic rhinitis as more of a nuisance, it can impact your life in ways you may not be aware of, even affecting your brain function. (See Table 1)

---∞---

Table 1
Effects of Allergic Rhinitis
Outside the Nose

Sleep disorders:
    78% suffer from lack of good night's sleep
    75% are unable to fall asleep
    64% wake up during the night
Fatigue
Learning problems
Cognitive function deterioration:
    Vigilance (sustained attention)
    Concentration
    Nonverbal learning (i.e., learning a new direction)
    Processing speed (response time)
    Mental flexibility
    Visual perceptual speed (i.e., reading speed)

There are two basic types of allergic rhinitis: seasonal and perennial (year around), and these are treated slightly differently by both conventional and alternative approaches.

Be Cautious of Allergy Testing

If you are unsure what you are allergic to, you can obtain testing from an allergy specialist. However, the technical aspects of allergy testing and the validity of the skin-scratch tests have been studied and questioned for years. The results may not be very reproducible, and the production of reliable, standardized allergens for use in testing has been difficult. Frequently patients are found to be allergic to everything on a panel or to nothing on a panel, both of which may not be accurate.

Treatments for Allergic Rhinitis

The Preventive Approaches
Eliminate or avoid contact with the allergens from your environment that may be causing your allergies, or reduce contact with them.

The Conventional Approaches
Medications. These include first-generation and second-generation antihistamines, decongestants, corticosteroids, leukotriene antagonists, and mast cell stabilizers. Each has different effects on symptoms, as seen in Table 2.

Table 2
Allergy Medication Effects on Symptoms

Agent	Sneezing	Itching	Congestion	Drainage	Eye
Oral antihistamines	++	++	+/--	++	++
Nasal antihistamines	+	+	+/--	+	--
Intranasal steroids	++	++	++	++	+
Oral decongestants	--	--	+	--	--
Intranasal decongestants	--	--	++	--	--
Mast cell stabilizers	+	+	+	+	--
Leukotriene inhibitors	+	+	+	+	--

Here's a brief rundown on these medications.

First-generation antihistamines, including Benadryl, Tavist, Drixoral, and Dimetapp, can cause sedation (20 percent of patients), dry mouth, urinary hesitancy (difficulty starting the stream), or cognitive problems. However, they are much less expensive than the second-generation antihistamines, so if you don't have bothersome side effects, these are a good first choice.

Second-generation antihistamines, including fenofenadine (Allegra), citirizine (Zyrtec), and loratadine (Claritin, Alavert), have fewer side effects but are more expensive than the first–generation medicines. Citirizine (Zyrtec) is the only one that may cause sedation (10 percent of people). Citirizine and loratadine are second-generation antihistamines that you can buy OTC, so they are cheaper than the others: (**Note**: Clarinex is a prescription version of Claritin, but is basically the same drug). There is only one intranasal antihistamine spray, azelastine (Astelin), but it can cause drowsiness in 11 percent of people, and 20 percent may experience an initial bad taste from the medication.

Helpful tip: Store-brand antihistamines are usually just as effective but are much cheaper than OTC trade-name antihistamines. Just look for the generic name listed in the ingredients to compare prices.

Corticosteroid intranasal sprays: Although most people with allergic rhinitis use antihistamines, prescription nasal steroid sprays are actually thought to be better for "as-needed" allergic symptoms during allergy season because they provide longer-lasting relief and work better and faster with repeated exposure to allergens. Prescription steroid nasal sprays, including Nasocort, Vancenase, Beconase, and Flonase (the latter is reported to have less stinging sensation), also have minimal side effects. Intranasal steroids are not significantly absorbed into the body, so they are relatively safe over the short-term; however, they do not provide complete relief in about 40 percent of patients. Nasocort and Flonase have both become available OTC, so they will be less expensive.

Warning: Steroid nasal sprays may cause cataracts with long-term use, so be sure to use them only when necessary (usually allergy "season"), and have your eyes checked regularly if you must use them long term.

Helpful tip: A recent study showed that a combination of intranasal steroid and intranasal antihistamine is more effective than either one alone. The combination is indicated in severe allergies or with uncontrolled symptoms.

Decongestants: These drugs constrict blood vessels and are commonly used to relieve congestion. They include pseudoephedrine (Sudafed) or phenylephrine. Side effects include insomnia, nervousness, headache, fast heartbeat, high blood pressure, and urinary retention. Some states do not allow or have restricted sales of pseudoephedrine due to its use in making methamphetamines; as a result, more products contain phenylephrine but a 2015 study showed that it is no better than placebo. Most decongestants are found in combination products with antihistamines. As with antihistamines, store-brand combination products may be as effective as, but less expensive than, trade-name brands.

Inhaled decongestants such as oxymetazoline (Afrin, Dristan and many others, including generic versions) basically have the same mechanism as the above decongestants and work very quickly, and they are especially useful for nighttime congestion. However, prolonged use has been associated with rebound congestion lasting up to a week. *Helpful Tip*: A 2011 study published in the *Journal of Allergy and Clinical Immunology* showed that if taken with inhaled steroids, the rebound effect is mitigated, so it can be taken long-term in combination.

Leukotriene inhibitors (Montelukast): This drug blocks one pathway in the allergic response, primarily the one causing congestion. It is as effective as second-generation antihistamines but less effective than nasal steroids. It may take three days to a week to have an effect.

Mast cell stabilizers (cromolyn sodium) stabilize the mast cells, which can be damaged in allergic reactions and release histamine, which in turn can cause allergy symptoms. They must be given before allergic reactions take place, and they have very limited use because they are less effective than nasal steroids. They also may take three weeks to have an effect. They can be obtained OTC.

Immunotherapy (allergy "shots") works by injecting increasingly larger amounts of allergens into your body so that your system becomes desensitized to them and no longer overreacts in response to them. It treats the cause of the allergy, not the symptoms. However, it may take up to one year to know if it will work and if it does, you will need to take the shots for 3 to 5 years. It may lose its effectiveness with chronic use but in many people, the symptoms may not return for years after stopping the injections.

Important note: Immunotherapy is also effective sublingually (under the tongue) and is commonly used in Europe, but US products are poorly standardized, and the units of potency differ from those used in Europe. The one product approved by the FDA is Ragwitek (short ragweed pollen allergen extract for ragweed allergies), and it is prescribed for use twelve weeks before ragweed season and you use it until the end of the season.

Hope in the Future?

Researchers have discovered that administering carbon dioxide for sixty seconds into each nostril, without inhalation, can reduce symptoms of allergic rhinitis within minutes and last for at least twenty-four hours. The method is not yet approved and requires more research, but in the future, you may be able to treat yourself at home for two minutes and be free of symptoms for days.

The Alternative Approaches
Acupuncture*:* The best alternative treatment for allergies is acupuncture, which has the potential to resolve it completely for years or at least significantly reduce the symptoms. Even one acupuncture treatment may be able to drain congested sinuses and help prevent sinus infection, although more may be needed for longer-lasting relief. Because acupuncture addresses the underlying cause, it can provide long-term relief.

Chinese herbs*:* Along with acupuncture, Chinese herbal formulas are commonly used, again to enhance and accelerate the effects. Various formulas are beneficial, depending on whether you have asthma, a stuffy or runny nose, sinus congestion, colored sputum, or other symptoms. A commonly prescribed formula is *Bi Yan Pian*, used for stuffy runny nose but not for dryness. Other formulas include *Bi Yan Pian, Cang Er Zi San, Qing Bi Tang, Xiao Qing Long Tang, or Yu Ping Feng Sang*, depending on your pulse and tongue diagnosis and symptoms.

Low level energy laser can also be very useful to reduce or resolve symptoms and can potentiate the benefits from acupuncture. This type of laser reduces sinus and nasal inflammation and is applied directly over the sinuses. It has no known side effects when treating allergies. Because LLEL addresses the underlying cause, it can provide long-term relief.

Nasal irrigation: An excellent natural (and inexpensive) treatment is the neti pot, which is used for nasal irrigation, although you can also use a bulb syringe with a mixture of a teaspoon of salt and half a teaspoon of baking soda in two cups of warm water. There are also nasal irrigation kits that can be found in any drugstore. Studies have shown that short-term irrigation for seasonal allergies can be helpful, but there is some debate regarding long-term use. A Cochrane review in 2009 showed

long-term irrigation to be beneficial without harmful effects, but other studies suggest that routine cleansings for more than a year may cause more frequent sinus infections. *Important Note*: Use filtered water only and clean the Neti pot frequently.

Western herbs*:* There are numerous western herbs and supplements that mimic the actions of conventional drugs and have been used for allergic rhinitis. These include:

- *Leukotriene inhibitor*: Butterbur, an herb from Europe (7.5 mg total petasine and isopetasine taken four times daily), has recently been shown to be as effective as conventional antihistamines but without causing drowsiness.
- *Mast cell stabilizers*: Quercetin, spirulina (blue-green algae), vitamin C, stinging nettle. Stinging nettle has been proven effective for rhinitis. You should use freeze-dried (cryogenic) preparations (one, three times daily, 300–600 mg daily).
- *Antihistamines*: Grapeseed extract and pycnogenol, which are not very effective for allergic rhinitis.
- *Decongestants*: Bitter orange (has replaced ephedra, which was banned in 2004 due to serious side effects and deaths). *Caution*: Bitter orange does have side effects on heart function, much like ephedra did. Read the labels for other names, including Citrus arantium, Zhi Shi, or Fructus arantii.
- *Immunotherapy*: Echinacea is often used but is ineffective.
- *Ayurvedic herb*: Tinospora cordifolia (300 mg three times a day) may be able to decrease allergy symptoms.
- *Others*: MSM and capsaicin (intranasally) has some initial research indicating possible benefits.

Homeopathy has also been used successfully for allergies, with each formula dependent on the particular symptoms. Arsenicum album (6c) can be used for runny nose, itchy throat, and sneezing; Pulsatilla (6c) can be used for chronic, thick mucus; and Allium cepa (6c) can be used for runny nose and itchy eyes. You should experience improvement in one to two months.

Your Empowered Patient Action Plan for Allergic Rhinitis

Step #1: Undergo acupuncture. This is the one approach that has the greatest potential to resolve allergies long term or significantly reduce the need for medications or injections.

Step #2: Undergo low-level energy laser on the sinuses and nose, either alone or with acupuncture.

Step #3: Take homeopathic remedies. These are preferred before the following steps because there are minimal side effects, and they may also potentially give long-lasting relief or resolution of allergies.

*Step #4: **Use a neti pot*** for short-term relief—and hopefully to avoid the need for herbs or drugs.

*Step #5: **Take stinging nettle or butterbur.*** These herbs can be as effective as and much less expensive than conventional drugs, but without the side effects.

*Step #6: **Take Chinese herbal remedies*** based on your Chinese tongue and pulse diagnosis and symptoms. These can be taken with acupuncture to enhance its effectiveness or if acupuncture is not effective.

*Step #7: **Take conventional drugs if the above steps are not beneficial.***

- For seasonal allergies, start with a nasal steroid one to two weeks before the season starts and throughout the season.
- For nighttime congestion, add inhaled oxymetazoline (OTC nasal spray) to inhaled steroids.
- For continued symptoms, use an oral antihistamine, with or without an oral decongestant.
- For perennial allergies, take nasal steroids and/or oral antihistamines (with or without decongestants).
- For both seasonal and perennial allergies, if severe, take both nasal steroids and oral antihistamines together.
- If symptoms persist, try a topical nasal antihistamine.
- If you still have severe symptoms, consider discussing with your doctor whether to prescribe a short course (three to ten days) of oral steroids.

*Step #8: **Try immunotherapy*** (allergy shots or sublingual). Consult an allergy specialist for testing and prescription. Sublingual treatment may work as well as injections if you have ragweed allergies. Over the long-term, immunotherapy may be more expensive than the previous conventional treatments.

Expected Outcome

With successful treatment using acupuncture, you have the potential to resolve your allergies for the long term. If not, there are many methods, both conventional and alternative, that can control your symptoms adequately and improve your quality of life.

Alzheimer's Disease and Dementia

What You Need to Know

Dementia is a progressive deterioration of nerve tissue in the brain. There are many different types of dementia, but over 50 percent involve the form called Alzheimer's.

There are also different magnitudes of dementia, from mild cognitive impairment to full-blown dementia.

The frequency of dementia increases with rising age from less than 2 percent for sixty-five to sixty-nine year-olds, to 5 percent for seventy-five to seventy-nine year-olds, and to more than 20 percent for the eighty-five to eighty-nine year-olds. Over the age of ninety, 41 percent of women and 28 percent of men suffer from dementia. Although there is no cure, there are many treatments that can slow the disease process.

Survival after Dementia Onset

A recent study showed that the median survival time for people diagnosed with dementia is 4.5 years. Factors associated with shorter survival included older age at onset, being a male, and having a disability before onset. Scores on mental status and education did not make a difference.

Important Note: Be aware that older patients with sleep apnea can be mistaken to have dementia because loss of sleep affects brain function. If you snore at night, have breathing problems, stop breathing at night for short periods of time, have restless sleep, or have excess daytime sleepiness, you should be checked for sleep apnea before being treated for dementia (see section on *Insomnia and Sleep Apnea*).

The Most Common Symptoms of Dementia

- Memory loss
- Repeating oneself
- Forgetting recent events
- Forgetting appointments
- Failure of "new" learning

A simple screening test for dementia, called the Sweet Sixteen, involves a sixteen-item test that requires only two to three minutes. If positive, more extensive testing is necessary. It does have a few false positives but is generally very reliable. You should know that there are no laboratory tests that can diagnose dementia, which is best diagnosed based on history (including mental status exam) and physical exam. However, a CT scan of the head and B$_{12}$ and thyroid function testing should be done to rule out other causes.

It is important to realize that over half of Alzheimer's patients are not told their diagnosis. According to the Alzheimer's Association, only 45 percent of patients with medical claims indicating a diagnosis of Alzheimer's were told of the diagnosis by their doctor. These statistics may even be worse for other types of dementia. Since the earlier the diagnosis, the better patients are able to make important decisions for their future care, you should make sure to review your diagnoses with your doctor.

Dr. A's Suggestions:
Should Alzheimer's Be Screened?

There is a lot of controversy regarding whether older people should be screened for Alzheimer's. Some doctors think that early detection would give patients the best shot at successful treatment, but there is no data yet showing that screening people who have no memory complaints leads to better outcomes. In fact, existing medications appear to help only those who already have dementia.

Screening can involve just a few tests for word recall, but a recent study showed that only one out of five people screened positive was referred to a specialist or given medication. If you or your loved ones have memory problems, you should be screened, but make sure you get proper treatment if the test is positive.

Rarely, doctors may perform brain biopsies in patients who have rapid decline in their mental capacity. A recent study in *Neurology* showed that such an invasive procedure can diagnose unknown causes in 35 percent of people, but in only 4 percent do these findings alter therapy. Brain biopsy should be considered only after careful examination of the potential harms versus benefits.

Important Information:
Tube Feedings, Dialysis Not Helpful in Dementia

Studies have shown that dialysis in elderly patients with dementia or heart dysfunction does not offer significant advantages compared with not performing dialysis. It is also recognized that tube feeding does not prolong life in severely demented patients (and is more frequently done in for-profit hospitals).

Treatments for Alzheimer's and Dementia

The Preventive Approaches

Keep your brain active and engaged as you age. Information-processing activities seem the most helpful; these include watching television; listening to the radio; reading newspapers, magazines, or books; playing games or solving puzzles; and visiting museums. However, you should frequently alter your activities because repetitive, habitual actions do not improve brain function (see chapter 2 regarding neuroplasticity).

Good Sleep has recently been shown to be protective against Alzheimer's; the study showed that a lack of deep sleep contributes to the deposition of a protein called beta amyloid, found to be increased (and may be causative) in the brains of Alzheimer patients. Another study from Berkeley showed that watching TV for four hours daily could also increase Alzheimer's risk.

Smoking increases oxidative stress and inflammation and should be stopped. A study in the *Archives of Internal Medicine* revealed that heavy smoking in midlife doubles the risk for dementia in older age.

Another study revealed that a deficiency of the B vitamin **folate** may triple the risk of dementia. This correlates with the findings that people with high serum folate levels have decreased risk of Alzheimer's. Have your folate level tested through a blood test, and if low, take supplemental folate and eat foods fortified in folate.

Another study in 2015 showed that several **medications** may increase the risk of dementia. Those who took the highest dosage had a 54 percent higher dementia risk than those who took the lowest doses. These included the older antihistamines (first generation, such as chlorpheneramine or Benadryl) so it is advised to use the second line generation instead (see section on *Allergies*). Other drugs that had this effect included tricyclic antihistamines (Sinequan) and oxybutynin (Ditropan, used for incontinence).

Technology for the Brain?

Several companies have designed products to improve memory and cognition through listening exercises or vision. These exercises are contained in software that can help support decision making, fine motor control, and gross motor control (balance). Although some studies have found long-lasting benefit by undergoing training for memory, reasoning, or speed of mental processing, another study showed that presently existing computer "brain-training" programs are not adequate to *prevent* dementia.

Diet: Antioxidants, which are found in certain foods, especially fruits and vegetables, have been shown to slow and even reverse the memory loss caused by the free-radical damage in Alzheimer's. Foods containing vitamin E and vitamin C have been shown to reduce the risk of dementia. B vitamins, especially folate, are also important, so green leafy vegetables are especially good, as well as eggs, low-fat dairy, and low-fat meats.

Researchers have shown that the Mediterranean diet, which is high in fruits and vegetables, not only can help prevent or delay Alzheimer's but can also add several years of life to those who are already diagnosed with the disease. The MIND diet, a hybrid of the Mediterranean and the DASH (Dietary Approaches to Stop Hypertension) diets, has shown to slow cognitive decline in elderly adults if rigorously followed. Another study showed that drinking fruit and vegetable juices at least three times week can delay the onset of Alzheimer's (*Caution*: watch the sugar content! Look for products that are 100% vegetable and/or juice, with no added high fructose corn syrup). Finally, a 2013 study showed that a high-fat diet (high glycemic index) could interrupt the clearance of beta amyloid, whereas a low glycemic diet reduced levels, so the latter is much preferred. (For a complete listing of glycemic values for all foods, go to www. mendosa.com.)

Omega-3 fatty acids from freshwater fish (such as mackerel, tuna, halibut, cod, trout, and salmon) may help fight inflammation in the brain caused by the beta amyloid.

Drinking four to six cups of green tea a week has been shown in small studies to reduce the risk of cognitive impairment.

Light-to-moderate intake of alcohol may lower the risk of dementia. Any type of alcohol (not only red wine) has this effect. However, high alcohol intake does more harm than good, so you should limit your intake to not more than one drink per night for women and two drinks per night for men (see appropriate alcohol doses in chapter 2).

Walking: A recent observational study published in *Neurology* revealed that older adults who walk frequently have lower risk for cognitive decline years later. It apparently prevents age-related shrinkage and improves special memory.

Treatments for certain concurrent diseases may be able to help prevent dementia. These include:

- *High cholesterol*: use of statin medications may dramatically reduce the risk of dementia (see section on *Cholesterol* for medication information).
- *High blood pressure* (especially the systolic or higher reading) also increases the risk of Alzheimer's, but low blood pressure (the diastolic or lower reading, less than 70 mm Hg) has been shown to double the risk for Alzheimer's, so correct blood pressure control will help prevent dementia.
- *Depression* nearly doubles the risk for dementia in older age, so controlling depression is essential.

BENZODIAZEPINES MAY RAISE THE RISK OF ALZHEIMER'S

A 2014 study in *BMJ* suggests that benzodiazepines (alprazolam o[Xanax], diazepam] [Valium], lorazepam [Ativan], etc.) are associated with excess risk for developing Alzheimer's. This is primarily when using these drugs chronically for five to ten years. Because these drugs can reduce certain receptors in the brain, they potentially could make you worse if you have Alzheimer's.

The Conventional Approaches

Medications are the mainstay of conventional treatment for dementia and Alzheimer's disease. Unfortunately, there is actually little information to guide doctors on which drugs to use. The authors of guidelines published in the *Annals of Internal Medicine* in 2008 pointed out that although many studies found statistically significant improvement in measures of cognition (brain function), many improvements "were not clinically important." They also revealed that the evidence is insufficient to compare the effectiveness of different drugs. They recommended that treatment choices should be made based on the drug's tolerability, side effects, ease of use, and cost.

Acetylcholinesterase inhibitors (Donepezil [Aricept], galantamine [Razadyne], and rivastigmine [Exelon]) are the primary drugs prescribed. However, a recent study in *Neurology* showed that donepezil was not effective for mild impairment, and the others also have only modest cognitive benefits. Donepezil can be obtained as a generic. Rivastigmine is now available in a patch, which has the advantage of fewer side effects and does not require swallowing a pill. If these are not effective, your doctor may recommend metrifonate as the next conventional drug to take.

Warning: The above drugs do have increased risks of falls, injury, and the possible need for pacemaker placement. They should be stopped if you have repeated falls, slow heart rate, or fainting spells.

Memantine (Namenda) is a newer drug. Although it will not stop the disease, it may temporarily reverse some symptoms or slow the disease development. In studies with Namenda alone, about 29 percent of patients showed improvement in symptoms such as behavior, attention, language, memory, orientation, social interaction, and activities of daily living. When Namenda was given to patients already on Aricept, patients showed major improvement over Aricept alone. Namenda has also been shown to reduce the number of hours caregivers work. Full effect may take anywhere from four to eight weeks. Although it is not a miracle cure, some patients have improved and progression of the disease has slowed.

Hydergine is an older drug that may provide some symptomatic relief in some people with dementia. The symptoms helped may include mental alertness, confusion, recent memory, orientation, emotional lability, appetite and anxiety/fears. Hydergine has very few side effects, most commonly occasional short-lasting nausea.

Tacrine hydrochloride (Cognex) is a conventional drug that has been shown to delay progression of Alzheimer's by six months. **Warning**: This drug can cause liver toxicity, which must be monitored closely. You might try this medication only if you're dealing with dementia that is resistant to other drugs and treatments.

In the future, a Russian drug called *dimebon* (Medivation), originally marketed as an antihistamine, may provide benefit for all symptoms of Alzheimer's. A study done by the manufacturer showed that these benefits were sustained over time, but it has not been approved in the United States yet.

Inappropriate Medications for Dementia Patients

A recent report revealed that thousands of nursing homes nationwide are using powerful antipsychotic drugs to quiet disruptive people with dementia. In fact, these drugs are the primary drugs paid for by Medicaid. Although some people may benefit from these drugs, they can also cause more confusion, falls, and even death. A study published in the *Archives of Internal Medicine* showed that "even short-term use of these medications is often followed by adverse events leading to hospitalization or death."

Experts say that there are almost always better ways to control disruptive behavior. Unfortunately, giving a pill is much easier, despite being contraindicated in most people.

In addition, a study published in *Lancet* in July, 2011, revealed that using antidepressants for depressed patients with Alzheimer's is no more effective than placebo.

In *advanced* dementia, many of the above medications have marginal benefit but can have significant side effects. In addition, many of these patients are taking other medications, such as statin drugs for cholesterol and blood thinners. All of these drugs are considered inappropriate and simply add to the cost of care. It is important to understand that as these patients worsen, these drugs should be discontinued.

Reality orientation therapy improves thinking functions. This is a process that strives to reorient the person to time, place, and person. It is often effective in people who have moderate to severe dementia, in combination with the above steps. Consult a doctor or clinic that specializes in Alzheimer's treatment for this type of therapy.

The Alternative Approaches
Herbs and supplements are the primary alternative approach to dementia and many have similar actions to conventional drugs.

Huperzine A (50–200 mcg twice daily), derived from Chinese club moss, has been shown to improve memory, cognitive function, and behavioral function in patients with Alzheimer's, multi-infarct, and senile dementia.

Folate deficiency is associated with depression and dementia in the elderly and may help improve cognitive function and memory using higher doses. L-methylfolate (Cerefolin) is a form commonly prescribed.

Vitamin E (2000 IU daily) is associated with slower functional decline in patients with mild-to-moderate Alzheimer's, according to a 2103 *JAMA* study.

Phosphatidylserine (100 mg three times a day), has been shown to improve mental performance, behavior, and mood in people who have dementia or Alzheimer's. However, phosphatidylcholine and lecithin, often used for Alzheimer's, do not seem to have a beneficial effect. Unfortunately, phosphatidylserine may have only a short-lived effect, only lasting for about sixteen weeks. It is not known whether discontinuing it at that time and then restarting a month or two later would continue to provide benefit.

Acetyl-L-carnitine (1500–4000 mg divided into two to three doses daily) may provide Alzheimer's patients some benefit in memory, behavioral performance, and a delayed progression of deterioration. It may be more likely to show some benefit in patients under sixty-six years of age with early onset and a fast rate of disease progression. ***Important note***: Don't confuse this with L-carnitine, which doesn't get into the brain.

Ginkgo leaf extract (120–240 mg per day of ginkgo leaf extract, divided in two or three doses) may stabilize or improve some measures of cognitive function and social functioning in patients with multiple types of dementia.

Vinpocetine (5–10 mg three times a day) increases cerebral blood flow like Gingko and has been shown in older studies to have a modest effect on cognitive impairment in most dementias.

Vitamin E (alpha-tocopherol; 2000 IU daily) may delay the progression of disease from the moderate stage to the severe stage by about six months. It has also been found to help slow cognitive decline when used in combination with donezepil (Aricept) or selegiline.

Important Information:
Avoid Combination Antioxidant *Supplements*

Animal studies showed that antioxidants decrease the formation of amyloid, but a recent human study showed that most antioxidant *supplements* alone did not change the progress of Alzheimer's. Instead, the study showed that treating patients with a *combination* of high-dose antioxidants (including vitamins C and E, Co-Q10, and alpha lipoic acid) actually *decreased* cognition and functional ability. Note that foods containing antioxidants appear to be beneficial, but the supplements do not.

Gotu kola and *cat's claw* contain substances that researchers think might block formation of beta amyloid. However, research has not yet shown benefit in Alzheimer's.

Fish oil (1,500–3,000 mg daily) supplements have a beneficial effect on brain function but have not been studied enough in dementia. Although a recent study purported to show that fish oil does not slow cognitive decline in Alzheimer's, the dosage used was well below recommended values.

Curcumin (1.5 grams twice daily with food) may have benefits against Alzheimer's disease.

Lemon balm may be useful for dementia symptoms but also to help control anxiety and agitation. It can be taken orally, applied as a lotion, or used as an essential oil in a diffuser.

Bright lighting has been shown by a study to provide reduced cognitive deficits, depression, and functional deficits in women with dementia. Giving melatonin (0.3 mg daily) had an adverse effect on mood and withdrawn behavior, but this affect was reversed when patients received both bright light and melatonin.

Golf Outing Can Help Dementia Patients

A form of therapy that can be helpful for dementia patients is called behavioral therapy. Caregivers have begun to search for activities patients enjoyed when they were younger and to allow patients to experience them again. However, even new experiences can help.

In one Alzheimer's facility, residents are taken on golf outings, which results in their being more content and lucid. From simply putting to swinging the club (in those who have played before), these actions seem to spark a startling transformation that makes these patients act almost normal again.

Your Empowered Patient Action Plan for Alzheimer's and Dementia

Step #1: Take nutritional supplements. You may want to try each alone to see if they work, but each may take six to eight weeks to show benefit. The best supplements appear to be Huperzine A, Phosphatidylserine, Acetyl-L-carnitine, Gingko, Vinpocetine, and vitamin E. These supplements are much less expensive and generally have fewer side effects than conventional drugs and may work as well or better. Lemon balm has few to no side effects and can be used at any time.

Step #2: Enroll in reality orientation therapy. This will help memory and orientation and can be done along with the above steps.

Step #3: Try prescription drugs if the supplements have not helped. There are many drugs available, and you need to discuss the benefits and potential side effects with your doctor. Take vitamin E along with the drugs for potentiation. If these drugs haven't shown benefit in two to three months, you may be wasting your money. Hydergine has the fewest side effects of conventional drugs.

Step #4: Use bright light and take melatonin to reduce depression and improve cognition and function.

Step #5: Take krill oil and vitamins and minerals. A multivitamin with at least 100 percent of the RDA values should suffice. Make sure you obtain at least 800 mg of vitamin D_3. However, eating nutritious foods with vitamins and minerals is more effective than taking supplements.

Expected Outcome

Dementia and Alzheimer's cannot be cured, but the above methods may help prevent and slow down their progression, as well as help control the symptoms and prolong survival. More research is being conducted that hopefully will provide breakthroughs as baby boomers age.

Anemia

What You Need to Know

Anemia is quite prevalent in the older population, occurring in almost 11 percent of people over the age of sixty-five. There are many causes of anemia, most commonly loss of blood, vitamin deficiencies (iron, B_{12}, folate), and chronic diseases (especially cancer, inflammatory diseases, and kidney failure). There are also rarer syndromes such as myelodysplastic disease, which can be genetic or caused by toxins including chemotherapy. A recent report documented that a frequent yet often missed cause of anemia is from "diagnostic blood loss," that is, taking blood repeatedly for lab tests if you are hospitalized for an extended period of time.

Your doctor may be able to diagnose the cause by obtaining a CBC (complete blood count) and looking at your blood indices (see sidebar below). Sometimes, however, the reason for your anemia may not be revealed by these tests, and it will be necessary to perform a bone marrow biopsy/aspiration. The bone marrow is where your blood cells are manufactured, and examining a sample of the contents may be helpful.

Diagnosing Anemia: Hints from a Complete Blood Count (CBC)

Obtaining a CBC can often give your doctor hints regarding what is causing your anemia, based on indices that evaluate your hemoglobin. Hemoglobin (abbreviated Hgb) is an iron-containing protein in the red blood cells that transports oxygen from the lungs to the tissues, where it releases the oxygen for cell use and then collects carbon dioxide to bring back to the lungs. It is the amount of Hgb that determines whether you are anemic (normal values vary depending on gender and age, but generally a Hgb of less than 12 indicates anemia). Below are descriptions of the various blood indices and possible conditions causing the anemia.

Indices:	Normal Values
MCV (average red blood cell size)	80–100
MCH (amount of Hgb per red blood cell)	27–31

Abnormalities   **Conditions Causing Anemia**

Normal MCV/MCH: sudden blood loss, sepsis, tumor, long-term disease, prosthetic heart valve

Low MCV/low MCH: iron deficiency, lead poisoning, thalassemia

Low MCV/normal MCH: kidney failure

Elevated MCV/normal MCH: chemotherapy, folate or vitamin B_{12} deficiency

If suspecting a nutrient deficiency (iron, folate, B_{12}), you should always measure the specific level of those nutrients in your blood to confirm the diagnosis and to make sure supplementation returns the level to normal. The diagnosis of iron deficiency anemia mandates an immediate search for potential sources of blood loss such as gastrointestinal bleeding from ulcers, cancer or other GI conditions.

Another test often used in evaluating anemia is the *ferritin* level. Ferritin stores iron and releases it when blood levels are low. Low blood ferritin in anemia usually indicates iron deficiency although it can also be low in hypothyroidism, vitamin C deficiency or celiac disease. Vegetarians may have low ferritin (caused by iron deficiency) and this can occur in up to 19 percent of such diets. Elevated ferritin is noted in patients with too much iron or in certain diseases with inflammation, including infections.

Anemia can also be a consequence of aging. You need a substance called erythropoetin, which is made in the kidneys, to maintain your red blood cell stores. Poor kidney function caused by aging or various conditions that cause resistance to its actions can result in anemia.

Anemia is more worrisome in the elderly as it can lead to increased falls, worsening cardiac function, causing poorer brain function, as well as increasing mortality.

It is important to realize that you can be significantly anemic yet have few symptoms (such as weakness, dizziness or light headedness, fatigue, shortness of breath); this usually occurs if blood loss or other dysfunctions have occurred very slowly (over months or even up to a year or longer). In such cases, your body has adjusted and compensated for the losses. However, sooner or later you will develop symptoms. You should see your doctor if these symptoms occur more frequently than normal or you have a definite change in your normal activities.

Treatments for Anemia

The Preventive Approaches

Correctable Causes: Obviously, if another medical condition is causing anemia, you must treat that condition to resolve the anemia. Conditions that commonly cause loss of blood include menstruation, GI problems such as ulcers, inflammatory bowel disease, cancer, and the use of various medications, especially nonsteroidal anti-inflammatories (NSAIDs) or aspirin.

If you lack iron or various vitamins, simply replacing those nutrients can prevent the anemia. Iron deficiency is commonly caused by menstruation, endurance training, surgical removal of part of the intestines (gastric bypass, etc.), certain foods (such as fiber or large amounts of calcium), drugs, caffeinated drinks (which can decrease iron absorption), and various chronic conditions. Eating iron-supplemented and vitamin-fortified foods can help prevent anemia. Eating little or no meat may cause a lack vitamin B_{12}, and overcooking or eating too few vegetables may cause a folate deficiency.

Certain types of vegetarianism also can cause anemia from lack of nutrient intake. This usually occurs if you don't eat meat (especially red meat), which is high in iron. However, vegetarians don't always develop anemia; there are many vegetables that contain iron (such as broccoli and spinach).

The Conventional Approaches
There are many different treatments for anemia, and the treatment depends on the severity and cause.

Iron supplementation treats mild to moderate iron-deficiency anemia. There are several forms, such as ferrous sulfate or ferrous glycinate, but ferrous bisglycinate may be the best tolerated. If toxicity occurs (usually stomach irritation), you can take it with food or take carbonyl iron (elemental iron). Vitamin C can increase the absorption of iron; 200 mg of vitamin C is necessary to increase the absorption of 30 mg of elemental iron. It may take several months for your iron stores to return to normal. *Caution*: Taking oral iron can decrease the absorption of other drugs and vitamins so take it at least two hours apart. If you have severe iron-deficiency anemia, intravenous iron may be necessary initially, followed by oral supplementation.

Vitamin supplements are indicated if you have nutritional deficiencies (folic acid, 250–1,000 mcg daily if mild, 1–5 mg daily if severe; vitamin B_{12}, 600–1,000 mcg daily). They both can be taken orally, but some people obtain better absorption of vitamin B_{12} using a subcutaneous injection or sublingually (under the tongue) if you don't absorb B_{12} (absorption may be decreased in patients with gastric bypass, decreased stomach acidity and some intestinal disorders).

Important note: In *anemia of chronic disease*, anemia associated with chemotherapy, or anemia associated with kidney disease, replacement of nutrients will not increase red blood cell count.

Recombinant erythropoietin (epoetin alfa) may be prescribed to stimulate red blood cell production. *Caution*: This drug has been controversial because a major study showed that it could increase mortality in cancer patients (although some cancers had worse outcomes than others). It is also not recommended in many patients with heart disease. Another study revealed that human erythro-poietin in critically ill anemic patients did not reduce the need for blood trans-fusion and was associated with an increase in thrombotic (blood clot) events. However, investigators also found that it reduced mortality for trauma patients, so it is indicated in such cases. However, it needs to be used cautiously in other conditions.

A **blood transfusion** may be necessary in severe cases of anemia, or with on-going blood loss. Doctors attempt to avoid blood transfusion in general as adverse patient outcomes can occur with more intensive transfusion strategies. Conservative approaches are indicated (watch and wait) unless your life is at stake or you are actively bleeding. *Important note*: With cancer, heart disease, and postsurgical patients, for example, transfusions may not currently be recommended until your hemoglobin level is below 7, unless you have certain symptoms caused by the anemia (see above) and/or have other specific indications or conditions.

Hyperbaric oxygen (HBO) is indicated when oxygen delivery to tissue is not sufficient in patients who cannot be transfused for medical or religious reasons. HBO may be used for medical reasons if blood product incompatibility is possible or if there is concern for transmissible disease. Studies have shown HBO to have beneficial re-sults in most people.

The Alternative Approaches

Herbs and supplements can be helpful if there are various nutrient deficiencies.

Vitamin C (1,000–2,000 mg daily) makes the stomach more acidic and can improve the absorption of iron in your diet.

Supplemental B$_{12}$ and folate (see dosages above) can alleviate anemia caused by defi-ciencies of these vitamins.

Iron supplements should be used only when a deficiency is found. Naturopathic doctors often use iron citrate, which is less constipating than other forms of iron. *Caution*: Taking iron supplements can cause inflammation in the body and be harmful if a person is not iron deficient.

Acupuncture may be quite beneficial for rebuilding the bone-marrow stores and accelerating the production of blood cells, as well as improving anemia of chronic disease. It usually takes six to twelve sessions to obtain benefit, although intermittent maintenance acupuncture may be necessary.

Chinese herbal formulas can also stimulate production of new blood cells. Several herbs in these formulas can stimulate blood cell regeneration, including *Ji Xue Teng* (spatholobus), *Dang Shen* (codonopsis), and *Huang Qi* (astragalus). A spe-cific formula is *Ba Zhen Tang*, and *Ren Shen Shou Wu W*an can be used for general anemia.

Your Empowered Patient Action Plan for Anemia

- *Important note: If you have acute blood loss or if your hemoglobin is critically low, your doctor may order a blood transfusion. You can then follow the next steps.*

Step #1: Find and treat the underlying disease or condition causing your anemia. This is the most important action you can take as correcting the underlying condition often can resolve the anemia.

Step #2: Take iron or vitamin supplementation (folate, B$_{12}$), with vitamin C, if your CBC indices indicate deficiency and blood tests of those nutrients are below normal.

Step #3: Take Chinese herbs to build up blood stores, especially in anemia of chronic disease or acute blood loss.

Step #4: Undergo acupuncture to compliment the Chinese herbs and accelerate the production of red blood cells.

Step #5: Take erythropoetin only if necessary to increase blood stores, after consulting with your doctor. Be cautious if you have anemia from cancer or chronic kidney disease.

Step #6. Undergo hyperbaric oxygen treatment if you cannot or will not undergo blood transfusion.

Expected Outcome

There are many ways to treat anemia and control it enough to ensure a good quality of life. With some alternative methods, anemia of chronic disease may be able to be reversed.

Anxiety and Anxiety Disorders (Including PTSD, OCD, GAD, Panic Attacks, and Phobias)

What You Need to Know

Anxiety is an unpleasant emotional state that can range from mild unease to intense fear. When there is a threat of some type, anxiety is a normal response, but when there is no clear or realistic cause, it is not normal. Certainly, anxiety can occur as you age and are met with new problems, but it can continue even after those problems are resolved.

Serious anxiety *disorders* (which are much different, longer-lasting, and more severe) include panic attacks, phobias, obsessive-compulsive disorders (OCD), and post-traumatic stress disorder (PTSD), "free-floating" anxiety (an unexplainable feeling of apprehension that can last for months), and generalized anxiety disorder (GAD), defined as excessive worry on most days for at least six months.

Generalized anxiety disorder (GAD) may be the most common mental disorder among the elderly, affecting 7 percent of seniors, although little is known about how to treat the disorder among older adults since very little research has been done. Late-life anxiety disorders have been underestimated for several reasons; for example, older patients are less likely to report psychiatric symptoms and more likely to emphasize their physical complaints. Due to the lack of evidence, doctors often think that this disorder is rare in the elderly or that it is a normal part of aging, so they don't diagnose or treat anxiety in their older patients, when in fact, anxiety is quite common in the elderly and can have a serious impact on quality of life (QOL).

Of course anxiety can occur in anyone, at any age. This constant state of worry and anxiousness may seriously affect your QOL by causing you to limit your daily activities and having difficulty sleeping. GAD and other forms of anxiety may also lead to depression in about one quarter of patients.

Anxiety may affect twice as many adults as depression, according to new research. Anxiety in the elderly is also associated with poorer thinking—an effect that is opposite from what researchers see in younger adults with anxiety. In fact, a recent study showed that stress reversibly impairs brain function.

Dr. A's Suggestions:
Panic Attacks a Risk Factor for Cardiovascular Events and Death in Postmenopausal Women

A recent study followed 3,400 postmenopausal women, and those who had full-blown panic attacks had a greater risk of death from heart disease and all-cause mortality than those who didn't. Women who reported less severe panic attacks also showed higher risks, but not as much. It is important, therefore, to address the underlying cause of anxiety to help prevent other conditions and death.

Treatments for Anxiety

The Preventive Approaches
The most important aspect of preventing anxiety is to *recognize it*. Many doctors do not address these symptoms, so it may be up to you or a loved one to bring it to the doctor's attention.

Identifying and eliminating any sources of stress are the ideal ways to prevent anxiety, but this is unrealistic in most cases, as you may not have control over the stresses in your life. Therefore, it's important to learn how to cope with stress in a positive manner and protect your body from the harmful effects of stress.

Increased lactic acid levels may be an underlying factor in anxiety and panic attacks, so eliminating nutritional factors that increase lactic acid may help reduce anxiety significantly; these factors include caffeine, alcohol, and sugar.

Studies have shown that people who exercise are able to reduce their tensions and worries, improve mood, and improve the ability to handle stressful life situations. I recommend both aerobic and anaerobic exercises.

The Conventional Approaches

Medications are the mainstay of conventional medicine treatment. There are primarily two types:

Antianxiety drugs (called anxiolytics) such as buspirone (Buspar) have slower onset of action but fewer side effects than the benzodiazepines (such as diazepam [Valium], lorazepam [Ativan], or alprazolam [Xanax]) and may be preferred initially. ***Warning***: A 2014 study in *BMJ* revealed that the use on anxiolytic drugs is associated not only with daytime fatigue, accidents, and falls but also with elevated risk of death (which could be due to the other adverse effects). These are dose-response relations, meaning that the risk increases as the dose increases. These effects are also worsened when using other drugs, such as for insomnia.

Antidepressants may be more beneficial for GAD and other more severe forms of anxiety, and several (Tofranil, Desyrel, Paxil, Celexa) have been shown to be superior to anxiolytics. Your physician needs to determine which medications and what dosages are most likely to be effective for you because different ones may affect you differently (see chart below).

FDA-Approved Antidepressants for Specific Anxiety Disorders					
Drug	**GAD**	**Panic Disorder**	**OCD**	**PTSD**	**Social Anxiety**
Citalopram (*Celexa*)			X	X	
Duloxetine (*Cymbalta*)	X				
Escitalopram (*Lexapro*)	X				
Fluvoxamine (*Luvox*)			X		
Fluvoxamine extended release (*Luvox CR*)			X		X
Venlafaxine (*Effexor XR*)	X	X			X
Fluoxetine (*Prozac*)		X	X		
Sertraline (*Zoloft*)		X	X	X	X
Paroxetine (*Paxil*)	X	X	X	X	X

Important notes: With antianxiety drugs, relief is usually very fast, but with antidepressants, it may take one to three or more weeks to have an effect. It is also important to realize however, that these medications do not work in all people, and you may need to try different types to find the one that works.

Psychotherapy is an important treatment for anxiety and is highly recommended, since it may provide long-term benefit rather than just treat symptoms. You should undergo counseling in conjunction with, not in place of, taking medications, especially as medications may not be that helpful and can have problematic side effects. The most common form of counseling is *cognitive-behavioral therapy*, also known as "talk" therapy. This therapy attempts to change unproductive or harmful thought patterns. You learn to examine your feelings and separate realistic from unrealistic thoughts. There are other forms that can also be helpful, including *thought field therapy* if traumatic events in the past are causing anxiety. Psychotherapy may take several months or even years to help reduce anxiety, but it is essential for long-term relief as you must understand and learn to deal with the underlying causes.

The Alternative Approaches

Nutritional Supplements: Deficiency of several B vitamins (especially folate), calcium, and/or magnesium can occur from the increased lactic acid caused by stress, so supplement these if your anxiety is chronic and/or your blood levels of these nutrients are low. A good multivitamin may also be of benefit.

Acupuncture can be very helpful in controlling anxiety. As acupuncture works directly on the brain, it is thought to help balance neurotransmitters. However, there may be only a few styles of acupuncture that are effective for anxiety, so check with your acupuncturist to make sure they have experience treating this condition. There are acupuncture points in the ear (auricular acupuncture) that are specific for general anxiety as well as some anxiety disorders such as OCD. Because acupuncture addresses the underlying cause, it may provide long-term relief.

Chinese herbal medicine can also be very useful for controlling symptoms of anxiety. A Chinese herbal formula called *Ding Xin Wan*, taken one to three tabs three times daily, can be very helpful in controlling generalized anxiety and help with sleep. It has minimal to no side effects. *Chai Hu Mu Li Long Gu Tang* is beneficial if your anxiety causes physical manifestations such as tense neck/shoulders, tension headaches, or upset stomach. *An Mien Pian* (meaning "peaceful sleep tablets") is another formula that may be recommended. An advantage of Chinese herbs over conventional drugs is that they usually do not affect thinking or make you drowsy, so you can perform your daily activities.

Herbs and supplements may help reduce anxiety. Anxiolytic (for anxiety alone) type herbs are described below.

Valerian root (up to 400 mg per night) can both help with sleep at night and reduce anxiety during the day, so is recommended if you can't sleep at night because of anxiety.

Passion flower (0.25-2 grams of the dried above ground parts or one cup of the tea two to three times daily) is often used as a bedtime tea to help relieve stress and anxiety and facilitate sleep. For generalized anxiety disorder (GAD), 45 drops of passionflower liquid extract has been used daily. A specific tablet formulation 90 mg/day has also been used.

Skullcap (1-2 grams or as a tea three times daily) is commonly used for relieving stress and tension and helping people feel calm and relaxed.

Theanine (200 mg/day), a major component of green tea, may help people feel more tranquil.

Kava kava (70 percent kavalactones three times daily) is helpful and effective for general anxiety. **Warning**: Some countries have banned kava due to liver toxicity but such cases are primarily from certain concentrated extracts. Nevertheless, it is important to not take kava with other drugs that cause liver problems (including alcohol and acetaminophen) and/or obtain liver tests. Toxicity can occur as early as three to four weeks of use.

For anxiety disorders, several herbs mimic the effects of conventional antidepressants.

St. John's wort (300 mg three times daily, containing 0.3 percent hypericin or 0.1–0.2 mg of total hypericin daily) is primarily for depression but can be used for some anxiety disorders or combinations of anxiety and depression. **Caution**: St. John's wort interacts with many medications and should not be taken without first checking with your doctor or pharmacist.

SAM-e, 5-HTP and *L-tryptophan* are also commonly used herbal antidepressants, but very few studies have been conducted to show benefit in anxiety disorders.

If you have both anxiety and depression, there are some herbal combinations containing kava, valerian, and St. John's wort that can be found in most health-food stores. All these herbs work by stabilizing various neurotransmitters in the brain. These herbs (and combinations) should work within a few days to a week.

Flaxseed oil (2–6 tablespoons daily of *freshly ground* flaxseed for two to three months) may be beneficial for some phobias, such as agoraphobia (fear of being alone or in public places). Agoraphobia is thought to be due to a deficiency in alpha-linoleic acid (omega-3), which can also cause dry skin, dandruff, brittle fingernails, and nerve disorders in people who have agoraphobia. It may take several weeks to a few months to observe benefits. **Helpful tip**: Flaxseed capsules and the bottled oil deteriorate very quickly, which is why freshly ground is the form recommended.

Meditation: Any type of meditation is helpful to reduce anxiety. Not only does meditation relax you, it also helps prevent the deleterious physical effects of anxiety on the body. It also allows you to better understand what is causing the stress and how to deal with it more effectively. The more anxious you are, the longer or more frequent you should meditate.

Interactive imagery is another very effective alternative method, which is akin to psychotherapy but may be more powerful. This is a mind-body method in which you mentally interact with images that represent your emotions, including anxiety. It is a powerful method to uncover and deal with subconscious psychological issues of which you may not be aware. The advantage of interactive imagery over psychotherapy is that it goes directly to the source of the emotions and works very quickly, often with benefits obtained in just a few sessions. It is also very beneficial and fast-acting if you have phobias. It can be used in conjunction with psychotherapy (se chapter 4 for more discussion on this type of imagery and the Appendix for an online resource).

Nature Walks Help Rumination

Many people with anxiety are beleaguered by endlessly ruminating on negative thoughts…interminably dwelling on any number of personal problems. However, a study conducted at Stanford University in 2015 demonstrated that just taking a walk in the woods can stave off the tendency to ruminate.

In the study, participants strolled for 90 minutes through an unspoiled landscape surrounded by greenery. Compared to participants that walked down a busy street, the nature walkers brooded less and their brain scans revealed decreased activity in a part of the brain that regulates negative emotions.

Massage is excellent for reducing mild anxiety states and can be used with all other treatments. Swedish massage is the form with which most Americans are familiar. It uses gentle pressure to relax the muscles. Another popular form of massage is shiatsu (Shi = finger, atsu = pressure). I recommend either one for general anxiety, but there are other forms that can be just as effective. Massage can give you immediate relief, but it is usually short-lived.

Hypnosis can be very effective for phobias and some general anxiety states. Two to six sessions are usually adequate to observe results. Results should be evident almost immediately after hypnosis.

Bach flower remedies or **aromatherapy** are other natural "sense" treatments that may help reduce mild anxiety. Bach remedies are designed to treat a particular emotional condition using essences from specific flowers. Aromatherapy uses your sense of smell to affect your emotions. Oil of lavender, jasmine, and blue chamomile are the most common aromatherapy products used for anxiety. Although these products can be found in health food and beauty stores, there are practitioners who have been trained specifically in aromatherapy treatment to provide more specific treatment using combinations of ingredients that cannot be found in stores. For flower remedies, many herbalists have such expertise, and I recommend consultation with them. Although you can expect to experience some benefits immediately, long-term relief may take several weeks.

Your Empowered Patient Action Plan for Anxiety

- **Important note**: *For anxiety that is significantly interfering with your daily activities, start with steps 1 and 4 or 5, and then return to step 2.*

Step #1: *Use interactive imagery techniques or psychotherapy*. Such therapy is essential for dealing with the anxiety and its underlying causes, not just treating symptoms. I recommend interactive imagery first because it is much faster at resolving anxiety, but there are very few qualified practitioners.

Step #2: *Use meditation* every day to help prevent the harmful effects of stress on your body as well as reduce your anxiety levels.

Step #3: *Undergo acupuncture*: Acupuncture can provide fast relief for anxiety and also can give long-term relief. Auricular (ear) acupuncture is especially effective. It can be used along with the above steps.

Step #4: *Take the Chinese herbal formula* Ding Xin Wan or Chai Hu Mu Li Long Gu Tang for short-term relief. These Chinese herbal formulas work as well as or better than conventional drugs without the side effects.

Step #5: *Take prescription anxiolytics* if the above steps have not helped. These medications work well but start with low doses because the older you are, the more sensitive you may be.

Step #6: *Take the Western herbal remedies valerian root or kava kava*, if you don't want to take conventional medications, they are too strong, or they have unacceptable side effects. Valerian can be beneficial for sleep as well as anxiety.

Step #7: ***Receive massage***: This will provide temporary relief and can be used with any of the above steps.

Step #8: ***Take Bach flower remedies*** or undergo ***aromatherapy*** for relaxation. These can, of course, be done with any of the above steps.

Your Empowered Patient Action Plan for Anxiety Disorders

Step #1: ***Use interactive imagery techniques or psychotherapy***. Such therapy is essential for dealing with the anxiety disorder and its underlying causes, not just treating symptoms. I recommend interactive imagery first because it is much faster at resolving anxiety and understanding the basis of the disorder, but there are very few qualified practitioners. It is especially beneficial for phobias.

Step #2: ***Use meditation*** every day to help prevent the harmful effects of stress on your body as well as reduce your anxiety levels.

Step #3: ***Take prescription antidepressants***. These medications can work well, but start with low doses to minimize side effects. It may take several weeks to obtain benefits.

Step #4: ***Undergo acupuncture***. Acupuncture can provide relief for anxiety disorders and can give long-term relief if an effective style or auricular acupuncture is available. It can be used along with the above steps.

Step #5: ***Use hypnosis for phobias and GAD***. This method may resolve the phobias completely and help reduce GAD symptoms long term.

Step #6: ***Take flaxseed oil for phobias***. This herb can help control phobias if the above steps haven't helped and can be used along with the above steps.

Expected Outcome

Anxiety is difficult to resolve completely, but if recognized, there are many methods, both conventional and alternative, that can control symptoms and improve your quality of life. Anxiety disorders are much more difficult to resolve but can be controlled sufficiently to provide a normal life.

Arteries: Aneurysm/Dissection

What You Need to Know

An aneurysm is a bulging of an artery wall. Aneurysms occur from weakening in the walls of the artery, and if they rupture, death can occur rapidly. Arteries can also develop "dissection": the inner lining tears, and blood surges through the tear, creating a new false channel and separating (dissecting) the middle layer of the artery from the outer layer. About three-fourths of aortic dissections occur in men and in people forty to seventy years of age.

Aneurysms can occur in any area of the body, but the most common is aortic aneurysm in the abdomen (called AAA). However, they can occur in the upper (thoracic) aorta (chest area) and brain blood vessels as well. Dissections also occur more frequently in the aorta, but primarily the thoracic aorta.

Most aneurysms are small and slow growing and rarely rupture. However, fifteen thousand people die of aortic aneurysms every year. If you are a smoker, you should definitely be screened on a regular basis.

Signs of a worsening abdominal aneurysm include a pulsating sensation near the navel, tenderness in the abdomen, and/or back pain. Signs of a brain aneurysm are sudden headache, vision loss, or loss of consciousness. Unfortunately, most brain aneurysms have no symptoms and rupture without warning. They occur in 2 percent of the population. If you survive however, there are actions you can take to prevent re-rupture.

Screening for aneurysms of the brain should be done for people with family histories of aneurysms (you should check with a geneticist) or who have a condition called coarctation of the aorta.

⸺◦◼◦⸺

Increased and Decreased Risks Associated with Aortic Dissection and Aneurysms

Aortic dissection and aneurysms are caused by a weakness of the connective tissue of the artery. Factors that increase this risk include:

- High blood pressure (10.8-fold increase)
- Smoking (2.2-fold)
- Kidney cysts (3.4-fold)
- Male gender
- Family history of dissection
- Over age eighty-five

If you have any of these risk factors, especially the top three, you should undergo screening. A protective effect occurs from:

- Exercising at least once a week
- Consuming nuts at least four times a week
- African-American or Hispanic ethnicity

Treatments for Aneurysms/Dissections

The Preventive Approaches

Stop bad habits: Since smoking cigarettes is a major contributing cause of aneurysms, the best way to prevent one is to stop smoking. Those who quit smoking for more than five to ten years have a dramatic decrease in risk.

Correctable causes: Besides high blood pressure (see above), high cholesterol worsens atherosclerosis, a major factor in weakening the walls of arteries, so it should be controlled as well (see section on cholesterol).

Nutrition is a major factor in causing, preventing, and reversing atherosclerosis. High fat content, processed and fried foods, fast foods, and high-cholesterol foods all worsen the atherosclerotic process. Even minor improvements in diet can help a great deal. Eating three to five servings of fruits and vegetables daily can increase your fiber intake and also provide other ingredients that protect the arteries, such as antioxidants. Green leafy vegetables and vitamin-C rich fruits and vegetables are especially protective. One meal per week of cold-water fish (mackerel, tuna, herring, salmon, cod, trout, or halibut) can reduce the risk of atherosclerosis by increasing HDL (the "good" cholesterol) and decreasing LDL (the "bad" cholesterol), but several times a week is better, of course. Consuming a handful of nuts daily is also recommended.

Moderate alcohol intake: Drinking one glass of wine daily has been shown to help prevent the development of atherosclerosis due to its antioxidant and anti-inflammatory properties. Red wine is the best choice because it contains antioxidants called polyphenols, but beer, white wine, and grape juice can provide almost as much benefit. To avoid weight gain from drinking alcoholic beverages, drink them *during* meals.

Exercising at least once a week decreases the risk of developing aneurysms.

The Conventional Approaches

For abdominal aneurysms

Medications such as *beta blockers* (such as atenolol or metoprolol) decrease the force of blood ejection from the heart to minimize the expansion of the aneurysm. *Calcium channel blockers usually* are used if you can't take beta blockers.

Surgery is indicated if the abdominal aneurysm is large (usually greater than 4.5 cm). For small aneurysms (less than 4 cm or 2 inches), watchful waiting rather than surgery is an option, with six-month or yearly ultrasounds being done to monitor any enlargement.

There are two types of surgery. *Traditional ("open") surgery* removes the damaged section of the aorta and replaces it with a synthetic tube (*graft*), which is sewn into place. This procedure requires open-abdominal surgery involving a large incision and lengthy recover time.

Endovascular surgery is less invasive. A synthetic graft is attached to the end of a thin tube (catheter) that's inserted through an artery in your leg and threaded up into your aorta. The graft (a woven tube covered by a metal mesh support) is deployed at the site of the aneurysm and fastened in place with small hooks or pins. The graft reinforces the weakened section of the aorta to prevent rupture of the aneurysm.

Comparison of surgeries: Studies have shown endovascular surgery to have better short-term survival than traditional but no advantage in long-term survival. However, the need for additional surgeries is significantly higher with the endovascular approach, although this technique is improving. Two-thirds of the repairs done in the United States are endovascular, so careful follow-up is needed. A 2015 study in the *NEJM* showed that both types of surgeries have similar long-term mortality rates (50 percent at 8 years). Late rupture occurred in 5.4 percent after endovascular repair and 1.4 percent after open repair.

Stent placement in the aorta is another method to prevent the bulging from rupturing. However, the FDA has reported a higher five-year death rate in patients treated with such a stent than with traditional surgeries.

For brain aneurysms

Surgery depends on several factors. Most unruptured aneurysms (less than 7 mm) don't have much risk of rupture, and sometimes treating the aneurysm can be more risky. If it is a large aneurysm causing symptoms, surgery may be necessary. Surgery is also dependent on the location.

There are two surgeries, *microvascular clipping* (requires opening the skull) and the less invasive *endovascular coiling*, in which the blood vessel is blocked by a coil so that blood cannot flow through it. The latter has a higher risk of rebleeding, but the risks involved with clipping increase substantially over the age of fifty. A 2014 study in *Lancet* showed that overall, coiling leads to better chances of survival after ten years of follow-up.

The Pipeline embolization device is a new device approved by the FDA in March 2011 to help avoid invasive surgery. It is a mesh tube that is threaded up into the brain without actually entering the aneurysm and diverts and reduces blood flow from the aneurysm. The aneurysm usually shuts off completely within 6 weeks to 6 months. In studies, 70 percent of aneurysms treated with this device remained blocked off without obstructing the artery.

For dissections of the arteries

This condition is considered an emergency because once they become symptomatic; they can rupture and cause death very quickly. Treatment is geared toward reducing blood pressure with intravenous beta blockers or calcium channel blockers, followed by surgery.

The Alternative Approaches

Nutritional supplements can be helpful to prevent the atherosclerosis that weakens the walls if the aneurysm is small and doesn't need surgery.

Flaxseed (freshly ground) *or fish oil* (1,500–3,000 mg daily) is the best supplement to help prevent deposition of fats into the arteries. Regular fish oil in high doses (3,000–4,000 mg daily) may decrease HDL cholesterol (the good cholesterol) in some people. If you take fish oil, and your HDL is reduced to below normal, you can try taking vitamin E (200 IU daily) and garlic (4,000 mg daily) or niacin (1–3 grams daily) to raise HDL.

Important notes: Niacin may cause flushing: but there are nonflushing products. Fish oil also can be prescribed, but the prescription form is much more expensive and may not have any advantage over OTC forms.

Intravenous chelation is recommended by many alternative practitioners, who believe that various metals accumulate in our bodies and cause atherosclerosis. In chelation, a specific substance (called EDTA) is injected into your bloodstream and binds to these metals and helps the body dispose of them. However, intravenous chelation is expensive and has not been proven effective to prevent progression of aneurysms or dissections. It is also very expensive ($2,500 to $4,000).

If you want chelation, you can take some herbs orally that can chelate (see recipe below). Although no studies have been done on these herbs, they are generally not harmful, so are worth a try. Malic acid (800–1,200 mg daily) is particularly useful for removing aluminum from the body. Cilantro is excellent for cleaning heavy metals out of the gastrointestinal tract, but it has not been found to chelate the stored metals that are found in other areas of the body.

───

Oral Chelation: Cilantro Recipe

Blend one cup of fresh cilantro with six tablespoons of olive oil until the cilantro is completely chopped. Add one clove of garlic, half a cup of nuts (cashews or almonds are the best), and two tablespoons of lemon juice. Blend these into a paste (which will be lumpy), adding hot water if necessary. Take two to three teaspoons per day for two to three weeks, every few months. If you make large amounts, you can freeze it for later use. You should see benefits within two to three weeks.

Your Empowered Patient Plan for Aneurysms/Dissection

- *Warning: A dissection is considered an emergency and requires immediate hospitalization and surgery.*
- *If an abdominal aneurysm is detected that is more than 4.5 cm, go directly to Step #4, but also follow Steps #1 and #2.*

Step #1: Stop smoking and maintain a good diet to prevent the progression of aneurysms and retard atherosclerosis.

Step #2: Take fish oil to prevent progression of atherosclerosis.

Step #3: Undergo ultrasound of the abdomen every six to twelve months if the aneurysm is less than 4.5 cm.

Step #4: Undergo surgery to repair the aneurysm when indicated.

Expected Outcome

Abdominal aneurysms and dissections are very dangerous and can cause sudden death, so it is important to detect and prevent their progression. With proper preventive measures and surgery, death can be avoided.

Arteries: Peripheral Artery Disease (PAD)/Stenosis(Carotid, Aortic, Renal)

What You Need to Know

Any artery can become clogged from the deposition of plaques of fatty material on their inner walls (called atherosclerosis), resulting in narrowing of the artery (referred to as stenosis) and thus decreasing blood flow to the areas of the body to which it provides blood. The most important arteries that can be involved (besides the heart; see "Angina") are the carotid arteries in the neck (providing blood to the brain) and the aortic and iliac arteries in the abdomen, supplying blood to the lower extremities, kidneys, and intestines.

The danger of carotid stenosis is that fragments can break off and go to the brain, causing TIAs (transient ischemic attacks, or ministrokes) or actual strokes. The danger of iliac or aortic stenosis is gangrene of the legs and death to the tissues of the intestines or kidneys.

You should understand that many people with stenosis do not have symptoms, with the disease being found when your doctor hears a particular sound over the artery (called a "bruit," pronounced "bru-ee"). Treatment can be dependent on whether you have symptoms or not.

Blockage in these peripheral arteries may be a sign that you have heart disease. In fact, more people who have peripheral artery stenosis die of heart disease than of stroke or require limb amputation.

Note: A term that is frequently confused with PAD is peripheral vascular disease (PVD), meaning disease in any blood vessel, *both* arteries and veins. This section only discusses disease in the arteries. (For vein disease, see sections on *Varicose Veins* and *Venous Thrombosis/Venous Insufficiency*).

Treatments for Arterial Stenosis

The Preventive Approaches

Stop bad habits: Smoking is a major cause of arterial blockage and should be stopped. The arteries cannot heal if you continue smoking.

Correctable causes: If you have high cholesterol or high blood pressure, you must reduce it to normal to stop clogging your arteries (see sections on cholesterol and hypertension for guidelines).

Nutrition is a major cause of peripheral artery disease when it's poor. You need to increase dietary fiber (eat more veggies) and eat at least two meals of fish per week (cold-water fish such as mackerel, salmon, halibut, tuna, herring, or cod) to reduce or prevent cholesterol buildup in the heart arteries. Avoid, or at least limit, saturated fats, foods high in cholesterol, and animal proteins, all of which increase cholesterol buildup in the heart arteries. Consuming a handful of nuts daily is also recommended.

Alcohol: Drinking one glass of wine daily with meals may help retard the progression of atherosclerosis. Red wine especially, has powerful antioxidant properties and can help prevent the buildup of atherosclerosis. However, any alcoholic drink can help as long as your intake is moderate (see chapter 2 for recommendations).

Exercise is a key way to improve blood flow in clogged arteries and helps you improve the ability of your cells to use oxygen efficiently, which reduces symptoms. Before starting an exercise program, however, you should undergo an exercise tolerance test (ETT) to determine your safe exercise level. Based on the ETT results, your doctor can advise you on a carefully graded, progressive aerobic exercise program.

Important Information:
Exercise the Arms…The Legs Benefit

A recent study published in the *Journal of Vascular Surgery* revealed that in patients who have difficulty walking or have impediments such as arthritis, upper extremity exercise can improve lower extremity performance. So if you can't exercise your legs, exercising your arms will still help your legs.

The Conventional Approaches

Medications for other medical conditions: In people with heart disease, drugs such as statins (to control high cholesterol), aspirin, and ACE inhibitors and beta blockers (for blood pressure) can help prevent heart attacks and strokes. Small studies show that they may do the same for people with PAD. If you have these concurrent conditions, these drugs may be helpful at slowing the progression of the disease. For high cholesterol, you need to lower your LDL ("bad" cholesterol) to below 100.

Medications for stenosis, both *blood thinners* (such as warfarin [Coumadin] and others; see section on *Venous Thrombosis)* and *antiplatelet agents* (such as aspirin, dipyridamole [with aspirin], or clopidogrel [Plavix]) may prevent further progression of stenosis and prevent blood clots and are used for those who have symptoms or have had a stroke already. With aspirin, 81 mg (baby aspirin) is sufficient for blood thinning. *Important note*: If you do not have symptoms, aspirin is usually recommended as the drug of choice, and Coumadin, clopidogrel, and combination aspirin with dipyridamole are usually not recommended.

Caution: Be aware that ibuprofen blocks the blood-thinning effects of aspirin. If you must take ibuprofen, take the aspirin first and wait at least two hours to take the ibuprofen so that the aspirin has time to exert its beneficial effects. Take the lowest dose of ibuprofen necessary. Aspirin use can deplete body stores of vitamin C, so make sure you get 600 mg a day through diet or by taking a supplement. It also can cause stomach irritation and bleeding in some people. Ordinarily, OTC proton pump inhibitors (such as Prilosec, Prevacid, Pepcid, Nexium) can protect the stomach if this occurs, but recent studies show that they can interfere with aspirin, so consider an H_2 blocker (Zantac, Axid, Pepcid) instead.

Important note: Clopidogrel (Plavix) may not work in 20 percent of people due to genetic variations. If indicated for long term use, CYP2C19 genetic testing should be considered.

Aspirin Resistance: Real or Not?

Some patients are found to have aspirin resistance, meaning that aspirin does not have the antiplatelet effect to prevent clots. People who are nonresponsive to aspirin have a fourfold increased risk of adverse events. However, a recent study revealed that 90 percent of patients who are unresponsive to aspirin have simply not taken their aspirin on a regular basis. You can find out if you are truly aspirin resistant by undergoing arachidonic acid testing.

Medications for symptoms can be used to reduce claudication (pain on walking) caused by aortic/iliac artery stenosis.

- *Cilostazol* (Pletal) increases blood flow to the limbs by preventing clots and widening blood vessels.
- *Pentoxifylline* is an alternative but is less effective.
- *Ramipril*, a blood-pressure medication, has been shown to substantially improve pain-free walking time and maximum walking time much better than all other drugs. It should be used with an exercise program for best results.

Thrombolytic therapy (injecting a clot dissolving substance directly into the stenosis) can be done to dissolve the clot. This may be especially beneficial in patients who have contraindications to blood thinners and/or have clots in dangerous areas.

Minimally invasive procedures (called *endovascular repair*) can be done if the above doesn't help. These repairs are done through an incision in the skin and include *angioplasty* (enlarging the opening through the artery with a balloon catheter), endarterectomy (cleaning out the artery), and *stenting* (placing a device in the artery that keeps it open.

Bypass grafting is commonly done for severe, symptomatic stenosis. In this procedure, a vein from another part of the body can be used to "bypass" and re-route blood around the clogged artery.

Comparison of surgeries: In the past decade, endovascular repairs have tripled while bypass grafting has decreased almost by half. This is because side effects and time in the hospital are much less with the former. However, bypass is indicated in patients with acceptable surgical risk who require a more durable repair, in those with lesions technically unsuitable for endovascular repair, and in patients who experienced failure of endovascular repair.

For carotid stenosis

Two types of **surgeries** may be indicated. *Endarterectomy* is indicated for *symptomatic* people with greater than 50 percent stenosis. Men who have moderate stenosis (50 percent) may also benefit from surgery, but the benefit is less pronounced for women, and they should be considered individually. *Stent* placement to keep the carotid artery open is another surgery option, but controversy exists as to whether endarterectomy or stenting is the best. Here are what the studies show:

- There is no difference in long-term outcomes between stenting and endarterectomy, and both increase brain function by 50 percent.
- Stenting may result in deterioration in average psychomotor speed while endarterectomy may produce a decrease in average memory.
- There is a higher risk of heart attack after endarterectomy but a higher risk of stroke and death with stenting.
- It has also been determined that younger patients may do better with stenting whereas older patients do better with endarterectomy. In fact, Medicare restricts coverage for stenting.
- ***Caution***: Many authorities feel that stenting is used inappropriately in many patients who are low risk and don't have symptoms.

Medication versus surgery comparison:

A recent study published in the *Archives of Neurology* showed that intensive medication therapy for carotid stenosis *without symptoms* can prevent complications more than surgery and works just as well, if not better. Medical management with the above mentioned drugs produces mildly improved outcomes for stenosis between 50 percent and 69 percent (medications decrease stroke risk 22 percent vs. 16 percent for surgery). Another study in the *NEJM* in 2011 showed that medical management is much more effective than angioplasty and stenting for reducing *recurrent* stroke or death in asymptomatic patients. However, some patients may still require surgery in special circumstances.

For renal (kidney) artery stenosis

A recent study from the *Annals of Internal Medicine* states that both stenting and drug therapy have the same effectiveness, but there is more risk with stenting. It also does not control blood pressure and may actually harm as many people as it helps in terms of kidney function. Stenting thus is not usually recommended for most people, especially if kidney function has remained stable for six months to a year and high blood pressure can be controlled.

The Alternative Approaches

Nutritional Supplements: Studies have shown that following angioplasty or stenting, certain vitamins and fish oil reduce the risk of the artery reclogging. These include:

- *Fish oil*, 1,500–3,000 mg daily
- *Folic acid*, 1 mg daily
- *Vitamin B_{12}*, 400 mcg daily
- *Vitamin B_6*, 10 mg daily

Warning: Antioxidant vitamins C, E, and beta carotene *should not be taken* after angioplasty for at least six months because they interfere with the artery repair process following these procedures.

L-arginine (3–6 gm three times a day; 8 gm twice daily IV for three weeks) is a supplement that improves symptoms in peripheral artery disease by augmenting nitric oxide in the blood (thus helping open your arteries). *Caution*: L-arginine may worsen herpes infection (cold sores).

Policosanol (10 mg twice daily) seems to significantly improve walking distance in patients with intermittent claudication.

Ginkgo leaf taken orally also appears to increase pain-free walking distance in patients with intermittent claudication. Although significant benefit has been found with doses as low as 120–160 mg per day, there is some evidence that a higher dose of 240 mg per day might be more beneficial in some patients.

Intravenous chelation: Many alternative practitioners believe that various metals accumulate in our bodies and cause atherosclerosis and peripheral artery disease. They recommend intravenous chelation, a process in which a specific substance (called EDTA) is injected into your bloodstream and binds to these metals and helps the body dispose of them. However, intravenous chelation has not been proven effective for this indication. It is also very expensive ($2,500 to $4,000).

Herbs that can chelate: Although no studies have been done on these herbs, they are generally not harmful, so they are worth a try. *Malic acid* (800–1,200 mg daily) is particularly useful for removing aluminum from the body. *Cilantro* is excellent for cleaning heavy metals out of the gastrointestinal tract.

Cilantro Recipe for Oral Chelation

Blend one cup of fresh cilantro with six tablespoons of olive oil until the cilantro is completely chopped. Add one clove of garlic, half a cup of nuts (cashews or almonds are the best), and two tablespoons of lemon juice. Blend these into a paste (which will be lumpy), adding hot water if necessary. Take two to three teaspoons per day for two to three weeks, every few months. If you make large amounts, you can freeze it for later use. You should see benefits within two to three weeks.

Your Empowered Patient Action Plan for Peripheral Artery Disease
Warning: For severe symptoms (TIAs/mini strokes, severe claudication), go to Step #7 or #9 and then return to Step #1.

Step #1: Change bad lifestyle behaviors by eating a balanced diet with more vegetables, exercising daily, and not smoking. This will help prevent progression.

Step #2: Take oral chelation to prevent further progression of disease.

Step #3: Take aspirin (81 mg) daily to prevent progression of atherosclerosis.

Step #4: Take fish oil to prevent further progression of atherosclerosis.

Step #5: Take L-arginine, policosanol, and/or ginkgo biloba for symptoms of claudication and to prevent further progression of disease.

Step #6: Take Cilostazol (Pletal) to decrease claudication symptoms if step #5 is not effective.

Step #7: Undergo minimally invasive surgery (angioplasty or stenting) if the above steps are not beneficial or for severe disease or otherwise when indicated.

Step #8: Take B vitamins after undergoing angioplasty or stenting.

Step #9: Undergo more invasive surgery (endarterectomy for carotid stenosis; bypass grafting for leg/kidney/abdominal symptoms) if indicated.

Expected Outcome
Peripheral artery disease and stenosis can be very dangerous and even deadly, so it is important to obtain appropriate treatment and prevent further progression. With adequate treatment, you should be able to prevent symptoms, complications, and death.

Arthritis (Osteoarthritis)

What You Need to Know
The number of people with arthritis is steadily increasing with the aging of the baby boomers, with 46.4 million people, or 21 percent of the population, having this

condition. Of this group, 27 million have *osteo*arthritis. Arthritis is the leading cause of disability in the country, costing more than obesity. (**Note**: For *Rheumatoid Arthritis* see that specific section).

Osteoarthritis (or degenerative joint disease) is the most common type of arthritis and is especially prevalent as we age. It can affect any joint in the body, but the hands, hips, knees, and spine are the most commonly involved. If arthritis progresses, it can limit and actually destroy the joint. (Note: for arthritis of the spine, see the section on *Back and Neck Pain*).

Genetics Influence Osteoarthritis

A recent study in *Arthritis and Rheumatism* revealed that people whose index fingers are shorter than their ring fingers (type 3 finger-length pattern) are at increased risk of developing osteoarthritis of the knee. As index finger length drops relative to ring finger length, the risk increases.

A study published in *BMJ* in March 2011 revealed that patients with osteoarthritis of the hip or knee have a higher risk for death than the general population. Speculation of cause included less physical activity, smoldering inflammation (thought to be a factor in cardiovascular disease), and use of NSAIDs (which can cause higher cardio-vascular risk). Thus, proper and effective treatment is of utmost concern, which is corroborated by a study published in *BMJ* in 2013; this study revealed that total hip and knee replacements are associated with subsequent lower heart-disease risk, due to being able to increase activity and decrease medications. Although this study refers to the benefits of surgery, any treatment that ameliorates arthritis and its symptoms can do the same.

Important Information:
MRI Overused in Assessing Knee Osteoarthritis

MRIs are commonly ordered by doctors before being referred for total knee replacement, yet studies show that MRI offers minimal or no benefit compared to taking simple weight-bearing x-rays. Since MRIs cost many times what x-rays do, this is wasteful spending and may be due to doctor ownership of MRI facilities (see chapter 3).

Hip X-rays May Not Show Arthritis

You might think that if you have chronic hip pain, x-rays will reveal arthritis, but symptoms do not often correlate with x-ray findings. A 2015 study from *BMJ* showed that only 9 percent to 16 percent of patients with frequent hip pain have x-ray evidence of osteoarthritis. The opposite was also noted: only 24 percent of patients with x-ray evidence of arthritis had pain.

The lack of x-ray evidence may lead doctors to not prescribe appropriate treatment. If your pain is persistent, MRI scanning may be necessary or you should see if a trial of treatment would benefit your pain.

It should be noted that the gold standard for diagnosing osteoarthritis is defined as "hip pain localized to the groin or anteriorly [in front]" or provoked by internal rotation [turning your foot inward].

Treatments for Osteoarthritis

The Preventive Approaches
Diet: Some people with osteoarthritis can have flare-ups of pain when eating shrimp, milk, or nitrates. It has been thought that some people can obtain pain relief by eliminating foods from the nightshade family, including tomatoes, potatoes, eggplant, and peppers, but no studies have shown this to be true, and these foods contain important nutrients. Some people however, have obtained significant relief by eliminating red meat, fruit, dairy products, additives, preservatives, herbs, spices, or alcohol. It is worth eliminating some of these foods to see if they affect your arthritis.

On the other hand, some spices, such as turmeric and ginger, have anti-inflammatory effects and may help reduce pain. Some people have done well on a vegetarian diet rich in lactobacilli, although this can cause side effects of nausea and diarrhea.

Vitamin K Deficiency May Play a Role in Arthritis

A recent multicenter study revealed that vitamin K deficiency may increase the risk (two or threefold) for developing knee osteoarthritis. It is not known, however, if vitamin K supplementation will help prevent or improve osteoarthritis in patients if they are not vitamin K deficient. You should also be aware that vitamin K can cause blood clotting and especially should not be given to patients on blood thinners except under the supervision of a doctor.

The best way to increase your vitamin K without potential side effects is to eat green, leafy vegetables, the best being kale, spinach, turnip greens, collards, Brussels sprouts, and broccoli.

***

Weight loss is very important for helping reduce osteoarthritic symptoms. Studies reveal that for every five pounds lost, patients experience an improvement in quality of life. People with stiff, achy knees can find relief if they shed as little as fifteen pounds.

Exercise: It is important for you to be active. Your osteoarthritic joints are like rusty hinges; if not used, they stiffen up until they freeze altogether. Exercise has definitely been proven to relieve arthritis pain. There are particular exercises (both aerobic and resistance) that are beneficial, especially for knee and back arthritis. Studies show that exercise has the potential to prevent disability and possibly slow disease progression. Exercise actually stimulates cartilage to take up more nutrients and help repair damage. *Caution*: If your joints are unstable, you need to exercise with caution or use braces. I recommend that you consult with your doctor or a registered physical therapist, who can teach you the best exercises for the joints involved in your particular condition. I do not recommend jogging, as runners are prone to develop or worsen osteoarthritis.

***

Dr. A's Suggestions:
Leg Length Discrepancies Can Cause Osteoarthritis

Unequal leg length is common, and a recent study published in the *Annals of Internal Medicine* showed that leg length inequality of greater than one centimeter was associated with symptomatic and progressive knee osteoarthritis, favoring the shorter leg.

Often, leg length discrepancies are due to pelvic dysfunction and can both be diagnosed and corrected by an osteopath or chiropractor.

———— ⬥ ————

The Conventional Approaches

Medications: Over-the-counter *NSAIDs* are usually the first treatment for mild arthritis, especially knee and hip. These include ibuprofen and naproxen (like Aleve). Even at low doses, these drugs may still cause stomach irritation. NSAIDs may take several days to a week to achieve pain relief.

Many patients may take *acetaminophen* (Tylenol) for pain relief, but the NSAIDs are more effective. In fact, a 2014 meta-analysis demonstrated that acetaminophen does not show clinical improvement for arthritis.

If your joints remain stiff and/or painful, a *stronger NSAID* is prescribed, such as naproxen [Naprosyn], meloxicam [Mobic], piroxicam [Feldene], oxaprozin [Daypro], nabumatone [Relafen], ketoprofen [Orudis], diclofenac [Cataflam], or diclofenac/misoprostol [Arthrotec]). These drugs are all equally effective, although one may work better for you than another. You may have to try several to see which one is the most effective for you (ask your doctor for samples). Prescription NSAIDs are stronger than over-the-counter products but also have a higher risk of side effects, primarily stomach irritation and bleeding. If stomach irritation occurs, NSAIDs known as Cox-2 inhibitors (celecoxib [Celebrex]) have less risk of stomach problems, although they are more expensive, not covered by many insurance plans, and may slightly increase your risk of heart attack if you already have heart disease. Prescription NSAIDs may take three weeks or longer to give you full relief. Often, one product will work for several months and then stop being effective: usually, switching to another brand will continue your pain relief.

Caution: In July, 2015, the FDA started requiring NSAIDs to carry a warning of increased risk of heart attacks, stroke and heart failure. This is especially evident when taken long term, at higher doses, or by people with pre-existing heart disease. The risks can increase as early as the first weeks of NSAID use. However, ibuprofen and naproxen do not appear to increase the risk, so are the safest and preferred NSAIDs.

Caution: Be aware that ibuprofen and other NSAIDs can block the blood-thinning effects of aspirin. If you must take ibuprofen, take the aspirin first and wait at least two hours to take the ibuprofen so that the aspirin has time to exert its beneficial effects. Aspirin use can deplete body stores of vitamin C, so make sure you get 600 mg per day through diet or by taking a supplement. All these drugs can also cause stomach irritation and bleeding in some people. Ordinarily, OTC proton pump inhibitors (PPIs, generically end in "prazole, such as omeprazole: most popular name brands include Prilosec, Prevacid, Nexium, Dexilant, Protonix and Aciphex) can protect the stomach if this occurs, but recent studies show that they interfere with aspirin, so consider an H$_2$ blocker (Zantac, Axid, Pepcid) instead.

Tramadol (Ultram) is a pain reliever that is often added to the treatment regimen if NSAIDs are not working. However, it has no anti-inflammatory properties.

A new product released in 2011 called *flavocoxid* (brand name Limbrel) is actually a dietary supplement, but it requires a doctor's prescription (which is why it's included here). Flavocoxid is a combination of flavonoids, a large group of plant chemicals that have anti-inflammatory effects and thus may help reduce arthritis pain. They are plentiful in fruits, vegetables, red wine, and green tea, but you cannot consume enough from foods to get a significant effect. Studies are preliminary, but some researchers think it may prove superior to NSAIDs, with fewer side effects. Understand that not all insurance covers it, and it is expensive, costing about $4 a day, although discounts are often offered.

Recently, *duloxetine* (Cymbalta), an antidepressant, has been approved by the FDA for chronic musculoskeletal pain, including osteoarthritis.

Topical Gels: Many doctors try topicals made from conventional drugs and mixed in a gel that is absorbed into the soft tissues to provide short-term relief. This is often the first line of therapy for arthritis of the hands. The topical form of these drugs usually doesn't have the side effects that can occur if you take them orally. These drugs include gabapentin (neurontin), amitriptyline, ketamine, and baclofen, but the most common are NSAIDs, including ketoprofen, voltaren, and others. A topical commonly used by doctors and physical therapists is *Biofreeze*. Its main ingredient is actually an herbal extract made from a South American holly shrub. It is fast-acting and can give several hours of relief. These topicals can relieve pain in many patients, but they do not resolve the condition or prevent further deterioration.

Another topical that has provided relief is *glyceryl trinitrate*, better known as nitroglycerin. Studies have shown that this substance can reduce arthritis pain and stiffness, although it is not used very commonly. In some studies, it has been combined with capsaicin, an herbal preparation derived from chili peppers; while nitroglycerin is effective by itself, when combined with capsaicin, it is even more effective.

Braces or taping: Many doctors prescribe either one of these to reduce pain, primarily in the knee joint. Both methods are used to provide support and take pressure off the joint. There are many different types of brace designs, and they can provide some reduction of pain. The primary problem is that they are bulky and may restrict motion, and they have no benefit after the brace is removed. Taping involves a rigid strapping of tape over the affected joint. The tape is applied every day for three weeks, but it can provide pain relief for up to three weeks after it is removed.

Lateral wedge insoles in the shoe of the affected leg may be recommended for knee arthritis on the inside of the knee (medial). These insoles are designed to shift the pressure on the knee to the outside. ***Important note***: However, studies show this not to be beneficial, at least when comparing it to simple cushioning insoles, which are much less expensive and can be bought in drug or grocery stores.

Physical therapy is a common treatment and usually involves exercises and modalities such as ultrasound, electrical stimulation, whirlpool, and TNS unit. Overall, physical therapy modalities do not help most people with osteoarthritis in the long term; self-administered exercise programs are just as effective. However, specific exercise programs designed by physical therapists have been shown to be beneficial in reducing pain and enhancing function.

Injection of steroids into the affected joint is a common conventional treatment and may provide relief that lasts several weeks to several months. However, you should only receive these injections three to four times a year because of their potential side effects, which include softening of the bone and weight gain. ***Important note***: Many studies have shown that such injections *work no better than placebo injections* but have many more side effects. ***Important Note***: Many doctors give steroid injections to reduce pain and inflammation before physical therapy. However, a 2015 study showed that steroids do not enhance the effectiveness of physical therapy in patients with osteoarthritis.

Viscosupplementation is another common injection, which uses hyaluronic acid derivatives (Synvisc or Hyalgan). Many people know this as "rooster comb," from which this substance is derived. Hyaluronic acid is what lubricates and maintains the joint and is usually deficient in osteoarthritis joints. Although these derivatives do not retard the progression of the arthritis, one study shwoed that it may delay the need for replacement surgery *if they are effective*; the caveat, however, is that the delay is only for an average of 233 days; in only 16 percent of people who undergo a second round of treatment (three to six injections), surgery can be delayed another seven months (reported at the 2013 annual meeting of *American College of Rheumatology* but sponsored by the company that makes the product). ***Important note***: More recent studies have shown that these injections *offer no better relief than placebo injections*, calling their effectiveness into question. A 2015 meta-analysis demonstrated that intra-articular injections of either steroids or hyaluronic acid appear to be superior to anti-inflammatory medications, but this is primarily because of the placebo effect.

Botox for Osteoarthritis?

Recently, a study was done showing that Botox injections could reduce osteoarthritis shoulder pain. However, it is not known how long this will last or if there are long-term side effects. Studies on larger numbers of patients are needed to answer these questions before it is recommended.

Surgeries are often done if no other conventional treatments have helped. There are several types of surgeries that can be done, and some are less invasive than others and can be done for specific patients. For knees, these include the *Unispacer* insert, *osteotomy*, and *arthroscopic debridement and lavage*. The latter is used to delay joint replacement by cleaning out the joint, but this is simply a temporary fix at best and can not only accelerate the arthritic process but also worsen your pain. ***Important note***: Several studies show that *arthroscopic debridement is no better than placebo*, so this is not recommended, even by many orthopedic associations; but it is a huge money-maker for orthopedists, so they are done routinely. ***Caution***: If you do undergo arthroscopy, it is advisable to take low-molecular-weight heparin injections to prevent deep vein thrombosis following the procedure.

Dr. A's Suggestions:
Meniscal Tears with or without Arthritis: Surgery Not Needed for Most

In many patients, knee osteoarthritis coexists with meniscal tears, which are tears of the cartilage that cushions your knees. Many meniscal tears don't cause symptoms, but when found, surgery is often done anyway. A study published in the *NEJM* showed that even with symptoms, most patients don't need surgery, and physical therapy is just as beneficial.

Another study corroborated this, finding that a three-month program of carefully designed exercise and education in patients with cartilage lesions eliminated the need for surgery in 64 percent of the patients. As surgeries for cartilage lesions are not long-lasting and are frequently ineffective, rehab should be tried initially.

Many meniscal tears are caused by aging (degenerative) without signs of arthritis. A *NEJM* study in late 2013 showed that arthroscopic surgery for these patients is no better than sham surgery and therefore should not be done.

Joint replacement is a common surgery for osteoarthritis and is considered a "last resort". Ninety percent of hip replacements are done due to osteoarthritis. Such surgery is recommended if your joint has been completely worn down by arthritis, but too often, it is done before other potentially effective alternative methods are tried. The most common joints replaced are the knee and hip.

Doctors Often Do Not Discuss Joint Replacement
With Elderly Patients Who May Benefit

Although an increased number of younger patients are receiving joint replacements, some older people who should receive them are not. A recent study published in the *Archives of Internal Medicine* revealed that elderly patients (over sixty-five years of age) take several weeks to recover from joint replacements but experience excellent long term outcomes. However, it was determined that many physicians don't discuss joint replacement with older patients who may benefit, thinking that they are too old.

At present, artificial joints last eight to twelve years on average, but some can last much longer, depending on factors such as weight, joint use, and replacement material. A joint can be replaced a second or third time, but it is not as successful; so the longer you can avoid the first surgery, the better. That is why most surgeons recommend waiting until you are sixty-five to seventy years old. However, many studies have shown that surgeons are more willing to perform replacements on younger patients, even though considered inappropriate for many of them.

Baby Boomers Getting Earlier Knee Replacement
But May Not Like the Results

The number of baby boomers choosing knee replacement for arthritis is growing steadily. The number has risen from 300,000 a year to nearly 500,000. It is estimated that 3.2 million annual knee replacements per year may occur a decade from now. The reason for this is that younger patients are experiencing an earlier onset of arthritis but want to maintain an active lifestyle.

However, the first study done to evaluate knee replacement surgery after the first five years revealed a discrepancy between patients' expectations and their actual abilities to engage in sports and recreational activities. They can perform activities of daily living but have diminished capacity beyond those activities.

Many of these patients also have to undergo revisions when the replacements wear out, usually in eight to twelve years; and patients have even more disabilities then, as revisions do not work as well as the original surgery.

Caution: There are several different types of knee replacement materials. Metal-on-polyethylene is the standard, but there are also ceramic-on-ceramic and metal-on-metal prostheses. The latter have been shown to expose patients to toxic metals and cause more failures (10 percent risk). Studies have shown that metal-on-polyethylene is as good as the others but much less expensive and requires fewer revisions. A 2014 study in *BMJ* advised *against* using five newer types of joint implants, stating that existing devices appear to be safer; those that are not recommended include: for *total hip replacement*; ceramic-on-ceramic, modular femoral necks and uncemented monoblock cups; for *knee replacements*; high-flexion knee replacement and gender-specific knee replacement.

Bisphosphonates Help Extend Life of Implants

A study from the *BMJ* showed that taking bisphosphonate drugs (usually used for osteoporosis) during and after knee and hip replacements can extend the life of the implant, thus reducing the need for expensive revisions. However, you should be aware that there are many downsides of bisphosphonates (refer to section on *Osteoporosis*). In addition, OTC strontium may be just as beneficial, although studies have not been conducted using this supplement.

Almost half the joint replacements done involve "minimally invasive" joint replacement, with an incision half that of regular surgery. The advantage is shorter recuperation time, but there are many disadvantages: surgeons have a harder time seeing what they are doing and thus there is a higher rate of mistakes, including uneven leg lengths, broken hipbones, off-kilter knee joints, and cement left in the wound that causes pain. You should always use a surgeon who has done at least twenty-five such procedures if you undergo this modified replacement surgery.

Dr. A's Suggestions:
Blood Thinners a Must after Joint Replacement

One of the most frequent complications of knee and hip joint replacement is deep-venous thrombosis (DVT or leg blood clots), which can cause significant problems and even death. At present, most doctors will prescribe low-molecular-weight heparin (LMWH), a daily injection, for a week to a month. In July 2011, rivaroxaban (Xarelto) was approved by the FDA and has been shown to offer better protection from blood clots. In addition, it is taken orally and requires no monitoring. Xarelto should be taken for twelve days after knee replacement and thirty-five days after hip replacement.

A recent study researched whether physical therapy after knee replacement is beneficial. Findings indicated that it may speed recovery to a minor degree, but it is no better than self-administered home exercises for long term benefits.

Joint Replacement versus Nonsurgical Treatment: Which is Better?

Joint replacements are very common but few studies have compared them to nonsurgical treatment. A 2015 study compared total knee replacement followed by nonsurgical treatment versus nonsurgical treatment alone. Findings were that knee replacement patients had greater improvements in pain, function and quality of life. However, there were a few caveats.

First, nonsurgical patients also experienced clinically important improvement and also sustained fewer serious adverse events. Second, the nonsurgical treatment consisted of supervised exercise, education, weight-loss advice, use of insoles, and pain medications; these did not include other potentially beneficial conventional treatments or alternative measures, yet they still showed significant improvement.

Regarding other benefits, in a 2013 observational study, investigators stated that total joint replacement lowered risk for heart problems. However, in a newer observational study in 2015, patients undergoing surgery had no significant difference in long-term heart events compared to nonsurgical patients, but did have an increased risk of heart attack in the first month after surgery.

The *bottom line* is that many patients might prefer a nonsurgical approach, especially if undergoing alternatives that were not included in these studies.

Hip resurfacing is another newer surgery that offers an alternative to hip replacement, covering the damage with smooth metal rather than cutting away worn bone and replacing it. This is an option primarily for younger patients. Even newer is **joint**

distraction, which has been shown in Europe to possibly reverse cartilage damage and delay the need for replacement.

The Alternative Approaches

Low level energy lasers (*LLELs* or "cold" lasers) have been a godsend for treating osteoarthritis. The laser appears to reduce the inflammatory response and may actually regenerate new cartilage, thus giving long-lasting relief and preventing further deterioration of the joint. These lasers are called cold lasers because they do not produce heat like the hot lasers used in surgical procedures. Since laser treatment addresses the underlying cause, it provides long-lasting relief rather than just providing temporary symptom relief. You should feel better within one to nine treatments (two to three weeks). With the use of cold lasers, joint replacements can be decreased substantially: In my thirty years of LLEL research, the majority of patients with osteoarthritis did not need joint replacements after laser treatment (see chapter 4 for more in depth discussion and recommendations).

Infrasound is another device that is helpful for treating osteoarthritis. Infrasound is low-frequency sound (6–14 Hz) versus ultrasound, which is high-frequency sound (20,000 Hz). Infrasound works by increasing the local circulation of blood and lymph, and it also stimulates the production of hyaluronic acid, which lubricates joints. It can not only reduce pain but also decrease stiffness and swelling. Numerous chiropractors, naturopaths, acupuncturists, and a few doctors use infrasound.

Acupuncture has been proven in numerous (well-done) studies to benefit osteoarthritic joints. You should notice less pain, stiffness, and swelling within six to seven treatments, although you might need ten to twelve treatments followed by maintenance treatments several times a year for maximum and long-lasting benefits.

Chinese herbal formulas may also be beneficial, especially when used with acupuncture. TCM practitioners call osteoarthritis "Bi Syndrome." A formula for Cold Damp Bi is *Duo Huo Ji Sheng Wan*, to help stiff joints relieved by warmth. Other formulas include *Shu Jing Huo Xue Tang*, *Du Huo Ji Sheng Wa*n and *Huo Luo Xiao Ling Dan*. You should feel better within three weeks but may need to take them longer for full relief. Consult a certified TCM practitioner to find out which one is best for you.

Herbal topical solutions can give you short-term relief, reducing pain and inflammation. Natural topicals include capsaicin, the Chinese herbal Zheng Gu Shui, EMU oil (usually with aloe vera and MSM), long crystal menthol, glucosamine/MSM, sea cucumber, and other herbs.

Some topicals may work better than others, so you may have to try several to find the best one for you. You can also mix several different topicals for better results. These topicals should provide you with pain relief in just a few minutes. In my clinic, I applied samples to my patients so they'd know whether the products worked before purchasing them. Encourage your doctor or practitioner to do the same. Although they don't cure the underlying problem, these products can provide pain relief for two to eight hours or longer.

Nutritional supplements: There are several that have been found very effective for osteoarthritis. *Glucosamine sulfate* (1,500 mg per day) is the most commonly used and is primarily beneficial for peripheral joints, not the spine. ***Important Note***: This supplement has been controversial due to studies showing it to be ineffective in arthritis. However, the studies that show negative results have primarily used glucosamine *hydrochloride*. The positive ones have primarily used glucosamine *sulfate*, which is the recommended kind (see sidebar below). You should notice improvement in pain or stiffness within four to eight weeks; if you don't, you are either taking a poor-quality brand or it won't work for you; there is no reason to take it longer than eight weeks if it isn't working.

Dr. A's Suggestions:
Research on Glucosamine Poor and Misleading

Lately, several research studies have concluded that glucosamine does not ease joint pain or improve other arthritis symptoms, but these are examples of poor research. In two major, multimillion-dollar studies (the last in 2014), the form of glucosamine used was the hydrochloride, which has been found previously to be ineffective in most patients. (You should use the sulfate form.) Unfortunately, many doctors and the media hyped up these negative findings.

Another study was a meta-analysis of ten studies, but each study was different. Meta-analyses can be very misleading, as in this case, because some of the trials used nonstandardized supplements, some studies had differing concentrations, and a few studies had questionable supplement quality. Despite the "apples-to-oranges" comparisons, the authors still concluded that glucosamine did not ease joint pain.

These authors would lead you to believe that glucosamine benefits are a placebo effect. However, veterinarians use glucosamine for dogs, cats, and horses, and it works very well for arthritis in these animals: animals don't have the placebo response. My recommendation is that if glucosamine *sulfate* works for you, keep taking it. If it hasn't worked in eight weeks, it probably won't be effective.

Other supplements may also be of value and can be as effective as glucosamine sulfate. These include:

- *Methylsulfonurea*, or MSM (1,000–3,000 mg per day). MSM is itself an anti-inflammatory, but it also can help glucosamine get into the joints.
- *Cetyl myristoleate* (1,000 mg twice daily) is an immunomodulator, which shuts off production of immune-system cells that irritate the tissue. Its advantage is that you only take it for one to three months, but its effects are long-lasting.
- *Sea cucumber* (500 mg, two to four times per day) has anti-inflammatory properties and is effective within four to six weeks.

Chondroitin Not Effective?

Chondroitin (200–400 mg, two to three times daily) is the most common supplement added to glucosamine, but many studies have declared it to be ineffective for arthritis. However, a study in 2011 showed that it did in fact decrease structural deterioration of joints (based on MRI), so it may be a valuable adjunct.

Other supplements that also have research support are listed below.

- *Collagenix* has been shown effective in 25–72 percent of patients in just seven days of use.
- *Phlogenzym* is a combination product containing proteolytic enzymes rutin (100 mg), trypsin (48 mg), and bromelain (90 mg) and has been shown to be effective in several studies.
- *Guggal* (500 mg three times daily), an herb from India, has evidence to show effectiveness in reducing arthritic symptoms.
- *Lyprinol* (100 mg twice daily), which comes from a New Zealand mussel, contains several anti-inflammatory compounds.
- *SAM-e* (200 mg three times a day) is a supplement imported from Germany that has been shown to be effective for reducing symptoms of osteoarthritis, but it is expensive for the high quality brands. You should notice improvement within three to four weeks.
- *Pycnogenol* (100–250 mg daily in two doses) is a powerful antioxidant that has anti-inflammatory properties and has been shown in studies to decrease

analgesic use after about three months. ***Helpful tip***: Pycnogenol contains the same active ingredients as grape-seed extract (200–400 mg daily), the latter of which is much less expensive.

- *ASU* (avocado-soybean unsaponifiables) was shown in a recent to not only help decrease pain and improve function in osteoarthritis patients but also reduce disease progression as noted on x-rays.
- *Cat's claw* (100 mg freeze-dried daily) has been shown to reduce knee pain associated with physical activity, but it doesn't work for knee pain that occurs while the knee is at rest.
- *Devil's claw* (2,400–2,600 mg/day providing 56–60 mg/day of the harpagoside constituent) appears to provide relief, but only when used in conjunction with NSAIDs.
- *Stinging nettle* (crude stinging nettle leaf, 9 g daily), an herb used commonly for allergies, has also shown some effectiveness, but only when used with NSAIDs.
- *Ginger* is known to inhibit the inflammatory response. Studies have shown this herb to be as effective as cortisone or phenylbutazone, a very powerful anti-inflammatory drug.
- *Guggul* or *turmeric* has potent anti-inflammatory effects.
- *Boswellia* appears to inhibit inflammation, prevent decreased cartilage production, and improve blood supply to joint tissue.
- Two other beneficial herbs, *willow bark* and *phytodolor* (used in Germany since 1963), contain ingredients found in aspirin.
- *Superoxide dismutase* (SOD) prevents oxygen-related damage to the join tissues. Oral SOD supplements are rapidly broken down in the stomach and thus are not beneficial. Only injections into the joint are effective.

You can take any of these supplements individually or in various combinations with or without glucosamine. There are several products, in fact, that combine glucosamine with many of the above herbs.

Warning: *Limbrel* (flavocoxid) is marketed for osteoarthritis as a medical food but has been reported to cause liver damage, albeit rarely. If you take this product and have abdominal pain, jaundice, or fatigue, check your liver enzymes. Fortunately, the damage is reversible.

Biomagnets, which are applied to the affected joint (either taped or contained in a brace), have been found useful by many people and have been supported by some research. Biomagnets can relieve your pain symptoms but can't cure the underlying cause of them; their relief disappears when the magnet is removed. There are many different types and strengths of magnets, as well as unipole, dipole, and north- or south-directed, all of which can make a difference in whether they are effective for your condition. Biomagnets should give you relief almost immediately.

Balneotherapy, the medicinal use of mineral baths and mud packs, is used by massage and health therapists in spas worldwide. It is very soothing and relaxing and can benefit almost any medical condition, including osteoarthritis. The minerals in the mud packs, not the mud itself, are the key ingredients that provide relief; people using mud compresses without minerals have very little relief, but those using compresses that are rich in magnesium, sodium, calcium, potassium, and chloride may find significant relief from the symptoms of osteoarthritis.

Your Empowered Patient Action Plan for Osteoarthritis

Step #1: Undergo LLEL (cold laser) treatment, which is the best treatment for long-term resolution or relief.

Step #2: Undergo acupuncture, which can also provide long-lasting resolution and relief. It can be used with Step #1 if both are available.

———

As a young man, Paul played football and sustained numerous injuries to his knees. Now fifty-seven years old, he always had some swelling in his knees, and they cracked and popped all the time. He had tried various anti-inflammatory drugs and had several debridement surgeries on both knees. He tried to exercise but couldn't because his pain and swelling would get worse. I started him on LLEL treatment. After just three treatments, his swelling was completely gone. After nine treatments, nearly all of his pain was gone, too. He was able to return to almost all activities that he had stopped (golf, tennis, skiing). To eliminate the remainder of his pain, I performed acupuncture, which took only eight treatments to give Paul something he hadn't experienced for decades: pain-free knees.

———

Step #3: Apply topical herbal or prescription solutions for temporary relief. These are a lot safer than oral supplements and medications.

Step #4: Take Glucosamine sulfate with MSM, Cetyl Myristoleate, sea cucumber, and/or other nutritional supplements for temporary relief. These are preferred over medications due to fewer side effects and less expense.

Step #5: Try other herbs or herbal combinations (listed above) for temporary relief if the above have not helped.

———

Louise had pain from osteoarthritis in her fingers, knees, hips, and shoulders. She had been placed on numerous medications, including prescription NSAIDs, and had been given several steroid injections (Step #11) in her hips and knees, which lasted only a few months. She had also undergone hyalgan injections (Step #12), which also failed to relieve her pain very long. Her doctor recommended joint replacements of her hips and knees (Step #13), but Louise was afraid of undergoing surgery because of her age (seventy-eight). I suggested using a combination of glucosamine and sea cucumber along with cetyl myristoleate. Within six weeks most of her pain was gone, and she actually went out dancing for the first time in fifteen years.

Step #6: **Take the Chinese herbal remedies** for temporary relief if you still have pain and stiffness. Consult with a TCM practitioner.

Step #7: **Apply biomagnets** for temporary relief.

Step #8: **Take an over-the-counter NSAID** for temporary relief if none of the above has helped.

Step #9: **Take flavocoxid** (by prescription) if the above steps have not relieved your pain. It may work better than some of the herbs in the above steps, but it is more expensive. However, it has fewer side effects than the drugs in the following steps.

Step #10: **Take a stronger prescription NSAID** for temporary relief if the milder NSAIDs haven't worked.

Step #11: **Receive corticosteroid injections** for temporary relief only if the above have not helped. Limit the number to three injections in one year.

Step #12: **Receive viscosupplementation** for temporary relief. Three to five injections are required.

Step #13: **Undergo surgery** only as a last resort and only after undergoing the previous steps.

Step #14: **Use the LLEL after surgery** to accelerate the healing process and minimize scarring.

Expected Outcome

Osteoarthritis is a very common condition as we age, but you really don't have to suffer. There are several alternative methods that can resolve symptoms long term and a myriad of other treatments that can control symptoms well enough to provide an excellent quality of life. Although more and more young people are receiving knee replacements, the need for surgery can be prevented in most cases by using alternative methods.

Back and Neck Pain, Acute (Recent Onset)

What You Need to Know

Acute spine pain can be a result of many different causes, including infections and cancer. However, trauma is by far the main cause. As we get older, we not only suffer more serious consequences of injuries but also take much longer to heal because our tissues degenerate over time.

Certainly, there are many sources of spine injuries, but commonly, as we age, many of us still think we can do activities we've always been able to do. Unfortunately, the tolerance of our bodies to the same activities decreases steadily as we age, especially if we do not keep active and well-conditioned. Many spine injuries are caused by just moderate lifting or twisting or simply "overdoing." Of course even if you are younger, you can be injured more easily if you are not in good condition.

Acute or recent spine injuries are different than chronic spine problems and thus are treated differently (see next section, "Chronic Back and Neck Pain," if you've had spine pain for more than six months). Fortunately, most acute spine injuries can heal with time; in fact, researchers have shown that 90 percent of people recover in six weeks. In fact, even with ruptured (herniated) discs, studies show that most can heal within a year. Too often, however, patients are in a hurry to eliminate their pain and opt for surgery and other invasive treatments, only to find out they may not be effective and/or have long-term side effects—as well as being very expensive.

Important Information:
Trends in Spine Pain Management Go Against Guidelines

There have been numerous studies on treating neck and back (spine) pain, and recent reports show that doctors commonly mismanage, overuse, and abuse treatments for the pain. In fact, most completely ignore guidelines. The unnecessary care includes:

- A 106 percent increase in the number of referrals to specialists (most for surgery) while referrals for physical therapy remain unchanged.
- A 56.9 percent increase in the use of advanced imaging (e.g., MRI).

- A 50.8 percent increase in the use of narcotics: use of nonsteroidal anti-inflammatory drugs has dropped from 37 percent to 25 percent while narcotic use has increased from 7 percent to 14 percent
- Increased use of spinal injections, even though proven no better than placebo.
- Increase in spinal fusion surgery, despite poor evidence that it works, high costs and increased side effects, disability, and mortality.

This is one condition for which you definitely need to become empowered. Many people want quick results and think that getting "more" equates to better care and satisfaction, but it may not. Spine-related pain costs $86 billion annually, much of it unnecessary and ineffective.

It is common to undergo an MRI scan to evaluate acute spine injuries, but most of the time, it is not indicated (see sidebar below). A major reason is that disc "bulging" is often seen on MRI, and if you have pain and these abnormalities are found, you get treatments for it that frequently do not help. Studies have shown that 75 percent of people with *no* neck or back pain will have abnormalities on MRI. The *bottom line* is that too many doctors treat the MRI, not the patient, and the MRI "findings" may not be causing the symptoms. Unfortunately, this may be the actual reason why more back surgeries are being performed…many unnecessary and ineffective, and many causing even worse problems as well as disability.

Dr. A's Suggestions:
Most Doctors Ignore National Guidelines for MRI Scans

MRI scans are performed and repeated much too often. Studies show that there is a minimal chance of any significant change within a year of doing an MRI scan for neck and back pain or for sciatica, but many doctors repeat them before then because they own their own MRI scan centers or simply because treatments are not working.

The first national guidelines for spine pain recommend against ordering imaging or other diagnostic tests unless severe or progressive neurological defects (such as paralysis or loss of bladder/rectal control) are present or a condition such as cancer is suspected. Furthermore, MRI is recommended only if surgery or epidural injections are considered.

The main concern with new back pain is fracture or cancer. A 2013 study in *BMJ* documented some "red flags" that might be useful in determining who should undergo testing. These include (probabilities in parentheses):

For cancer:

- History of cancer (7% in primary care, 33% in emergency care)
- Old age (< 3%)
- Unexplained weight loss (< 3%)
- Failure to improve after one month (< 3%)

For fracture:

- Presence of contusion or abrasion (62%)
- Prolonged use of steroids (33%)
- Trauma (11%)
- Age older than 64 (9%)

It should be noted, however, that many guidelines recommend imaging with *any* red flag, which results in many unnecessary tests. However, if more than two or three red flags are present, imaging is indicated.

⁂

MRI scans are not the only test that is overused and misused to determine spine treatment. In a recent guideline by the *American Pain Society*, it was determined that invasive diagnostic tests such as *discography, facet joint block, and sacroiliac joint block* have not been proven to be accurate for diagnosing various spinal conditions; and their use to guide therapeutic choices (such as surgery) is uncertain, again leading to unnecessary surgeries and a high failure rate from surgery.

Another test is the *myelogram*, during which dye is injected into the spinal column, outlining the spinal nerves as they leave the spinal cord and go to the leg. If the dye is seen to be obstructed, this may mean that the nerve is being compressed by a ruptured disc. This test can reveal abnormalities not observed on MRI or confirm abnormalities that are seen on MRI.

Sometimes, an injection called a *selective nerve root block* is used to test whether a particular nerve is involved. If you get temporary relief from the injection, it often means that nerve is irritated. Like discogram, however, there is no corroborative evidence that this test will lead to positive outcomes.

The *EMG* (electromyogram) is a very common (but painful) test if you have pain going down your arm or leg. This test is often worthless because 70 percent damage to the nerve must be present for it to be positive. Few doctors base recommendations for surgery or other treatments on EMG, and often, surgery is done even when the EMG is negative. Nevertheless, it is commonly ordered, at a cost of about $1,400 (see chapter 3 for more discussion on EMG).

Does Most Spine Pain Really Resolve Spontaneously?

Most studies have shown that *acute* spine pain nearly always resolves spontaneously. However, this is usually based on results showing that the majority of patients discontinue seeking medical care. Other studies have shown that up to 80 percent of patients with acute spine pain may continue to experience some pain or disability at one year following their initial doctor visit, so they would be considered to have chronic spine pain. If this occurs to you, see the next section on chronic spine pain.

Treatments for Acute Spine Pain

The Preventive Approaches
Being in good physical shape is the best preventive for spine injuries. Good posture and good lifting techniques are invaluable in preventing injuries, especially when doing manual lifting and pushing and pulling activities. Consultation with a physical therapist or attending a back school will help you learn proper techniques. Unfortunately, most industries do not participate in such programs.

Falls Common as We Age

One of the most common problems as we age is falling, which most commonly occurs due to weakness, poor balance, blood pressure (too high or too low), and even wearing multifocal glasses. About one in six adults over the age of sixty-five falls every three months and one-third sustain injuries. Therefore, in general, preventing falls is a good way to prevent injuries.

The CDC describes fourteen effective fall-prevention strategies in a new publication, *Preventing Falls: What Works* (http://www.cdc.gov/ncipc/

PreventingFalls/). In addition, taking vitamin D$_3$ (800 mg daily) has been shown to prevent falls as well.

One unusual cause of falls is decreased blood pressure only after eating, which occurs to many elderly patients. If that should occur, increased water intake before eating or eating six smaller meals a day rather than three large ones can help prevent this.

A recent study showed that elderly people who fell and had access to an alarm system did not use the alarm in 80 percent of cases…this is "alarming" in itself because prolonged time on the floor after falling is associated with greater injury and hospitalization.

***

Helpful tip: Many people use lumbar supports when lifting or carrying heavy objects to prevent back injuries. A meta-analysis of fifteen studies shows that back belts or braces do little or nothing to prevent back pain, so they are usually unnecessary.

***

Dr. A's Suggestions:
Neck and Back Braces for Pain: Help or Hindrance?

Back and neck braces also are often prescribed or used by people who have acute spine pain. Although they can provide needed support and protection and lessen pain, they can also prolong healing and cause stiffness and loss of muscle tone. Only use a back brace when needed for support or when prescribed by your doctor for specific instability in the spine. Use it as infrequently as possible.

***

The Conventional Approaches

***

Dr. A's Suggestions:
Conventional Treatments to Avoid

Many treatments are given for acute low back pain that have never been supported by research and therefore are not recommended here. These include traction, prescription antidepressants, lumbar supports, and TENS units (small devices that conduct electricity to the superficial soft tissues). Neck braces are commonly used for neck injuries, but can actually increase your pain and disability if overused (see above in Preventive Approaches). I also recommend against spinal injections, for reasons detailed below.

Important note: You should understand that many conventional treatments are ineffective. A recent study revealed that nonsurgical treatment for neck/back pain averages $16,000, yet it is often not beneficial. This is also why many patients may stop seeing their doctor, who then may think that your pain has resolved. In addition, you should realize that many surgeries are done because these other conventional treatments have failed to relieve the pain. The *bottom line* is that alternative methods are frequently more effective than conventional methods, at much less expense, and should be considered before surgery (see below under *Alternative Approaches* for further details).

⁂

Medications are the first treatment given by most conventional doctors, to relieve your pain and decrease inflammation while allowing your body tissues to heal themselves.

Analgesics, such as Tylenol (acetaminophen), or over-the-counter NSAIDs, such as Advil, Aleve, and Ibuprofen, are often recommended first. *Important Note*: However, a 2014 study in *Lancet* revealed that acetaminophen for low back pain is no better than placebo. *Caution*: Acetaminophen can cause liver damage if you drink excessive alcohol or the proper dose is exceeded (greater than four grams per day). The latter may occur if you take other products that contain acetaminophen, such as cold medicines and other pain medications.

Stronger NSAIDs (such as naproxen [Naprosyn], meloxicam [Mobic], piroxicam [Feldene], oxaprozin [Daypro], nabumatone [Relafen], ketoprofen [Orudis], diclofenac [Cataflam], and diclofenac/misoprostol [Arthrotec]) may be prescribed if the above drugs do not control your pain. These drugs may cause stomach irritation and bleeding, and if this occurs, you can try the Cox-2 inhibitor, Celebrex, which has a lower risk of these side effects. *Caution*: In July, 2015, the FDA started requiring NSAIDs to carry a warning of increased risk of heart attacks, stroke and heart failure. This is especially evident when taken long term, at higher doses, or by people with pre-existing heart disease. The risks can increase as early as the first weeks of NSAID use. However, ibuprofen and naproxen do not appear to increase the risk, so are the safest and preferred NSAIDs.

Muscle relaxants (Flexeril, Robaxin, Zanaflex, Parafon Forte, or Soma) are commonly prescribed, but in fact they do not affect skeletal muscle and they also cause drowsiness in many people. They are beneficial primarily in the first few days after an injury, although studies reveal that they add little benefit to NSAIDs.

Narcotics (usually hydrocodone or oxycodone) can be prescribed for severe pain but should only be taken for a short period of time to avoid addiction. Like muscle relaxants, they do not add much benefit beyond NSAIDs.

Gabapentin (Neurontin) or *pregabalin* (Lyrica) is often given for pain that radiates down the legs (radicular pain or sciatica) but no large randomized studies have been conducted to prove their efficacy. One study showed that gabapentin was no better than epidural steroid injections (see below).

Physical therapy is the most common initial conventional treatment, and there are two approaches. The first, and most common, are *formal exercises*. Such exercises can help many people but it needs to be done with your spine in neutral position, so a physical therapist is definitely needed to help guide you; you should see a therapist as soon as possible because the longer the delay, the longer it will take to improve your condition. Complete rest is not advised, as it may cause more stiffness, loss of muscular tone, and disability. You should continue doing as many physical activities as you can tolerate, but don't overdo them. Let the pain be your guide; some soreness is to be expected, but if you have severe pain, don't continue the activity.

Physical therapy *modalities*, such as electrical current (applying low-voltage current to the area of pain), ultrasound (applying high-frequency sound that projects heat to the deep tissues), infrasound (low-frequency sound that increases local blood and lymph circulation and activity of the nervous system), hot/cold packs, alternating current, and therapeutic massage can help accelerate the healing process often better than exercise in acute cases. Ultrasound is sometimes helpful but can be irritating if there is inflammation, but is usually the most valuable. These treatments can be provided by PCPs who have the necessary equipment, but registered physical therapists are more experienced and trained. You should feel better after six to twelve treatments.

Psychological factors are an important aspect of back pain and can hinder healing, even if you are not aware of them. This does not mean that you are "crazy" or have a mental problem. Many people simply do not realize that other psychosocial factors (such as job dissatisfaction, family problems, or financial difficulties) can prolong back pain, but once you are aware of these factors and how to deal with them, you can heal properly by going to a psychologist or counselor who specializes in such therapy for pain.

Epidural steroid injections (injection of cortisone into the lining of the spinal column) is a very common, although off-label, procedure done for spine pain, but it is *significantly abused and overused*, simply making lots of money for the doctor and costing you a lot (average cost is $7,500 for three, and your co-pay may be over $2,500). **Helpful tips**: *This procedure should be considered only if the MRI reveals disc or nerve abnormalities that correlate with the symptoms and do not yet require surgery, it has been less than two months since the start of your symptoms, and other therapies have not relieved your pain.* **Important Notes**: Usually three injections, a week apart, are recommended, but the effectiveness of this "series" has never been supported by research. If you obtain pain relief from the first injection, but the relief lasts only a few hours or days, further injections will usually not be beneficial, and I don't recommend proceeding with more. If these injections are effective, pain relief may last four to six months, perhaps up to a year; but studies show that most people who obtain relief only maintain it for an average of three weeks. Epidural injections are not beneficial if you have normal test findings or if you have spine pain alone. *Warning*: In rare cases, epidurals can cause blindness, stroke, paralysis or death.

Spinal Injections (ESI) Are Often Unnecessary, Ineffective, and Harmful

Numerous studies have shown that epidural steroid injections are no better than placebo (salt water) injections: the latest studies showed this to be true with sciatica, with arm pain originating from the neck (cervical radiculopathy), or from leg pain originating from the back (lumbar radiculopathy). In fact, of all the guidelines on spine pain in the world, only one country (Belgium) recommends spinal injections. In addition, some doctors recommend injection of etanaercept, a tumor-necrosis factor used in rheumatoid arthritis, but this is even less effective than steroids.

Furthermore, a 2012 study in *Spine* showed that postmenopausal women who receive ESI had a decline in bone density of the hip six months later. A 2013 study in the *Journal of Bone and Joint Surgery* found a modestly increased risk of vertebral fractures in older women who had undergone ESI.

Based on the available studies and literature, steroid injection therapy for spine pain and sciatica can be regarded as having limited clinical benefit. As other, less invasive and more cost-effective therapies are available, you should become empowered and seek these first.

Other injections are also commonly tried, depending on your symptoms, physical findings, and MRI results. These include trigger point injections (injection of cortisone into "tender" muscle areas), facet joint injections (injection of cortisone in the joint[s] that connect the bones of the spine), or selective nerve root blocks (injections of cortisone around the nerves coming from the spinal cord and going to the legs). Like ESI, these injections are usually effective only temporarily, but they are hypothesized to allow time for the body to heal itself. If they are not effective, don't continue undergoing them—they are not cumulative.

Depending on what further diagnostic tests show, other methods may be recommended. **IDET** (intradiscal electrothermal therapy) is a procedure that is used when there is a tear in the covering of a spinal disc (annular tear). It involves placing a wire around the disc and heating it, which seals the tear. IDET is most effective when you have only one damaged disc with a limited area of damage; it should not be done otherwise. Healing may take four to six months following the procedure, and you are not allowed to engage in any activity during that time. ***Important note***: *Studies have shown long-term effectiveness to be very poor.*

Spinal surgery should be your treatment of last resort, or performed if you have unrelenting leg or arm pain or neurological signs (paralysis, inability to urinate or have a bowel movement) that correlate with the above testing. If done appropriately, surgery is often beneficial for reducing the pain that radiates into your legs, but it may not be as helpful for reducing the neck and back pain. The optimum time for surgery is within three to six months of symptom onset, although beneficial results may still be achieved at longer intervals. In general, however, the longer the symptoms have been present, the poorer the results. In fact, surgery can sometimes make your pain and other symptoms worse in the future, requiring additional spine surgeries to relieve the additional symptoms. ***Important Note***: Unfortunately, spinal surgery is overused and abused and is often done for monetary reasons.

There are several different types of back surgeries, the least invasive being a simple *discectomy* (removal of the herniated fragment of disc) with or without laminectomy or laminotomy (enlarging the "hole" in the bone through which the nerve goes). Many surgeons, however, recommend *fusion* surgery. There are two types of fusion surgery: if performed by a neurosurgeon, cadaver bone is used to fuse the vertebra together; if performed by an orthopedist, the vertebra will be fixated with rods and screws. No studies have compared the two types. ***Cautions***: This surgery, no matter which type of doctor does it, *has a very high failure rate*, and a one-level fusion frequently causes increased stress on the other discs, causing their accelerated degeneration and requiring additional surgeries…each one having a substantially decreased success rate. Independent, nonbiased studies reveal only a 15 percent two-year success rate with fusions. Fusions of the neck have a better outcome than fusions of the back. In addition, fusions can lead to the development or acceleration of spine arthritis. ***Helpful tip***: For acute spine injuries, discectomies are preferred if you have to undergo surgery. They are easier to do, less expensive, and cause less long-term side effects and harm.

The Alternative Approaches

Low level energy laser *(LLEL or "cold" laser)* is probably one of the most effective yet underused therapies for spine pain. Since it addresses the underlying cause, it provides long-lasting relief rather than just temporary symptom relief. It is very beneficial for healing disc problems and can even resolve ruptured discs without surgery, often within six to eight treatments. The laser appears to directly stimulate repair and healing of the disc and has no long-term side effects. Once your pain resolves, it doesn't reoccur unless you reinjure the spine because it addresses the underlying cause rather than treating the symptoms. As a leading researcher on cold lasers for thirty years and having used it to resolve my own ruptured disc, I can attest to its effectiveness in the vast majority of acute spine injuries.

Manual therapy: Very often, injuries cause a misalignment of the spine, which is what may cause your pain. Unfortunately, most doctors are not trained in misalignment diagnosis, and x-rays and MRIs do not reveal these abnormalities. Too often, doctors rely on spinal tests and rush into therapies that will not help if misalignment is present. Manual therapy is indicated first if there are underlying structural problems (bones, ligaments, tendons, joints, and/or muscles not working correctly), which needs to be determined by a chiropractic or osteopathic exam. Common symptoms include popping or cracking when you move your neck or back, or locking up. *Helpful tip*: If your pain comes and goes, various positions make your pain better or worse, or you feel as if your spine needs to be popped, misalignment is likely. If structural problems are evident, then they must be corrected first or your symptoms will probably not improve, or if they do, they may recur.

Osteopathic mobilization and *chiropractic manipulation* are the manual therapy methods most likely to be helpful in uncomplicated back problems (that is, if you don't have significant preexisting back problems, such as severe arthritis, spinal stenosis, ruptured disc, or previous back surgeries), especially in the first one or two months of an injury. Your pain should start decreasing in six to eight treatments, although additional treatments may be necessary to achieve maximum benefit. If pain is still present after ten to twelve treatments, any structural problems are probably not the primary cause of your pain and further evaluation or a different method may be necessary.

Acupuncture is effective for reducing acute muscle spasms and trigger points (small areas of muscle that become inflamed and are very painful when you push on them) but is also useful for pain caused by discs pressing on nerves (radicular pain down the leg or arm). In my clinic, we also were able to relieve pain from bulging and herniated discs using acupuncture in combination with the LLEL. However, acupuncture alone may be effective for reducing symptoms enough to avoid surgery. You should feel better within six to eight acupuncture treatments but might need additional sessions for maximum benefit.

Topical solutions are helpful for short-term relief while the above methods have time to heal. Natural topicals that can reduce pain and inflammation include the Chinese herbal Zheng Gu Shui, EMU oil (usually with aloe vera and MSM), long crystal menthol, Biofreeze, capsaicin, glucosamine/MSM, sea cucumber, and other herbs.

Some topicals may work better than others, so you may have to try several to find the best one for you. You can also mix several different topicals for better results. These topicals should provide you with pain relief in just a few minutes. In my clinic, I applied samples to my patients so they'd know whether the products work before purchasing them. Encourage your doctor or practitioner to do the same. Although they don't cure the underlying problem, these products can provide pain relief for two to eight hours or longer.

There are some **oral supplements** that have anti-inflammatory actions, but for acute neck and back pain, they are not very helpful, and conventional medications work better and faster for temporary relief.

Your Empowered Patient Action Plan for Acute Spine Injuries

- *Warning: Worsening severe back pain with radiation down the arm or leg, paralysis, or inability to urinate or have a bowel movement requires emergency medical attention and diagnostic testing, as well as surgical consultation.*

Step #1: Use topical solutions for temporary relief of pain. Start with Zhen Gu Shui or EMU oil products. These are the safest and quickest remedies.

Step #2: Take over-the-counter pain relievers or NSAIDs for temporary relief of pain while undergoing the following treatments that heal the tissue.

Step #3: Take prescription medications to relieve pain and inflammation or relax muscles temporarily if the above steps have not helped.

Step #4: Undergo LLEL treatment to accelerate healing, decrease inflammation and resolve the pain long term. You should observe reduction in pain and increase in mobility within four to eight treatments. LLEL can be used along with the following treatments to heal the tissues more quickly.

Step #5: Undergo acupuncture for long-term resolution, especially if you have arm or leg pain accompanying the neck/back pain. Use with the laser if both are available for faster resolution.

Michael is a forty-seven-year-old man who hurt his back lifting a heavy object. He had already been seen by an orthopedist and neurosurgeon, and an MRI had shown a ruptured disc. He was prescribed physical therapy, had chiropractic treatment, and also underwent three epidural steroid injections, none of which was beneficial. Initially, his doctors did not recommend surgery, because he was not having leg pain or other severe symptoms. However, they changed their minds because the therapy and injections had not helped, but Michael wanted to try other methods before surgery. After nine treatments with the LLEL and acupuncture in combination, his back pain was reduced 90 percent, and he did not require surgery. Within six months, his back pain completely resolved.

◦◦◦

Step #6: *Undergo physical therapy* using modalities and specific exercises under the guidance of a physical therapist.

Step #7: *Undergo osteopathic or chiropractic evaluation* to rule out misalignment causes if the previous steps have not been beneficial. If present, proceed with ***mobilization therapy (OMT)*** or ***chiropractic manipulation***. Do not continue if you have no relief within six to eight treatments or if the pain is made worse.

◦◦◦

Jane was fifty-six when she slipped and fell, landing on her buttocks. She went through the usual conventional treatments of physical therapy, medications (anti-inflammatories), and epidural steroid injections, none of which gave her much relief. MRI revealed some bulging discs, and a fusion surgery was recommended, using plates and screws at two levels. Jane had heard that fusions had a high failure rate and sought alternative treatments. She had told her doctors that her back popped and locked up on her, but they ignored those complaints and urged the surgery. When I examined her, her right pelvis was one inch higher than her left, and her pelvis and lumbar spine were rotated abnormally. Osteopathic manipulation was performed on three occasions, resolving her symptoms completely and saving her a surgery that would have been costly and most likely have failed.

◦◦◦

Step #8: *Undergo MRI* to discover more severe disc or nerve problems only if the above steps have not resolved your symptoms.

Step #9: *Seek counseling* if the MRI is normal or is consistent with aging to find and treat any underlying and unrecognized psychological factors.

◦◦◦

When Jo Ann slipped and fell, hurting her back, her doctor prescribed physical therapy and gave her narcotic medications, but neither helped. Her MRI was normal. Jo Ann became frustrated and demanded that something be done. Her doctor sent her for epidural injections (despite her normal MRI), but they did not give her any symptom relief. She was referred to me for acupuncture and laser. When I talked with Jo Ann, she revealed that her mother, whom she'd been taking care of for ten years, had just died after an extended illness. During this time Jo Ann also had been raising her children and been a full-time wife. I sent her to a psychotherapist, who helped Jo Ann realize that she just wanted to be taken care of after all these years of taking care of everyone else. After continued psychotherapy, her back pain went away.

Step #10: *Consider epidural steroid (ESI) and/or other injections* if the MRI is abnormal *and* you have radicular symptoms (arm or leg pain) and the above steps have not helped you. Do not undergo ESI if you have neck or back pain only. If the first injection is not beneficial, additional injections are unlikely to help.

Step #11: *Undergo additional diagnostic testing* (discogram or myelogram) if you still have neck or back pain.

Step #12: *Undergo surgery* as a last resort if the above steps have not resolved your pain. Be sure to obtain a second opinion to make sure that the type of surgery is the least complicated and most effective for your diagnosis.

Step #13: *Use the LLEL after surgery* to accelerate healing and reduce scarring.

Expected Outcome

Most acute spine pain and injuries receive too much testing and conventional treatments that are not necessary, thus wasting your time and money. By utilizing the alternative methods listed, the vast majority of people will not require expensive tests, injections or surgery.

Back and Neck Pain (Chronic)

What You Need to Know

Acute spine pain (see above section) is usually self-limiting, meaning that 90 percent of people recover in six weeks. Chronic pain and disability are the primary results when recovery does not occur. In addition, of course, it is common to develop neck and back pain as a result of degeneration of discs from aging. As a result, chronic spine pain is the most common physical complaint in the United States. About 26 percent of Americans have moderate to serious neck or back problems, which has increased 5 percent since 1997.

— ∞ —

Important Information:
Does Most Acute Spine Pain Really Resolve Spontaneously?

Most studies have shown that *acute* spine pain nearly always resolves spontaneously. However, this is usually based on results showing that the majority of patients discontinue seeking medical care. In reality, 80 percent of patients with acute spine pain continue to experience some pain or disability at one year following their initial doctor visit, and are now considered to have chronic spine pain.

— ∞ —

Most chronic back and neck pain is a result of the development of arthritis, which can occur from numerous causes, most often trauma or aging. The spine can become weaker and result in herniated (ruptured or slipped) discs, fractures, or spinal stenosis (narrowing of the spinal column) as you age.

— ∞ —

Neck Spurs: Symptom, Not Cause

If chronic spine inflammation has been present for a long time, spurs may result. Spurs are made of calcium, which is deposited in areas of chronic inflammation. They can continue growing unless the inflammation (arthritis) is curtailed and may impinge upon other body structures, causing more problems. In the past, surgery has been done to remove spurs but may have a high failure rate because the spurs are a *result* of inflammation and not the *cause* of your pain. It is the inflammation that must be addressed, whether surgery is performed or not.

— ∞ —

Although they can be caused by injury and age, many chronic spine problems are a result of lack of exercise, poor posture, use of vibratory tools, anxiety, depression, job dissatisfaction, and mental stress at work. Therefore, it is very important to discover if you have such underlying reasons for your spine pain; if you have these causes and don't identify them, you may end up undergoing treatments that are either not effective or make you worse.

Many people want to undergo surgery to get relief of their chronic pain, but patience is the key: Even pain that has been present for decades can be relieved with other methods, but if you rush into surgery, you may end up taking pain medications for the rest of your life or even have more pain, as well as disability.

MRI Scans: Misused, Overused, and Abused

MRI scans are performed and repeated much too often. Studies show that 75 percent of people with no neck or back pain will have abnormalities on MRI, meaning that *just because you have an abnormality does not mean that is what is causing your spine pain.* Unfortunately, many invasive procedures and surgeries are done based on the MRI, resulting in high failure rates and often worsening of chronic pain.

Furthermore, if your pain continues, studies show that there still is a minimal chance of any significant change within a year of doing an MRI scan. Yet, many doctors repeat them before then because they own their own MRI scan centers or simply because treatments are not working. In fact, a 2007 study in the *NEJM* showed that a year after onset of sciatica, patients with favorable outcomes were as likely to have herniated disks as those with unfavorable. Nevertheless, many surgeries are done or repeated due to continued pain, yet those may have an even higher failure rate.

National guidelines for spine pain recommend against ordering imaging or other diagnostic tests unless severe or progressive neurological defects (paralysis, loss of bladder/rectal control) are present or a condition such as cancer is suspected. Furthermore, MRI is recommended to be done only if surgery or epidural injections are considered. Based on the steps below, most MRIs will not be needed for chronic spine pain.

MRI scans are not the only tests overused and misused to determine spine treatment. In recent guidelines by the *American Pain Society*, it was determined that invasive diagnostic tests such as discography, facet joint block, and sacroiliac joint block have not been proven to be accurate for diagnosing various spinal conditions, and their use to guide therapeutic choices (such as surgery) is uncertain, again leading to unnecessary surgeries and a high failure rate from surgery.

Many doctors may tell you that there is nothing more they can do to relieve your pain and that you will just have to learn to live with it. I do not believe this is true for most people, especially if you use the following steps. Overall, the goal should be elimination of the pain, but complete relief may not be possible, especially if you have already undergone spinal surgery. A more reasonable goal is to lessen the pain enough to be able to enjoy life and be able to participate in most activities of daily living. That is certainly attainable based on my experience treating thousands of patients with chronic back pain.

Important Information:
Costs Rising for Spine Problems Despite Fewer Benefits

A recent study shows that health care expenditures for back and neck problems have increased substantially over time. Even worse, there has been no improvement in health outcomes commensurate with increasing costs. Self-reported measures of mental health, physical functioning, work or school limitations, and social limitations are also worse. The rise in costs without benefit is due primarily due to using expensive conventional tests, procedures and surgeries that are often unnecessary and may worsen your condition rather than using lower-cost methods that can significantly diminish or alleviate spine pain.

Treatments for Chronic Spine Pain

The Preventive Approaches

Exercise is a mainstay of prevention and also of reducing the pain and preventing further deterioration. Exercise stimulates large neurons (brain cells) to help reduce the perception of pain and stimulate the production of natural painkillers from the brain. Exercises are recommended for all patients with chronic spine pain. Stretching and resistance exercises are the main forms, along with exercises specifically designed for the spine. However, because your pain may be caused by different underlying problems, you should consult a physical therapist to help you design an exercise program for your particular condition.

Back schools that teach proper posture and techniques can benefit most people with chronic spine pain. Sitting, lifting, and performing other activities properly are very important factors in both preventing and treating back problems. For example, many people walk hunched over or sit stooped over a computer. You might lift without using your legs. Back schools teach you dozens of ways to avoid worsening of back pain and to prevent further injuries.

Ergonomic Products and Appliances: There are many products that can help reduce neck and back pain. This is in the realm of ergonomics, which is the design of such things as safe furniture and easy-to-use interfaces to machines and equipment. Proper ergonomic design is necessary to prevent repetitive strain injuries and other musculoskeletal disorders, which can develop over time and can lead to long-term disability. Such equipment includes special beds, mattresses, and pillows; back supports; and ergonomic chairs, desks, and recliners. ***Important Note:*** Many companies make such products and you should always comparison shop to obtain the best product for you. These products can make your life much easier and less painful. ***Helpful tip***: When purchasing such products, make sure you can return them if they don't help.

Dr. A's Suggestions:
Mattresses: Hard or Soft?

A study in *Spine* showed that people with low back pain reported increased pain when sleeping on a hard mattress, compared to softer, body-conforming foam mattresses or waterbeds. Hard beds may increase pressure on certain body parts, leading to tossing and turning at night. However, other studies have shown soft beds to cause more pain.

Comfort is really the key, and most studies show a *firm* mattress—not too hard, not too soft—is the best. Adjustable beds may be the best for finding the most comfortable firmness.

The Conventional Approaches
Medications: Chronic pain does not usually respond to basic OTC medications such as ibuprofen or acetaminophen. Although stronger *NSAIDs* (naproxen [Naprosyn], meloxicam [Mobic], piroxicam [Feldene], oxaprozin [Daypro], nabumatone [Relafen], ketoprofen [Orudis], diclofenac [Cataflam], and diclofenac/misoprostol [Arthrotec]) are usually tried first, many people require narcotic medication to control their pain.

Narcotic medications are usually given for severe, unrelenting back pain that has not responded to any other treatment approaches. They vary in potency from tramadol (the mildest) to oxycodone, morphine, dilaudid, fentanyl (Duragesic), and others. Narcotics are highly addictive and have strong side effects, affecting cognition as well as causing constipation. ***Helpful tip***: They should be prescribed and monitored only by a physician specializing in pain management. ***Warning***: Death from accidental narcotic overdose is becoming more common, especially in middle aged people, so be sure to comply with your doctor's instructions.

Low-dose antidepressants, such as amitriptyline (Elavil) 25–50 mg daily or trazadone (Desyrel) 50 to 150 mg daily, may decrease chronic spine pain through effects on the pain center (hypothalamus) and neurotransmitters in the brain. However, they do not improve your ability to perform activities, and most studies show them to be ineffective for most patients.

Physical therapy involving supervised exercises may help increase strength and mobility. In fact, a study has shown that lumbar fusion surgery is only slightly better than exercise. Another study revealed that physical therapy may achieve the same symptom relief as surgical decompression in patients with lumbar stenosis. Physical therapy *modalities* such as ultrasound or traction usually do not help *chronic* pain at all. However, electrical stimulation (e-stim) may be beneficial in many patients.

TENS units (transcutaneous electrical nerve stimulator) are commonly prescribed for temporary relief of pain. This involves wearing a small electrical generator strapped to your belt, which is attached by wires to small pads placed around the area of pain. These units can be worn continuously to control pain, although sometimes they can lose effectiveness over time.

Multidisciplinary pain programs are often recommended for chronic pain, and they provide a combination of treatments, including physical therapy, occupational therapy, and counseling. Although such programs are not designed to reduce back pain specifically, they do improve function and the ability to return to work and teach you how to cope better with your pain.

Epidural steroid injections(ESI): Although studies have proven them to be *ineffective* for chronic pain, especially if there is no pain down the arms or legs, ESI into the spine or discs continues to be one of the most common, although off-label, conventional treatments provided. Furthermore, most doctors who provide the injections will tell you three injections are required, but in fact, no study has proven that if the first one doesn't work, the next two will. If it works at all, the average patient generally may obtain up to three weeks of relief from these injections although rarely, some patients will get relief for several months to a year: eventually they will wear off in most people. They are also very expensive, costing about $2,500 for a fifteen-minute procedure. *Warning*: In rare cases, epidurals can cause blindness, stroke, paralysis, or death.

Important Information:
Studies Shows Epidural Steroid Injection to Be No Better than Placebo

Despite epidural steroid injections being routinely performed off-label, a study performed in Canada was the first one to compare these injections to one using only salt water (placebo). The results showed that the placebo injection was just as effective as the steroid injection. This study was totally ignored by pain doctors and neurologists because ESIs are tremendous money-makers, costing up to $2,500 for a fifteen-minute procedure. The study was criticized for not including a series of three injections, yet no high quality study has proven that three injections are superior to one.

A 2013 study in *Spine* showed that patients with spinal stenosis who received ESI had significantly less improvement in physical functioning and pain over four years of follow-up, and the injections did not help them avoid surgery. A 2014 study published in the *NEJM* and a 2015 study in the *Annals Int Med* also showed that ESI is generally ineffective for lumbar spinal stenosis. Another 2014 meta-analysis showed that it was also ineffective for sciatica.

ESI is largely a wasteful, unnecessary, and ineffective procedure for most people with chronic spine pain, especially since there are alternatives that are much more effective and less costly. But it is a huge money-maker for pain management doctors, and insurance and Medicare still pay for it, which is why it is done so frequently.

Other invasive therapies include the following:

- *Selective nerve root blocks*, which are given to deaden a nerve but, again, usually only give you temporary relief.
- *Facet joint injections* (into the joints where one vertebra hooks into the next) have not been shown to benefit chronic spine pain.
- *Rhizotomy* is another procedure in which your nerve root is destroyed, either by cutting it, using radio waves to destroy it, or injecting a chemical that destroys the nerve. This interrupts the pain message going to your brain. However, your nerve will eventually grow back, and the pain will return. Rhizotomy is considered successful if you get 50 percent relief of pain for one year.
- *Intradiscal electrothermal therapy* (IDET) is a procedure in which electrical current is produced in a wire placed around the disk to "seal" tears, but you have to relinquish all physical activities for six months afterward, and the success rate is negligible.

Important Information:
Many Other Medical Procedures Ineffective for Spine Pain

In the 2008 guidelines established by the *American Pain Society*, it was stated that local injections, Botox injections, facet joint injections, sacroiliac joint injections, and radiofrequency ablation "are not supported by convincing consistent evidence." However, they continue to be done nevertheless.

Spine Surgeries: Since most of the above conventional treatments usually don't work or give long lasting relief, spine surgeries are very commonly done as "a last resort." There are several types, each having different indications and costs.

Dr. A's Suggestions:
Be Careful What You Hear from Spine Surgeons:
The Last Resort Fallacy and More

Spine surgeons commonly give you several reasons for undergoing spine surgery that may be, in fact, untrue. The most common is that surgery is a "last resort" because "conservative treatment hasn't helped." First, does a "last resort" mean it's effective? If it was that effective, it wouldn't be a last resort! Second, the treatments usually done before surgery don't include alternative treatments, which could help avoid most back surgeries.

Another common warning is that if you don't have the surgery, you could become paralyzed. This complication is extremely rare, and I have never seen it happen in thirty-nine years of practice. The *bottom line* is that surgery, especially fusion, is very lucrative, costing upward of $100,000. If you were a spine surgeon, that's what you would want to do. But don't rush into surgery, especially if they try to scare you.

An increasingly common surgery for chronic back pain is *spinal fusion*, in which your spinal bones (vertebra) are fused together using bone from your hip (done by neurosurgeons) or with instrumentation (rods, screws, and/or cages, done by orthopedists). Sometimes, a 360-degree fusion is done, fusing the vertebra from front *and* back. Unfortunately, despite the frequency of this type of surgery (about half a million done every year), it has an extremely high failure rate for chronic spine pain, especially when done on the lower back.

Spinal Fusion: Overused and Abused

Spinal fusions have witnessed an explosive increase—134 percent between 1993 and 2003. More lately, estimates have placed the increase at 200 percent. The reasons for this increase include lingering symptoms, new surgical techniques, and, above all, high profit.

Several studies have been done on spinal fusions, most with poor results. For specific abnormalities such as spondylolisthesis and spinal stenosis, surgery may improve pain, function, and disability at two years, but *not* in a majority of cases. For degenerative disc disease without radicular symptoms, less than half of patients experience optimal outcomes (optimal defined as reducing pain and increasing function by 50 percent). The rate of repeat surgery after the initial surgery is around 25 percent over four years, even with no adverse events reported through one year post-surgery.

It should be noted that these studies did not compare fusion to nonsurgical treatments. In a landmark study published in February 2011 in the *Annals of Rheumatic Disease*, it was proven that the invasive and high cost fusion procedure did not afford better outcomes as compared with a significantly lower-cost conservative treatment approach (education, support, and physical training sessions over three weeks). It should further be noted that fusion surgery has never been compared to alternative methods.

The *bottom line* is that spinal fusion is tremendously overused and abused and may be unnecessary in the majority of cases, not to mention being extremely expensive. It can also cause significant disability in and of itself. Unfortunately, it is considered standard practice and continues to be paid for by Medicare and insurance, simply (and unnecessarily) increasing the costs of medical care.

Fusion surgery is not recommended if more than three levels are involved, but even a fusion done at one or two levels exerts more pressure on the spinal disks above and below the fusion, often causing them to deteriorate within two to five years. This is why many people have persistent or recurrent spine pain after such surgeries and end up undergoing many more surgeries. Additional fusion surgeries usually have very poor outcomes. *Helpful tip*: Fusions for chronic spine pain should be done *only* for unrelenting pain with evidence of structural deterioration of the discs and/or additional or worsening neurological signs. It is also indicated for severe spondylolisthesis, in which one vertebra slides over another, causing destabilization of the spine.

Prosthetic disc replacement is another more recent type of surgery, which can be used at one or two levels. It takes much less time to perform but is not indicated in seniors with stenosis. However, studies show that, much like with fusion, rehabilitation and other methods have similar results and are much less expensive.

Other surgeries: For other spine conditions, less complex and less expensive surgeries can be done. For ruptured discs, *discectomy* with *laminectomy* (taking out the disc and cutting bone away to free the nerve: also referred to as "decompression") are common, although studies show that non-surgical, alternative interventions (see below) are just as effective.

This surgery can be done "open" or via microdecompression (taking out a smaller piece of the bone/disc): a 2015 study showed that *microdecompression* surgery is as effective as laminectomy for spinal stenosis but has much less side effects. It may be effective for spinal stenosis, in which there is a narrowing of the spine, although studies have only compared the surgery's effectiveness against physical therapy and drugs, not against alternative methods.

Decompression Vs Fusion: Profit is the Key

Surgeons primarily use two surgical methods for spinal stenosis, a very common condition causing chronic low back pain. One is spinal fusion, and the other is decompression. A study in *JAMA* found that decompressions have declined, and fusions have increased. They also found that fusions had double the rate of major complications and double the thirty-day death rate compared to decompression. In addition, fusions cost $80,000 compared to $24,000 for decompression. They concluded that economic (money) incentives were at work because surgeons can make ten times as much from a fusion than from decompression.

Many surgeons advertise *minimally invasive spine surgery*, in which a smaller incision is made; it can be utilized for any of the above surgeries. Although proponents state that this technique is advantageous, there are pros and cons, as follows:

Advantages:

- Smaller incisions, usually a few smaller scars instead of one larger scar
- Less tissue dissection
- Less damage to surrounding muscles

- Potential for less blood loss, quicker healing, shorter hospital stay, and less pain
- Quicker return to daily activities

Disadvantages:

- Potential for prolonged operative time
- Usually associated with increased radiation exposure
- Not appropriate for every case
- Less surface area of bone exposed for fusion cases
- May be difficult to repair a spinal fluid leak if one occurs

Placement of a **dorsal column stimulator** (DCS) into the spine is often tried when spine surgeries are not successful. A DCS can control chronic, severe spine pain but is effective in only a small percentage of people and has a high failure rate over time, even among those who do receive initial relief. DCS should be used as a last resort only for continued severe back pain not helped by other treatments. A new spinal cord stimulator used in Europe was cleared by the FDA for use in 2015 and is the first to be wireless (it is comprised of an implantable stimulator and externally worn power device). According to the company, results are consistent with other neurostimulators, in which 60–80 percent of patients may sustain pain relief of 50 percent. However, this device may be easier to use and less invasive than other stimulators. ***Important note***: The success of neurostimulators depends on choosing the correct patients; unfortunately, they are placed in many patients who are not good candidates and thus fail to provide relief.

Cognitive-behavioral therapy is one other treatment that does have benefit and is low cost. This is a form of psychotherapy that changes unproductive or harmful thought patterns. You learn to examine your feelings and separate realistic from unrealistic thoughts. Studies show that the combination of cognitive-behavioral therapy and exercise is as effective as lumbar fusion surgery, but significantly less costly. Nevertheless, it is rarely done as often as fusion, and few doctors (especially spine surgeons) refer patients for such therapy.

The Alternative Approaches

Helpful tip: If you want to decrease or even resolve your chronic spine pain long-term, several alternative approaches have the potential to do so. If such methods are used first, most injections and surgeries might be avoided.

Low level energy laser *(LLEL or "cold" laser)* is one of the best and most effective methods. This is not the "hot" laser used in surgery to coagulate blood and cut tissues. The cold laser helps heal the tissue, reduces inflammation, and gives long-lasting relief for arthritic, nerve, and disc problems. It also appears to heal the disc and make new cells to re-expand it. It may take from three to fifteen treatments to obtain relief with most cold lasers. Pain relief is long term, often lasting ten to twenty years or longer, because it corrects the underlying cause rather than just treating symptoms. My research studies done for over thirty years show that it works in the majority of patients with chronic spine pain.

Acupuncture is also very effective for chronic spine problems and can be used with the laser for faster results. Acupuncture is especially useful if you have nerve pain (radicular pain down the arm or leg) and often resolves the nerve pain before the neck or back pain. I have also used it successfully in patients with spinal stenosis and degenerative disc disease. Most people obtain initial relief within six treatments, although you may need more to obtain maximum benefit. If done correctly, acupuncture also provides long-lasting relief, although occasional sessions may be needed for flare-ups.

Several **Chinese herbal formulations** can reduce back pain and increase mobility, and can safely be used with the above steps. Formulas commonly used include *Wan Du Hua Yu Tang*, *Shu Jing Huo Xue Tang*, or *Huo Luo Xiao Ling Dan*, which is used more for trauma. *Juan Bi Wan* helps with heaviness and stiffness but cannot be used with red, hot, swollen joint stiffness. It may be useful for arthritis in the upper body that is relieved by warmth. These formulas are often used with acupuncture. *Zheng Gu Shui* is a Chinese herbal topical that can be quite effective in relieving pain temporarily for bone-level pain. If the pain is more of a muscular pain, *white flower oil* may be more effective.

Manual manipulation may be useful if underlying structural ("misalignment") problems (bones, ligaments, tendons, joints, and/or muscles not working correctly) are either causing your chronic back pain or not allowing proper healing to take place.

Important Information:
Sacroiliac Joint, Spine Misalignment Problems
Often Misdiagnosed and Not Treated Correctly

MDs are not trained in diagnosing or treating problems that involve misalignment of the spine or pelvis, which is a common cause of chronic spine pain. Often, doctors rely solely on MRIs, which may not detect misalignment, so treatment is provided that may not be effective, even leading to unnecessary surgery.

Besides misalignment of the spine, other so-called "structural" problems are also commonly misdiagnosed. This includes sacroiliac joint inflammation, which is frequently caused by shifting of the pelvis. Most doctors simply inject steroids, which help only a small minority of patients because, again, the underlying misalignment is not corrected.

The treatment for these problems is manual therapy, which resolves the underlying misalignment in the majority of cases.

Osteopathic is the manual therapy of choice for *chronic* spine problems because it is done more holistically and extensively, usually not requiring "popping" the spine. You should obtain benefits within one to six sessions using osteopathic methods. *Chiropractic manipulation* can also be done and can help some people, but studies have not proven long-term effectiveness. However, there are many more chiropractors than osteopaths who perform manipulation, and chiropractic can be helpful. If you choose chiropractic care, you should observe initial benefits within six to eight treatments. If you do have a structural cause for your spine pain, occasional maintenance adjustments may be necessary. I see many patients who have received chiropractic adjustments every week (sometimes several times a week) for years, with pain relief only lasting a few hours or days; these perpetual, frequent adjustments may not be appropriate because they can lead to long-term problems and can be very costly.

Leg Length Discrepancy: Often Overtreated

Often, patients will be told by practitioners that one leg is shorter than the other, causing posture and gait changes and contributing to knee, hip, foot or back pain. Many practitioners will attempt to treat this discrepancy with shoe lifts or orthotic devices. It is important to know that many people have leg length discrepancies, but it may not be what is causing the pain, so these treatments may be ineffective in such cases.

It is always important to find out if the discrepancy is significant, and if so, what is causing it. Leg or foot fractures, hip replacements, muscle imbalance, and pelvis asymmetry can all cause this and must be corrected in order to alleviate the pain.

Bodywork is another type of manual therapy that involves realigning, rebalancing, and retraining the structures of the body that have become dysfunctional due to pain, injury, disuse, or misuse. There are several types; the most common are listed below.

- The *Feldenkrais method* focuses on retraining how you move your body to interrupt unhealthy patterns of movement that have become habits.
- The *Alexander technique* concentrates on correcting faulty posture in daily activities (sitting, standing, and moving).

- *Rolfing* involves manipulating and stretching the body's fascial tissues (deep connective tissues that hold your body together), allowing correct realigning of the body.

These bodywork methods require a therapist certified in these techniques and may take several months to obtain benefit.

Herbal remedies may be helpful in reducing inflammation and pain. These include curcumin, boswellia, ginger, fish oil, and digestive enzymes (taken separately from food).

Herbal topical solutions can be helpful for temporary relief when applied over the painful area. These include EMU oil, long crystal menthol, Biofreeze, capsaicin, and other herbal combinations. These topicals are not curative, but they may provide pain relief for two to eight hours, and have minimal side effects (skin allergy or sensitivity most commonly). Some of these may work better than others on different people, so you may have to try several to find the best one.

Glucosamine May Not Be As Helpful for Spine Pain

Many people use glucosamine-chondroitin to reduce inflammation in arthritis but also for other musculoskeletal pain, including spine pain. Two studies published in *JAMA* demonstrated that glucosamine had no benefit for pain, disability, or quality of life. However, if you have tried it and it helps relieve your pain, you can safely continue using it. If it hasn't helped in a month, stop taking it.

Reconstructive therapy (also known as sclerotherapy or prolotherapy) is another common alternative method. This method involves the injection of a mildly irritating solution (usually dextrose, glycerin, and phenol) into the injured tissues, strengthening the ligaments and tendons in the spine. Two studies using prolotherapy with manipulation and exercise demonstrated benefits. However, one study has shown that saline injections are as effective as prolotherapy. You should improve within six treatments and will usually notice improvement during the first week of treatment.

Yoga is often successful in reducing chronic spine symptoms. Yoga promotes relaxation and stretching, both of which are important in healing and preventing back pain. Because there are many different types of yoga, with some better for spine pain than others, you should work with a qualified yoga instructor.

Inversion Therapy/VAX-D: Good or Bad?

Many people have "gravitated" to inversion therapy, which involves lying at a downward slant, hanging upside down, or using gravity boots. The idea is that the pull of gravity will allow your spine to decompress and elongate, thus relieving pressure on disks, ligaments, and nerves. Unfortunately, the effects may be temporary at best and could even worsen back pain in some cases. It can also have serious side effects, including increased blood pressure, retinal bleeding, headaches, and blurred vision.

Another alternative method is VAX-D, a computerized system that provides traction to your spine. Its purpose is, again, to elongate the spine, allowing the body to heal the disks. This method works in some people but may be temporary in most and is very expensive, often costing $4,000. It is not covered by insurance.

Your Empowered Patient Action Plan for Chronic Neck and Back Pain

Step #1: Apply Zheng Gu Shui, EMU oil, long crystal menthol, Biofreeze, or capsaicin for temporary pain relief while undergoing the following longer-lasting treatments. Try these topicals before medications as they have less potential for side effects or harm. If you are already taking medications, these topicals may provide additional relief or help you decrease the medications you are already taking.

Step #2: Try a TENS unit to obtain temporary relief while undergoing the next steps. A TENS may provide relief without the side effects/harm of medications.

Step #3: Most of you with chronic neck or back pain may have already have been *prescribed medications*. If you must take medications, start with the ones that have the least potential for side effects or harm, such as NSAIDs. Avoid narcotics if at all possible. If the medications are helping, continue taking them while undergoing the following steps and discontinue them when the steps are effective. If they have not helped, the following steps should help relieve your pain.

Step #4: Go to back school: If you know proper posture and lifting techniques, you can prevent spine injuries or lessen existing spine pain.

Step #5: Use appropriate ergonomically designed appliances and products to ease or reduce your pain. This step can be helpful no matter what other treatments you receive.

Step #6: ***Receive LLEL therapy:*** Cold laser can potentially resolve your spine pain long term by healing the discs and nerves directly. It is the most cost-effective treatment available.

Step# 7: ***Undergo acupuncture:*** This method can also potentially resolve spine pain long-term and is especially effective for pain down the arm or leg.

Step #8: ***Receive osteopathic or chiropractic manipulation*** if an evaluation finds misalignment or if your spine pops, cracks, catches, or locks up or certain positions increase or decrease the pain.

Step #9: ***Undergo physical therapy*** for exercises and electrical stimulation.

Step #10: ***Undergo cognitive therapy*** with a counselor trained in pain treatment. Even if your pain is being caused by a physical/structural problem, cognitive therapy can help you lessen your pain.

Step #11: ***Undergo bodywork,*** using Feldenkrais, Alexander, Rolfing, or other forms if the above steps are not beneficial. These methods can retrain your body and thus reduce pain and disability.

Step #12: ***Practice yoga*** postures for back and neck.

Step #13: ***Take Chinese herbal remedies*** for temporary relief if you still have pain.

Step #14: ***Undergo sclerotherapy or prolotherapy*** if the above steps still have not worked. These injections are more effective than conventional injections.

Jesse had injured his back fifteen years previously, subsequently having had four surgeries, each one giving him relief for only four to eight months. The first surgery was to repair a ruptured disc, the second to clean out scar tissue, the third to fuse two spinal levels, and the fourth because of another disc rupture above the fusion. He had undergone numerous epidural steroid injections, selective nerve root blocks, used a TENS unit, and was on narcotic medications, but still had constant pain. I sent him first for an osteopathic exam, which revealed that part of his pain was from problems with his sacroiliac joint (which is part of the pelvis), and his sacrum (the lowest bony part of the spine) was in an abnormal position (called sacral torsion). Osteopathic treatment gave him considerable relief, but he still had residual pain. I then started him on acupuncture with LLEL. After twelve treatments, nearly all of his pain was gone, and he was able to stop taking his narcotic medications.

Step #15: ***Enter a multidisciplinary pain program*** to learn how to cope with chronic spine pain and improve your quality of life if your pain continues.

Step #16: ***Undergo ESI*** if none of the above method have helped and only if you have arm or leg pain that has not been relieved. However, if the first one doesn't work, don't undergo additional injections.

Step #17: ***Consider selective nerve root blocks, or rhizotomy*** if indicated, if you still have chronic spine pain and nothing else has worked.

Step #18: ***Undergo surgery*** as a true last resort. Undergo decompression or laminectomy and discectomy if indicated *instead of* fusion, especially for ruptured discs or spinal stenosis. If you undergo fusion, and the first fusion does not work, repeat fusions are unlikely to benefit you. If you smoke, you should definitely stop because there is a higher failure rate if you smoke.

Step #19: ***Use the LLEL after surgery*** to accelerate healing and decrease scarring.

Step #20: ***Try a dorsal column stimulator*** to control your pain if it is still present and unbearable.

Step #21: ***Take prescription narcotics***: This will be necessary for the rest of your life if none of the above steps has helped you. This step is recommended last because it can interfere with the effectiveness of the above treatments, leads to addiction and disability, and is usually not necessary.

Expected Outcome

Chronic spine pain is one of the most common medical conditions and can definitely interfere with your quality of life. Although conventional methods are the most commonly used, they are the most expensive and least successful. With alternative methods, most chronic spine pain can be controlled adequately or resolved completely.

Bell's Palsy

What You Need to Know

Each year, about forty thousand Americans develop Bell's palsy, a condition that occurs when the nerve that controls the facial muscles becomes swollen or compressed. This condition often makes people think they are having a stroke, but if your muscle weakness or paralysis affects only your face, a more likely cause is Bell's palsy.

For most people, Bell's palsy symptoms begin to improve within a few weeks and resolve in three to six months. About 10 percent will experience a recurrence of the symptoms, sometimes on the opposite side of the face. Some people never recover and continue to have some symptoms for life. If the damage to your facial nerve is severe, the fibers may be permanently damaged or cause other symptoms such as involuntary contraction of certain muscles when you're trying to move others: for example, when you smile, the eye on the affected side may close.

The most common cause of Bell's palsy appears to be the herpes simplex virus, but other viruses have been linked to it as well.

Treatments for Bell's Palsy

The Preventive Approaches

There is no actual preventive measure for Bell's palsy, other than to avoid close contact with others who may have the herpes simplex virus (which *also* causes cold sores). Paralyzed muscles can shrink and shorten, causing permanent contractures, so massaging and exercising your facial muscles may help prevent this.

The Conventional Approaches

Medications: Doctors usually prescribe *corticosteroids*, such as prednisone, which are powerful anti-inflammatory agents. Their effect is to reduce the swelling of the facial nerve, so it will fit more comfortably within the bony tunnel that surrounds it. As this condition is thought to be caused by a virus, *antiviral drugs*, usually acyclovir or valacyclovir, are commonly prescribed.

Important note: Some clinical studies show benefit from early treatment with corticosteroids, antivirals, or a combination of both types of drugs. Other studies do not. Evidence of the effectiveness of corticosteroids appears to be stronger than that for antiviral drugs.

Hyperbaric oxygen therapy (oxygen given under pressure) has also been shown in studies to produce significantly faster recovery (twenty-two versus thirty-four days) compared to steroids.

Occasionally, **surgery** is done to relieve the pressure on the facial nerve. This decompression surgery is controversial and rarely recommended. In some cases, however, plastic surgery may be needed to make your face look and work better.

The Alternative Approaches

Acupuncture is potentially the best treatment for Bell's palsy, and it can be effective even if it has been present an extended period of time and thought to be permanent. However, the faster after diagnosis it is done, the more effective it is. Consider adding cupping, which can also help. You should observe benefits within six to eight treatments. In TCM, palsy is considered wind getting into the system, so stay away from fans and windows. Also, it is a sign of a lack of nourishment, so eat naturally colored foods and get some rest. Because acupuncture addresses the underlying cause, it can provide long-term relief.

Low level energy laser (LLEL or "cold" laser) is a laser that does not produce heat and has minimal to no side effects. It may accelerate healing of the damaged nerves and decrease inflammation. Because LLEL addresses the underlying cause, it can provide long-term relief.

Vitamin B$_{12}$ is known to benefit nerves, and a recent study showed that people given an injection of 500 mcg (methylcobalamin) three times a week for eight weeks showed faster recovery rate than people given steroids. Oral vitamin B$_{12}$ is not effective, however.

Biofeedback techniques seem to help limit the deterioration of muscle function as well as speeding recovery. Using a mirror as a feedback has been shown to improve facial symmetry and muscle function as well as using a mirror plus electrical biofeedback.

Your Empowered Patient Action Plan for Bell's Palsy
Helpful tip: I do not recommend antivirals or surgery, which have poor results.

*Step #1: **Undergo acupuncture*** for complete or faster resolution of the condition, even if the condition is chronic.

Step #2: Undergo treatment with ***low level energy laser***, which can be used with acupuncture for better effectiveness.

*Step #3: **Take vitamin B$_{12}$ injections*** to accelerate healing.

*Step #4: **Undergo hyperbaric oxygen therapy*** to accelerate healing. This step can be used with the above steps.

*Step #5: **Take corticosteroids*** to accelerate healing.

*Step #6: **Undergo biofeedback*** to prevent muscle deterioration if the condition becomes chronic.

Expected Outcome
Most cases of Bell's palsy will resolve, but may take several months. With the above steps, especially using alternative medicine, you may be able to resolve the condition completely without permanent damage, whether acute or chronic.

Bursitis, Tendonitis

What You Need to Know
When you hear the term "-itis," it means inflammation. Bursitis is inflammation of a bursa, a saclike membrane pouch that lubricates joints. There are 150 different bursa sacs throughout the body, but the most commonly affected are the hip and shoulder.

Tendonitis (also spelled tendinitis) is inflammation of a tendon, the fibrous tissue that connects muscles to bones. The most common tendons affected include the Achilles (heel), elbow (tennis elbow or lateral epicondylitis), and wrist (DeQuervain's tenosynovitis). Tendinopathy is similar and also causes pain and swelling, but it is due to degeneration from overuse rather than inflammation. However, treatment is usually the same as for tendonitis.

Both tendinitis and bursitis occur more frequently as we age, and the effects can be much different than when they occur at a younger age. Because tissues degenerate over time, there may be more serious consequences from such conditions, but they may take much longer to heal as well.

Injuries causing tendinitis and bursitis can occur from numerous sources, and even minor objects can cause injuries, the most common being beds and bedding, household containers, sofas, and footwear. Of course, as we age, many of us still think we can do activities we've always been able to do, so these conditions are often caused by overuse.

Both of these conditions are difficult to treat and resolve because the bursa and tendons of the body do not receive a large blood supply. These conditions are notorious for lasting months and even years.

Treatments for Bursitis/Tendinitis

The Preventive Approaches

Warming up and stretching properly before and after sports activities or exercise is the primary method of preventing tendinitis and bursitis caused by overuse or injury.

Caution: Many exercise trainers advise against stretching *before* exercise and recommend doing it *after* exercise for best results. Some still advise stretching before exercise, but you should do so only after you have first warmed up your muscles by doing aerobic activities.

As we age, one of the most common problems is falling, due to weakness, balance problems, blood pressure problems, and other causes, including wearing multifocal glasses. About one in six adults over the age of sixty-five fall every three months, and one-third sustain injuries. Therefore, in general, preventing falls is the best way to prevent injuries that cause bursitis and tendinitis. The CDC describes fourteen effective fall-prevention strategies in a new publication, *Preventing Falls: What Works* (http://www.cdc.gov/ncipc/PreventingFalls/). In addition, taking vitamin D_3 (800 mg daily) has been shown to prevent falls as well.

One unusual cause of falls is decreased blood pressure after eating, which occurs in many elderly patients. If that should occur, increased water intake before eating or eating six smaller meals a day rather than three large ones can help prevent this.

The Conventional Approaches

For mild to moderate problems, conventional methods start with the **RICE protocol**:

- *Rest* the joint: avoid using it, especially for strenuous activities such as lifting (shoulder) or walking/climbing (knee, hip).
- Apply *ice* to the affected area: you can use commercial ice packs sold in drug-stores or wrap a towel around some ice. Do not apply it for more than twenty minutes every hour.
- *Compress* the joint: wrap the joint with an elastic bandage such as an ACE wrap, but don't tighten it to the degree your circulation is cut off. Tennis elbow straps are available OTC.
- *Elevate* the affected limb. Keep the joint elevated, such as placing your knee on some pillows.

Dr. A's Suggestions:
Ice versus Heat

Should you use heat or ice if you've sustained an injury? In general, ice is recommended for an acute injury with swelling. Heat is usually applied after the swelling has subsided and if you are sore or achy; it can potentially worsen inflammation if applied too soon. For *chronic* inflammation, either one may relieve pain; you just have to try each to see which is most effective. Whichever one is used, do so for only twenty minutes every two to three hours while awake.

Medications: Over-the-counter *NSAIDs*, such as ibuprofen or naproxen (Aleve), are commonly prescribed for short-term pain relief and to reduce inflammation while the tissues heal naturally. You should obtain temporary relief quickly from these drugs.

If these are not effective, *prescription NSAIDs* (such as naproxen [Naprosyn], meloxicam [Mobic], piroxicam [Feldene], oxaprozin [Daypro], nabumatone [Relafen], ketoprofen [Orudis], diclofenac [Cataflam], and diclofenac/misoprostol [Arthrotec]) are more powerful and may work if the OTC drugs don't. *Warning*: These drugs may cause stomach irritation and bleeding, and if this occurs, you can try the Cox-2 inhibitor, Celebrex, which has a lower risk of these side effects, or take proton pump inhibitors (PPIs) with them. However, recent studies show a small increased risk of heart attack in patients who use Cox-2 inhibitors, especially if you have heart disease. All these drugs should be used short term to relieve pain and swelling.

Caution: In July, 2015, the FDA started requiring NSAIDs to carry a warning of increased risk of heart attacks, stroke and heart failure. This is especially evident when taken long term, at higher doses, or by people with pre-existing heart disease. The risks can increase as early as the first weeks of NSAID use. However, ibuprofen and naproxen do not appear to increase the risk, so are the safest and preferred NSAIDs.

Nitroglycerin paste is a novel treatment and applied to the joint once daily. This appears to increase joint mobility and reduce pain in both acute and chronic tendinopathies. However, it commonly causes headaches. Studies show that such applications help patients recover twenty weeks earlier than those not using the drug.

Injection of *polidocanol*, a sclerosing agent, into the tendon had been shown to be beneficial in two small pilot studies in 2002. This appeared to be a promising therapy but has not been supported by replicable and more recent studies.

Physical therapy modality treatments are often done for these conditions but have a high failure rate. However, eccentric training protocols have been shown to be beneficial.

Local steroid injection is a common but unnecessary treatment for tendinitis and bursitis. These *are not recommended*, even though they are performed frequently. One study showed that such injections improve pain for tennis elbow at four weeks but lose their effect after that. In fact, after one year, the outcomes were worse, and it can increase the risk of recurrence and decrease recovery. Another study showed that steroid injection for rotator cuff (shoulder) tendinitis is ineffective as well. It has also been proven that physical therapy and specific exercise therapy helps patients in the short term much better than injections. *Warning*: If you undergo more than three injections per year, the steroids can soften the bone and damage the joint. If one injection is not helpful, they won't work, so don't repeat them.

Dr. A's Suggestions:
Avoid "Special" Injections for Tendinopathy

Many elite athletes, such as Tiger Woods, undergo injections of "platelet-rich" plasma into the affected tendon, which supposedly contains elements that promote healing. Although its use has increased during the past few years and it has been endorsed by athletes, the first controlled study ever done (published in *JAMA*) demonstrated that such injections are no better than placebo and are not recommended.

Other practitioners recommend injections of autologous blood, which contains growth factors and cytokines that might promote healing. A study in the *BMJ* revealed that such injections provide no benefit.

So don't get injections into your tendons. They are a waste of time and money.

Surgery is a treatment of last resort. For bursitis, surgery removes the offending bursa sac. For tendinitis, it debrides (cleans) the tendons. I have found surgery to help only a small percentage of people in bursitis, and be only slightly more helpful in tendinitis. Furthermore, it can cause permanent problems, such as decreased strength and range of motion as well as nerve injuries.

Extracorporeal shock-wave therapy (ESWT) is another treatment sometimes done for tendinitis and used primarily in the shoulder, elbow, and heel. ESWT can be done with high energy and low energy. Even so, ESWT can be quite painful, and it has not been well supported by most research, even though it has been highly marketed by its manufacturers. A study published in the *BMJ* revealed that supervised exercise is more effective than ESWT, with only one-third of those patients receiving benefit (compared to two-thirds with exercise).

The Alternative Approaches

Acupuncture is by far the best treatment: because it addresses the underlying cause, it can provide long-term relief. You should feel better within six to eight acupuncture treatments, but you might need additional sessions for maximum benefit.

Along with acupuncture, a **Chinese herbal formula** called *Shen Tong Zhu Yu Tang* may be useful in relieving pain. *Warning*: This formula should not be used during pregnancy.

Low level energy laser (LLEL or "cold" laser) therapy helps heal the tissue, reduce the inflammatory response, and give long-lasting relief. You should feel better within six to nine treatments with laser alone, but I often use this laser in conjunction with acupuncture for better and faster results. Laser alone may only work in about 50 percent of patients. Because LLEL addresses the underlying cause, it can provide long-term relief.

Topical lotions can provide temporary relief, and there are several that can provide reduction of pain and inflammation for several hours. These include the Chinese herbal formulas Zhen Gu Shui or White Flower oil, Biofreeze, capsaicin, EMU oil, and many others.

Nutritional Supplements are more effective than conventional drugs with fewer side effects. *Bromelain* (250–750 mg three times per day between meals) and *curcumin* (200–400 mg three times per day between meals) can decrease inflammation and bruising. To cut healing time by half, add *citrus flavonoids* (600–1,000 mg three times daily) to these two supplements. You should observe benefits with two to three weeks.

Infrasound (low-frequency sound) appears to work better than ultrasound (high-frequency sound). Infrasound works by increasing the local circulation of blood and lymph, thereby accelerating the healing process. It not only can reduce pain but can decrease swelling as well. Infrasound is used by numerous chiropractors, naturopaths, acupuncturists, and a few doctors.

Counter strain is an osteopathic technique that may help relieve tendinitis. Your nerves may be over stimulating your tendons in certain positions, causing your pain. Counter strain is used to "rewire" your nerve-tendon communications to reduce the stimulation. It is done by first finding the area that has the most tenderness and the position that causes the most pain. Then you use your other surrounding muscles to find a position that immediately relieves the pain. You repeat that position as often as you can, thus establishing a different pattern of nerve firing, which doesn't cause pain. You can be taught this technique by an osteopathic physician and perform it at home.

Your Empowered Patient Action Plan for Bursitis/Tendonitis
Helpful Tip: *Injections are not helpful and are not recommended.*

Step #1: Use the RICE Protocol for mild symptoms.

Step #2: Apply herbal topicals for temporary control of pain and inflammation while the following steps are healing the inflammation. Start with Zhen Gu Shui or White Flower oil and use the others described above if you still have pain.

Step #3: Undergo acupuncture for long-term resolution. This is the most cost-effective treatment.

Leslie was a competitive tennis player, even at age sixty-two. Unfortunately, she injured her elbow, and the pain had continued for six months, without any relief. She had been prescribed anti-inflammatory medications, underwent physical therapy, and had three steroid injections by three different doctors, even though none of them ever worked. I started her on acupuncture. By the third treatment, she had significant improvement; and by the fifth treatment, her pain was completely gone.

Step #4: Undergo LLEL therapy for long-term resolution, which is also very cost-effective and has no side effects. Use with acupuncture, if possible, for faster results.

Nick, a sixty-five-year old man with bursitis of his hip, had undergone two steroid injections and physical therapy that had not helped. He took numerous types of NSAIDs, but his bursitis continued for over a year. His doctor recommended bursectomy (removal of the bursa sac), but he wanted to avoid surgery. I treated him with acupuncture and LLEL. His symptoms were gone within seven treatments.

Step #5: ***Learn and practice counter strain*** for resistant symptoms.

Step #6: ***Apply nitric oxide topical*** to reduce pain temporarily and accelerate healing if the above steps have not worked.

Step #7: ***Try sclerotherapy*** if the above steps still have not improved your condition.

Step #8: ***Take bromelain, curcumin, and citrus flavonoids*** to promote healing if symptoms continue.

Step #9: ***Take an NSAID*** for temporary relief if pain and swelling continue. Do not continue these drugs if they do not relieve your pain quickly.

Step #10: ***Try eccentric training protocols*** if you still have symptoms.

Step #11: ***Try corticosteroid injections*** to reduce symptoms and swelling *only if* the previous steps have not been effective. If one doesn't help, don't repeat them.

Step #12: ***Try ESWT*** if you still have not improved.

Step #13: ***Undergo surgery*** as a last resort.

Step #14: ***Use the LLEL after surgery*** to accelerate healing and decrease scarring.

Expected Outcome

Tendonitis and bursitis are difficult to resolve, but with the use of alternative methods, faster resolution is probable.

Cancer

What You Need to Know

The four leading types of malignant cancer are lung, breast, prostate, and colorectal, with lung cancer having the highest death rate in men and non-Hispanic women. Many types of cancer are decreasing in incidence, but others are increasing: The latter include melanoma, esophageal, kidney, anus, pancreas, and HPV (virus)-related head and neck cancers. The largest increases in both genders are thyroid and liver cancers.

Currently in the United States, more than 1.6 million new cases of cancer are diagnosed each year. It is estimated that cancer rates will double by 2050, primarily because the population will be larger and will be living longer due to better control of other chronic diseases; the fact is that as fewer and fewer people die from heart disease, strokes, and accidents, more and more people live long enough to develop cancer.

That's the bad news. There is good news, however: *deaths* from cancer have decreased 20 percent since 1991. This is attributed to decreased smoking rates, increased screening, and improved treatments. So, overall, with the substantial increase in cancer incidence yet decrease in overall deaths, we are making substantial strides in fighting cancer.

What Causes Cancer? "Bad Luck"?

There is no question that certain human habits contribute to certain types of cancer. These would include inherited factors, smoking, poor diet/obesity, sun overexposure, and other environmental causes.

A 2015 study from *Science*, however, showed that "two-thirds of the difference in risk of cancer between the different cancers is due to bad-luck mutations." Unfortunately, this study was misinterpreted by the press to mean that 65% of cancers are caused simply by "bad luck."

Certainly, cancers can occur spontaneously but because of this faulty conclusion, many of you may think that there is nothing you can do to decrease the risk of cancer, which is untrue. In fact, the study was trying to identify why some organ's tissues produce more cancers than other tissues, *before* considering environmental and lifestyle factors.

The American Cancer Society states that about half of all cancers are due to lifestyle issues and that percentage increases significantly with environmental factors.

A cancer diagnosis is not necessarily a death sentence. Some cancers are now curable, and there can be long-term remission from treatments. In fact, even if some cancers are incurable, they can often be treated as a chronic condition with years of survival.

The latest available statistics (March 2011) from *MMWR* revealed that the percentage of the nation's population that has survived a cancer diagnosis increased from 1.5 percent in 1971 to 3.5 percent in 2007. Accounting for over half those diagnoses were breast (22 percent), prostate (19 percent), and colorectal (10 percent). If you have not had a recurrence of your cancer within five years, you have a lower risk that it will return and thus a very good likelihood of long survival.

<hr>

Cancer Myths

- Pollution is a greater risk for lung cancer than smoking (smoking is responsible for 87 percent of lung-cancer deaths).
- Eating lots of antioxidants will negate the effects of smoking.
- Low-tar cigarettes are safer.
- Electronic devices (cell phones, etc.) can cause cancer (research is negative so far).
- Shampoos and antiperspirants cause cancer.
- How social you are has a lot to do with cancer risk.

<hr>

One of the most important aspects of treating cancer is the oncologist (cancer specialist). Although there are some who practice solo, most are either in group practices, work for hospitals, or are at large cancer centers. It is very important that you have good rapport and communication with your oncologist; otherwise, you may not respond as well to treatment, and many more complications can occur. It is also important that they provide the care that *you* need and that *you* desire.

<hr>

Dr. A's Suggestions:
Not All Cancer Centers/Oncology Groups Are as Good as Advertised

In this day and age, cancer centers and oncologists must compete for patients, and marketing is very important. Be very careful with what you hear, because some cancer centers and oncologists may not deliver what they promise. Some things you may hear might include:

- There are many cancer centers that label themselves as "comprehensive," yet they differ widely in their approach to evaluation and treatment. Be sure you understand what their definition of "comprehensive" really is.

- The types of technology that they have available may vary widely, and some technologies may be outdated.
- Each may have a different approach or model of care for the patients. For example, some may provide little support while others support *all* aspects of your life, not just the treatment part (such as psychological, social, family, financial, and work aspects). Some may treat you as a "person" and some as a "number."
- Many expect you to do only what they recommend and many others will help you decide on various options (i.e., *empower you*).
- Some prefer patients with early diagnosed cancers yet don't treat the more difficult ones, or literally "abandon" you or give up on you when the cancer progresses.
- Some communicate with you well, and others have poor communication and poor follow-up. Some centers may have "teams" that work with you, and others are more fragmented, causing delays in treatment.
- Some are more interested in you for research, and others focus on standard treatments that can still be beneficial.
- Many do not adequately address side effects of the cancer and its treatment while others make quality of life (QOL) a priority.
- Some may tell you that they have alternative methods, but they either really don't have them, have only a few minor methods, or do not use them effectively or frequently. The majority don't even consider alternative methods.
- Some will tell you there is nothing more that can be done, whereas a few think "outside the box," are hopeful, and don't "give up" on you.

You always need to check out the oncologist or cancer center and talk with other patients if you can. You should also get a second opinion to compare the differences. Finally, ask them if they participate in the quality measurement programs from the CoC (Commission on Cancer), which has rigid standards to make sure patients are receiving optimal care.

Caring for the "Whole Person": Lip Service versus Reality

A big "buzzword" in cancer care is addressing the needs of the "whole person." In fact, the Institute of Medicine has released a number of reports over the past several years addressing this need, and several different cancer commissions have issued recommendations. Most cancer centers commonly market this approach, but do they really deliver on their promise?

According to an editorial published in the December 2013 issue of the *Journal of the NCCN*, the standards of caring for the whole person includes distress screening, incorporating navigation, better communication between patient and doctor and the use of survivor care plans. These are all beneficial actions and do improve patient-centered care, but many oncologists and centers do not provide these services or only minimally address them.

Furthermore, addressing the "whole person" involves more than the above: it should also include mind and spirit approaches and taking care of other medical conditions and QOL issues. The above editorial represents a limited conventional approach and doesn't include an integrative approach, which is fundamental to treating the whole person. Even fewer cancer doctors and centers use these methods.

The *bottom line* is that many oncologists and cancer groups use the catchphrases, "We treat the whole person," or "We provide patient-centered care" but in fact they do the same things they have always done, that is, just treat the cancer rather than the person. Be sure to become empowered and make sure what a doctor or cancer center define as treating the "whole person".

Helpful tip: Because cancer treatment options and approaches can vary widely, I recommend that you always consider *obtaining a second opinion*. Many oncologists will only recommend the treatments they have available, but other options may exist that they may not tell you about. In addition, different oncologists may have different beliefs in their philosophy of treatment. For example, if you have stage 4 cancer (spread or metastasized to other organs), some oncologists will recommend no treatment, even though the cancer may still be responsive. Some oncologists may be too timid to prescribe aggressive treatments that may have benefit and prolong survival. The *bottom line* is that you need to become empowered and find out all the information you can.

Important Note: Although chemotherapy may still be beneficial in late stage cancer, its use is discouraged for end-stage patients who only have a few weeks of life left; in fact, such therapy can actually harm those patients and make QOL worse.

Important Information:
Don't Be Fooled by Cancer Hospital Ratings

You may have read magazines that rate cancer hospitals, but in fact, those ratings are often based on measures that may be capricious, unrelated to quality, easily manipulated and/or incentivize the wrong attributes. What they also don't tell you is that only the hospitals that fall under certain pre-determined categories are rated, whereas others that may be just as good or better for you are not listed or even considered.

For example, one of the most familiar ratings are from *US News and World Report*, which bases 40 percent of its ratings on reputation, yet reputation is an error-prone variable and is easily manipulated. Furthermore, to be in their rankings requires (1) being a member of the Council of Teaching Hospitals, which leaves out many private hospitals and cancer centers, and (2) being directly affiliated with a medical school, which again leaves out many private centers as well as excellent community cancer centers.

You should also realize that these ratings may not incorporate survival rates or satisfaction reports, both of which are very important. In fact, survival rates may not be provided by some of the top-rated cancer centers.

It is advisable to get second opinions from other cancer centers, whether ranked or not. Rather than focus on ratings, make sure you go to a center that cares about you first and foremost, communicates well, addresses quality of life issues, has integrative services that are readily available, and has a friendly, hopeful and healing atmosphere. They should treat you as a person, not a number or research statistic.

The *bottom line* is that ratings are based on whatever factors the magazine or other rating entities think are important; but they may not be what are most important to *you*. Make sure, wherever you go, that they empower you so that you can take an active role in your care. Cancer can be a challenging disease; you need all the support you can get.

———

A major problem with diagnosing and treating cancer is *delays*. Most cancer patients may need several different types of doctors treating them, including surgeons, radiation oncologists, medical oncologists, GI specialists, and so on, as well as numerous tests that are also performed by other doctors. What occurs is that it takes time to make appointments and be evaluated or tested by these doctors, and then it takes more time for the reports to be interpreted and sent back to the ordering physician, and then it takes even more time for that physician to reschedule you to discuss the findings and treatment recommendations. Such events may take weeks or even months before you begin treatment, and the same occurrences may transpire after beginning treatment.

Certainly, if you go to a cancer *center*, it may shorten the time, but even some cancer centers may use doctors and services outside the facility or still have delays referring you to specialists within their own system. It is important that you obtain proper diagnosis and treatment as soon as possible, so become empowered and make sure your care is provided in a timely and efficient manner. Ask the facility how much time it will take: if you are not receiving timely care, seek out a second opinion.

Related to the problem of time is that of communication among providers. A team approach is highly recommended. Otherwise, different doctors may have different opinions and may not arrive at a proper consensus for your treatment. You need to realize that there may be several options available for you, each of which may be provided by a different specialist (such as surgeon, medical oncologist, radiation oncologist), who may want to use only the treatments they specialize in. However, if all these specialists are "under the same roof" and/or have meetings with each other to discuss your particular situation, it will be more conducive to considering the best options and developing an appropriate treatment plan for your specific condition.

A good example is a patient with newly diagnosed head/neck cancer. A radiation oncologist told him he absolutely needed radiation only but the oncologist told him he needed to be in a chemotherapy study instead. The patient found out that each of the doctors was conducting a different research study and they received money for every patient in their particular study. The patient became empowered and went to another cancer center. After consultation with the entire team, his best option was actually surgery, which was never considered or recommended by the first doctors. Fortunately he is now cancer-free.

As mentioned above, another important aspect of cancer care is addressing QOL issues. Cancer, as well as its treatment, can cause many side effects and complications, which can adversely affect your work and social life. Unfortunately, many cancer doctors and centers do not address these problems adequately (some not at all), so patients may suffer unnecessarily; there are many treatments that can help you live life better, even during cancer treatment. It is important to realize, however, that many of the best treatments for QOL involve alternative methods, so it benefits you if your doctor or cancer center offers these approaches.

Quality of Life (QOL) of Utmost Importance

Your QOL is one of the most important aspects of cancer and its treatment. Numerous studies have shown that the better you feel, the better you can tolerate cancer and treatment side effects. But QOL is not just about feeling good; it may also help survival. In fact, two recent studies revealed that QOL parameters such as pain, physical function, and appetite loss can be predictive of better outcomes.

Unfortunately, many cancer doctors do not address QOL issues. For example, many studies show that pain medications are under prescribed in cancer patients. At the 2011 ASCO (American Society of Clinical Oncology) meeting, it was noted that greater than two-thirds of oncologists are not even trained in addressing QOL issues. Even those that are may still not address these aspects. Many large cancer centers have QOL programs, but only when you are hospitalized, not as an outpatient. Even fewer use alternative methods, which can be more beneficial for many QOL issues (see below under *Alternative Approaches*)

Treatments should be directed at the symptoms caused by the cancer, as well as at the side effects of cancer treatment, including those that continue even after a remission or cure has been achieved. Some of the most common symptoms and side effects are fatigue, pain, weakness, decreased appetite, lack of energy, nausea, and weight loss.

It should be realized that many medical providers refer to QOL as palliative care. Unfortunately, this may have the connotation that you are at the end of your life when, in fact, palliative care is basically the same as QOL care. Recent studies reveal that palliative care/QOL should be addressed at the very start of diagnosis and treatment and not just at the end of life. In fact, these studies show that patients who receive this care from the beginning require less chemotherapy and make fewer emergency room visits. A more recent study done on stage 4 lung-cancer patients found that those on palliative care lived longer, spent less time in the hospital, and had a better quality of life.

QOL can make a huge difference in your fight against cancer. So become empowered and make sure your physician or cancer center addresses these problems.

Even if you've conquered cancer, you still may have residual effects and complications from the cancer and/or its treatment, even decades later. Many people experience anxiety, depression, sexual concerns, and fear after surviving the cancer, and oncologists may not address these problems after successful treatment. This is an area called *survivorship*, and you should make sure your oncologist, PCP, or cancer center addresses these issues.

Dr. A's Suggestions:
Adult Cancer Survivors Not Receiving Good Follow-Up

A recent report showed that 61 percent of primary care physicians were unsure about their role in follow-up care (surveillance) for the most common types of cancer, including lung, breast, prostate, colorectal, bladder, melanoma, non-Hodgkin's lymphoma, kidney/renal cell, leukemia, and uterine cancers. Half were unaware of side effects and concurrent problems caused by long-term side effects of treatment. Thirty-one percent were uncertain as to what medical interventions are recommended for preventing or treating such side effects and problems.

One of the authors stated that "post treatment cancer care is at best fragmented and at worst nonexistent." Therefore, it is important to ask your PCP what he or she knows, and if not knowledgeable, make sure you receive follow-up from your oncologist or provide your PCP with guidelines from your oncologist. (***Important Note***: I have developed a program designed to teach PCPs how to follow-up the care of cancer patients, which is available to any physician group).

You should also realize that many cancer survivors do not eventually die from their cancer, but from other conditions, especially heart disease. In fact, studies show that cancer survivors are very lax at improving their lifestyles after surviving cancer and many doctors are also lax at making sure your other medical conditions are addressed.

Fighting cancer is not an easy task and is a condition for which you need to know the best options and obtain the greatest support possible. The *bottom line* is that when choosing an oncologist, cancer group, or cancer center, become empowered and make sure that you receive the best care throughout *all* facets of cancer care, including testing, diagnosis, treatment, follow-up care, social and psychological support, quality of life issues, and survivorship. If you don't think you are receiving the care you need or desire at any point in the process, be sure to get another opinion.

Treatments for Cancer and the Side Effects of Cancer and Cancer Therapies

You need to understand that cancer is a complex disease and each type of cancer can act quite differently than other types or even in the same type in different people. There are numerous mechanisms by which cancer cells protect themselves from eradication, such as "hiding" from the immune system, which allows it to continue to grow and spread. Because of these mechanisms, it is often necessary to consider a variety of treatments.

The barriers created by the cancer itself are not the only problems when trying to find effective treatments: there are also daunting barriers to *providing* those treatments. The Institute of Medicine in 2012 issued a report that concluded that the cancer care delivery system is in crisis: care is often not patient-centered, many patients don't receive palliative or QOL care to manage their symptoms and side effects from treatment, and decisions about care are often not based on the latest scientific evidence.

Because of those factors, you must become empowered: *What you need is excellent care, compassion, and hope.* The following will help guide you in understanding your options.

The Preventive Approaches

—∞—

Dr. A's Suggestions:
Marital Status Impacts Cancer Outcomes

A study published in September 2013 revealed that married cancer patients have better outcomes than unmarried patients, for three reasons:

- *Usually diagnosed earlier and thus have less advanced tumors.* This is likely due to the spouse making sure the patient gets cancer screening and/ or sees a doctor sooner for worrisome symptoms.
- *Comply with treatment better,* which increases the odds of response. This is likely due to spousal support to help the patient get through difficult treatments, take all their medications and make all their appointments with doctors on a timely basis
- *Have longer survival.* Married patients have more psychological support and thus display less anxiety, stress, and depression, all of which may impact cancer survival.

The authors recommend that cancer doctors and centers focus on supporting unmarried patients more, but unfortunately, this doesn't happen in the majority of cases. In addition, what the authors did not say is that it is necessary to support the spouse as well, who often has as much or more stress than the patient. In fact, a recent study showed that the spouses of survivors have more anxiety than the patient. Become empowered and find a doctor or cancer center that provides such support, whether you're married or not.

—∞—

Preventive testing and early detection are some of the best deterrents against cancer (see chapter 2). For women, annual pap smears and breast exams are essential and routine mammograms should be done after age forty to help prevent breast cancer. For men, prostate exams and testing (PSA) are important for prevention of prostate cancer. For both men and women, screening for blood in the stool should be done routinely, and a colonoscopy (placing a fiberoptic scope into the colon to look for polyps or cancer) should be done after the age of fifty to help prevent colon cancer.

Dr. A's Suggestions:
For Certain Female Cancers, Check Your Genes

Certain cancers have a family predilection, which means that your children may be at higher risk for developing the same type of cancer as you have and sometimes additional types of cancer. This is especially true in women with ovarian or breast cancer. If you have these cancers (especially at a younger age) or a strong family history, you may need to be tested for the BRCA1 and BRCA2 genes and, if positive, have your daughters tested as well. ***Important Note***: These tests have now been expanded and include many more genetic tests (called MyRisk). However, there are other genetic syndromes that can increase the risk of cancer as well, including in males (such as Li Fraumeni and Lynch syndrome) so be aware if you have a strong family history, even of different types of cancer.

It is important to note that the father's side of the family should be checked as well because both men and women are equally likely to pass these genes to their offspring. Unfortunately, women are five times more likely to be referred for genetic testing with a maternal than a paternal family history of cancer.

If these tests are positive, you and/or your family will require specific screening, surveillance, or prophylactic treatments to prevent cancer. I highly recommend consultation with a certified geneticist if you have a strong family history of cancer or have such genes.

Discontinuing smoking is one of the primary ways to prevent cancer. Smoking is the most common environmental pollutant and can cause a variety of cancers, including lung, breast, stomach, throat, bladder, esophagus, and prostate. Cancers related to smoking are more likely to affect women than men.

Dr. A's Suggestions:
Survivors of Childhood Cancer Face Increased Death Risk, Yet Are Screened at "Alarmingly Low" Rates

A study published in the *Annals of Internal Medicine* show that childhood cancer survivors face an increased risk for later cancers, chronic conditions and heart and lung complications. Later cancers were highest five to nine years after diagnosis and declined after thirty years had passed since diagnosis. Reduction in lifespan ranged from four years for kidney tumors to more than seventeen years for brain and bone cancer survivors, with an average of ten years.

Another study from the *Annals* found that women who had chest radiation for pediatric or young adult cancer were at 13 to 20 percent greater risk of developing breast cancer by age forty to forty-five. Radiation can also cause an increased risk of skin cancer (both melanoma and nonmelanoma), colorectal, and other types of gastrointestinal cancer.

Yet another study in the *Annals* showed that survivors of childhood cancer are too often not getting recommended screenings for second malignancies, especially those at the highest risk.

The latest study published in the *Annals* in January 2014 showed that despite half of all internists caring for a childhood cancer survivor, at least 75 percent never received a summary from the pediatric oncologist. Less than 20 percent were familiar with the need for breast cancer and heart dysfunction surveillance for those receiving chemotherapy or radiation. Only 10 percent had any familiarity with follow-up guidelines.

If you had a childhood cancer, you should be aware of these findings and receive more frequent health exams and screenings (especially pap smears, colonoscopy, and skin exams) and women should undergo yearly mammograms starting earlier than age forty. You can find the guidelines for what you and your doctor need at: http://www.survivorshipguidelines.org/pdf/ltfu-guidelines.pdf.

Medications to avoid: Some blood pressure medications may *increase* the risk of breast cancer. If you have a high risk, you may need to avoid thiazide diuretics (40 percent increased risk), and potassium sparing diuretics (60 percent increased risk). Calcium channel blockers were originally thought to increase risk, but a newer study has disputed this. The diabetes drug, pioglitazone, was found in a 2015 study to potentially increase the risk of pancreatic and prostate cancer.

Dr. A's Suggestions:
Diabetes Associated with Increased Incidence
of Cancer and Poorer Outcome

A study presented at the annual scientific session of the American Diabetes Association revealed that diabetics have a 25 percent increased risk for developing cancer, a 30 percent greater risk of mortality from any cancer, as well as having a shorter survival time after cancer diagnosis. The *bottom line* is that better diabetes care can both help prevent cancer and, if you already have cancer, may improve cancer survival.

Two other studies showed that metformin, typically the first medication used for adult-onset diabetes, may help prevent certain cancers, as well as slow cancer growth and increase survival as an adjunct to standard therapies; these cancers include lung, breast, ovarian, colon, prostate, and breast. It is known that metformin lowers blood-sugar levels and increases insulin sensitivity, two factors that are associated with cancer growth when abnormal. It is too early to recommend this to all patients with these cancers, but if you have diabetes, this is one drug you should consider taking. However, many doctors use some of the newer drugs first, even though they may not be any more effective, are much costlier and do not have anti-tumor potential.

Helpful medications: There are some medications that may *decrease* the risk of cancer. Low-dose aspirin (81 mg) has been shown in several recent studies to potentially reduce the risk of numerous cancers as well as reducing its spread if it does occur, most likely due to its effects on reducing chronic inflammation, which is thought to be an underlying cause of cancer. (See sidebar below). *Important note*: These studies are not yet conclusive enough for general recommendations but hold significant promise. *Caution*: Be aware that aspirin can cause harm, such as GI bleeding, which needs to be taken into account, especially in older people (taking aspirin for ten years increases the risk of bleeding to 3.6 percent).

Can Aspirin Help Prevent and Restrict Cancer?

Several specific studies have shown reduction in cancer growth, metastasis, recurrence and mortality for colon, breast and now prostate cancers by taking low dose aspirin. Other studies include pancreatic and liver cancers.

These studies include one from the *Journal of Clinical Oncology*, showing that aspirin reduces the likelihood of recurrence and death in prostate cancer. Another study published in *JAMA* demonstrated that aspirin can lengthen survival in non-metastatic colorectal cancer. Another report from the *Journal of the NCI* showed that aspirin users were 16 percent less likely to die from cancer than nonusers. A 2011 study from *Lancet* showed that taking daily aspirin decreases mortality from solid cancers and reaches its most significant benefit at five years.

For cancer *prevention*, a study in 2014 from Queen Mary University of London, showed that bowel cancer rates were decreased by 35 percent and death by 40 percent, and rates of esophageal and stomach cancer were cut by 30 percent and deaths from these cancers by 35 to 50 percent. No benefit was seen while taking aspirin for three years; lower death rates were seen only after five years, especially between the ages of fifty and sixty. A 2015 study in the *Annals Intern Med* showed that continuous use of low-dose aspirin for greater than five years was associated with a 27 percent reduction in colorectal cancer risk. A previous study in 2012 in *Lancet Oncology* showed that it decreased risk in numerous GI cancers as well as breast. Another study in 2012 showed the same observation with prostate cancer prevention.

Important note As mentioned above, again be aware that aspirin has not yet been recommended for general prevention of cancer. In addition, these findings may be applicable only to certain patients with these cancers as determined by genomic testing of the tumor.

Can Statins and Beta Blockers Help Decrease Mortality from Cancer?

An intriguing study from Finland showed that patients taking statin drugs (used to lower cholesterol) for four or more years during the study had significantly decreased overall cancer deaths, especially deaths from lung and colorectal cancer. Like aspirin, statins have anti-inflammatory properties. A 2015 study showed that statins decrease the risk of prostate cancer.

Beta blockers, usually used in heart disease and hypertension, have also been shown to reduce risk, recurrence, and death from melanoma and some other cancers. The mechanism proposed is that it decreases the negative effects of stress on the body.

Because these are observational studies, they may not be as accurate as randomized, prospective studies, but they suggest a potential use for these drugs as an adjunct in cancer prevention and treatment. Further studies are needed to document this effect.

Diet: Almost one-third of all cancers may be related to being overweight, especially cancers of the breast, colon, uterus, prostate, kidney, and gall bladder. There is no question that diet plays a significant role in both preventing and causing cancer. Animal fats and processed foods are the main foods that contain cancer-causing substances (called carcinogens), and they should be limited. In fact, high intake of processed meat (cured, salted, fermented, or smoked) and bacon has been declared carcinogenic by WHO and has been linked to increased deaths from cancer. Red meat might be carcinogenic, but not as much as processed meats. Citrus fruits and especially cruciferous vegetables are foods that can protect against cancer, and these should be increased in the diet; a 2015 study in the *J of Clin Nutrition* showed that women with the highest levels of carotenoids (found in fruits and veggies) had a 23 percent reduction in breast cancer risk. Onions, garlic, berries, tomatoes, and autumn olives (an Asian fruit that tastes like cranberries) also have cancer-fighting properties. Various spices, including basil, rosemary, turmeric, ginger, and parsley, all contain flavonoids that can help against cancer, but fresh herbs are preferred. Flaxseed (fresh ground) has been found to potentially help prevent breast cancer. Foods containing boron, such as wine, almonds, coffee, peanut butter, raisins, legumes, low-fat milk, and certain fruits and nuts, may help stave off cancer, especially prostate.

Dr. A's Suggestions:
Nutrition of Utmost Importance

Nutrition is especially important when treating cancer. Not only can cancer treatment cause weight loss due to side effects, the cancer itself can cause loss of appetite and can "steal" nutrients from your body. The weight loss is often not from fat but from protein; since protein comes from your muscles, you can become weaker as well.

Malnutrition in cancer patients can increase the risk of infection, toxicity from treatment, and costs while decreasing treatment response and quality of life. Studies have shown that patients who are well nourished not only have fewer side effects from conventional cancer treatments but also may have longer survival. A significant percentage of cancer mortality is related to poor nutrition, and a large number of cancer patients die of malnutrition rather than their cancer.

Important note: A 2014 study showed that up to 50 percent of overweight cancer patients may have or be at risk for malnutrition, which is not addressed because they appear to be well nourished.

Unfortunately, a large percentage of oncologists and cancer centers do not make nutrition a priority or address it at all, but if not, you should seek out a registered dietician on your own or find a cancer center that does.

———— ⬥ ————

There are no specific diets that will cure cancer, but, as mentioned, limiting saturated fats, high-fat dairy, and processed foods and increasing whole grains, fruits, and vegetables may help slow the progression of cancer and protect the body against toxic cancer treatments. Polyphenols (antioxidants) found in red wine have been found to keep prostate cancer cells from proliferating and may do the same for other cancers. Lycopene, contained in watermelon and tomatoes, also helps fight prostate cancer. Green tea has potent compounds that can not only prevent cancer but can help retard its growth as well. Apple peels seem to have an anticancer effect, so eat the whole apple. Peaches that contain the most "red" contain cancer-fighting compounds.

Soy products can provide high-quality protein and phytoestrogens (natural estrogen produced by plants) are especially beneficial for hormonal-related cancers such as prostate and breast (do not exceed 30–35 grams per day). Soy and red grapes have antiangiogenic effects (may reduce new blood-vessel growth in tumors). *Caution*: If you already eat soy products (tofu, edamame), you can continue eating them if you have cancer. However, many dieticians advise not to start eating them if you have hormone-related cancer and haven't eaten them before.

———— ⬥ ————

Some Cancer Attributable to Alcohol Consumption

A recent study published in April 2011 in *BMJ* revealed that 10 percent of cancers in men and 3 percent on women are attributable to alcohol consumption. It was noted that consuming more than the recommended upper limit of alcohol accounted for the majority of alcohol-related cancers.

These percentages were higher for specific cancers: 44 percent male; 25 percent female for upper aerodigestive tract cancers; 33 percent male, 18 percent female for liver cancer; 17 percent male, 4 percent female for colorectal cancer; and 4 percent for breast cancer.

Another study, in 2015, showed that even light-to-moderate drinking is associated with increased risk for these cancers in patients who smoke.

Thus, drinking *moderately* may confer benefits, but overdrinking can increase cancer risk (see chapter 2 for recommended alcohol limits). And if you smoke along with drinking too much alcohol, the risk is even higher.

———— ⬥ ————

Side effects of cancer and its treatment can significantly affect nutrition. Some of these related problems include sores in the mouth, swallowing problems, feeling full quickly, loss of appetite, and taste changes. All of these can be addressed, but you need to seek out the help of a registered dietician, especially one who treats cancer patients frequently. There are also many alternative methods that can alleviate these side effects as well. Again, good nutrition is of utmost importance in fighting cancer, but again, only a minority of oncologists and cancer centers may address these issues adequately.

Do Multivitamins Help Prevent or Treat Cancer?

There have been several studies to determine whether taking multivitamins may have an effect on preventing cancer or lowering the mortality rate once you get cancer. In fact, two recent studies do show promise: The Physician's Health Study suggested that MVIs may have some cancer prevention benefits in middle-aged men. In the Women's Health Initiative, older women who developed invasive breast cancer while taking MVIs had a 30 percent lower rate of mortality. However, other studies do not show benefits from taking MVIs. Furthermore, some of these results may be because patients who take MVIs also have better lifestyle habits. If you are not obtaining adequate nourishment, taking an MVI may still be advisable (see chapter 2 for additional discussion on MVIs).

Regular **physical exercise** helps protect against several types of cancer, noted by studies especially in cancer of the lung, breast, colorectal, and prostate. Once cancer occurs, exercise is invaluable for reducing fatigue, lessening anxiety and depression, increasing physical capacity, and helping to provide a better overall quality of life. Cancer patients who are able to exercise regularly also have better outcomes from cancer treatments. A 2015 study showed that men in midlife who are more fit have less incidence of colorectal and lung cancer and have better survival if they get those cancers. Another recent study showed that moderate exercise improved survival and reduced side effects in post-diagnosis and post-treatment colon cancer patients.

Exercise Recommendations for Cancer Patients

- It is safe. There have been no reported adverse effects.
- There will be "down days" that you don't feel like exercising. Don't feel guilty.

- Avoid high-intensity workouts during treatment: They may suppress your immune system.
- Walking and cycling are preferred.
- Moderate intensity is adequate (heart rate 50 percent of maximum).
- Exercise three to five days a week, twenty to thirty minutes per session.

The Conventional Approaches

Conventional treatments for cancer are the ones proven to destroy cancer cells and prolong survival. There are numerous types of treatments, each indicated for specific cancers or groups of cancers. These include, but are not limited to, chemotherapy (oral, intravenous, intrathecal, intraperitoneal), several different types of radiation (see below), surgery, hyperthermia (elevating body temperature), chemoembolization, photodynamic therapy, radiofrequency ablation, therasphere, hormonal therapy, cryotherapy, and others. Proven conventional methods are your best bet for a cure, remission, and/or to prolong survival.

Much of cancer treatment is determined by guidelines developed by the National Comprehensive Cancer Network (NCCN). In fact, most testing and treatment reimbursement by Medicare and insurers is based on these guidelines. You should realize, however, that within the guidelines, there may be several options available that are equally acceptable, so depending on what oncologist or cancer center is treating you, treatment may differ based on their experience or what therapies they have available. You also need to realize that many of these therapies are more toxic than others and costs vary as well. You also need to understand that if your cancer progresses, these guidelines may not be able to provide additional recommendations. Thus, it behooves you to become empowered and make sure you know all the options, so you can make the best choice for your needs and desires. Here is a brief overview of the major types of treatments:

Chemotherapy is a common form of therapy for most cancers. It is especially indicated if your cancer has spread to other parts of your body but also may be used to prevent its spread or recurrence. There are many chemotherapy drugs that have been used for decades and are still beneficial and there are many standard combinations of chemotherapy drugs that have proven effective for many cancers. Over the past decade, however, numerous discoveries have led to drugs that target specific mechanisms that promote cancer growth and thereby have potential to slow or stop the growth. However, many of the targeted drugs only work on a small percentage of cancers, they may be very expensive, and they may only provide a survival benefit of a few months. Nevertheless, the more we discover, the more successful the treatments can become.

Dr. A's Suggestions:
Problems with Oral Chemotherapy Drugs

Up until this decade, chemotherapy drugs were always given intravenously (IV). Many of the newer chemotherapy drugs can now be taken orally. However, there are several caveats noted with oral chemotherapies.

First, you should realize that even if taken orally, these drugs may still have significant side effects.

A recent study also showed that many patients on oral chemotherapy do not take the drug as prescribed, either taking too much or not enough. This was particularly noted in breast cancer patients. The incidence increased when the regimen was more complex.

Another study showed that a variety of common drugs for other conditions can cut the potency or increase the toxicity of the oral cancer drugs. These cancer drugs were in the class of "kinase inhibitors," and the common drugs included heartburn drugs, steroids, calcium channel blockers (for heart disease and high blood pressure), and some antibiotics and antifungal drugs. The chemotherapy drugs were prescribed by oncologists and the others by PCPs.

It is important that you be empowered and have good communication with your oncologist and make sure you are correctly taking the drug as it is prescribed. It is also important to make sure your oncologist and PCP communicate with each other and that both know all the medications (and any nutritional supplements) that you are taking.

Because chemotherapy can be quite toxic and affect normal tissue, it can cause "collateral damage", causing numerous side effects, including some that can be lethal. So it is important to know what complications can occur and make sure your oncologist tries to prevent or will address these side effects. You also need to know, again, that there may be several different drugs or combinations of drugs that are recommended by the NCCN, each of which may have different side effects.

Cost May Affect Choice of Cancer Drug

Unlike in other conditions for which doctors write prescriptions for drugs, many oncologists must buy drugs up front so they can deliver them intravenously. Thus, oncologists are out the money until insurers or patients pay the bill. One problem is that many cancer drugs are so expensive that insurers are delaying and denying claims, and many patients cannot afford the high co-pays (often up to $11,000 per month). This is especially true of the new cancer drugs made through gene therapy.

For these reasons, cost may be an important factor in what chemotherapy you receive, and many oncologists may not even bring up the option for the more expensive agents. They also worry that they'll lose business because patients may not like to discuss these issues, not to mention the liability issue if they push lower-cost treatments that don't work.

Understand that just because your physician orders it doesn't mean it will be paid for, and you should always check with your carrier first (some cancer centers and oncologists check for you). Otherwise, you will have to pay for it out of pocket. Even if covered by your carrier, the co-pays for expensive drugs can be thousands or tens of thousands of dollars.

In fact, financial hardship is common in cancer patients. A recent report found that 28 percent of patients, especially with advanced disease, were in danger of losing their homes, and 64 percent had limited or very limited financial resources left as a result of their disease. Unfortunately, many patients delay treatment because of the financial constraints, leading to worse outcomes.

You also need to consider that many of the newer, more expensive drugs may only provide a few additional weeks or months of life and they may also have significant side effects. Many oncologists have decried the high price of these drugs, stating that the prices may not reflect the true value of the drug. There is now a website (www.drugabacus, org) that uses a calculator that compares the cost of more than 50 cancer drugs with what the prices would be if side effects and survival were considered.

The *bottom line* is that you should always discuss the costs versus the effectiveness of these drugs with your oncologist. Sometimes, the best treatment may be the most expensive, but there may be other options available. There also may be discounts available, or you may qualify under a "hardship" classification, both of which may help you afford these drugs.

Dr. A's Suggestions:
Obese Patients May Be Shorted on Chemotherapy

Obese people have been shown to be less likely to survive cancer, and one reason may be that they are often undertreated. Oncologists may short them on chemotherapy by not basing the dose on size. Instead, they use ideal weight or cap the dose out of fear of increasing side effects. Studies suggest that as many as 40 percent of obese cancer patients have been getting less than 85 percent of the right dose for their size.

As even a little less chemo may worsen the odds of survival, if you are overweight, you must be empowered and make sure you are getting a dose based on *your* weight.

Unfortunately, many cancers can become resistant or don't respond to certain chemotherapy drugs, and the cancer recurs or spreads. Although many oncologists may tell you there is no hope, and the NCCN guidelines have run out of recommendations, that doesn't mean you should give up. There actually may be other drugs or methods that can still benefit you, and you need to become empowered and get other opinions. In fact, there are genetic tests available that may be able to determine mutations that are driving the growth of the tumor and may be able to uncover other chemotherapies (many unpredicted) that may be effective against the cancer. There are numerous patients I have seen who have been told they only have a few months to live and there is no more treatments available, and yet we have been able to find treatments that may help them survive much longer or even go into remission.

Genetics: Personalizing Cancer Prevention and Treatment

Our genes determine and regulate everything that happens in our bodies. More commonly than you may realize, those genes can mutate and, as a result, cause various diseases, including cancer. There has been a great renaissance in cancer treatment in discovering these "genomic" mutations and developing treatments to reverse or block their negative effects.

In cancer, there are two basic areas of genetics: germ line and tumor genomics. Knowing about both can be essential in fighting your cancer.

Germ line mutations run in families and can be passed from generation to generation. If you have breast, ovarian, or colon cancer, or several of your family members (including aunts, uncles, and grandparents) have these tumors, you may be carrying genes that have predisposed you or your children to developing these and other cancers (see above in *Preventive Approaches*).

In addition, however, there can be genomic mutations within tumors themselves, causing them to grow uncontrollably. These mutations are rapidly being discovered, and already there have been numerous drugs developed to block their actions. Many of these mutations may exist in tumor types that would not otherwise be expected. Furthermore, there are some mutations that can implicate whether a standard chemotherapy drug may work or not, so you won't waste time and money on a drug that may be ineffective. In fact, many oncologists are now treating some cancers based on their genetic mutations rather than the cancer type. This is a very promising development that truly makes cancer treatment individualized and is a great hope for the future.

There are now numerous companies that test for these mutations. It is very important, therefore, to ask your doctor about these tests and whether you are a candidate for them. Unfortunately, a 2014 study in the *Journal of Clinical Oncology* reports that only 25 percent of oncologists and surgeons would use genomic testing frequently. Again, you need to become empowered and ask about this aspect of cancer care and/or find a cancer center that has expertise in genetic testing and treatment.

Most insurance companies and Medicare cover these tests if they are indicated, although some require consultation by a certified geneticist. Such testing may make a significant difference in the outcome of your fight against cancer. ***Important Notes***: However, be aware that even if testing is positive, there may not yet be treatments available for that particular mutation. In addition, the existing treatment(s) may not offer significant benefit.

On the other hand, studies have shown that over 50 percent of cancer patients whose life expectancy is less than 6 months continue to receive chemotherapy. The studies revealed that chemotherapy use was not associated with longer survival but was associated with poorer QOL near death for those with good performance status.

So obviously there is a quandary; when and how do you know if chemotherapy will prolong life or instead will not improve survival while making QOL worse? In general, if there are chemotherapy drugs that have not been tried and have been proven to be beneficial and prolong life appreciably, they should be considered (along with their possible side effects and complications). However, if you've taken numerous rounds of different chemotherapies that have not worked, additional chemo may not help either and may cause additional suffering. The *bottom line* is to be empowered and communicate with your oncologist to make sure the benefits of continued chemotherapy outweigh the harm, and/or obtain a second opinion.

Palliative versus Curative Chemotherapy: Misunderstood

Unfortunately, some cancers are incurable no matter what treatment is provided. Often, chemotherapy is given as a "palliative" treatment, that is, to prolong life as long as possible but not to cure. Unfortunately, many of these cancer patients continue to undergo chemotherapy thinking that it will cure them. In a 2012 study in the *NEJM*, fully 69 percent of lung-cancer patients and 81 percent of colon-cancer patients felt that chemotherapy was very or somewhat likely to cure their cancer.

These perceptions are most likely due to a combination of the oncologist's tendency to skirt the detail of poor prognoses as well as patients' unwillingness to believe the word "incurable."

We all want cancer to be cured, and patients should still hold out hope. However, you must also be realistic, so that you can live the rest of your life as you deem important.

Immunotherapy or biologic therapy is currently another tact being used to fight cancer. Rather than use chemotherapy to directly destroy tumors, immunotherapy is designed to help the immune system recognize and destroy tumor cells (remember, most cancers are able to "hide" from the immune system). Immunotherapy can be used in several ways:

- Stimulating your own immune system to work harder or smarter to attack cancer cells, including cancer vaccines.
- Using personalized cell-based therapies that use a patient's own white blood cells to attack tumors.
- Giving you immune system components, such as manmade immune system proteins (for example, monoclonal antibodies).
- Injecting a substance (such as a virus) into the tumor that causes a general immune system response to the substance that also kills the tumor cells.
- Stimulate the immune system in a general manner (these therapies often have more and significant side effects and are not used as often).

Immunotherapy has been recognized since the 1980's but only recently has scientific knowledge and technology advanced enough to be able to refine the techniques and avoid the many setbacks that occurred during the past decades. Immunotherapy is now one of the main thrusts and promises in cancer research, but much research is yet to be done.

Surgery in cancer is performed for various purposes. If your cancer is localized (early stage disease), removal of the tumor may be indicated and may even be curative, depending on the type. If the cancer has already spread (metastasis), surgery may still be able to help (called "debulking"), depending on where it has spread and to how many areas; in some types of cancer, even if it has spread, removing the primary tumor can still affect outcome.

Sometimes cancers can block vital organs and may need to be removed or bypassed. In some cancers, various organs or parts of organs must be removed with the cancer. For cancers that have caused spine fractures or compressions, a procedure called balloon kyphoplasty has been shown to be effective in relieving pain.

A few cancer centers perform HIPEC, in which heated chemotherapy is directly applied to the open abdomen after debulking surgery. This is most often indicated in patients whose cancer has spread onto the inner lining of their abdomen (called carcinomatosis). However, not all such patients are good candidates for this procedure and there can be more complications and longer recovery associated with it.

Important Information:
Not All Cancer Surgeries Are Done the Same

You may think that standard surgeries are performed for specific cancer diagnoses, but that is not always true. For example, there has been a recent trend in this country to perform more limited procedures, especially in cases such as breast cancer (e.g., lumpectomy rather than mastectomy), for cosmetic reasons and because the surgeon may feel that other treatments (chemo, radiation) can kill any cancer cells left behind. However, some patients who undergo limited procedures are not good candidates and thus the cancer may recur.

In addition, some surgeons may *not* make the effort or take the time to remove tumors that are close to nerves or blood vessels, again thinking that other treatments will help kill the cancer left behind. Sometimes, it is too dangerous to remove such tumors, but at other times, it can be done but requires more time and skill. In fact, some surgeons may tell you that surgery is not possible, but other surgeons actually may be able to perform the surgery. In addition, sometimes the surgeon may remove or damage nerves along with the cancer (causing loss of function in that area) rather than sparing the nerve by using intraoperative nerve monitoring.

It is important to undergo cancer surgery by an *oncologic* surgeon when possible. These surgeons are specialized in operating only on cancer patients and understand how cancers spread and recur. In addition, these surgeons are more likely to take the extra time (sometimes hours) to remove cancers from difficult areas. There are also surgeons who specialize in removing specific cancers, such as breast, head/neck, and lung (thoracic). Especially with the latter two, there are more generalized surgeons who include cancer in their scope of practice but don't focus their surgeries to just cancer, and so may miss important characteristics; for this reason, it is important to find a surgeon that specializes in resecting your specific type of cancer.

You should also know that there are several cancer surgery techniques that are not supported by evidence and should not be done, according to the American College of Surgeons. There also may be several different types of surgery that can be done for the same situation (such as laparoscopic, robotic or open), with each having different complications and outcomes. Due to these issues, it may be important to obtain a second opinion.

Radiation may be done in conjunction with chemotherapy for better effectiveness or after (and sometimes during) surgery to kill remaining cancer cells. In some cancers (e.g., prostate), it can be the sole treatment. It may be used to shrink tumors that are compressing or obstructing vital organs or that are in locations which are difficult to access with surgery. It also may be used as a palliative measure to treat pain-causing metastases.

What you need to know is that there are many different types of radiation, including brachytherapy, tomotherapy, IMRT, SBRT, therasphere, proton, Calypso (moves with the organ), IORT (intraoperative), hyperthermia, gamma or cyber knife, and so on. It is very important to explore your options and get second opinions: radiation oncologists may only have available some of these types of equipment, but that doesn't mean it's the best one for you.

Proton Therapy: Real Benefit or Just More Expense?

There are several different types of radiation therapy, one being proton-beam radiation. It is advertised as sparing normal surrounding tissues and thus reducing side effects. It is beneficial for some cancers in difficult places, such as eyes and in some pediatric patients.

Proton therapy has been heavily marketed for other cancers, especially prostate, yet most clinical trials have not shown that it is more effective or has fewer side effects than other radiation therapies. In fact, there have been some reports revealing poorer outcomes in some patients; a 2012 study showed that prostate cancer patients experienced more bowel problems, such as bleeding and blockage, than those treated with conventional radiation (called IMRT, Intensity Modulated Radiation Therapy). A health technology assessment by the state of Washington in 2014 found that proton-beam therapy was not advantageous compared to IMRT in prostate patients.

A major issue is that proton-beam radiation costs much more than conventional radiation therapy because the facilities cost so much (about $200 million initially, now about $50 to $100 million). Investors of these facilities thus want to treat every cancer they can. In fact, Medicare still pays more than twice as much ($50,000 vs. $20,000) despite no evidence of superiority. Many insurance companies won't pay for proton therapy and in many states, owners of these centers are organizing patients to help pass legislation to require them to do so. So the end result for you may be a lot more expense (and more side effects) without better outcomes.

Despite the problems noted, more proton-beam centers are in the planning stages. However, the newer proton machines are better designed and use "pencil beam" photons, which are superior to the mechanism of the older proton machines. Theoretically, the newer machines should have fewer side effects than the older machines and should be as efficacious as IMRT. However, few studies on the newer machines have been conducted as of yet. If you decide to use proton therapy, seek out a facility that has the more advanced machine, but be sure to compare other types of radiation first.

———

When radiation is given, there is a total dose calculated, which is then divided into smaller doses given each day for several weeks (called *fractionation*). Many radiation oncologists are now providing *hypofractionation*, which involves higher doses given over fewer days (3 weeks versus 5-7 weeks). Hypofractionation is more convenient, less expensive and initial studies show no difference in outcome or side effects over 10 years, as compared to standard fractionation. ***Caution***: However, the studies were done in particular patients (over age 50, had tumors smaller than 5 centimeters, had no cancer in their lymph nodes, and did not receive chemotherapy), so it is not known if the same benefits will occur if you don't fit this criteria.

You need to understand that radiation, just like chemotherapy, can have significant side effects and complications. Radiation burns the tumor but can also burn normal tissue, so side effects can occur. For example, radiation of the chest can lead to increased heart disease as well as lung or skin fibrosis (scarring of tissues), radiation to the prostate may cause inflammation of the anus or rectum, and radiation to the head/neck can cause mucositis (sores in the mouth and esophagus) and dry mouth, as well as scarring of soft tissues.

Fortunately, there are therapies that can help prevent or treat these side effects, but not all oncologists or cancer centers address them successfully. Again, this is an area for which a second opinion may be valuable.

Other Treatments. As mentioned above, there are other treatments that may be done in place of the above or as an adjunct to them (to help them kill more tumor cells), such as photodynamic therapy (PDT) and hyperthermia (both superficial and deep). It is not my purpose to describe all the other potential treatments here: what you need to realize is that many of these are only done in major cancer centers, which is why again I always recommend obtaining a second opinion.

⸺⸙⸺

The Team Approach: A Valuable Adjunct

I have already mentioned that delays may be common in cancer diagnosis and treatment, especially when numerous doctors are involved. This is because it takes time to obtain appointments and testing, as well as doctors communicating with each other. For these reasons, it is often advisable to go to a cancer center in which physicians are "under one roof", even though sometimes there may still be delays.

There is another reason why this may be an advantage. In many cancers, it helps to have different doctors present when evaluating or treating a patient. For example, it may be expedient for a surgeon to be present when a GI doctor does a colonoscopy for a mass in the colon, so that the surgeon knows beforehand what to expect. Or a surgeon and radiation oncologist may do a pelvic exam together for a cervical cancer since both may be treating the patient. A third example is a radiation oncologist being available to perform radiation during an operation (IORT) if a surgeon finds that he cannot remove all the cancer.

Although doctors can team up in any hospital, it needs to be coordinated and is more likely to occur if the doctors are located close to each other.

⸺⸙⸺

Treatments for Quality of Life Issues

As conventional cancer treatments can be quite toxic, other treatments should be tried to prevent or treat side effects. A major side effect of many chemotherapy drugs is a *significant decrease in your blood cells (called pancytopenia)*, leading to anemia, decrease in platelets (causing increased tendency to bleed), and decreased white cells (causing increased risk for infection). There are several conventional treatments that may stimulate more production of these cells, such as Neulasta or Neupogen for white cells and NPlate for platelets. For severe anemia and low platelets, blood transfusions may be needed. ***Warning***: Erythropoietin, given to increase red blood cells, may cause additional harm, including blood clots, tumor progression, and death if given for mild anemias.

Pain is a common side effect of cancer that can and should be well controlled, although many physicians are wary of giving adequate medication to truly control it. In fact, the majority of oncologists are not trained in pain management and significantly under-treat pain (for example, they may prescribe a medication every six hours but the medication only lasts three hours, so you are always "chasing" your pain"). There are a large number of medications that can be helpful, and there are many routes of administration, including oral, IV, sublingual (under the tongue), buccal (melts in your mouth), sprays, suckers, and skin patches. ***Caution***: If you must take potent narcotics, constipation is usually a problem, and you should always be prescribed laxatives at the same time.

It is important for you to control pain. Many patients are afraid to become "addicted" or don't want the side effects, such as drowsiness. However, there are enough types of pain medications so that you can find one that gives you relief while minimizing side effects. Furthermore, if you *need* pain drugs, addiction should not be an issue. What you should realize is that having pain may cause the body to secrete substances that can adversely affect your immune system. In addition, several studies have shown that patients who control their pain are able to fight their cancer better and may have better overall outcomes. It helps to find a cancer center or hospital that has a pain specialist on staff.

For *fatigue, weakness, and lack of energy*, there are few conventional treatments that may be beneficial. Often, exercise and rest (energy conservation) are prescribed. That may seem to be contradictory, but both are important. Otherwise, methylphenidate (Ritalin), Provigil, and steroids are sometimes tried, but they do have potential serious side effects.

Up to 50 percent of patients receiving chemotherapy have *nausea and vomiting* and it can also occur after treatment. Zofran, Compazine, Phenergan, Ativan, and Kytril are the most commonly used during and after chemotherapy. A Sancuso patch (long-acting Kytril) may decrease nausea for up to a week. Other drugs include metoclopramide, haloperidol, Zyprexa, and steroids, depending on the cause. A new drug (rolapitant [Varubi]), works differently than the above medications and has just been approved for nausea and vomiting; it may be effective in up to 70 percent of patients.

Many side effects, such as *neuropathy*, are treated with the conventional drugs commonly used for neuropathy from other causes (gabapentin [Neurontin] or pregabalin [Lyrica]). However, studies reveal that less than 15 percent of cancer patients obtain relief from such drugs. Other side effects that may respond to drugs include constipation, diarrhea, thrush (yeast infection of tongue and throat), skin reactions, and dyspnea (perception of impaired breathing).

Many patients are *unable to eat* well after chemotherapy, radiation, or surgery or their cancer suppresses their appetite. Megace and dronabinol are drugs that can improve appetite and increase caloric intake. Remeron (an antidepressant also used for insomnia), periactin (an old anti-itch drug), and steroids may also increase appetite. If patients cannot eat over a prolonged period of time, it may be necessary to use other forms of nutritional support. These include TPN (total parenteral nutrition), which is liquid food given through a large vein or PPN (partial parenteral nutrition), which can be given through a smaller vein. Other methods include placing a tube from the stomach (PEG) or small intestines (PEJ) to the outside of the body, so that food and even medications can be placed through the tube and go directly to the stomach or intestines. ***Helpful tip***: You should always consult with a registered dietician if you can't eat, have no appetite, and/or continue to lose weight.

Some side effects, such as mouth sores (*mucositis, stomatitis*), have few adequate conventional remedies, although solutions containing anti-inflammatory compounds, antacids, and analgesics may help ease throat pain and swallowing difficulties. Any chemotherapy drug can cause allergic reactions, including anaphylaxis (rash, throat swelling and/or low blood pressure).

If your cancer spreads to bones, fractures and pain can occur frequently. Several drugs can help both problems, including Zometa (by infusion) and denosumab (Xgeva), a once-monthly injection. Radiation is commonly done to decrease bone pain caused by metastases. Pain from collapsed vertebrae can also be helped by a surgery called kyphoplasty.

Some chemotherapy drugs and radiation can cause damage to the heart, especially when used in breast cancer patients and need to be closely monitored with a heart test (MUGA scan or echocardiogram) performed before and after treatment. One study showed that a blood pressure medication (candasartan) prevented heart decline, although the benefit was small (improvement of only two to three percent).

Lymphedema may also occur in some women treated for breast cancer and can be helped by specialized types of massage (usually done by physical therapists trained in that procedure.) Some women with lymphedema will get cellulitis, an infection/inflammation of the affected arm. A new device (Flexitouch System by Tactile Medical) has shown an 80 percent reduction in cellulitis episodes and a decrease in physical therapy costs. This device is a pneumatic compression device that can be used at home.

Chemotherapy for breast cancer also frequently causes *hair loss*. It has been demonstrated that cooling the scalp to near freezing may often prevent such hair loss and many patients bring gel-filled cold caps to use during chemotherapy sessions. There are cooling cap products available and the FDA has now approved one version called the DigniCap, which is leased to cancer centers and costs around $1500 to $3000 depending on how many rounds of chemotherapy are given; the company's studies show that more than two-thirds of the treated women kept more than half their hair. Side effects included cold-induced headaches and neck/shoulder discomfort, chills and pain.

Survivorship

More and more patients are surviving cancer; there are presently almost 20 million cancer survivors. As a survivor of cancer, it is important for you continue to be followed closely by your doctor, either your oncologist or primary care physician, for several reasons: first, to detect if the original cancer reoccurs or a secondary cancer occurs; second, to address side effects or complications that can persist due to treatment; and third, to treat other conditions unrelated to cancer that can still affect your life. Unfortunately, studies show that only 20 percent of oncologists speak to survivors about lifestyle guidelines, and even fewer address long-term side effects and complications. Even fewer PCPs may do so, because they often don't know what to look for.

This is one area that is very important. Many cancer survivors die from something other than their cancer, and many have medical problems that decrease their quality of life. You must become empowered because of this. The following are actions that should be taken:

- Stop smoking and decrease exposure to secondhand smoke.
- Integrate physical activity (there are certified cancer exercise trainers).
- Avoid weight gain.
- Decrease time in front of the TV and computer.
- Increase intake of fruits and veggies; focus on legumes and eat chicken rather than red meat (see additional suggestions in chapter 2, under "Diet").
- Drink alcohol in moderation.
- Stay connected with friends, family, and other survivors.
- Get necessary screening and regular check-ups. Make sure you find out the recommendations for follow-up testing.
- Make sure any other medical condition you have is treated appropriately.

Hospice

If cancer has spread and is no longer amenable to treatment, doctors usually recommend *hospice*. Hospice is a type and philosophy of care that focuses on the symptoms of patients who are terminally ill. These symptoms can be physical, emotional, spiritual, and/or social in nature. The modern concept of hospice includes care given in such institutions as hospitals, nursing homes or self-standing hospice facilities, but it also includes care provided to those who would rather die in their own homes.

End-of-life decisions are significant when you have cancer that has progressed. Many cancer patients want to try to find anything that can prolong life, and cancer doctors don't want patients to die, so treatments may continue. However, many cancer patients die in ways they don't really want to…in a hospital or ICU, unaware of loved ones or suffering through continued painful treatments that are futile.

With cancer, there are always promising treatments being developed, so there can always be hope; but you shouldn't be given "false" hope. It is important to ask and understand what additional treatments will or will not do; studies show that two-thirds of patients who receive treatments for palliation (symptom control only) think that the treatment is to cure their cancer. In addition, many patients receive intensive and invasive treatments that have no hope of prolonging life and thus decrease their chances of having greater comfort in the time they have left.

It is important to get accurate information from your physician before you and your loved ones can make a decision on how to proceed. Even toward the end of life, being empowered is important.

The Alternative Approaches

Alternative methods alone have not been proven to cure cancer, but they can potentially enhance conventional treatments and are exceptional at preventing and treating side effects, thus improving quality of life. As mentioned above, since improved QOL can help patients fight cancer, alternative methods are important adjuncts to conventional treatment. According to various surveys, up to 88 percent of all cancer patients use alternative methods.

Many alternative methods are effective, but many are a waste of time and money. Unfortunately, even the beneficial methods are not commonly used or even understood by most oncologists, even at major cancer centers, so most patients may not be able to receive the potential benefits. On the other hand, most cancer patients use alternative methods and may be using ones that are actually interfering with proper treatment. Therefore, *it is most important to seek care from alternative practitioners who are qualified in treating cancer patients.*

Important Note: The following alternative methods are evidence based, but some studies have been small so larger studies may not demonstrate similar results. It is highly recommended that you undergo evaluation by an alternative medicine practitioner certified in that particular approach.

Acupuncture is one of the most important alternative methods for cancer patients. It is excellent for preventing or treating the nausea and vomiting side effects of chemotherapy, as well as resolving or diminishing other side effects of either the cancer or cancer treatment such as pain, fatigue, neuropathy, lymphedema, salivary problems from head/neck irradiation (dry mouth, difficulty swallowing, taste), GI problems (gas, bloating, nausea, diarrhea, constipation, appetite loss), breathing difficulties (shortness of breath), incontinence (from bladder or prostate treatment), skin rashes (including hand-foot syndrome), anxiety and depression, and many other complications. A 2015 study demonstrated acupuncture is better than drugs for hot flashes in breast cancer survivors (it may also be beneficial for hot flashes in men treated with hormone suppression for prostate cancer). Frequently, acupuncture is more effective than conventional treatments for such QOL issues.

Chinese herbal formulas can help conventional treatments work better, reduce or prevent side effects, and help survival, much like Western herbs and supplements (see Table 1). For ***cautions***, see section on Chinese herbs in chapter 4. Again, it is very important to obtain recommendations and treatment for Chinese herbs from TCM practitioners who are certified in Chinese herbs and have experience working with cancer patients.

Table 1
Chinese Herbs for Cancer Treatment and Side Effects

- *Zuo Gui Wan/You Gui Yin* is given before and after any surgery or cancer treatment to prevent or treat fatigue and reduce other side effects. It may also speed up recovery from surgery if taken afterward.
- *Coriolus* (also known as turkey tail) is a mushroom extract that over 400 studies have shown may prolong survival time in people with stomach, uterine, colon, lung, colorectal, prostate, breast, and liver cancers, when taken *with* chemotherapy.
- *Ba Zhen Tang* may help build up blood cells and be beneficial when chemotherapy suppresses the bone marrow.
- Several **Chinese mushrooms** (Wild red ganoderma [Reishi], tremella, poria, maitake, and polyporus) may improve outcome when used with chemotherapy and radiation and have antitumor properties. Polyporus (Grifola umbellatae) has been shown to decrease recurrences of bladder cancer after surgery. Agaricus blazei has been shown to be beneficial in gynecologic cancers.
- *Astragalus** (15–25 grams powdered form daily) with ligustrum, a Chinese herb also known as Chinese privet (10–15 grams powdered form daily or 3–5 ml of tincture three times daily) may increase survival rate when undergoing radiation therapy for breast cancer or chemotherapy for lung cancer.
- *American Ginseng** (1,000–2,000 mg twice daily) has been shown to decrease cancer fatigue in a third of patients. Korean (Asian) ginseng is stronger than the American ginseng and may be as or more beneficial.

***Important note**: Although the single Chinese herbs above have been supported by studies, single herbs are actually rarely used. Mushrooms are usually balanced in and of themselves, but it is recommended to use formulas that contain these herbs, especially "boosting" formulas like *Dang Gui Bu Xue Tang* (Astragalus and Gan Cao) or *Gui Pi Tang* (contains ginseng).

In several clinical studies, daily consumption of a traditional Chinese soup containing vegetables and herbs was associated with regression and prolonged survival in patients with small cell tumors of the lung. The soup has ostensibly been used successfully in other cancers. See chart below for ingredients.

Cancer "Soup" Ingredients

Soybean	Ginseng	Shiitake mushrooms	Sesame seed
Mung bean	Red date	Angelica root	Hawthorn fruit
Scallion	Licorice	Dandelion root	Parsley
Garlic	Senegal root	Lentil bean	Onion
Ginger	Leek	Olive	

For further information on this soup, contact Alexander Sun, PhD, the Connecticut Institute for Aging and Cancer, 203-882-9672, or go to www. Sunfarmcorp.com.)

Western Herbs and supplements may enhance the beneficial effects of conventional treatments and help prevent and/or treat side effects of cancer treatments. Although most of these can be used without interfering with conventional treatment, some supplements may interfere and should be avoided or monitored closely (see Table 2).

Many Oncologists Don't Talk to Their Patients About Herbs and Supplements

In a national survey in 2010 and published in 2014, fewer than half of cancer doctors bring up the subject of herbs or supplements with their patients. Many doctors cited their own lack of information as a major reason why they don't. As over 80 percent of cancer patients may use supplements, and some supplements may interfere with cancer treatment, this is not a beneficial scenario.

In addition, what the survey did not address was that, of the oncologists who do discuss herbs and supplements with their patients, many of them still may lack accurate and appropriate knowledge and often simply tell the patient not to take any supplements at all.

Helpful tip: It is highly recommended that for Western herbs, you *consult with a naturopathic doctor* who has expertise working with cancer patients and is familiar with the type of treatment you are getting. There are well-trained naturopathic doctors who obtain FABNO certification (Fellow of American Board of Naturopathic Oncology), who specialize in oncology and can guide the individual, depending on the type of cancer they have and the conventional treatment they are prescribed. Many naturopaths are also expert in Chinese medicine and herbs as well.

Table 2
Supplements to Be Cautious With

- **St John's wort**: This herb may interfere with the metabolism of many chemotherapy and other drugs.
- **Garlic**: May theoretically also interfere with chemotherapy drug metabolism.
- **Echinacea**: Should *not* be taken if you have lymphoma or are immuno-suppressed due to adverse immune function actions.
- **Blood-thinning herbs**: Gingko, ginger, garlic and saw palmetto can thin the blood and may increase risk for bleeding if you take warfarin (Coumadin) or other blood thinners, although studies do not show major bleeding complications.
- **Antioxidants**: *Theoretically*, antioxidant vitamins (such as vitamin C) may interfere with the action of chemotherapy drugs, but again there is no definitive research proof. (In fact, some naturopaths recommend IV vitamin C and some research supports its benefits in fighting cancer.) Antioxidants may also interfere with radiation therapy.
- **Hormonal herbs**: Black cohosh, saw palmetto, and soy may interfere with hormonal therapies for breast, prostate, and ovarian cancers, but most studies show no adverse activity, and some studies show benefits.
- **Selenium and vitamin E supplements** in high doses may double the risk of prostate cancer in patients with high concentrations of selenium in their bodies.

Many supplements and herbs may help protect normal cells from harm by specific chemotherapy agents, hyperthermia, or radiation damage and thus help prevent damaging these tissues (see Table 3).

Table 3
Herbs/Supplements That May Protect Normal Tissues from Conventional Treatments

- *Glutathione* (600 mg on days 2–5 of chemotherapy, intramuscularly) may reduce the kidney and neurological toxicity of Cisplatin, a chemotherapy drug used in cancers of the testicles, bladder, and ovaries.
- *L-Glutamine* (10 gms powder three times daily) may protect the GI tract and nerves. Use 24 hours after chemo, then for 5 days only.
- *L-Carnitine* (1–2 grams daily) and CoQ10 (50 mg daily) may protect the heart against damage from chemotherapy using Adriamycin, a drug used in many solid and blood cancers in which a small cell type is dominant, and Herceptin and Perjeta, drugs used for cancers (breast and upper GI) that are positive for a gene called Her-2-Neu.
- *Garlic* (4 grams, or one clove, containing at least 10 percent alliin) and/or onions (50 grams fresh onion) daily may protect the liver from toxic damage.
- *Milk thistle (silymarin)*: Based on the results of studies using methods of molecular biology, silymarin can significantly reduce tumor cell proliferation and angiogenesis (blood vessel proliferation in the cancer) and help suppress alpha-induced tumor necrosis factor protein production. Milk thistle also appears to protect liver cells from being damaged and may regenerate liver cells.
- *Vitamins C, E, and selenium* may decrease the rate of kidney and hearing problems with chemotherapy.

Selenium: Preventive or Harmful?

Many studies have shown that people living in areas where the soil has a high concentration of selenium have a lower incidence of cancer. Selenium also appears to increase cancer cell death and reduce the formation of free radicals. As a result, many people take selenium as a supplement.

However, only one study has shown a correlation between selenium levels in the blood and lower cancer mortality. In addition, taking too much selenium may *increase* cancer and overall mortality and increase the risk of diabetes and cause other side effects. The best way to acquire it is through food, but if you do take a supplement, take less than 200 mcg a day.

It should be realized that cancer drugs and radiation may not kill all the cancer cells, which can predispose to reoccurrences and relapses. There are several herbs and supplements that that may help potentiate these conventional treatments (see Tables 4 and 5)

Table 4
Herbs/Supplements That May Potentiate Conventional Treatments

- **Quercetin** (400–500 mg three times daily) may increase the amount of tumor cells killed when using cisplatin. It can also be given by IV, 420–1,400 mg/m2, weekly or every three weeks. Quercetin may also increase the amount of tumor cells killed when *hyperthermia* is performed. It can also be given by IV, 420–1,400 mg/m2, weekly or every three weeks. **Caution**: However, it may interfere with other chemotherapy given at the same time, such as Taxol.
- **Selenium** (200 mcg daily) may increase the tumor-killing effects of cisplatin in the presence of EDTA (a chelating agent). **Caution**: However, I do not recommend chelation therapy or detox *during* treatment. Also, be careful of how much selenium is prescribed.
- **Melatonin** (20–50 mg per day with chemotherapy, beginning one week before therapy is begun) may be especially beneficial in hormone sensitive cancers such as breast and ovarian. It appears to boost your immune system. It can be used even without chemotherapy: studies indicate that it also may improve survival when undergoing chemotherapy using the following:
  - *Interleukin-2* is called a cytokine, a protein that helps regulate your immune system. It may be used to treat cancers of the lung, GI tract, liver, kidney, breast, and melanoma.
  - *Triptorelin*, a drug used in prostate cancer.
  - If you undergo *radiation* therapy for glioblastoma, the most common malignant tumor of the brain.
- **Niacin** (100–300 mg per day) may help make radiation therapy more effective by depleting the oxygen used by cancer cells, thus killing them.
- **Bromelain** (80–320 mg per day for ten days) may improve the effectiveness of:
  - *Vincristine*, a drug used in leukemia and Hodgkin's and other lymphomas.
  - *5-FU*, a drug used primarily in cancers of the gastrointestinal tract (stomach, colon, rectum, pancreas).

- *Curcumin* (500 mg twice daily or turmeric extract, 36-180 mg curcumin) has been the focus of numerous studies and may potentiate 5-FU, xeloda, and gemcitabine. It has also been shown to intervene at each stage in the sequence of events that enable cancer cells to develop, proliferate and metastasize
- *Fish oil* (1500 mg daily) may potentiate doxyrubicin and platinum-based chemotherapies, according to several studies. ***Important Note***: A 2015 study found that fish oil may cause chemo-resistance and should not be taken during the days around chemotherapy until further studies are done. However, another 2015 study in the *Journal of Parenteral and Enteral Nutrition* showed that omega-3 fatty acids added to chemotherapy may improve treatment response and quality of life (fish oil was used with gemcitabine for pancreatic cancer).
- *Astragalus* (600 mg twice daily) may potentiate cisplatin.
- *Berberine* may enhance the effects of cisplatin in ovarian cancer.

Table 5
Additional Supplements That May Help Fight Cancer

- *Green tea* (average of 4 cups per day, providing 240–320 mg of polyphenols, or standardized extracts containing up to 97 percent polyphenols) may inhibit the growth of cancer. ***Caution***: It may interfere with the drug bortezomid (Velcade), used to treat multiple myeloma.
- *Ellagic acid* (200 mg daily), derived from red raspberries, has antitumor potential.
- *Vitamin K* (5 mg) with vitamin C (250 mg) twice daily to inhibit prostate and breast cancer. Vitamin K (45 mg) alone has been shown to inhibit the progression of liver cancer. ***Caution***: Due to vitamin K's effects of clotting blood, take it only under supervision of a doctor.
- *Flaxseed* (2 tsp daily, freshly ground) may deter prostate cancer growth.
- *Curcumin* (can be given in high dosages of up to 12 g without toxicity), besides enhancing conventional treatment, may also have a direct inhibitory effect on cancer, especially noted in multiple myeloma and pancreatic cancer. If combined with piperine, bioavailability is significantly increased.
- *Vitamin D* (2000-5000 IU daily, D_3 form preferred; need blood levels between 40-60 ng/ml). Lab studies show inhibition of growth and spread of tumors. Cell culture studies suggest that vitamin D promotes cell differentiation, inhibits cancer cell proliferation, and exhibits anti-inflammatory and anti-angiogenic properties.

—∞∞—

There are also many herbs and nutritional supplements that may help reduce or even prevent the side effects of chemotherapy and radiation (see Table 6).

—∞∞—

Table 6
Western Herbs/Supplements That May Help Reduce or Prevent Side Effects of Conventional Treatments

- *"Chemo brain"* (cognitive dysfunction due to chemo): Gingko biloba (240 mg daily with chemotherapy) may protect normal brain cells and stimulate production of new cells. ***Caution***: Some studies suggest that it can interfere with the metabolism of some chemotherapies and other conventional medications depending on its concentration. It may also increase blood thinning. Fish oil may be more helpful.
- *Immune modulation*: Medicinal mushrooms, especially Trametes versicolor (also known as Coriolus, also known as turkey tail), 3 grams daily. Fermented wheat germ.
- *Neuropathy*: This occurs as a side effect of many chemotherapy drugs. L-glutamine (30 grams daily) appears to work well for neuropathy. Vitamin E taken orally (300–600 mg daily) appears to work better if the neuropathy is caused by platinum drugs. ***Caution***: Vitamin E can thin the blood and should be used cautiously with radiation).
- *GI dysfunction* (common with many chemotherapies or antibiotic use, causing diarrhea): Probiotics may be useful, but they should be discontinued if white blood cell count is less than 2.5.
- *Nausea* (from chemotherapies): Try ginger (1 gram per day during chemo).
- *Dermatitis* (from radiation): Use calendula lotion or chamomile skin cream. However, it should be removed completely each day before radiation treatment.
- *Cachexia* (weight loss): High-dose fish oil (3,000–4,000 grams daily) may maintain weight and increase dietary intake. L-carnitine (500–1,000 mg daily) may also be helpful.
- *Lymphedema*: In breast cancer, head and neck, or pelvic cancers. Try selenium under direction of a naturopath or doctor (loading dose 1,000 mcg for one week, then 300 mcg per day,), gingko biloba (240 mg daily), or bioflavones.

- *Vasomotor symptoms* (hot flashes, night sweats): In breast cancer, black cohosh (20 mg herbal drug daily). Magnesium and fish oil have been shown to be beneficial as well.
- *Fatigue* (from all cancer treatments): Carnitine (especially if carnitine deficient), 6 grams daily; high-dose fish oil (krill, 2 grams daily); vitamin B_{12}.
- *Mucositis/stomatitis* (from radiation and chemotherapy): Zinc (25–50 mg three times a day) and proteolytic enzymes (head and neck radiation); Arnica Montana (Traumeel), or glutamine (improves nutrition and decreases pain), 0.4 g/kg daily; German chamomile as a rinse (extracts or flowers standardized to 1.2 percent apigenin three to four times daily) can be beneficial. Honey is also very good for healing the sores.

Medical Marijuana and Derivatives May Be Helpful for Quality of Life

As of March, 2015, 23 states and the District of Columbia had medical marijuana laws in place. These laws allow the use of marijuana for a variety of medical conditions, which vary among the states. However, it is approved in all of these states for treating nausea and vomiting in cancer patients (due to chemotherapy) and for appetite stimulation. It is also used for neuropathic pain. There is high-quality research evidence to support these uses.

There are also two FDA-approved drugs that are derivatives of marijuana, dronabinol and nabilone. Although they may be effective for many patients, marijuana is more potent, being comprised of more than 400 compounds, of which 70 are cannabinoids. Cannabinoids appear to be the active compounds and have individual, interactive and entourage effects (entourage means that a compound has an effect only in the presence of other compounds).

Cautions: Although medical marijuana may be beneficial, you can develop a tolerance requiring higher doses and you may also have withdrawal symptoms. It may also interfere with the action of opioid medications for pain, which are commonly prescribed to cancer patients. Approximately 1 out of 10 people will develop an addiction to marijuana. It should be avoided in patients with psychoses such as schizophrenia or bipolar disorder.

Low level energy laser (*LLEL)* is a very effective device for numerous side effects of cancer treatment, including mucositis, fatigue, xerostomia (decreased salivation), dysgeusia (decreased taste), neuropathy, pain, and lymphedema, and can be used to stimulate acupuncture points. It is also very effective for accelerating wound healing. The laser often provides long lasting relief and may prevent worsening of these conditions despite continued treatment. (See Chapter 4 for more detailed discussion). I have recently completed and presented research on the benefits of LLEL for treating mucositis secondary to radiation of head and neck cancers. Frequently, LLEL is more effective than conventional treatments for the above QOL issues.

Qigong has been shown to help prevent, reduce, or eliminate the side effects of cancer treatment, including radiation and chemotherapy, and it appears to improve immune function. A 2013 study in the *Journal of Cancer Survival* showed that it improves fatigue in prostate cancer, but I have observed the same benefits with other cancers as well. It can be done before, during, and after conventional treatment. There are many qigong exercises designed specifically for cancer patients and many are easy to do (see chapter 4), even while sitting or lying down.

Mind-body interventions, primarily meditation, guided imagery and interactive imagery/active imagination can improve quality of life and reduce the side effects of conventional cancer treatment. Interactive imagery is especially beneficial for cancer patients and can improve mood and reduce anxiety. More importantly, it can positively and significantly change patients' outlook on their life and even help them avoid fearing the possibility death (see chapter 4 for more in-depth discussion).

Psychedelic Drugs: Helping Patients Cope

Scientists are taking a second look at psychedelic drugs for treating severe distress and emotional suffering in cancer patients. Researchers at Johns Hopkins, UCLA and NYU have used psilocybin to help individuals "transcend their primary identification with their bodies and experience ego-free states . . . and return with a new perspective and profound acceptance".

Patients have experienced improved personal well being as well as significantly decreased anxiety and fearfulness. Many patients describe the experience as one of the most meaningful of their lives. As such, this is a new type of mind-body medicine and one whose effects can last for long periods of time, even up to a year or longer.

It appears that such drugs act on a part of the brain called the default-network mode (DNM), which narrows and constrains thought processes. Psilocybin reduces this activity, freeing the mind to release long-held repressed thoughts, feelings, fears and memories.

This type of therapy is still in research and these drugs are still illegal. In addition, a trained therapist must be present during the entire experience because what is released from the mind must be interpreted and negative reactions controlled. To obtain benefits, any and all material that comes forward must be addressed.

Certainly such a drug may be beneficial in such a setting. However, interactive imagery/active imagination can produce *exactly the same results*, in much less time and without using illegal drugs. The limitation is that there are very few practitioners who are trained in this technique (For reference sources, see Appendix).

Meditation, prayer and spiritual belief can also reduce side effects, anxiety and depression. These techniques also benefit family members who are dealing with their own worries, fears, and concerns.

Support groups during or after your cancer treatment have been noted to help prolong survival in most cancers, especially breast cancer and melanoma, and also provide a great deal of support and information to help you cope with cancer. Most hospitals or cancer centers have such support groups or can refer you to one.

Both **massage** and just **touching** advanced cancer patients have been shown to improve pain and mood almost immediately, although a thirty-minute massage showed slightly better results.

Yoga is also beneficial for cancer patients. Studies show that it improves physical function and general health, as well as decreasing daytime sleepiness and fatigue, and getting better nighttime sleep. A November 2015 study (not published yet) showed that yoga may help maintain QOL and alleviate some side effects for men undergoing radiation therapy for prostate cancer.

Beware of Alternative Cancer Treatments Not Proven Effective

There are many alternative treatments purported to cure or control cancer, and these flood the Internet. Many cancer patients may wonder if they are missing out by not taking these treatments that sound so promising. The fact is that no high-quality studies have proven their effectiveness (in fact, many have had no studies performed) although there are many testimonials that support each, and some ingredients have been noted to have antitumor potential in test-tube research. The following are the best-known.

- *Essiac (or Flor Essence)*, based on an Ojibwa Indian formula, containing four herbs: burdock root, sheep sorrel, slippery elm bark, and turkey (Indian) rhubarb. Although some of these herbs have anti-cancer potential, there has been no clear research evidence of efficacy.

- *Antineoplastons*, which are made from your own urine. Phase 1 and Phase 2 trials have been conducted but Phase 3 trials have not been done and effectiveness has not been proven.
- *Laetrile*, derived from apricot seeds. It has shown no anticancer activity in human trials. ***Warning***: Laetrile contains cyanide, which can cause numerous side effects and death.
- *Hoxsey therapy*, which consists of two remedies; two external mixtures containing antimony trisulfide, zinc chloride, and bloodroot (red paste), and arsenic sulfide, sulfur, and talc (yellow paste), as well as an internal liquid mixture containing licorice, red clover, burdock root, stillingia root, barberry, cascara, prickly ash bark, buckthorn bark, and potassium iodide; seven herbs have antitumor activity. Reviews by major cancer centers and the NCI have found no evidence of benefit.
- *Insulin potentiation therapy* (IPT) uses insulin as an adjunct to low-dose chemotherapy. IPT is closely related to Insulin Potentiation Targeted Low Dose (IPTLD); however, IPTLD is used specifically to treat cancer with 10-25% of the traditional dose of chemotherapy drugs. Long-term outcomes, such as survival, have never been published. Four individual case studies, one small, uncontrolled clinical trial and one small prospective, randomized controlled trial have shown temporary reductions in the size of tumors for some patients. It costs $2000 per session. ***Warning***: this technique lowers blood sugar to potentially dangerous levels.
- The "*Greece Test*", also called RGCC, uses blood or tissue to find circulating tumor cells and cancer stem cells. It then tests these cells against 49 chemotherapy drugs, 64 tumor related genes (looking for mutations) and 50 biologics (including many listed above such as green tea extract, melatonin, curcumin, and so on), purportedly to see what chemotherapies are most likely to work. Although used since the mid 1990's, there have been no randomized clinical trials providing evidence of its reliability. In addition, there are many laboratories that provide such testing (both in the US and Europe) but results are not consistent from lab to lab.
- *Mistletoe*, used primarily in Europe; only 5 out of 333 studies showed benefit
- *714X*, a homeopathic camphor compound: no RCT has found effectiveness.
- *Hydrazine sulfate*, an anticachexia drug (prevents weight loss and debilitation), which ostensibly stabilizes or regresses tumors. RCTs have been conducted, showing no benefit for cancer or cachexia (severe weight loss) and some have actually shown an increase in cancer.

- *Shark cartilage*, which contains compounds that ostensibly slow blood vessel growth in cancers. One RCT and other case studies have generally found no benefit, with cancers recurring in most within a few months.
- *Gerson therapy*, which uses a radical diet, nutritional manipulation, and coffee enemas to rid the body of toxins. Most trials have been retrospective but reviews of those studies have shown no benefit.
- *Pancreatic enzyme therapy (Gonzalez regimen)*, which uses numerous pancreatic enzymes to fight pancreatic cancer by eliminating the body of toxins. One clinical trial showed that patients had worse QOL and less survival on this regimen.
- *Others* include coffee enemas, ozone therapy, blue scorpion poison, dendritic cell therapy, kangaroo stem cells, and bone marrow stem cells, none of which have been supported by any research.

A few of these alternative therapies are currently under investigation by the NCCAM. However, until the results of the research are available, I cannot recommend any of them. I have also evaluated numerous patients who have tried one or many of these methods: although in a few instances their cancers appears to have stabilized for short periods of time, the cancer has always recurred at some point and has been more aggressive when it has. It is not known whether the stabilization was due to the treatment or a natural consequence of the cancer. In addition, some are very expensive, costing over $50,000 per year.

Special note: *For comprehensive information on cancer and its treatment from "live" oncology information specialists available 24/7, call toll-free 888-242-6536.*

Your Empowered Patient Action Plan for Treating Cancer

- *Important note: Each type of cancer has specific treatments. The following are general suggestions for all cancers, with additional information for specific cancers at the end of the section.*

Step #1: Choose your oncologist or cancer center carefully. This choice can make a significant difference in your outcome as well as your QOL. A second opinion is highly recommended to discover your best options.

Step #2: Start with proven conventional treatments: Chemotherapy, radiation, surgery, hyperthermia, hormonal, or others; these are the treatments most researched and proven to fight cancer and are your best hope for a possible cure or remission.

Step #3: ***Practice guided imagery, interactive imagery, prayer, meditation, and/or other mind-body techniques*** every day during and after treatment to help fight your cancer and lessen side effects of treatment.

Interactive imagery can sometimes lead you to information that has eluded conventional detection. When Diane was diagnosed with breast cancer, she was told that the cancer was very tiny and only in one spot. Her doctors recommended surgery, but she wondered if she could cure the cancer by natural means and just watch it to make sure it didn't grow. I directed her in interactive imagery, during which she saw the image of a wise man (her "inner-healer" figure). She heard him say that she needed to undergo the surgery and that everything would be all right. Diane still didn't want to go through surgery, but she underwent interactive imagery once more and again heard from other images that she needed to have surgery. She finally agreed to have surgery, at which time several more areas of cancer were found as well as some in her lymph nodes. The surgery is the reason Diane is alive today, with important direction from her mind.

Step #4. ***Practice qigong*** before, during and after conventional cancer treatment, to prevent side effects, increase energy to fight the cancer, and enhance the immune system.

Step #5: ***Take the Chinese herbal formula Zuo Gui Wan/You Gui Yin*** before and during conventional cancer treatments (including surgery) to prevent side effects and accelerate healing and recovery. Continue taking Zuo Gui Wan/You Gui Yin after cancer treatment if fatigue persists.

Step #6: ***Take various western herbs and supplements*** listed in Table 3 under the guidance of a certified naturopathic doctor (ND) to protect specific body tissues from damage during cancer treatment, to strengthen your immune system and to improve QOL.

Step #7: ***Take the Chinese herb Coriolus*** during and after conventional cancer treatments to enhance the effectiveness of your treatment.

Step #8: ***Take mucopolysaccharide-containing mushrooms*** during and after cancer treatment to help prevent fatigue and enhance the immune system.

Ellen was diagnosed with stage 3 (advanced) colon cancer. She was to undergo surgery to remove the mass, followed by chemotherapy. She was quite concerned about the side effects of the chemotherapy. I instructed her first in meditation and qigong exercises, and then started her on Zuo Gui Wan/You Gui Yin Chinese herbal formula. Following surgery, her surgeon was very surprised when she recovered twice as fast as expected and she was able to start chemotherapy sooner. During chemotherapy, I started her on Coriolus to extend survival and Ba Zheng for bone-marrow support. She had no nausea or vomiting from the chemotherapy. She also maintained her energy level. She was able to complete all her chemotherapy treatments as scheduled. After her treatments were finished, she took green tea and mucopolysaccharide-containing mushrooms for over a year. She never had fatigue or other problems. Five years later, she was still cancer-free with excellent QOL.

∞

Step #9: ***Take proven prescription medications*** for side effects of cancer treatment and complications of cancer as listed above, for immediate relief, if the above steps are not effective or do not completely alleviate your QOL issues.

Step #10: ***Undergo acupuncture*** after conventional treatment for side effects of treatment and complications of cancer as listed above for both short-term and long-term relief. If beneficial, you can reduce or discontinue the drugs in Step 9.

Step #11: ***Undergo cold laser*** therapy for specific side effects of cancer treatment for immediate and long-term relief as described above.

Step #12: ***Take various Western herbs and supplements*** listed in Table 4 to treat side effects of cancer and its treatment with step 11 or if that step is not effective.

Step #13: ***Join a support group.***

Step #14: ***Avoid alternative therapies*** that have no research support. You will be wasting your time and money.

Special Notes on Treating Specific Cancers

In addition to the general steps above, there are specific factors and research findings that you need to know about regarding specific cancers, as detailed below.

Breast Cancer

- DCIS (ductal cancer in situ) is referred to as a "borderline" breast lesion and is difficult to diagnose correctly. Some experts state that needle biopsies of low-grade DCIS may be misread 20 percent of the time, leading to unnecessary surgery, so review by another pathologist may be necessary. The treatment of DCIS is controversial; many women may not need aggressive treatment but there are some women who may progress without such treatment (***Note***: low-grade or non-aggressive DCIS represents about 15 percent of those detected by screening). However, another study has shown that women under 40 with

DCIS should be treated aggressively since they have twice the mortality rate. For all women with DCIS, intensive follow-up screening is imperative.

- Hormonal and genomic testing of breast cancers is very important for all patients. Hormonal testing (estrogen receptor [ER], progesterone receptor [PR]) and Her2Neu, as well as perhaps luminal or basal subtyping should be done. Although the results of these tests can help determine what treatments are appropriate, additional tests such as *Oncotype Dx* or *Mammaprint/Blueprint* can provide further information on how aggressive the cancer may be and whether chemotherapy may be necessary. Especially with cancers that appear to be slow growing or non-aggressive, these tests may help direct proper treatment and avoid unnecessary surgery and chemotherapy.

- Women with the specific abnormality in their cancer (called Her2Neu) can obtain double the cure rate by taking specific targeting drugs. However, 10 percent of tumors reported as positive are in fact negative; 20 percent of those that are reported as negative are in fact positive. ***Helpful tip***: Have another pathologist confirm the findings.

- Vitamin D deficiency at the time of breast cancer diagnosis is common and is associated with increased risk of cancer spread and death, so make sure your vitamin D levels are normal (the level can be determined by a simple blood test). ***Important note***: For cancer, many naturopathic doctors recommend a vitamin D level of at least 50 ng/dl. If taking vitamin D, take the D_3 form

- ***Warning***: Beware of "rejuvenating" creams. There are many "youth-enhancing" and "rejuvenating" creams on the market, but realize that about one-third contain estrogens. Cosmetic laws are based on an untrue concept that intact skin forms a barrier to topically applied hormones. Such estrogen-containing creams can cause an increased risk to breast cancer patients with estrogen-positive (ER+) receptors. ***Warning***: There may be no mention of the estrogen on the ingredient list.

- Some women diagnosed with breast cancer who use low dose aspirin (81 mg) regularly appear to be less likely to die from the cancer (70 percent less likely) and have fewer recurrences in other body tissues. ***Note***: The NCCN guidelines have not yet recommended aspirin use for breast cancer patients.

- Certain chemotherapies can cause significant bone loss and joint pain in premenopausal women. Refer to the sections on osteoporosis and arthritis for prevention and proper treatments.

- Because older women with breast cancer may have other conditions, more complications from treatment and a shorter life expectancy independent of the cancer, less aggressive treatment is a consideration.

- Mastectomy rates are rising. For localized breast cancer, survival after breast-conserving therapy (lumpectomy followed by radiation) may be equivalent to survival after mastectomy. However, a study in BMJ showed that 20 percent of women with DCIS or invasive cancer who undergo lumpectomy will require another operation with three months.

- It is recommended that most women with certain types of breast cancer (ER positive) take Tamoxifen (estrogen blocker) for at least five years after completion of chemotherapy, to prolong survival and remission (40 percent decreased risk). However, almost 50 percent of older women with breast cancer do not complete the five years due to side effects (such as hot flashes or bone and joint pain) or other reasons. Most of these side effects can be resolved using step 10 (acupuncture) although most doctors give SSRI antidepressants. ***Caution***: The SSRI antidepressants paroxetine (Paxil) and fluoxetine (Prozak) can reduce Tamoxifen's effects and should be avoided—use the other SSRIs instead.

  - There are other hormone-suppression drugs called aromatase inhibitors (anastozole [Arimidex], letrozole [Femara], exemestane [Aromasin]) and an estrogen receptor blocker (fulvestrant [Faslodex], a monthly injection) that have an effect similar to Tamoxifen's on reducing recurrence but can only be used if you are postmenopausal. Some studies have shown them to decrease recurrence if replacing Tamoxifen after two or three years (the recurrence rate is reduced by 30 percent versus tamoxifen). Major side effects are joint/bone pain and constipation, again which may be relieved by using step 10 (acupuncture).

  - ***Important notes***: Half of all women stop taking estrogen blockers within the five years due to side effects. Some oncologists recommend that women take these drugs for more than ten years to prevent recurrence. They do significantly decrease recurrence risk, so if you have side effects, it is better to reduce them than to discontinue the medications. Again, see the steps above for doing so.

- A 2015 study showed that taking bisphosphonates (used in osteoporosis and bone metastases) conferred highly significant reductions in breast cancer recurrence and mortality, but only among postmenopausal women. However, the role of bisphosphonates for this purpose is still considered controversial because of research inconsistencies.

Ovarian and other Gynecological Cancers

- A 2014 report revealed that almost two-thirds of ovarian cancers are not treated appropriately. The primary reason for this was that ovarian cancers are not very common and thus oncologists may not have enough experience to know about updated treatments. You should always get a second opinion before starting treatment.

- There is a validated test called ChemoFx which may determine what chemotherapy drugs the cancer is most sensitive to. This allows you to be treated with the chemotherapy that is most likely to benefit you and avoid the drugs that may not work. This test is applicable to gynecologic cancers and primary peritoneal (lining of abdomen) cancers only.

Colon Cancer

- A recent 2008 study published in the *Journal of the National Cancer Institute* revealed that nearly two-thirds of hospitals fail to check colon cancer patients well enough for signs that their tumor is spreading. By not doing so, proper treatment may be delayed, and survival may be shortened. Doctors should always check lymph nodes (via testing such as CT scan) to detect spread. If they don't, make sure they do.
- If colon cancer spreads, a genetic test called K-ras should always be done because it can indicate chemotherapy drugs that will not be effective.

Lung Cancer

- A study published in *BMJ* showed that smoking cessation after diagnosis of early stage lung cancer does improve outcome.
- Genomic testing is very important in certain types of lung cancer (non-small-cell), in order to find specific, targeted therapy, but some oncologists and lung doctors do not order these. At this time, there are 7 mutations for which there are targeted therapies available.

Prostate Cancer

- Men who regularly eat cruciferous vegetables, such as broccoli and cauliflower, have a reduced risk of aggressive prostate cancer.
- Men over the age of seventy-five with localized, low-grade cancers may not need aggressive treatment.
- Many studies have pointed out that many prostate cancers are over-treated, especially those with low PSA levels (less than 7). Many patients with prostate cancer can be watched (called "active surveillance") if they have PSA levels less than 10, are less than a stage T2a and Gleason score is less than 6. Be sure to get a second opinion if you fall into these categories. Don't rush into surgery! ***Important note***: The majority of urologists will recommend surgery with the above findings and

tell you that if the cancer recurs after other treatments, you can't get radiation. This is very misleading and not completely accurate and recurrence after either surgery or radiation often requires completely different treatments anyway.

- Understand that active surveillance requires PSA testing every three months for two years, then every six months and you will need another biopsy within twelve months and then every three to four years.
- A recent study showed that radical prostatectomy has been shown to *not* reduce cancer-related mortality any better than observation in patients with PSA levels less than 10, but may improve survival in those with PSA's greater than 20.
- PSA levels can be monitored after treatment to detect any recurrence of the cancer. However, a few patients that have prostate cancer will have normal PSA levels and will need other testing to detect recurrence.
- In patients with clinically localized cancer (within the prostate), androgen deprivation therapy does not improve survival and is unnecessary.
- There are several different treatments for prostate cancer, each having different side effects, as follows:
  - Brachytherapy (radioactive seeds) causes more urinary problems (pain, increased frequency), although this is temporary.
  - Brachytherapy and external beam radiation has worse bowel function, which improved after one year.
  - Hormonal therapy given with radiation or seeds has lower vitality scores and lower sexual function (hormonal therapy is given too often in less severe cases, which is unnecessary; it should primarily be given if the cancer has spread to other organs or there is a rise in PSA after initial treatment).
  - Surgery causes significantly more incontinence and ED. Sometimes those side effects will be temporary but most often they are permanent.
  - Radiation causes more fatigue and depression a year after treatment
  - Cyberknife and proton-beam therapy have the fewest side effects of radiation. Proton therapy is much more expensive without added benefit.
- There are effective alternative methods for side effects of treatment, including incontinence, bowel dysfunction, fatigue and others. See above section, "Alternative Treatments," for details.
- A recent study in 2011 showed that behavioral therapy with pelvic floor exercises decreases episodes of incontinence by half.
- Following hormonal suppression treatment, you should be regularly checked for calcium, vitamin D levels, bone-density, and anemia.

- You should also make sure your cholesterol and triglyceride levels are normal. A 2014 study at Duke showed that elevated levels of these two blood fats may be linked with greater risk of the cancer's return.

Dr. A's Suggestions:
Treatment of Prostate Cancer Depends on Doctor

A recent *Archives of Internal Medicine* study corroborated that prostate cancer is treated differently depending on what type of doctor you see. Consulting only urologists, men were much more likely to undergo radical prostatectomy, while those consulting both urologists and radiation oncologists were more likely to receive radiation therapy. Financial incentives (of the doctor) were a reason why this occurred. Make sure you get opinions from both types of doctors before making a decision.

Expected Outcome

Cancer incidence will continue to increase, but cancer deaths may continue to decrease due to better treatments and prevention. It is important to realize that you have a much greater chance at present to conquer your cancer than in previous years. You also have a much better ability to prevent side effects and long-term complications from cancer, especially using alternative methods; since initial studies show that feeling better may overall translate to better survival, such treatments are very important. If your cancer is cured, it does not mean that you won't have long-term residual side effects, but those can also be conquered. My goals are first to prolong life and second to improve quality of life; both of these goals may be achievable.

Compressive Neuropathies: (Carpal Tunnel, Cubital Tunnel, Guyon Canal, Radial Tunnel, Tarsal Tunnel)

What You Need to Know

A compressive neuropathy means that a peripheral nerve is being compressed by scarring or inflammation. The term "tunnel" identifies a compression that occurs where the nerve goes through a tunnel formed by ligaments and tendons.

The most common compressive neuropathy is carpal tunnel syndrome, compression of the median nerve at the wrist. There are several others as well, including radial tunnel (radial nerve in the forearm), cubital tunnel (ulnar nerve at the elbow), guyon canal (ulnar nerve at wrist), and tarsal tunnel (posterior tibial nerve in the ankle).

Many people are prone to developing compressive neuropathies and should avoid any type of repetitive work, if possible. Many people who have been treated successfully for these syndromes often return to the same type of work that caused it in the first place and, as a result, find that their symptoms return. However, there are other causes of compressive neuropathies, including diabetes, menopause, pregnancy, and thyroid dysfunction.

Important Information:
EMG Often Unnecessary for Diagnosis

Most often, compressive neuropathies can be diagnosed adequately by physical examination and your description of pain or numbness along the path of the nerve. Doctors almost always order EMG/NCV (electromyogram/nerve conduction velocity) to corroborate the diagnosis, but this test is often ignored; if negative, surgeons will usually operate anyway if your symptoms suggest the diagnosis. The test also has high false positives: many people without any symptoms will have nerve dysfunction, but they don't need treatment. So, most of the time, the test may be unnecessary. It is also quite painful and expensive.

Treatments for Compressive Neuropathies

The Preventive Approaches

If your activities are causing the condition, obviously the best way to prevent them is to stop the activities. That being said, if this is not possible, there are other methods to reduce the symptoms and prevent progression.

Carpal tunnel is the most frequent type of compressive neuropathy, and if you are just starting to get symptoms, wearing a brace, especially at night, can help prevent further progression. However, the best way is to use stretching exercises, as detailed in the table below. ***Important note***: There are no specific splints or exercises designed for the other compressive neuropathies.

Stretching Exercises for Carpal Tunnel Syndrome

Stretching Exercise 1

Hold your arms with elbows bent. Gently let your elbows fall down, with your wrists relaxed and also falling toward the ground. Do not initiate the exercise with using your wrists—let the elbows do the work. This will allow a gentle stretch to your wrists. This will primarily benefit carpal tunnel but also radial and cubital tunnel. To help tarsal tunnel, slowly kick out using your knee, allowing your ankle to stretch gently.

Stretching Exercise 2

Extend one arm forward, palm up, while keeping your elbow straight. With the opposite hand, slowly pull down the fingers of your outstretched palm toward the floor, keeping the arm steady (don't pull the arm down). Hold the stretch for three seconds, and then stretch slightly farther. Rotate the outstretched fingers as far right as possible—without rotating the rest of the arm—and hold for three seconds. Repeat, rotating to the left.

Stretching Exercise 3

1. Start by warming up your fingers and hands:

- Massage the inside and outside of your hands with your opposite thumb and fingers.
- Grasp your fingers and gently bend your wrist backward. Hold for five seconds.
- Gently pull your thumb down and back until you feel the stretch. Hold for five seconds.
- Clench your fist tightly and then release, fanning out fingers. Repeat this five times.

2. Wrist Rotation

Sit with your elbows close to your waist. Extend your forearms in front of you, parallel to the floor, with your palms facing down. Make fists with both hands and make circles with your fists to the right. Do this ten times and then make circles to the left ten times. Open your hands, extend your fingers, and repeat the entire step.

3. Wrist Curl

Take the same position as with the wrist rotation. Then hold a one-pound dumbbell in each hand and slowly bend your wrists downward. Hold this position for five seconds; repeat ten times.

4. Sideways Bend

Take the same position as before. This time, with the one-pound dumbbells, slowly bend your wrists sideways in and out. Repeat ten times.

5. Wrist Twist

Take the same position as steps 3 and 4 and, with the one-pound dumbbell, slowly turn your wrists and forearms until your palms are face up and then turn them down again. Repeat ten times.

The Conventional Approaches

Splints or braces are the first conventional treatment usually offered. They are helpful in preventing symptoms and can also be worn during work, while asleep, and while undergoing treatment.

Physical therapy modalities can be helpful using ultrasound (high-frequency sound that projects heat into the deep tissues) and iontophoresis (application of steroids through the skin using electrical current).

NSAIDs and vitamin B$_6$ (100 mg daily) may help for mild symptoms, but for moderate to severe cases, they usually won't work at all. You should notice improvement within four to six weeks with these, although vitamin B$_6$ may take three months to be helpful.

Injection of corticosteroids just outside the specific "tunnel" is another common treatment. It is slightly more effective than placebo at ten weeks but not at one year, and most patients still end up undergoing surgery. *Helpful tip*: They are not highly recommended.

Surgery is performed as a last resort. However, because the above treatments are not helpful in the majority of cases, surgery is frequently performed. Although this is currently the most frequent treatment for compressive neuropathies in this country, surgeries have a high failure rate. One study has shown the five-year success rate at only 5 percent. Guidelines have established the need for surgery when the following apply:

- Failure of other *conventional* methods
- Age of fifty years or older

- Symptoms occurring for more than ten months
- Constant numbness and tingling
- "Catching" of fingers when flexed (called trigger fingering)
- Positive Phalen's sign (tingling in the fingers when extending the wrist backward for thirty seconds)

Surgical treatment is usually considered when four to six of these factors are present, but this does not necessarily mean it will be successful. However, many hand surgeons perform surgery even if only one or two are present. Many surgeries for compressive neuropathies will be successful for at least one year, but symptoms may return after that. You should realize, however, that surgery can make the symptoms worse as well.

There are two types of surgery done, and both have equal results. Older orthopedists tend to perform *open releases*, and younger doctors prefer *endoscopic release*, which is less invasive. However, sometimes an endoscopic surgery turns into an open release if the surgeon cannot get a clear view of the nerve or ligaments.

The Alternative Approaches

Two alternative treatments have the potential to resolve compressive neuropathies completely. The first is **Low level energy laser** ("cold" laser or *LLEL*), which has been approved by the FDA since 2002 specifically for compressive neuropathies. Studies show resolution of these conditions in the majority of patients, with few to no side effects. Despite this, few hand surgeons use the laser and few insurers pay for it. You should observe a decrease in symptoms within two to six laser treatments.

Acupuncture is the second alternative method that is quite successful. The NIH has supported acupuncture as effective for these syndromes since 1997, especially carpal tunnel. With acupuncture, you should feel improvement within six treatments, but you might need additional sessions for maximum benefit. At my clinic, I used the cold laser with acupuncture for faster results. Because acupuncture addresses the underlying cause, it can provide long-term relief.

Along with acupuncture, a **Chinese herbal formula** called *Shen Tong Zhu Yu Tang* may be useful to relieve pain. *Warning*: Do not use this formula if pregnant.

Your Empowered Patient Action Plan for Treating Compressive Neuropathies

Step #1: Use wrist braces and stretching exercises to prevent symptoms or halt progression initially and for temporary relief.

Step #2: Undergo LLEL, which is the best treatment to resolve the condition completely and long term.

Step #3: Undergo acupuncture to resolve the condition completely. It can be used with Step 2 if your acupuncturist has a laser.

Elena developed both carpal tunnel and cubital tunnel syndromes from using her hands and arms repetitively at work on an automobile assembly line. She had already undergone surgery for carpal tunnel of her right wrist, which had not helped. She went back to work, using splints, but redeveloped the right wrist problem along with the other neuropathies. She tried physical therapy and injections, but these did not help. Surgery was recommended by several hand surgeons, but she declined, as the first surgery hadn't helped. I recommended LLEL with acupuncture, which resolved her symptoms in all joints affected after eight treatments. I recommended that she then find another line of work and to perform stretching exercises whenever she used her hands and arms repetitively.

Step #4: Use stretching exercises during and after treatment: This will help heal you faster as well as prevent recurrence, especially if you return to the same repetitive work that caused the condition in the first place.

Step #5: Take vitamin B$_6$ and NSAIDs for temporary symptom if not improved. If the NSAIDs are not beneficial within a week, discontinue them as they will probably not work.

Step #6: Undergo physical therapy modalities, primarily iontophoresis. Although there is a high failure rate, it is worth a try before undergoing surgery.

Step #7: Receive corticosteroid injections: Similar to step 6, there is a high failure rate, but it may delay surgery.

Step #8: Undergo surgery: Surgery is your last option if none of the above steps has been effective.

Step #9: use the LLEL after surgery to accelerate healing and decrease scarring.

Expected Outcome

Compressive neuropathies can be resolved completely using alternative methods. Surgery should be considered only in the worst cases or if alternative methods do not help. Surgery may be helpful initially, but with time and/or return to repetitive activities, the condition commonly returns.

Cataracts

What You Need to Know

By age seventy-five, almost half of all Americans either have a cataract or have had surgery for a cataract. Although aging is the number-one cause, cataracts can also be caused by trauma to the eye, and you may be predisposed if you have certain diseases, such as diabetes.

Because cataracts cause a clouding of vision, you need to seek care when your vision interferes with your activities, such as reading, driving, or watching television. If caught early enough, you may be able to avoid surgery. In most cases, delaying cataract surgery will not cause long-term damage to your eye or make the surgery more difficult. So, you do not have to rush into surgery.

Treatments for Cataracts

The Preventive Approaches

Correctible Causes: Two major causes of cataracts, besides aging, are diabetes and smoking. By controlling your blood sugar and by stopping smoking, the risk and progression can be significantly decreased. If you have diabetes, *aldose reductase inhibitors* may help prevent or delay cataract formation. The only current one now available is epalrestat (Aldorin).

The symptoms of early cataracts can be improved by obtaining new eyeglasses, using brighter lighting, and wearing antiglare sunglasses.

Diet: Antioxidants may protect the lens of the eye against damage caused by free radicals. Dark leafy greens, orange and yellow vegetables, vitamins A and C, and beta-carotene are good sources of antioxidants. Dark berries, particularly blueberries, may also help protect the lens. People who take multivitamins or any supplements containing vitamins C or E for more than ten years have been reported to have a 60 percent lower risk of forming a cataract.

Cataracts Occur More with Antidepressant Use

A study in *Ophthalmology* revealed that SSRI antidepressants may lead to an increased risk of cataracts (15 percent). Previously, another antidepressant, amitriptyline, was found to have the same effect. People who were previous users of SSRI antidepressants did not have an increased risk; so once you stop, the risk apparently disappears.

The Conventional Approaches

Certain **eye drops** containing phenylephrine and homatropine dilate the pupil, thus providing better vision in some people, but do not prevent cataracts.

Surgery is the mainstay of cataract treatment and is very effective, involving removal and replacement of the lens of the eye. Sometimes, surgery is indicated even if your cataract is not severe but prevents examination for other eye problems. There are two types of cataract surgery: *Phacoemulsification* ("phaco" for short) is the most common form and requires only as small incision. *Extracapsular* requires a longer incision but is not used often. After the lens is removed, it is often replaced by an artificial lens, called an intraocular lens (IOL).

Cataract surgery slightly increases your risk of retinal detachment and other eye disorders, such as high myopia (nearsightedness). One sign of a retinal detachment is a sudden increase in flashes or floaters. Floaters are little "cobwebs" or specks that seem to float about in your field of vision. There can be complications of bleeding or infection, but these are rare.

Warning: If you undergo surgery, you should not take the drug Flomax (used for urinary retention symptoms in men and women), which interferes with cataract surgery and causes a higher risk for complications.

The Alternative Approaches

There are no alternative methods that can reverse cataracts, but they may delay or help slow the progression. The primary alternative treatments involve the use of **nutritional supplements**, which include:

- *Lutein* (6 mg daily) reduces damage from UV sunlight and is an antioxidant.
- *Bilberry with bioflavonoids*, 80 mg (containing 25 percent anthocyanidin content) three times daily.
- *Glutathionine* may protect against UV light; adding *selenium* (200 mcg daily) helps keep *glutathionine in its active form*.
- *Vitamins* B$_2$ and B$_3$ are necessary to protect glutathione, and vitamin B$_2$ deficiency has been linked to cataracts.
- *Vitamin E* (400 IU daily) may also protect the lens against free radical damage and activates glutathione.
- *Vitamin C* (1,000 mg daily) is needed to activate vitamin E in the eye.
- *Ginkgo biloba* (120–240 mg daily) increases blood flow to the eye.

A **Chinese herbal formula** called *Huang Lian Yang Gan Wan* may also be useful if heat symptoms are present. Other formulas that treat kidney deficiency are useful, such as *Jin Gui Shen Qi Wan*.

Your Empowered Patient Action Plan for Treating Cataracts

Step #1: *Stop smoking* if you are a smoker and ***control your diabetes*** if you have this condition. These actions will significantly decrease your risk of developing cataracts.

Step #2: *Take the nutritional supplements* listed above if you have early signs of cataracts to delay or prevent cataract development.

Step #3: *Take aldose reductase inhibitors* if you have diabetes.

Step #4: *Undergo surgery* if your vision interferes with daily activities.

Expected Outcome

Cataracts do not have to interfere with activities of daily living. If not preventable, surgery is usually able to return your sight to normal or near normal.

Cholesterol

What You Need to Know

In the blood, cholesterol binds to proteins to form lipoproteins, of which there are several varieties. These include high-density lipoproteins (HDL) and low-density lipoproteins (LDL). The HDL is regarded as protective against heart disease, and high LDL is considered harmful.

Dr. A's Suggestions:
Repeat Cholesterol Testing Done Too Much

Usually, doctors will test your cholesterol every year. However, a recent study revealed that cholesterol measurements often vary within the same person regardless of treatment, partially due to week-to-week fluctuations. The true, long-term increases in cholesterol occur very slowly and usually are not apparent until three years after treatment. The authors recommended that the guidelines be changed and that adherent patients be retested every three to five years once adequate response has been noted.

It should also be realized that cholesterol levels can vary as much as 7 percent from test to test, and this should be taken into consideration before making substantial changes to treatment.

In 2013, the American Heart Association AHA and American College of Cardiology abandoned the previous treatment goals of decreasing LDL cholesterol and increasing HDL because some drugs that "improve" the LDL and all drugs that increase HDL did not improve clinical outcomes. Instead, they issued new treatment guidelines based on risk of developing heart disease and treat if you fall into one of four high-risk groups (see chart below). (To find your risk, the AHA has a web-based calculator on its website, or you can go to ClinCalc.com. This will give you your ten-year and lifetime risk of heart disease). Sometimes, even if your ten-year risk is low, if your lifetime risk is high, treatment may be recommended. This new guideline uses the risk calculator instead of specific cholesterol levels. *Caution*: This calculator may have flaws – see sidebar below for more discussion.

Lipid Guidelines 2013

New guidelines suggest treating high cholesterol under these circumstances:

- Clinical heart disease
- LDL > 190
- Diabetic 40–75 years old with LDL 70–189
- Ten-year heart disease risk > 7.5% (using risk calculator: see sidebar below)

If you fit in one of these categories, it will then need to be determined by your doctor if you need high-intensity (larger dose) therapy or moderate intensity treatment.

If a treatment decision is uncertain or your risk is considered borderline, the following factors may place you in a treatment category:

- LDL > 160
- Family history of premature heart disease
- CRP > 2 (C-reactive protein, a measurement of inflammation)
- Coronary calcium score > 300 (done by CT scan of the heart)
- ABI (Ankle-Brachial Index) < 0.9 (measurement of peripheral artery disease, done by measuring blood pressure at ankle and in arm)
- Elevated lifetime risk for heart disease

Important Information:
The Risk Calculator: Controversial

It should be noted that there is controversy regarding use of the risk calculator. Under the guidelines using the calculator, millions of people who presently don't take medications will become candidates. In fact, overall, one billion people would be placed on statins based on these guidelines. The cumulative global sales of statins would approach $1 trillion by 2020. The controversies include:

- The calculator may overestimate risk by between 75 and 150 percent.
- Studies upon which risk was determined were conducted in the 1990s.
- It does not take LDL levels into account.
- The 7.5 percent threshold for starting medications is much lower than previous thresholds.
- Crucial evidence is still missing.
- There are no long-term studies documenting that such guidelines will significantly decrease heart disease better than previous guidelines.

One of the nation's leading endocrinology associations has rejected these guidelines, stating that the calculator is outdated and the guidelines are incompatible with the current guidelines. A 2014 study in *JAMA Intern Med* also showed significant discrepancies that could not be explained, and a 2015 study again showed significant overestimates of risk from the calculator.

On the other hand, two recent studies show benefit from the new guidelines, as compared to 2004 guidelines. One study showed that the AHA guideline is more efficient at identifying which patients will benefit most from statins and extrapolates that an estimated 41,000-63,000 heart "events:" would be prevented over a ten year period in the approximately ten million people who would be newly eligible for statins. Another study showed that this guideline is more cost-effective than previous guidelines.

In the future, additional studies should delineate whether more people would benefit from statins. Until then, you should confer with your doctor.

Important note: Although makers of cholesterol-lowering drugs have pushed doctors to decrease cholesterol as low as possible, a blood-cholesterol level below 160 may be harmful, causing depression, anxiety, and increased risk of bleeding strokes, so you don't want to over treat.

Different Blood Tests May Be Better than LDL/HDL Tests

Doctors have used LDL and HDL levels to determine response to drugs as well as to determine risk for heart attack, but this may be changing. First, a 2008 study published in *Lancet* showed that the ratio of LDL to HDL is more predictive than each level alone.

Second, a different test to determine the ratio between apolipoproteins (called apoA1 and apoB—ratio of apoB to apoA1) is a better predictor than LDL/HDL. There have not been any studies showing that this test will provide better *outcomes* than other tests, but it does appear to reveal more information.

A November 2014 study in the *NEJM* showed that another new test, called HDL efflux capacity may be much more predictable of heart disease than other measurements of HDL.

In the future, these tests may be the ones recommended, especially as the LDL/HDL tests are not considered as important in determining treatment, as discussed above.

Treatments for High Cholesterol

The Preventive Approaches

Although high cholesterol can be caused by heredity, the best prevention is a balanced **diet**. People differ in their responses to cholesterol-lowering diets, and some may not respond at all. *Just being overweight can prevent you from controlling your cholesterol by diet*, so losing weight is extremely helpful.

Calorie and Fat Consumption Up among Statin Users

According to a 2014 *JAMA Internal Medicine* study, calorie and fat consumption increased significantly among statin users (drugs for lowering cholesterol) from 1999 to 2010, but not among nonusers. What this means is that people with high cholesterol levels feel that if they take drugs to lower cholesterol, they can still eat unhealthy foods. Although these drugs are heart-protective, unhealthy foods can still cause damage to the body in other ways, so diet change should be the first treatment for high cholesterol.

The *Portfolio diet*, a vegetarian diet emphasizing plant sterols, soluble fibers, soy, and almonds has been shown to reduce LDL levels 30 percent after one month, much better than a standard very-low-saturated-fat diet (only 8 percent) and comparable to a standard diet plus a statin drug (33 percent). Although difficult to follow in the long term, using just some of the food guideline is beneficial.

If you want to follow another particular diet, the *DASH diet* (Dietary Approaches to Stop Hypertension) reduces levels of LDL and total cholesterol. (Go to www.nhlbi.nih.gov/health/public/heart/hbp/dash/ to obtain a copy of the DASH diet).According to a 2014 review in the *American Journal of Medicine*, the Mediterranean diet has proven to reduce cardiovascular events to a degree greater than low-fat diets and equal to or greater than the benefit of taking statin drugs.

For highly elevated cholesterol levels, the *Dean Ornish, MD program* has proven that a very-low-fat diet, in combination with stress reduction from yoga, relaxation techniques, breathing techniques, "heart healing" imagery, meditation, aerobic exercise, and group support, can significantly lower the levels and reverse medical diseases caused by increased cholesterol. His method requires great motivation, so I recommend it for the more severe elevations of cholesterol. However, it can be used by anyone with elevated cholesterol. (For details of the Ornish diet, buy his book, *Reversing Heart Disease* [Royal Publications, 1996]).

No matter what type of diet you choose, *avoid cholesterol-containing products.* However, certain foods contain stanols and sterols, which are plant compounds that *compete* with cholesterol for absorption and thus can lower cholesterol. Some foods are now being fortified with these compounds. Use plant-based butter spreads, which can reduce cholesterol by an additional 10 percent. In addition, soy products are excellent at reducing cholesterol levels, as are black tea and barley products. Avocado is very potent at reducing cholesterol levels.

Increasing the fiber in your diet can also decrease cholesterol levels. Almonds, walnuts, pecans, and pistachio nuts can lower total cholesterol and LDL cholesterol if they are natural or dry roasted (no added salts or oils), but eat only about 2.5 ounces per day. Oats reduce LDL without affecting HDL due to their fiber content. Soluble fiber also comes from beans, barley, apples, oranges, and carrots. A recent study revealed that berries (five ounces daily) increases HDL levels.

Factors That Affect HDL (The "Good" Cholesterol)

- Exercise: Boosts HDL modestly
- Losing weight: For every ten pounds lost, HDL rises 2 mg/dl
- Stop smoking: Smoking lowers HDL an average of 5 mg/dl

- Drink alcohol (moderately): Can raise HDL, but may increase triglycerides
- Omega-3s: Boost HDL

Note: It is more difficult to raise HDL than lower LDL.

In addition to diet, **exercise** can significantly lower blood-cholesterol levels and raise the HDL component. High-volume aerobic exercise is the preferred form of activity, with fast walking being the safest. Although resistance training does not increase HDL levels, it does decrease LDL, total cholesterol levels, and body fat, so it is also recommended.

The Conventional Approaches

Medication is the preferred conventional treatment and is used primarily to lower LDL. In fact, lipid regulators are the largest medication class prescribed in the United States, accounting for sales of over $18.4 billion. The primary drugs prescribed are called *statins* and they are listed below.

Statin Drugs

Natural (generic)	_Trade Name_
Atorvastin	Lipitor
Fluvastatin	Lescol
Lovastatin	Mevacor, Altoprev
Pitavastatin	Livalo
Pravastatin	Pravachol
Rosuvastatin	Crestor
Simvastatin	Zocor

Most statin drugs are expensive, but two statins—simvastatin and atorvastatin—are available as generics. Crestor and Zetia will become generics in 2016. ***Important note***: A 2014 study in *Annals of Internal Medicine* showed that people taking generic statins were more likely to take their pills and had slightly better outcomes than people prescribed a brand-name statin.

Dr. A's Suggestions:
Zetia (Ezetimbe) and Vytorin: Helpful or Unnecessary?

A 2008 study called the *Enhance Trial* revealed that taking the prescription drug Zetia (ezetimbe) failed to reduce atherosclerosis progression compared with simvastatin (a statin drug) alone. Zetia, which blocks cholesterol from being absorbed in the stomach, is combined with simvastatin in the prescription drug Vytorin. The study showed that there was no advantage to taking this combination versus simvastatin alone. (Simvastatin is also an OTC drug and thus is much cheaper than Zetia or the combination).

In addition, another study revealed that Zetia and Vytorin may increase cancer mortality (although not cancer incidence). In yet another study, Zetia was noted to be inferior to taking niacin.

Despite these findings, a 2014 study published in the *American Heart Journal* revealed that although its use declined in the United States after the 2008 study, it was still prescribed to the tune of $2.2 billion in 2009.

The drug company supported another study (IMPROVE-IT study), first reported in 2014, showing that ezitimbe improved outcomes if given with simvastatin after a coronary event in high-risk patients. Despite a guidelines committee chairman concluding it is now a proven therapy, the study revealed only a 2 percent difference in outcome compared to simvastatin alone (absolute outcome was that you would have to treat 100 patients with the combination for seven years to prevent two patients from having an ischemic stroke or heart attack). In addition, there were limitations to the study, including that the study population was very narrowed and stand-alone ezetimbe was not tested.

At this writing therefore, Zetia alone or in combination form (Vytorin) may not be indicated to be used first line and should be cautioned in patients with cancer. However, don't be surprised if doctors use it anyway after marketing by the drug company. Be sure to become empowered and question your doctor if prescribed these drugs.

A meta-analysis of ten studies published in April 2011 showed that statins could reduce heart attacks by 30 percent, strokes by 19 percent, and mortality rates by 12 percent in people with high cholesterol who do not have heart disease but have risk factors for it such as high cholesterol, obesity, hypertension, or diabetes. The benefits are even better in people who already have heart disease. However, some benefits of preventing or slowing heart disease may not be as significant as previously thought. Other studies show that the absolute number of people actually helped by statins is relatively low. Just because it changes blood tests (lowers LDL, raises HDL) doesn't necessarily mean it will translate into significantly protecting your heart.

You Don't Need Statins If You Don't Have High Cholesterol

The pharmaceutical companies making statins have tried to convince doctors that they should prescribe statins if you are at even low or moderate risk for heart disease even if you don't have high cholesterol. Two papers in the *Archives of Internal Medicine* show that there is no difference in all-cause mortality; thus the benefit is very small, if any.

Furthermore, recent studies have shown that statin drugs increase the risk of developing diabetes (see below). So if you don't need it, why take it?

Statins Overprescribed for the Very Elderly?

A 2015 study from *JAMA Intern Med* revealed that one third of very elderly people who do not have heart or blood vessel disease use statin drugs. However, it has never been determined if statins benefit this population and so they may be unnecessary.

Caution: Statins are known to have several side effects, although overall, only 6 percent of patients will have those complications. In general, statins are considered to have more benefit than harm, but you need to be aware of the side effects and either change to a different type of statin or another type of medication or alternative supplements (see below). Side effects to be aware of:

- *Muscle pain, weakness, cramps.* These are the most common side effects, with the worst complication being rhabdomyolysis, a destruction of muscle, but very rare.
- *Muscle injuries*, such as sprains, strains, and other injuries (19 percent higher risk).
- *Elevation of liver enzymes.* You should have your liver enzymes checked yearly.
- *Diabetes*: Statins can increase the risk for developing diabetes by at least 9 percent. A 2015 study showed that relative risk for diabetes was nearly 50 percent

higher in statin users (this higher risk needs to be balanced with the benefits of statins, so discuss with your doctor, especially if you are borderline diabetic).

- *Rhabdomyolysis* (severe inflammation of muscle) risk is increased when simvastatin is used with an antiarrhythmic drug called amiodarone (Cardarone, Pacerone).
- *Prostate cancer*: A 2008 study published in the *American Journal of Epidemiology* revealed that the use of statin drugs was associated with a 50 percent increased risk of prostate cancer among obese men, but not overweight or normal-weight men. In the latter, other studies have shown statins to be preventive of prostate cancer.
- *Acute kidney failure* (rare; high-potency statins).
- *Cataracts* (rare and minimal).

Statins and Muscle Pain: What to Do

The major side effect of statins is myalgia—pain or soreness in muscles, especially the legs. Approximately 5 percent of patients taking statins will have this side effect, according to pharmaceutical research. However, a recent report from the *Cleveland Clinic Journal* stated that the incidence of muscle pain caused by statins is higher in clinical practice than is reflected in studies.

There are several actions you can take if this occurs. First, some statins have this side effect less often than others. Lescol (fluvastatin) and Crestor (rosuvastatin) have the least occurrences. If you have this side effect, changing statins, lowering their doses, or using them on alternate days may help.

Be sure to check your TSH for thyroid function. Severe hypothyroidism can cause similar muscle weakness, as well as raising lipid levels. Reduced kidney or liver function, being on steroids, and vitamin deficiency are also causes of muscle symptoms.

Finally, try CoQ10. Studies vary on whether this helps, although it is known that statins can lower the levels of CoQ10 in the body. The studies that show no benefit may not have used a high enough dosage (see below).

Some statins have fewer side effects than others. Simvastatin and pravastatin have the best overall tolerability and lowest discontinuation rates. Atorvastatin and rosuvastatin have the highest discontinuation rates. Atorvastatin and fluvastatin have the highest risk of increasing liver enzymes. Thus, if one statin has intolerable side effects, you may be able to tolerate a different one.

Statins Can Possibly Adversely Affect the Brain

Although memory loss, concentration, and fuzzy thinking are not listed as side effects of statins, many doctors have seen these side effects in a small percentage of patients taking these drugs. Many doctors may dismiss these problems as many elderly people and those who take many medications or have multiple conditions may have these symptoms anyway. If you have developed such symptoms, simply discontinue the statin temporarily. If the effects go away and then return again when you retake the statin, you'll know it's the drug causing the problem.

Caution: Statins may have a suppression effect on the immune response to flu vaccine, thus decreasing your ability to fight the flu. This response is more dramatic with synthetic statins (lovastatin, pravastatin and simvastatin are all derivatives of a fungal compound and are sometimes termed 'natural' statins; atorvastatin, rosuvastatin, fluvastatin are synthetic).

Warning: Taking certain antibiotics (called Macrolides) with statins can increase toxic side effects. These include erythromycin and clarithromycin but not azithromycin.

Warning: If you take a statin, you should *not* take more than the RDA recommended amounts of antioxidants such as vitamins E, C, b-carotene, and selenium. These antioxidants blunt the beneficial effect of statins on raising the HDL levels (the "good" cholesterol). Most statins can also cause a decrease in coenzyme Q10, which is important for proper heart function.

Statin Drugs May Increase Risk for Diabetes

It is now recognized that statin drugs (for high cholesterol) may increase the risk of developing diabetes by at least 9 percent. Two 2015 studies showed the relative risk was nearly fifty percent higher in statin users. Since high cholesterol is part of the metabolic syndrome, taking statins may be valuable if you have a high risk of developing heart disease but in others, especially pre-diabetics, the risk may be greater than the benefit. So discuss this with your doctor.

Important note: Generally, you should take statin drugs in the evening as cholesterol synthesis occurs primarily at night. The exceptions are Lipitor and Crestor, which are the longest-acting and can be taken any time during the day.

Important Information:
Statins and Grapefruit Juice

Studies have shown that grapefruit and its juice may interfere with the metabolism of certain statins, raising their blood levels dangerously high. An occasional drink is not a problem, but regular consumption may be. You should avoid grapefruit or take it at a different time than you take the statin. Statins that are not affected by grapefruit include Pravachol, Crestor, and Lescol, as they are metabolized differently than the others.

Other medications: Another drug (actually a vitamin that some drug companies produce) commonly used with statins primarily to raise HDL is *niacin*. Initial studies showed that a combination of niacin and statins is more effective than either one alone at lowering cholesterol levels and stopping the progression of atherosclerosis. However, a trial published in the *NEJM* in 2014 showed that niacin was ineffective and caused serious side effects. *Caution*: Some people taking niacin can have the side effect of flushing. Niacin can be obtained as a prescription drug, but it can also be taken OTC. The OTC form is much cheaper and can have fewer side effects (look for nonflushing products).

Fibrates are also used to raise HDL but are also not very effective. In fact, a 2014 study in *BMJ* revealed that niacin and fibrates do not lower mortality rates or risk for stroke despite elevating HDL levels.

Dr. A's Suggestions:
Fibrates for Triglycerides May Be Unnecessary

Fibrate drugs (gemfibrozil [Lopid], fenofibrate [Tricor and others], and fenofibric acid [Trilipix]) are currently prescribed widely to lower triglyceride levels. However, their effectiveness in preventing heart disease, especially in statin-treated patients, is lacking and controversial.

The reason for the increased use of fibrates is aggressive marketing by the drug companies and confusion among doctors about the hard evidence to support adding these drugs to patients on statins. At this time, if you are on a statin, you would only rarely need a fibrate, and statins are far superior.

There are several other older conventional medications that can lower cholesterol, including *gemfibrozil* (Lopid), and *cholestyramine* (Questran). These medications are usually given when triglyceride levels are elevated alone or along with the cholesterol. However, they may have more side effects than the statins. Your doctor may prescribe these if your cholesterol level is not improving or if there are special circumstances regarding any other medical conditions you may have.

Two new cholesterol drugs have recently been approved by the FDA. Alirocumab (Praluent) and evolocumab (Repatha) are called monoclonal antibodies (called PCSK-9 inhibitors) and are injected bi-weekly or monthly (evolocumab). Although these drugs produce dramatic reductions in LDL cholesterol, they will be very expensive (Praluent is priced at $14,600 a year). In addition, they may not improve health outcomes any better than the above medications; in fact, the comparative clinical outcomes are not yet clear.

The Alternative Approaches

There are many **herbs and supplements** that can reduce cholesterol levels but may take several months to do so. The best supplement is *fish oil*, which has been shown to further lower heart disease risk (by 19 percent!) if taken with a statin drug.

Important notes: There are problems with fish oil that you need to be aware of. Although regular fish oil can decrease cholesterol levels and protect the heart, you must take *at least* 1,500 mg daily to obtain benefits. Many studies were done using 3,000–4,000 mg. Many fish oils also deteriorate very rapidly (three months), so by the time you buy them, they may already be partially deteriorated. Krill oil may be more potent and more stable, and it contains two natural antioxidants and has few to no side effects. However, krill oil products differ in their concentrations of omega-3s and combinations with other ingredients, so check the label. Decrease in cholesterol levels will take about two months when taking krill oil. *Warning*: In some patients, fish oil can raise LDL as well as HDL levels.

There are many other cholesterol-lowering herbs and supplements that can be taken alone or with fish oil. *Red yeast rice* (two 600 mg caps once or twice daily), which is a natural statin (it is actually equivalent to lovastatin), can lower cholesterol, but generic lovastatin is cheaper. You should not take more than four a day. It is best taken with CoQ10, the same as with a statin drug. **Warning**: A recent analysis of twelve red yeast rice products by consumerlab.com published in the *Archives of Internal Medicine* in late 2010 showed a "dramatic variation in active ingredients" among the products. The amount of lovastatin ranged from 0.2–14 mg, well below the usual dose of lovastatin of 20–40 mg.

As mentioned above, *niacin* (B_3 or nicotinic acid) can decrease cholesterol and triglyceride levels and increase HDL levels when given in large amounts (1–3 grams daily). There are prescription versions (Niaspan), but it can be purchased cheaper as a supplement. The main side effect is flushing, but taking aspirin and vitamin C before taking the niacin may prevent this side effect. The nonprescription extended-release form is more likely to cause flushing, but there are nonflushing forms as well. **Caution**: You need to check your liver enzymes when on niacin.

Other nutritional supplements that may lower cholesterol include:

- *Gamma-oryzanol* (150 mg twice daily) is derived from rice bran oil and is a prescription medication in Japan for high cholesterol. It can reduce cholesterol, LDL, and triglycerides 12–15 percent.
- *Flaxseed* (one tablespoon daily of freshly ground only) and *garlic* (equivalent to 4,000 mg of allicin daily). This combination alone can reduce cholesterol levels 50–75 mg/dl in about two months when your cholesterol is 250 mg/dl. If your cholesterol level is greater than 300 mg/dl, it may take six months.

Important Information:
Bad Research Downplays Garlic

Many studies have shown that garlic can help prevent heart disease, but a recent study showed that garlic does not decrease LDL levels at all and should not be used. However, this study did not measure LDL oxidation; it is when LDL is oxidized that it causes heart disease. In fact, garlic prevents or decreases the oxidation of LDL and thus may be protective. So it is not just lowering your LDL that is important.

- *Calcium citrate supplements* (1,000 mg daily) appear to lower cholesterol levels in postmenopausal women, increasing HDL and lowering LDL. Fiber supplements such as psyllium or beta glucan also help lower cholesterol.
- *Gugulipid* (100–500 mg per day), an herb from India, can decrease total cholesterol levels 14 to 27 percent and triglyceride and LDL levels 22 to 30

percent in four to twelve weeks, but *only* if you eat a well-balanced, nutritious diet.

- *Phytosterols*, derived from plants, are also commonly used and found in combination products. Several drug companies have included phytosterols in multivitamins for the heart. Most of these contain 400 mg, which lowers LDL cholesterol by only 5 percent if taken twice a day.
- *Policosanol* (10–20 mg once or twice daily) has been previously touted as cholesterol lowering, but all favorable studies have been derived from a Cuban company that makes the product from sugar cane. Studies from other parts of the world and using sugar cane as well as other plants, have found no benefit from taking this herb.

One **Chinese herbal formula** that has been shown to lower cholesterol in individuals who are compromised, weak, or elderly is *Shou Wu Pian*.

Intravenous **chelation** is another alternative method that has been used to lower cholesterol and prevent heart disease, the latter of which has been supported by a recent study (although still controversial). This type of chelation is also very expensive, costing around $4,000. An easier and simpler way of reducing your cholesterol (and helping clean your arteries) may be by using an oral, herbal chelation recipe:

Blend one cup of fresh cilantro with six tablespoons of olive oil until the cilantro is completely chopped. Then add one clove of garlic, half a cup of nuts (cashews or almonds are best), and two tablespoons of lemon juice. Blend these into a paste (which will be lumpy), adding hot water if necessary. Take one to three teaspoons per day. If you make large amounts, you can freeze it for later use.

Finally, I have mentioned taking *CoQ10* if you take statin drugs, because these drugs can deplete stores of this important energy nutrient in your muscles. Whether it works or not is controversial: There are two randomized studies that show significant improvement in the severity of muscle pain by using CoQ10, but according to a meta-analysis and a more recent trial, it had no effect on muscle symptoms. However, because statins are known to decrease CoQ10 levels, it may help other health aspects not presently recognized.

Another supplement shown to have possible improvements in muscle pain is *l-carnitine* (300–500 mg three times daily), and in fact, patients with statin myalgias frequently have carnitine abnormalities.

Your Empowered Patient Action Plan for Lowering Cholesterol

- *If your LDL cholesterol is greater than 190 and you have heart disease or a high risk of heart disease, start at step 5 and return to step 1.*

- *If each step does not reduce your cholesterol levels to normal in the indicated time period, proceed to the next step. These steps can be combined if necessary.*
- *You should take herbs or statins at night as this is when the body makes most of its cholesterol (see discussion above for exceptions).*

Step #1: Good diet and exercise are keys to preventing and treating high cholesterol.

Step #2: Try cilantro chelation: You should see reduction in cholesterol within two to four weeks.

Step #3: Take fish oil (or krill) to help long-term control of cholesterol and decreased risk of heart disease. Repeat your cholesterol test after two months to make sure it has decreased. However, even if your cholesterol is not lowered, fish oil is still recommended due to prevention of heart disease. Be sure to take at least 1,500 mg daily (1,000 mg krill).

Step #4: Try the nutritional supplements listed above that have been proven to lower cholesterol.

Step #5: Take a prescription statin drug. I prefer the above steps before statins due to fewer side effects. However, they may not be powerful enough to decrease your level to normal.

Step #6: Take red yeast rice if your cholesterol is not yet normal or you can't take statins. Repeat your cholesterol levels after six weeks. This supplement is equivalent to statins but generic statins are cheaper and don't require as many pills so they are preferred.

Step #7: Take nonflushing niacin (OTC) or Gamma-oryzanol if your triglycerides are elevated. Repeat your cholesterol testing after eight weeks.

Step #8: Try flaxseed oil, garlic, and/or calcium citrate if you still need to lower your cholesterol or to help lower the dose of statin medication. Repeat testing after two months.

Step #9: Take prescription gemfibrozil or cholestyramine if nothing else has worked.

Expected Outcome

Through the above steps, your cholesterol levels should be able to become and remain normal, and your risk of heart disease should decrease.

Colds and Flu

What You Need to Know

Colds and influenza (flu) are infections of the upper respiratory tract (called URIs). Most colds and all influenza infections are caused by viruses, with a minority of URIs being caused by bacteria. Influenza is a more potent respiratory infection than a cold and has an enormous impact worldwide and causes significant complications and death in older adults. Influenza is responsible for more than $1 billion in annual Medicare expenditures. Of deaths resulting from influenza, 80 to 90 percent occur in adults sixty-five years and older, but that also implies imply younger people can still die from the flu.

Bird and Pig Flu May Be More Dangerous

Flu caused by transmission from animals such as pigs or birds can cause the same symptoms of typical viral influenza, but they act differently in many ways. Depending on the type and strength, these viruses can be more lethal. In addition, they primarily affect infants, children, and adolescents rather than older people. The same treatments below apply to any kind of flu.

Older adults are more prone to severe and potentially fatal complications from influenza because of coexisting chronic disease and weakened immunity. Thus, if you are older, you can benefit most from vaccination, early detection and aggressive therapy.

Heart Attack/Stroke Can Occur after Respiratory Infection

A recent study published in the *European Heart Journal* revealed that in the month after respiratory infections, risks for heart attack and stroke are significantly increased. The risk is highest in the first three days and doubles within a week of infection. For this reason, prevention, immunization, and prompt treatment are important.

Important Information:
Colored Sputum: Not Necessarily What You May Think

Most people think that having colored drainage (yellow or green) means that they have a bacterial infection and they need antibiotics. This is not always true—viruses and noninfectious causes of drainage are just as apt to have colored phlegm or sputum.

—∞—

Tests for Determining Bacteria versus Virus

Several commercially produced rapid-diagnostic tests can detect influenza viruses within thirty minutes in your doctor's office. One such test (called Xtag Respiratory Viral Panel) can check simultaneously for twelve different viruses. Most of these tests are "rapid antigen tests," but they do produce false negative results (tests are negative but you do have a virus) in 25 to 30 percent of people.

The FDA in 2014 mandated better performance from these tests, requiring sensitivity of 90 percent for Influenza A and 80 percent for Influenza B. In January, 2014, the FDA approved an influenza test (Alere) that is highly sensitive (greater than 90 percent) and can now be provided in doctor's offices, emergency rooms, and health departments.

Other tests can quickly reveal if you have a bacterial infection, especially strep throat (Rapid Strep Test, which only misses 5% of strep infections). Although most colds and flu are due to viruses, if there is any doubt, you can undergo these tests to make sure.

—∞—

Note: This section pertains to treatment of *upper-respiratory* illnesses. Other infections, including sinus and lung infections (such as pneumonia), are discussed in other sections.

Treatments for Colds and Flu

The Preventive Approaches

All people who are debilitated, elderly, or have lung or heart diseases (including asthma) should get *flu vaccination* (flu shots) every year, as influenza can be fatal especially in those who are weakened by other health conditions. Influenza vaccines target the strains of influenza A and B that are most likely to cause illness during a particular season and reduce the risk of influenza infection by 30 to 70 percent among elderly persons in home settings.

Influenza vaccination has been shown to be about 58 percent effective in reducing influenza infection and has resulted in a 39 to 69 percent decrease in mortality from all causes during the influenza season in older adults. Vaccination for animal-related influenza (Type A) is also available but takes several months to develop after the type of infection is known. ***Helpful tip***: Many people state that they feel "bad" or have flu-like symptoms after receiving flu shots. This can be avoided by taking 800 mg of ibuprofen with the injection.

Important note: There are three types of flu vaccines. The first two are injections and can be either trivalent (protects against two type A viruses and one type B) or quadrivalent (protects against two type A viruses and two type B), the latter indicated more for those in health care or those who are older. There is also Flu Mist, a nasal spray (quadrivalent), which can be given from ages two through forty-nine. ***Warning***: Flu Mist should not be given to patients who are immunosuppressed, as it is a live vaccine.

Caution: Statin drugs used for high cholesterol may have a suppression effect on the immune response to flu vaccine, thus decreasing your ability to fight the flu. This response is more dramatic with synthetic statins (lovastatin, pravastatin and simvastatin are all derivatives of a fungal compound and are sometimes termed 'natural' statins; atorvastatin, rosuvastatin, fluvastatin are synthetic).

Preventive supplements: Some studies have shown that taking *panax ginseng* (Asian ginseng) at 100 mg daily starting four weeks before vaccination and for eight weeks after reduces the risk of contracting both colds and flu. *American ginseng* (200 mg twice a day) has been shown to reduce the risk of developing colds or flu and reducing repeat colds if taken over a three- to four-month period during the flu season. A supplement called *colostrum* has been found in one study to be more effective at preventing flu than vaccination. Colostrum supports the immune system and contains immunoglobulins and other antiviral substances.

Helpful Tip: Although the above nutritional supplements may help prevent colds and flu, you must take them for several months. This may not be cost-effective unless you have a high risk for developing these infections or have several every year.

Other herbs and supplements that are commonly taken for *preventing* colds, yet have not been adequately supported by studies, include brewer's yeast, andrographis, vitamin C, astragalus, Echinacea, vitamin E, and garlic. I do not recommend taking any of these preventively, but some are useful for treating respiratory infections once you get them (see below under "Alternative Approaches").

Dr. A's Suggestions:
**Combination Herbals May Prevent Colds
from Continuing or Worsening**

If you start getting a scratchy throat, having drainage, and feeling tired, you may be in the "prodromal" (initial) stage of a cold or flu. I have found that taking a combination of Yin Chao Jin (Chinese herbal formula) and elderberry at onset of these symptoms can help abort the further development of the cold or at least decrease symptoms and duration.

This combination is also helpful if you are around people who have a cold or flu or are around people who may have symptoms (such as on an airplane).

———⚬⚬⚬———

The best way to avoid transmission of influenza in your household is to **wash your hands** frequently (hand soap and alcohol hand rub after sneezing, coughing, or touching surfaces) and use face masks for at least seven days.

Diet: Avoid milk products, which increase mucous production. Avoid sugar, which competes with vitamin C and decreases immune function. Chicken soup has been proven to help relieve sore throats and runny nose by speeding up the movement of mucus and is highly recommended (homemade is best). Eating garlic is also helpful because it helps prevent viruses from invading and damaging your tissues.

Also, **drink lots of water**, which improves the function of the white blood cells and keeps the respiratory tract moist, which repels viruses. *Fruit juices* containing vitamin C are helpful but should be taken undiluted, as the processed variety contains sugars that retard the white blood cells from fighting the infection. Obtaining the juice from a juicer or eating the fruit itself are the best ways to obtain the benefits.

Exercise: A recent study from *Appalachian State University* showed that people who exercise aerobically at least five days a week during the fall and winter were about half as likely to get a respiratory infection as those who exercised one day or less per week. In addition, if they got a cold, it was milder. Previous research has shown that moderate exercise (3 days a week) improves immunity, whereas intense exercise can depress the immune system and cause more colds.

Adequate **sleep** has been shown to reduce susceptibility to the common cold; shorter sleep duration prior to viral exposure has been demonstrated to have an increased risk of getting a cold.

The Conventional Approaches

Most people start by taking **OTC medications** to control symptoms. *Ibuprofen* is the best analgesic to reduce fever and achiness. ***Caution***: Acetaminophen products (Tylenol) can increase mucous and in large amounts can cause liver damage, so they should be avoided.

———⚬⚬⚬———

Don't Treat Low-Grade Fevers

Low-grade fevers (< 101 degrees) without symptoms should not be treated as they are actually a protective mechanism of the body to help fight the infection. For moderate fevers (> 101 degrees), take ibuprofen if you feel feverish. For higher-grade fevers and/or severe symptoms (> 103 degrees), call your doctor.

There are many other OTC remedies for reducing symptoms of colds and flus, such as decongestants and cough suppressants. Take them only for short periods of time since they can make mucous thicker and harder after several days of use. OTC drugs containing guaifenesin, however, can reduce mucous. Most of these conventional remedies are designed to suppress the symptoms rather than assist the body to heal. Even if they improve your symptoms, they may prolong the *duration* of the cold.

Statin Use May Decrease Death in Influenza

Influenza kills around forty thousand people a year. In a recent study, it was observed that patients already on statin drugs (for lowering cholesterol) had a lower death rate than those not taking statins. Whether adding a statin to patients who have the flu but who don't already take statins makes the same difference is not known. ***Caution***: remember that statins may interfere with the immune response to flu vaccine (see above). If this occurs, take non-synthetic statins preferably.

Antiviral medications: Viruses are by far the most common cause of colds and flu and the vast majority *do not need to be treated* by antivirals or antibiotics. However, many doctors continue to prescribe them. There are four drugs that may kill viruses, amantadine (Symmetrel), rimantadine (Flumadine), zanamivir (Relenza), and oseltamivir (Tamiflu). The latter two are more effective for the more serious types of influenza. Rimantadine costs more than amantadine but has fewer adverse effects on the central nervous system (i.e., confusion, nervousness, anxiety) and is less dependent on kidney function (which is usually decreased in elderly people). The FDA approved the first intravenous antiviral in December 2014, called peramivir (Rapivab).

Warning: Side Effects with Antiviral Drugs

Recent post marketing studies have shown that the antiviral drugs may cause delirium and abnormal behavior, seizures, and hallucinations, with some cases resulting in self-injurious behavior.

In addition, these drugs may develop resistance to viruses. Amantadine and rimantadine have the highest resistance. Despite this fact, 25 percent of the prescriptions for flu are for these two drugs.

Important notes: You should realize that antivirals reduce the duration of colds and flu by only *one day or less*. A 2014 series of *BMJ* articles revealed that they relieve symptom duration at most by seventeen hours (peramivir by twenty-one hours) and do not reduce risk of pneumonia or hospital admissions. Another study in 2015 showed that oseltamivir decreased symptoms by twenty-five hours, and patients experienced fewer respiratory complications and hospitalizations (but only one fewer per hundred treated patients). However, this latter study also revealed that taking oseltamivir caused significantly more nausea and vomiting. The latest study (August, 2015) showed that oseltavivir did not decrease the risk for household transmission of flu, which is one of its primary uses.

In addition, these drugs must be taken within forty-eight hours of the onset of illness to be effective (the latter study used the drugs within thirty-six hours), which is difficult because most patients treat their illness at home for several days before seeking treatment from a physician. So they are not recommended if your symptoms have been present over two days. However, one study did show that if you do take these drugs within forty-eight hours, they may be effective in reducing flu-related complications of pneumonia, bronchitis, sinusitis, and pharyngitis (but only 25 percent reduction of risk).

The most recent *CDC* recommendations for taking antivirals to prevent and control flu include:

- Early treatment for those with suspected or confirmed influenza who have severe illness or are hospitalized.
- High-risk patients should be considered based on clinical judgment of their doctor.

- Less than two years of age or older than sixty-five.
- Chronic lung, heart, kidney, liver, hematological, and metabolic disorders (diabetes).
- Immunosuppression.
- Pregnant or postpartum women.
- American Indian and Alaska natives.
- Morbidly obese.
- Residents of nursing homes or chronic-care facilities.
- The CDC recommends oseltamivir and zanamivir but not amantadine or rimantidine.
- Health care workers should keep updated as to antiviral resistance patterns in your area.

Helpful tip: Despite these recommendations, many infectious disease experts still do not recommend taking antivirals due to poor effectiveness.

Important Information:
Antiviral Drugs: Marketing Wins

Despite the fact that oseltamivir (Tamiflu) has been used by sixty-eight million people worldwide during the last decade, and millions more doses have been stockpiled to combat future pandemics, this class of drugs is only mildly effective for typical flu (shortens symptoms by one day) and may not work at all in pandemics (such as bird flu). This is according to a study in the *BMJ*.

In fact, the *BMJ* and the Cochrane group requested that Roche, the maker of Tamiflu, release all its Tamiflu data, because 60 percent of the data had never been published or released. The latest Cochrane review (2014), incorporating thousands of pages of previously unavailable data, showed that these drugs reduce mean duration of flu symptoms by 14 to 17 hours only.

The company still makes tremendous profit convincing doctors, and patients, to use it despite minimal benefits and high costs. In addition, another study showed that Chinese herbs are more effective for flu. This is a prime example of hiding negative results and the success of marketing to promote a minimally effective drug.

Most colds last for several days to a week, but influenza can last for much longer. Many people think that if the symptoms do not resolve sooner, they need antibiotics. In most cases, this is untrue, but in some, bacteria can overgrow due to lowered resistance of the respiratory tissues. If your symptoms do not resolve or worsen, you should seek professional medical care and take antibiotics only if testing reveals bacterial overgrowth (see below).

Important Information:
Overuse of Antibiotics: A Significant Danger to All of Us

Because most colds and flu are caused by viruses, they do not require antibiotics unless testing clearly shows evidence of bacterial infection. If you take antibiotics for a virus, bacteria can build up resistance to those antibiotics, which then will no longer be able to be eradicated by those antibiotics. Unfortunately, we are already seeing the results; each year in the United States, two million people contract drug-resistant infections, and twenty-three thousand die.

Some of you who always take antibiotics if you have a cold think it is the antibiotic that gets rid of it, but in actuality, the cold usually goes away in the same period of time without antibiotics, as studies have documented again and again. Unfortunately, many doctors would rather just give you antibiotics than try to explain why they shouldn't or fight with you about demanding them. This is bad on both ends.

Even worse, many doctors prescribe antibiotics that are not recommended for bacterial infections of the upper-respiratory tract, including cephalosporins, azithromycin (Z-pack), and fluoroquinolones (such as cipro).

Medications for bacterial infections (upper respiratory): If you do develop a bacterial infection, there are numerous antibiotics on the market, with much overlap on the type of bacteria they can eradicate. Drug companies are notorious for marketing the newer, more expensive antibiotics, which are also broader spectrum (effective against many different strains of bacteria) but in most cases, the older antibiotics are just as effective and safer. To determine if your bacteria is susceptible to particular antibiotics, your doctor may culture your sputum or take a throat swab. There are also rapid antigen tests that can detect certain strains of bacteria.

Warning: One popular antibiotic, azithromycin ("Z-pack") is associated with a threefold increased risk for heart death and a twofold increase in overall death (absolute statistics show 1/110,000 occurrences in healthy people, 1/4100 at high risk for heart disease). Azithromycin should not be used as first line in uncomplicated upper-respiratory conditions.

Flouroquinolone Antibiotic *Caution*

In some upper-respiratory infections, antibiotics are indicated. However, one type of antibiotic, a class called flouroquinolones, may increase the risk for rupture of tendons when taken orally. These side effects are seen primarily in people over the age of sixty, those taking corticosteroids, or recipients of organ transplants. Flouroquinolones are antibiotics that end with the name "floxacin," such as ciprofloxacin ("cipro").

Another study in 2014 revealed that those taking flouroquinolones have twice the risk of developing polyneuropathy, which may not be fully reversible after discontinuation. Stop taking these drugs immediately if you start getting pain, numbness, tingling, or loss of strength in your hands or feet. Flouroquinolones are *not indicated* as a first line drug for URIs: there are many older antibiotics that work as well and are much cheaper.

Some people may develop a chronic cough after the cold has resolved, which is usually due to hyper-reactivity of your airways. Your doctor may prescribe β_2 agonists (such as an albuterol inhaler) or steroid sprays, but unfortunately, most conventional methods are not very effective for this type of cough. If you don't obtain benefits within a few days, it won't work, and it may take up to three months to dissipate on its own. However, a recent study showed that gabapentin (Neurontin) may be able to control such a cough.

The Alternative Approaches

Important Information:

In the elderly, supplemental vitamin E may lengthen recovery
and increase symptoms of colds/flu, so it should be avoided.

Chinese herbal formulas may be more powerful and more effective than the more expensive conventional drugs. In fact, a study published in the *Annals of*

Internal Medicine in August 2011 showed that Chinese herbs are more effective than Oseltamivir (Tamiflu) for shortening flu symptoms. However, there are many underlying syndromes that can cause colds, such as Wind, Damp, Heat, and Cold, so evaluation by a certified TCM practitioner is advised. *Yin Qiao Jin* is particularly effective in the early stages when fever, headache, cough, or sore throat may be present and can often prevent the full development of colds or flu if taken as soon as symptoms begin. *Xiao Qing Long Tang* is useful for colds that produce thin, watery drainage. *Chuan Xiong Cha Tiao Wan* treats Wind Cold. *Gan Mao Ling* is a more modern formula that treats Wind Heat with sore throat. *Bi Yan Pian* helps with clear or stuffy runny nose. There are several others that can shorten the duration of colds if you do contract one, such as *Gan Mao Ling*. Most of these contain antiviral herbs such as isatis, lonicera, and andrographis.

Chinese herbs can also help persistent coughs. One beneficial formula is called *Er Chen Tang*, but there are many other formulas, depending on other causes of cough. You should observe initial benefits within three to seven days (sometimes sooner) but may need to take them longer, depending on your condition(s).

Western herbs and supplements: There are numerous herbs and supplements that have antiviral and antibacterial properties and may be useful for fighting colds and flu. These include:

- *Elderberry* (Sambucus; 700 mg, two to six capsules a day in divided dosages), is very effective against both colds and flu. It shortens the duration of symptoms by about 56 percent and reduces the severity of symptoms such as fever and myalgia, according to studies. It can be used with the Chinese herbs for better effectiveness. Elderberry also has activity against bacteria.
- *Andrographis* seems to significantly improve symptoms of the common cold when started within seventy-two hours of symptom onset. Some symptoms seem to improve after two days of treatment, but it typically takes four to five days before maximal symptom relief.
- *Zinc lozenges* may reduce the severity and duration of colds, although studies have been inconsistent. A recent Cochrane review of fifteen studies showed that taking zinc within twenty-four hours of the start of symptoms significantly reduced the duration of colds. Use the gluconate or acetate forms, containing 9–24 mg of elemental zinc. **Important notes**: You must start within twenty-four hours of symptom onset for it to be effective and must take it every two to three hours while awake. Zinc can cause anosmia (loss of sense of smell) when used in nasal sprays, and the beneficial effects are minimal at best. Zinc can produce nausea and a dry or astringent feeling in the mouth.
- *Echinacea* is an herb that ostensibly decreases the severity and duration of colds and flu through its antibacterial and antiviral properties. However,

most studies show that it minimally reduces symptom severity and duration. There is a combination of echinacea with two other herbs, wild indigo root and white cedar leaf (called Esberitox), which is more potent than echinacea alone and has been used in Germany for several decades. ***Important notes***: There are numerous forms and dosages of echinacea, so many products are ineffective. Look for a standardized product. Echinacea has been found to reduce the duration of colds only by about one day, much like antivirals. ***Warnings***: Echinacea should not be used if you have systemic diseases (such as tuberculosis), collagen diseases (such as scleroderma), multiple sclerosis, and autoimmune disorders (such as AIDS, HIV, and lupus), as it can make all of these conditions worse. You should also not take echinacea prophylactically to prevent colds because, after taking it for eight consecutive weeks, it may suppress the immune system.

- *High-dose vitamin C*, 1–6 grams per day (in divided doses, because the body is unable to utilize more than 500–1,000 mg at once), can decrease the duration of a cold or flu by one to one and a half days and decrease the severity of symptoms through its antioxidant effects. It is more effective if taken naturally through fruit and fruit juices, and it can be taken along with other herbs. ***Caution***: The high doses used for treating the common cold can increase the risk of side effects, so the modest benefit may not be worth the risk. You should also know that there are different forms of vitamin C (liposomal vs. buffered vs. ascorbic acid). High doses of ascorbic acid can cause GI irritation. Liposomal is the best but is not easily found, so buffered is recommended.
- *N-acetylcysteine* (600 mg twice daily) can help alleviate cough and reduce flu symptoms by breaking up mucous. It is indicated for influenza only, not colds.
- *Garlic* (4 grams daily) helps prevent cold and flu viruses from invading and damaging your tissues, thus shortening the recovery period.
- *Larch arabinogalactan* (1 tsp in water two to three times per day) stimulates the immune system.
- *Eucalyptus leaf* (200 mg three times daily) is used more for lower respiratory tract infections and bronchitis and can be used as an essential oil.
- *Osha* (tincture 20–60 drops five times daily) helps decrease irritation of the lungs as well as congestion. It has antiviral and anti-influenza properties.
- *Thyme* is antibacterial and antiviral and is an excellent expectorant for bronchitis and cough.

Other herbs and supplements are used not to fight viruses but to *reduce symptoms*. These include:

- *Anise* (tea or 50–200 ml essential oil three times daily) to reduce mucus. ***Caution***: Essential oils taken orally may cause GI upset, especially at the high dose of 200 ml three times a day.
- *Bromelain* (80–320 mg daily) as an expectorant and also decreases bronchial secretions.
- *Slippery elm bark* (alcohol extract, 1:1 in 60 percent alcohol, 5 ml three times a day) for sore throat. ***Caution***: Using lozenges while taking other oral medications can affect absorption of certain drugs.
- *Honey* for sore throat.
- The inhalation of *aromatic vapors* from various herbs, such as sage or thyme (aromatherapy), can also reduce throat irritation and coughing.

Lots of other natural products have been tried for treating a cold or flu but there's no reliable studies showing that they relieve symptoms of cold or flu. Goldenseal, pau d'arco, astragalus, bee propolis, boneset, wild indigo, and Siberian ginseng are products marketed as "immune-system supporters." These supplements are commonly used alone or in combination with other natural products, such as echinacea. ***Caution***: Astragalus should not be used acutely during an upper respiratory infection because it can tonify the infection and make symptoms worse.

Airborne: Great Marketing, Not So Good Benefit?

You may be familiar with **Airborne**, which is very popular because most consumers think it can prevent or cure colds. It is now marketed OTC as an "immune booster", and contains various herbal extracts, amino acids, antioxidants, electrolytes, synthetic vitamins, and other ingredients.

The company agreed to refund customers $23.3 million in 2008 for false advertising and claims (***note***: the company did not admit wrongdoing). Although there are many testimonials of its benefits and it may work for some people, I am not aware of any good peer-reviewed studies that have documented its effectiveness and you should understand that most of its ingredients may be obtained with a good diet. ***Caution***: This product contains high levels of vitamins C and A. At the dosage recommendations, toxic side effects may occur primarily if you have chronic kidney disease..

Herbal Teas are often promoted for cold and flu symptoms as well, but again, they have no scientific support for effectiveness. These include goldenseal, peppermint, elderflower, rose hips, meadowsweet, chamomile, ginger, slippery elm, Mormon tea, and linden flowers.

There are several **homeopathic remedies** that may be effective, depending on the specific symptoms. In fact, several OTC products for colds contain homeopathic remedies. These remedies include:

- *Gelsemium* for chills, aching, weakness, fatigue, and sore throat.
- *Allium cepa* for burning, runny nose, sneezing, and eyes watering constantly.
- *Nux vomica* for a runny nose that becomes congested at night.
- *Aconite* for a barking cough, burning sore throat, and a bitter taste in your mouth.
- *Arsenicum album* for runny nose with nasal congestion.

Pulsatilla, hepar sulphuris, lycopodium, sulfur, and belladonna are other homeopathic remedies commonly used for upper respiratory illnesses. These are all given as a12C dosage potency and may be dosed every two hours for a maximum of four doses. Consult a qualified homeopathist for guidance on which remedies will be most beneficial and for proper dosages. Benefits should be observed in one to three days. Another common remedy used for colds is oscillococcinum. Some researchers claim it reduces duration of colds, but analysis of the data shows only an insignificant one-fourth of a day reduction. (***Note***: if you use this remedy, take separate from food and medications and avoid coffee, mint, and menthol products while taking).

⸺∘◯∘⸺

Dr. A's Suggestions:
Wet-Sock Treatment:
Home Remedy for Cutting Colds Short

A very easy and inexpensive way to help blunt colds is using the cold sock method. The basis of this technique is that by stimulating your blood circulation and lymphatics, your immune system is activated and congestion is decreased. Here's what you do:

1) Take some cotton socks and soak them in cold water (some people put them in the refrigerator).
2) Soak your feet in a warm bath tub for at least a few minutes (some for twenty minutes).

3) Put the cotton socks on and cover them with dry wool socks.
4) Go to bed.
5) By morning, the socks will be warm, and you'll feel much better.

An alternative is whole-body hydrotherapy ("Burrito wrap"), in which you take a warm bath and then place a well-wrung-out cold, wet sheet around you and then a wool blanket on top of that.

Acupuncture is excellent for reducing the duration of colds/flu as well as decreasing symptoms, including sore throat, congestion, fever and cough.

Dr. A's Suggestions:
Honey Good for Cough

An easy way to suppress cough is taking a teaspoon of honey thirty minutes before bedtime. Honey may be as or more effective than dextromethorphan for controlling cough and is a lot less expensive.

Your Empowered Patient Action Plan for Treating Colds and Flu

Step #1: Flu vaccine is recommended for everyone since the benefits far outweigh the potential harm. If you are prone to recurrent respiratory infections, take panax or American ginseng before and after your flu shot. If you usually feel "bad" after a flu shot, take 800 mg of ibuprofen with your injection.

Step #2: Take a combination of elderberry and Yin Chao Jin at the first signs of cold or flu to either prevent it or reduce its duration and severity. As these herbs have long shelf lives, have them available before cold/flu season begins.

Step #3: Rest, drink plenty of fluids and use a Humidifier: Rest and fluids are the major treatments for both colds and flu, allowing your body to heal itself faster. I also recommend using a cool air humidifier, which can help relieve congestion and loosen mucous; you can purchase one in any drugstore. Steam inhalation may also be helpful but should be done with caution as breathing in essential oils like thyme and eucalyptus can burn nasal passages if done too quickly.

Step #4: **Use the wet sock method** to halt the progression of the cold.

Step #5: **Take Chinese herbal formulas containing Isatis, Lonicera, and Andrographis** if your cold or flu continues. These herbs are more effective than antivirals and less expensive.

Step #6: **Take N-acetylcysteine and garlic** to reduce flu symptoms if you get the flu. These work better than antiviral medications, without side effects.

Step #7: **Undergo acupuncture** to shorten the duration of the cold/flu and reduce symptoms.

Step #8: **Take OTC herbal expectorants, anise, bromelain, or guaifenesin** to reduce mucous.

Step #9: **Take slippery elm bark or use aromatherapy** for sore throat.

Step #10: **Take appropriate homeopathic remedies** to speed recovery if your symptoms continue.

Step #11: **Take an appropriate Chinese herbal remedy or honey** if your cough persists.

Step #12: **Take appropriate conventional OTC medications** to relieve severe symptoms that have persisted despite the above steps.

Step #13: **Consider Taking antiviral medications** if you are at high risk or for your at-risk household members to prevent flu from spreading.

Step #14: **Take antibiotics** if your symptoms have persisted or worsened *and* you have tested positive for bacterial overgrowth or infection by your doctor.

Step #15: **Try prescription medications** for persistent cough if the above steps have not helped.

Manny is a forty-five-year-old man who caught a cold four weeks previously. The cold symptoms had resolved, except for a persistent cough. He stated that his throat felt ticklish, and he would start coughing even when he spoke. His doctor had prescribed an albuterol inhaler and inhaled steroids, but these only helped to a minimal degree. I recommended a Chinese herbal formula, which resolved the cough in five days.

Expected Outcome

Colds are inevitable, but they can be shortened in duration and frequency and even prevented from fully developing by using the above steps. Influenza is a more potent infection with more complications, especially in older people, but it can still be prevented or shortened by the above steps. If you do get a cold or flu, alternative methods (especially Chinese herbs) are more effective than conventional medications. For the vast majority of colds, avoid antibiotics unless bacterial infection is proven by testing.

Constipation

What You Need to Know

Constipation is an abnormal process when eliminating solid waste (stool) from the body, characterized by a slowing down and decreased frequency of bowel movements. The wastes from the food that you eat should be eliminated within two or three days, and the longer the fecal material stays in the colon, the worse the constipation becomes.

In actuality, it is normal to have more than one bowel movement per day, although what's regular for you can be normal, even if it's every few days. As we get older, however, constipation becomes more of a problem as our intestinal motility may slow and weaken.

There are two basic mechanisms of constipation: decreased water in the colon (which dries out the stool) and inactive or dysfunctional muscle contractions of the colon. Thus, treatments are designed to correct one or both of these factors.

Treatments for Constipation

The Preventive Approaches

Correctable Causes: There are many underlying causes of constipation that, if corrected, can resolve constipation. *Medical conditions* that cause constipation include irritable bowel syndrome (IBSO), diverticulosis, colorectal cancer, diabetes, Parkinson's disease, multiple sclerosis, pregnancy, and depression.

Drugs that can cause constipation include most narcotics (morphine, codeine, etc.), aluminum-containing antacids, some iron and calcium supplements, and some antihistamines, diuretics, antidepressants, and blood pressure medications. If you have constipation and are taking any medications, check the Physicians' Desk reference *PDR* to see if constipation is a side effect, or ask your pharmacist. If you have any conditions that require drugs that cause constipation, if you can resolve or better control those conditions, you can discontinue the drugs and the constipation should resolve as well.

Diet is one of the most important factors to prevent and treat constipation. Fiber is one important component of the diet for treating constipation as it increases water content and improves motility (movement) in the intestines. Increase your intake of foods that contain fiber, especially raw vegetables and fruits such as peas, beans, and broccoli. Bran cereals; barley (as an additive to stews, soups, and salads) or barley flour; whole wheat bread; and dried fruits such as figs, raisins, and especially prunes, are also beneficial (1.5 ounces of prunes a day is as effective as taking psyllium, a bulk laxative, twice a day). You should also drink lots of water, about eight to ten glasses a day (or half of your body weight in ounces of water), to improve the moisture content of the bowels.

Yogurt contains beneficial microorganisms, but these may not be the most important or potent (see probiotics, chapter 2). Also, many yogurt products are pasteurized after they are made, to increase shelf life, but this may destroy the benefits. Several yogurts are specifically made and advertised to help constipation (Activia, Dan Active, Align), and studies have supported their benefits for many people with mild to moderate constipation.

Exercising is another proven preventive measure. Walking for twenty to thirty minutes a day is very helpful for stimulating the colon and preventing or decreasing constipation. Don't forget to hydrate afterward.

The Conventional Approaches

Medications: The mainstay of conventional treatment involves *laxatives*. There are four main mechanisms:

- *Bulk-forming agents* stimulate the natural contractions of the bowel as well as making stools softer. They should be taken with plenty of fluids.
- *Stool softeners* increase the amount of water the stools can hold, thus also increasing the bulk.
- *Osmotic laxatives* pull large amounts of water into the large intestines making the stools loose and soft. Side effects of osmotic laxatives include bloating, cramps, gas, and nausea. These laxatives may cause dependency and can also deplete your system of important nutrients, especially potassium.
- *Stimulant laxatives* induce the muscles of the colon to contract and push stool out and are often used before diagnostic procedures and for constipation caused by narcotics. They can be taken orally (may take six to ten hours to work) or rectally (taking fifteen to sixty minutes to work).

The Most Common Laxatives

Stool Softeners
    Docusate sodium (Colace)

    Phosphate of soda

Bulk-Forming Agents
    Bran
    Psyllium

Osmotic Agents
    Milk of magnesia
    Magnesium citrate

    Lactulose
    Sorbitol
    Alumina-magnesium (Maalox,

Polycarbophil
Methylcellulose

Mylanta)
Polyethylene glycol (Miralax)
Linaclotide (Linzess)

Stimulants
Senna
Cascara
Bisacodyl (Dulcolax, Fleet)

Warnings: All laxatives can cause dependency if used regularly. Stimulant laxatives can interact with Coumadin (a common blood thinner), thus increasing the risk of bleeding. Prolonged use of stimulant laxatives can damage the large intestine.

Tegaserod (Zelnorm) is a prescription drug used for constipation in IBS and regular constipation. However, polyethylene glycol is less expensive, is OTC, and is more effective. *Caution*: Zelnorm has been found to have potentially harmful effects on the heart. At one point, it was taken off the market, but it is now available with a black-box warning. Over half the patients stop taking it due to side effects. IBS constipation can be resolved in most cases without using this medication (see section on IBS).

Amitiza is a drug with dual actions: it promotes fluid secretion in your intestines and increases intestinal muscle movement, which helps make it easier to pass stools (bowel movements). It is indicated for chronic constipation or for IBS constipation.

Linaclotide (Linzess), a newly approved drug (August 2012), is also indicated for IBS constipation but only works in 20 percent of patients.

For narcotic-induced constipation, *methylnaltrexone* (Relistor) can reduce constipation rapidly, but it is used primarily in those with terminal illness or cancer. It is given by injection every other day and works anywhere from within a few hours to a day. However, it works in only half the people who take it. In September, 2014, the FDA approved *naloxegol* (Movanik) for the same indications. It works in about 40 percent of patients (vs 29 percent placebo).

Enemas can provide immediate relief but can be irritating if used frequently. Fleet's enemas are the most commonly used, but Milk and Molasses enemas are more potent and effective in my opinion.

The Alternative Approaches
Perineal self-acupressure is a Chinese method that can help over 72 percent of patients, according to a study done at UCLA. In this technique, you press on the perineum (the area between your anus and genitals) with your middle and index fingers, pushing up toward your back repeatedly, before you defecate.

Colon cleansing: The first step is to clean out toxins and old fecal material that can collect in the colon. This is done utilizing formulas that can cleanse and detoxify your colon using osmotic substances. A good formula should contain most or all of the following: apple fruit pectin, slippery elm bark, bentonite clay (pharmaceutical grade), marshmallow root, fennel seed, activated willow charcoal, and psyllium seeds/husks. You take this formula for one week every three to four months. ***Important note***: Because this formula may actually *cause* constipation due to slowing of the colon's muscular movement while it works, you must take it with a stimulant formula.

Stimulant formulas also can be continued after cleansing and for intermittent use. Look for a formula that contains most or all of the following: cape aloe, cascara sagrada, barberry root, senna, ginger root, fennel, and African bird pepper. Use ***caution*** as prolonged use may cause irritation of the stomach and can cause reflux symptoms. With such a formula, you take one capsule in the evening and increase by one or two each succeeding night until your constipation is relieved. You then can reduce the dose back to one per night. ***Warning***: Stimulant herbs may interact with Coumadin, thus increasing the risk of bleeding. Prolonged use of stimulant laxatives can damage the large intestine.

Another way of conquering constipation is to start with the upper GI tract, where food is broken down. Poor digestion and incomplete breakdown of food, which stagnates in your colon, can cause or worsen constipation. **Digestive enzymes** help break down your food better. There are many products that contain digestive enzymes, and they should contain some or all of the following: ox bile, protease, papain, amylase, lipase, bromelain, cellulase, and lactase.

Probiotics, which contain beneficial microorganisms that aid in digestion, absorption, and the production of vitamins and enzymes, can also help reduce constipation. *L. acidophilus* and *Bifidobacteria* are the preeminent probiotics, but there are numerous other species that can be beneficial. Because the organisms in probiotics die off rapidly, however, you must be careful what you purchase. Some products must be refrigerated, and make sure you purchase them as close to the manufacture date as possible (at least within sixty days). Other products do not require refrigeration because they contain a prebiotic such as FOS (fructooligsaccharides), which preserves the bacteria (see chapter 2 for more information). ***Important note***: Because probiotics kill off harmful bacteria and yeast that are in your GI tract, you may have gas, bloating, and cramping for up to ten days. If so, decrease the amount you are taking (one-half to one pill per day) and increase slowly. Inclusion of FOS may be what causes gas and bloating. You should notice improvement in one to two weeks when taking probiotics.

Chinese herbs have long been used successfully for constipation and may include many of the above ingredients. Common formulas include *Tao Ren Wan* or *Ma Zi Ren Wan* for excessive constipation. *Fructus persica tea pills, peach kernel tea pills, Run Chang Tang, Tiao Wei Cheng Qi Tang* or *Ji Chuan Jian* can help deficiency- syndrome constipation. Consult a practitioner qualified in Chinese herbal medicine to determine which Chinese herbal formulas are the best for your particular syndromes. You should experience improvement within three weeks (sometimes sooner), but you may need to take them longer, depending on your condition.

Acupuncture is also effective in many people with chronic constipation and should be used in conjunction with the Chinese herbs. You should notice improvement within six acupuncture treatments, but you might need additional sessions for maximum benefit.

Yoga exercises, such as the cobra position and knee-to-chest pose, can activate and tone the abdominal organs and relieve gas.

- For the *cobra position*, lie on your stomach with the side of your head resting on the ground and your legs together. Place your hands palm down, just below your shoulders, and keep your elbows close to your body. As you inhale, lift your head and chest off the floor, keeping your face forward. Only your upper body should be raised. Your navel should still be touching the floor. Look up as high as you can and hold this position for five seconds. As you exhale, bring your head and chest back down. Repeat it several times a day.
- For the *knee-to-chest position*, stand straight with your arms at your sides. Lift your right knee up and grasp your right ankle with your right hand and your right knee with your left hand. Pull your leg in as close as you can to your chest. Hold this position for six to eight seconds and then do the same with the other leg. Repeat this three to four times a day.

These poses activate the colon and are most effective for long-term prevention of constipation. It can take several weeks or even several months to observe the benefits.

Your Empowered Patient Action Plan for Treating Constipation

Step #1: *Eat a better diet* with more fruits, vegetables, and grains and decrease intake of or eliminate processed foods. Also increase daily water intake. Within four to six weeks, your bowel movements should be improved.

Step #2: *Try Perineal Self-Acupressure*, which may be the fastest and is the least expensive treatment for constipation.

Step #3: *Take a colon detoxifier/cleanser* to get your bowels moving. Use it as needed but avoid prolonged use.

Step #4: *Take a stimulant formula (colon activator)* for maintenance after your bowels are moving and every four to six months, which may prevent constipation from occurring.

*Step #5: **Take probiotics and/or digestive enzymes** for maintenance and prevention. After taking probiotics for one to two weeks, you may be able to stop taking the colon activator. Continue taking them long term as they also have benefits for your immune system and can prevent yeast overgrowth (especially in women).*

*Step #6: **Undergo acupuncture**, which can provide long-term relief.*

*Step #7: **Practice the cobra and knee-to-chest yoga poses** to improve bowel motility.*

*Step #8: **Take the appropriate Chinese herbal remedies** along with acupuncture to obtain longer-term relief if the above steps have not helped*

*Step #9: **Take conventional laxatives** to relieve constipation short term if the above steps have not been effective. The best and safest laxatives are the bulk formers.*

*Step #10: **Try Amitiza or Tegaserod** (see warnings) if you have IBS constipation and the above steps have not been effective.*

*Step #11: **Try methylnaltrexone** or **naloxegol** if you have narcotic-induced constipation.*

When Noreen came to me, she had suffered with constipation for many years. She had tried numerous conventional and OTC laxatives but had become dependent on them, and her constipation had continued. I recommended probiotics and digestive enzymes along with a colon activator. I also recommended that she drink more water, eat more fiber (vegetables), and start walking one mile a day. After three weeks, her constipation was much improved. She was able to discontinue the colon activator formula and continued taking digestive enzymes only.

Expected Outcome

Constipation can sometimes be a very difficult condition to control or resolve. However, with the above steps, most people can return to regularity.

COPD and Bronchitis (Chronic Obstructive Pulmonary Disease, Emphysema)

What You Need to Know

Chronic obstructive pulmonary disease (COPD) is a so-called "silent killer" because half the people who have it do not know it. Although it is most commonly caused by smoking, there can be other causes, such as occupational dust, chemical exposure, or infections.

COPD is now the fourth leading cause of death in this country, and the mortality rate for COPD has increased 100 percent in the past three decades. For women, the death rate has increased 300 percent. Hospitalizations for COPD have increased more than 40 percent, so it is important to get this disease under control.

In COPD, the alveoli of the lung (where oxygen gets into the blood stream) become damaged and restrict airflow. Emphysema is the end result and cannot be reversed. Until that occurs, however, COPD has a reversible component that can be improved, much akin to asthma. It can also involve bronchitis, an inflammation of the lungs, but this can also be treated.

Check for Osteoporosis

Patients with advanced COPD are at high risk for developing osteoporosis. You should have a bone-density test and refer to the section on *osteoporosis* for treatment.

Because many people don't realize they have COPD, the best test to diagnose it is spirometry (pulmonary function test). Treatment should be considered if you have symptoms and your FEV_1 (the part that measures oxygen flow) is less than 60 percent of predicted for your weight and age. ***Caution***: A 2015 study revealed that spirometry alone may not be sufficient to rule out lung disease in current and former smokers (42 percent had normal spirometry). CT scan and 6-minute walk testing may also be required.

COPD Often Misdiagnosed

Many patients are given a diagnosis of COPD and are treated with inhalers, yet lack confirmation of the diagnosis. A 2015 study in *Chest* showed that of previously medicated patients, 38 percent showed no evidence of airflow obstruction and thus were treated inappropriately. These patients were more likely to be obese and have other conditions such as heart failure, sleep apnea and depression.

This is important because there may be other reasons for breathing problems or fatigue besides COPD. Thus it is always necessary to undergo spirometry before beginning treatment for COPD.

A common complication of COPD is bronchitis, an inflammation of the airway passages, which can be acute or chronic. Bronchitis symptoms include coughing with sputum production, and many doctors treat bronchitis as an infection. Although this can occur, much of the time it is not the causal factor, and *antibiotics usually do not help, especially in chronic situations.*

Treatments for COPD

The Preventive Approaches

The major preventive is to **stop smoking**. As soon as you stop, the progression of the disease stops, and some damage may be reversible.

Diet: COPD patients use a lot of energy in trying to breathe and may need to eat as much as ten times the calories of a healthy individual. COPD patients need lots of protein as well as a greater amount of fat—healthy fat—in their diet. Besides the proteins from fish, poultry, and other lean meat, fats, such as those found in olive oils and oily fish, are beneficial. In fact, a 2015 study in *BMJ* showed that high intakes of whole grains, polyunsaturated fatty acids, nuts, and long chain omega-3 fats while lowering intake of red/processed meats, refined grains, and sugar-sweetened drinks lowers the risk of COPD.

In addition, *antioxidants* are very important to maintain several lung functions. Studies have shown that a vegetarian diet, rich in vitamins E, A, and C, can provide benefit when there is a reversible component present. Broccoli contains selenium and magnesium, both of which are able to reduce asthma-like symptoms. Lycopene, found in tomatoes, autumn olives, pink grapefruit, and watermelon, may protect against asthma; and all contain powerful antioxidants.

Black tea contains chemicals related to the stimulant theophylline, which is an older drug used for asthma. Three or four cups of black tea can open airway passages and ease breathing.

Several *other eating tips* include:

- Limit your salt intake. Sodium causes fluid retention, which may interfere with breathing.
- Avoid foods that cause gas and bloating.
- Eat several small meals of high nutritional value. Large meals leaving you feeling full will restrict full inflation of the lungs, making it more difficult to breathe.

- Eat your main meal early in the day so that you will have more energy throughout the day.
- If you use oxygen, be sure to use it during meals. Your body will need the oxygen during eating and digestion because those activities expend energy.

Exercise, at most any level, benefits COPD for several reasons. It improves the oxygen utilization, work capacity, and state of mind of COPD patients. Low-impact activities place minimum stress on joints and are easier to perform than high-intensity activities. Some COPD patients may also benefit from exercise programs that target the upper body and are designed to increase the strength of the respiratory muscles. There are also lung exercises that can strengthen your breathing (called pulmonary rehabilitation; usually done by trained physical or occupational therapists).

Treat acid reflux: COPD and bronchitis can also be complicated by acid reflux (GERD or heartburn). The acid in the esophagus can be inhaled into the lungs, causing irritation as well as aspiration (which can lead to pneumonia). If you have GERD, obtaining appropriate treatment can reverse or reduce your bronchitis symptoms (see section on *GERD* for treatment guidelines).

The Conventional Approaches

There are several conventional treatments for COPD, but you need to realize that the benefits of proven treatments for most patients are small, with little to no effect on respiratory status or hospitalizations. As you will see below, medications can be very confusing, and there may be harmful side effects, which is why you need consultation with a pulmonologist (lung specialist) to find the best treatment for you.

Inhaled medications are the primary treatment for COPD. *Beta$_2$ agonists* (e.g., albuterol, salmeterol [long-acting, called an LABA]) and *anticholinergics* (e.g., ipatropium) are commonly the first prescribed drugs, either alone or in combination. Spiriva (tiatropium) is a newer anticholinergic drug used for COPD but is linked to an increased risk of stroke in 2 percent of patients. It can decrease symptoms of COPD but does not slow its progression. A study published in *NEJM* in 2011 showed that tiatropium was superior to salmeterol and should be used first, but in another study in the *Annals of Internal Medicine* in May 2011, mortality was higher in those taking tiatropium than those taking LABAs. In December 2013, the FDA approved Anoro Ellipta (a combination of a new anticholinergic and beta-2 agonist) as a long-acting medication.

Warning: Inhaled anticholinergics raise the risks for urinary retention in older men, especially those who have enlarged prostates. They can also increase risk for heart disease when given long-term. Anoro Ellipta can cause paradoxical bronchospasm (shouldn't be used in asthma), glaucoma, and some possible heart effects.

Dr. A's Suggestions:
Learn How to Use Your Inhaler

Most conventional drugs for COPD are given by inhalation, but many people do not use their inhalers correctly. A recent report from the *American College of Chest Physicians* revealed that when a clinician shows a patient how to use an inhaler, 77 percent use it correctly. Of those who rely only on a brochure, 53 percent failed to receive any medication. So ask your doctor or pulmonary technician how to properly use your inhaler. However, realize that many doctors, including lung specialists, do not know how to use them correctly either.

Another *warning* is that some inhalers use capsules containing powder. Many people mistakenly take these capsules orally rather than in their inhaler. Fortunately, side effects are minimal, but if you don't get your proper medication, it can be harmful in that respect.

Inhaled corticosteroids (ICS) are another option and are prescribed in as many as 85 percent of COPD patients. Several products (such as Advair, Serevent, Foradil, and Symbicort) contain both steroids and a long-acting $Beta_2$ agonist (LABAs). Systemic steroids can also be given, but they have significant side effects and are reserved for severe flare-ups. A recent study showed that a combination of Spiriva and Foradil (cholinergic agent plus long acting $beta_2$ agonist) may help more than a steroid plus Advair, thus decreasing the need to use steroids. It should be noted that none of these drugs can stop the decline of lung function, but they can provide symptom relief and improvement in breathing tests.

Caution: A 2015 study demonstrated that inhaled corticosteroids may increase the risk of pneumonia in COPD patients. Experts recommend that long-acting bronchodilators be used alone in many patients unless flare-ups continue to occur; the benefit of ICS is greatest among patients with COPD/asthma overlap syndrome.

Warnings: LABAs have been associated with an increased risk of severe asthma symptoms and hospitalizations as well as deaths in adults with asthma. They should only be used with an asthma-controller medication such as an inhaled corticosteroid or anticholinergic. If high doses of steroids are given systemically, they can cause bone loss.

―∞―

Inhaled Corticosteroids May Provoke Diabetes, Osteoporosis, and Cataracts

A study published in the *American Journal of Medicine* in 2010 revealed that there is a significantly higher incidence of diabetes as well as more rapid diabetes progression in patients who receive ICS. It has previously been known that they can also cause osteoporosis and cataracts. If you are on ICS, have your doctor monitor for these conditions, and be sure that pulmonary disease guidelines are followed as to when to initiate ICS therapy.

―∞―

In the past, it was thought that using **beta blockers** (commonly used in heart conditions and high blood pressure) would worsen breathing in COPD. However, that thinking has changed. In fact, a study published in *BMJ* in May 2011 showed that cardioselective beta blockers (atenolol, metoprolol) decreased all-cause deaths by 22 percent as well as decreasing oral steroid use and hospital admissions for respiratory disease. Beta blockers may be especially beneficial if you have both COPD and heart disease.

For flare-ups of COPD

Steroids are commonly prescribed. A five-day course of prednisone (40 mg) in addition to other standard therapies has been shown (*NEJM* June 2013) to be as effective as longer duration of treatment.

The FDA has recently approved a new drug called **roflumilast** (Daxas, Daliresp), used to treat excess mucus and cough. It is taken daily but does have some side effects, including diarrhea, nausea, headache, insomnia, back pain, reduced appetite, and vertigo.

Oxygen is commonly prescribed for severe COPD with low blood oxygen. Oxygen has been shown to prolong survival in such patients. This can be tested easily by placing a device on your thumb to measure oxygen saturation (usually, below 89-91 percent may be an indication for oxygen). Most oxygen is delivered through nasal cannula.

Antibiotics are often used for flare-ups because patients with COPD are prone to infections. Many doctors use the newer, more broad-spectrum antibiotics, but a study in 2010 showed that older antibiotics such as trimethoprim-sulfamethaxazole

(Bactrim, Septra) or doxycycline are just as good as cephalosporins, quinolones, or augmentin.

Dr. A's Suggestions:
Bronchitis: Conventional Treatment Ineffective

The primary "infection" found in patients with COPD is bronchitis. Usually the symptoms are cough and sputum production. If your sputum is yellow or green, it *does not necessarily mean* that you have a bacterial infection. Most patients with bronchitis don't need antibiotics and they usually are ineffective.

Nevertheless, doctors often prescribe antibiotics for uncomplicated bronchitis. Studies (*JAMA* 2013) have shown that the most common antibiotic, amoxicillin, is largely ineffective in bronchitis. A 2014 study in *JAMA* showed that during the past fifteen years, the overall rate of antibiotic prescribing was 71 percent, despite national education programs and guidelines focused on eliminating the use of antibiotics in chronic lung disease. Furthermore, the use of broad-spectrum antibiotics, which are definitely not indicated and can lead to bacterial resistance, were prescribed at 35 percent of visits.

Ibuprofen is often given for fever or discomfort in bronchitis but also has been shown to be ineffective, especially with cough resolution.

Most patients with bronchitis will respond best to acupuncture (see below), whether acute or chronic. Most of the time, you're wasting time and money taking antivirals, antibiotics, or anti-inflammatory medications.

The Alternative Approaches
Acupuncture is quite effective for bronchitis, flare-ups of COPD, and for improving airflow and can provide long-term relief as well as reducing the need for medication. In addition, a recent study published in the *Archives of Internal Medicine* revealed that acupuncture benefits COPD patients through relaxation of accessory respiratory muscles and especially helps the symptom of shortness of breath on exertion. You should see initial benefits within six to eight treatments.

Often, acupuncture is used with **Chinese herbs**, such as *Ren Shen Ge Jie San*. *BanXia Huo Po Wan* can be used if there is profuse phlegm (in Chinese terminology).

There are several **nutritional supplements and herbs** that have been used for COPD, but research support has been minimal.

- *N-acetylcysteine* (NAC, 1,200 mg three times daily) helps break down mucous and therefore may be beneficial if bronchitis is present. However, it does not seem to be effective if you are on inhaled steroids.
- Skeletal muscle wasting and dysfunction are strong predictors of mortality in patients with COPD, so *creatine* (20 g per day, or 0.3 g per kg) for five days followed by a maintenance dose (2 or more g, 0.03 g per kg daily) can help by producing increased muscle mass and exercise performance.
- *Panax ginseng* (100 mg containing 37 percent ginsenosides twice daily for three months) has been shown to improve lung function and oxygen capacity in patients with moderately severe COPD, with no side effects.
- Japanese researchers at Kagoshima University Hospital found that supplements of *omega-3 fatty acids* appeared to improve patients' breathing difficulties, possibly by countering the airway inflammation seen in the disease.

Relaxation techniques, including meditation and guided imagery, are important as anxiety and stress are common in COPD.

Massage can strengthen respiratory muscles, reduce heart rate, increase oxygen saturation in blood, decrease shortness of breath, and improve pulmonary functions.

Certain types of **yoga** can ease anxiety and provide relaxation and more oxygen to the bloodstream through controlled breathing. The exercises help open blocked airways caused by bronchitis or emphysema. Simple yoga moves can even aid those with advanced COPD.

- The *pigeon posture* may enhance breathing. Start at a kneeling position and slide your left leg straight behind you. Take a deep breath and stretch your torso while arching your back slightly. Hold this position for twenty to thirty seconds, breathing deeply during this time. Exhale and relax; then repeat with the other leg.
- The *cobra posture* can ease wheezing. Lie face down, placing both forearms on the floor, your elbows directly under your shoulders. Inhale and push your chest upward, straightening your arms while keeping your pelvis against the ground. Hold this posture for fifteen seconds, breathing deeply, and then slowly relax.

Some people, especially those with chronic neck and back pain or who have had chest injuries, may have structural abnormalities in their ribs. The ribs must expand for breathing to occur, and if your ribs are twisted or frozen, this can cause more breathing difficulties. This diagnosis is frequently overlooked, but **osteopathic manipulation** can help your breathing immensely if you have this problem.

Dr. A's Suggestions:
Singing Helpful for Bronchitis

Studies have found that singing helps people with reversible airway dis-ease (asthmatic component of COPD or bronchitis) because of the deep breathing involved and because a variety of the muscles of respiration are strengthened.

Your Empowered Patient Action Plan for Treating COPD/Emphysema

Step #1: **Stop smoking** if you have this habit (see chapter 2 for methods).

Step #2: **Use prescription inhalers/medications:** Try these first for immediate im-provement in breathing as they have the most research support. The choice of inhaler type should be made by your doctor or pulmonologist. Remember, however, that they may be of only minimal help, so don't continue them if there is no benefit.

Step #3: **Consider taking beta blockers**, especially if you have concurrent heart disease.

Step #4: **Undergo acupuncture** for COPD, especially if you have bronchitis or asthma-type symptoms, for longer lasting relief and reduce your need for medications.

Step #5: **Take nutritional supplements** including fish oil, panax ginseng, and/or N-acetylcysteine if you have a bronchitis component with mucous production.

Step #6: **Try a Chinese herbal remedy** if you still have breathing difficulties.

Step #7: **Undergo osteopathic evaluation** to evaluate for rib dysfunction and undergo rib mobilization to help improve your deep breathing, if abnormalities are found.

Step #8: **Obtain massage on a regular basis** to ease anxiety and reduce stress.

Step #9: **Practice the yoga pigeon and cobra postures** to reduce stress and improve breathing.

Step #10: **Use supplemental oxygen** if your oxygen level is low. Oxygen needs should be evaluated by your doctor, as unnecessary supplemental oxygen can cause problems as well.

Expected Outcome

COPD is a very difficult disease to treat effectively. Both conventional and alterna-tive methods may be necessary to improve your condition. Emphysema is end-stage disease and unfortunately, is not reversible. Therefore, it is important to prevent the continued progression of COPD.

Cosmetics (Corrective Eyesight, Skin, and Body Rejuvenation)

What You Need to Know

We all realize that our body structures deteriorate as we age. Our eyesight worsens, our skin wrinkles, and body fat starts gathering in unwanted places. There are many procedures, both surgical and nonsurgical, that can make us look younger by altering our body. Most of these procedures are safe and work well, but there are many different approaches and choices.

Most cosmetic procedures are quite expensive, and insurance does not cover them. However, there are alternatives that are less expensive and may be just as beneficial as some of the more costly procedures.

Helpful tip: One of the most important aspects of corrective cosmetics is to make sure you fully understand the procedure and what you can expect. Many failures occur because patients expect more results than they will actually obtain. For that reason, it is important to undergo any procedures with an experienced, reputable doctor, who will explain what results you should expect. You can shop around, but the cheapest prices may not ensure the best results.

Dr. A's Suggestions:
Obtain a Second Opinion!

There are many procedures performed by one specific specialist, but other procedures may be able to be performed by doctors from different specialties. For example, eyelid surgery can be performed by a dermatologist, a plastic surgeon, or an ophthalmologist.

What you need to know is that each of these specialties may have a different approach or technique for correcting the problem, each having different side effects, complications, and/or outcomes.

For this reason, it is important for you to become empowered, explore your options, and consider obtaining a second opinion.

Corrective Eyesight (PRK, LASIK, and More)

Eyesight is very important and certainly changes as we age, a term referred to as presbyopia, a condition where the eye exhibits a progressively diminished ability to focus on near objects with age. Normally, our near vision especially decreases, requiring reading glasses. Most people start developing presbyopia after the age of forty.

A very common eyesight problem as we age is the formation of cataracts, which is clouding of the lens in the eye (see section on cataracts for more information and treatment options).

Treatments for Poor Eyesight

The Preventive Approaches

Diet: It is possible to slow the impact on our eyes from aging. Certain foods containing antioxidants, especially carotenoids, can help improve your vision. Apricots, mangos, cantaloupe, blueberries, carrots, and yams are especially beneficial for the eyes. They are rich in vitamin A, which is vital for healthy eyes, preventing easy tiring, irritability, light sensitivity, and night blindness. Yams are a particularly good eye food because they also contain the antioxidants vitamin C and vitamin E, which fight cellular deterioration in the eyes. Corn and even popcorn contain nutrients (carotenoids) that are beneficial for the eyes. Consumption of 6.9–11.7 mg of lutein through diet has resulted in the lowest risk of developing cataracts.

Applying **good vision habits** while reading and doing close work will help maintain or improve your close-up vision. Adding brighter lights in more places around the house may help you see better. Staring is one of the principal poor vision habits to eliminate, so take frequent breaks from reading or using a computer screen.

Eye Exercise Programs Not Helpful

There are many books and programs that claim improvement in vision by exercising eye muscles. But the muscles that focus the lens do not need exercises. These programs will not help vision and should be avoided.

Screen for and treat other medical conditions: There are some diseases that can cause vision problems, primarily hypertension and diabetes, so you should be screened for them and treat them appropriately if you have them.

You should also **undergo a complete eye exam** with an ophthalmologist or optometrist every two to three years as vision problems can be slowed or corrected with eyeglasses and other treatments.

The Conventional Approaches

Obviously, **corrective eyewear** is the primary method of correcting poor eyesight. Most older people wear bifocal or multifocal (progressive) eyeglasses. *Caution*: You need to realize that multifocal lenses can impair depth perception and peripheral vision, making falls 40 percent more likely. If you engage in activities involving distance, you should wear single-lens glasses for those activities. However, if you spend almost all of your time indoors, switching between glasses actually increases the risk of falls outdoors.

There are now several **surgical procedures** that can correct vision by changing the shape of the cornea. The initial procedure, called RK, is no longer used as it caused several side effects, and there are now more advanced procedures, such as:

- *Laser-assisted in-situ Keratomileusis (LASIK)* is the most common procedure and is done by making a thin, hinged flap in the eye's surface. This flap is lifted, and then laser energy is applied underneath to reshape the eye. The flap is replaced and functions as a natural bandage. LASIK's main advantage over other procedures is that there is little or no discomfort immediately after the procedure, and vision is usually clear within hours rather than days. Different forms of LASIK exist, many depending on how the flap is created; these include LASEK, Epi-LASEK, Bladeless, and blade-free or all-laser LASIK.
- *Photorefractive Keratectomy (PRK)*, also known as surface ablation, is still commonly used, but LASIK is by far the most popular laser procedure today. However, PRK and LASIK produce similar outcomes. Also, nerve regeneration in the eye's surface appears to take place faster with PRK than with LASIK following a procedure, and there is also no risk of surgical flap complications. PRK does not involve creating a thin, hinged flap on the eye's surface, as occurs with LASIK. PRK also appears to be a safer procedure in cases when a person's cornea may be too thin for LASIK surgery.
- *Laser Epithelial Keratomileusis* (LASEK): The LASEK technique is actually a cross between LASIK and PRK. It avoids any corneal flap-related LASIK complications and lessens the likelihood of removing too much cornea and compromising the structural integrity of the eye. There also is slightly less risk of developing dry eyes after LASEK eye surgery. LASEK also may be a better option if you have a high degree of myopia (near-sightedness), which

requires more tissue removal from the central cornea to correct the refractive error, or if your occupation or hobbies puts you at high risk of an eye injury and dislodging the corneal flap created in LASIK surgery. It's important to note, however, that LASEK typically involves more discomfort and a longer recovery time compared with LASIK surgery.

In summary of these three procedures, the fundamental difference in how LASIK, PRK, and LASEK are performed concerns how the eye is prepared for the laser treatment. ***Important note***: LASIK, PRK, and LASEK all can utilize *wave-front-guided procedures*, which measure precisely how light travels through the eye. Studies suggest that wave-front-guided LASIK reduces the risk of night glare after LASIK surgery.

- *Conductive Keratoplasty* (CK) uses a tiny probe and low-heat radio waves to apply "spots" around the periphery of the eye's clear front surface. This relatively noninvasive method provides near vision correction for people who are farsighted. CK also can be used to correct presbyopia or enhance near vision for people who have already had LASIK or cataract surgery.
- *Implantable lenses* are another option for vision correction surgery. Similar to contact lenses, these surgically implanted lenses primarily are considered appropriate for higher levels of nearsightedness. When implantable lenses are used, your eye's natural lens is left in place. Both of these lenses have a long track record of use, including more than sixteen years in Europe.

Important Note: Some people have certain conditions or diseases that would make them poor candidates for certain vision correction procedures and better candidates for other procedures. For example, if you have diabetes or other diseases that affect wound healing, you might be a better candidate for PRK or LASEK than certain types of LASIK. If you have thin corneas, PRK, LASEK, or lens implantation may also be more appropriate for you than LASIK.

The average costs of these procedures in 2014 (per eye):

- $2,223 for all laser-based vision correction procedures in which a single price is quoted.
- $1,543 for noncustomized LASIK using a bladed instrument that is not guided by wave-front analysis.
- $2,177 for wave-front-guided LASIK using IntraLase.
- CK: $1,500 to $2,900.
- PRK, Epi-LASIK and LASEK: about the same as LASIK.
- Refractive lens exchange (RLE): $2,500 to $4,500 per eye or more, depending on extra costs such as facility fees.

Dr. A's Suggestions:
Beware of Hidden Costs

Prices for corrective eye surgery differ widely from one provider to another and depend on many factors. The only universal standard is that refractive surgery prices are quoted *per eye*. Remember that one procedure equals only one eye even if both eyes are corrected on the same day. So the price quoted for a procedure doubles if you intend to have both eyes corrected.

Surgeons also might add extra charges for new technologies, including wave-front analysis for extra precise corrections. You also might be charged extra for IntraLase, a LASIK procedure in which a laser is used instead of a bladed instrument to create the flap on the front of the eye. There are also many costs for testing as well as royalty fees to manufacturers.

It is also common to see advertisements for low prices, but when you are examined, you are told that you need a more expensive procedure, as the quoted one won't work as well. Typically, only a few select people are actually eligible for LASIK at prices that sound unusually low, because most eyes require more extensive correction or more follow-up after the surgery. Another reason for lower prices is the use of older equipment. In addition, the offer price may not cover all fees, including follow-up visits.

So ask plenty of questions related to what a procedure actually costs beyond what is advertised. Be sure to ask for an estimate, in writing, that details exactly what you are getting for that low price. Make sure you clearly know what the *total* cost of the procedure will or could be, including surgeon and facility fees or any other extras. One advertised price represented as a "bargain" might include those types of extra costs, whereas another might not.

You may be tempted to choose a surgeon based only on the fee charged, but that can turn out to be unwise. It's better to choose the best surgeon you can find and then, if you need it, get the most affordable financing you can.

If you are forty or older or have *severe* vision problems, LASIK, PRK, and other laser vision correction procedures may not be the best option for you. However, there are still other options, such as:

- *Monovision*: With this approach, LASIK may be used to correct one eye for distance vision and the other eye for near vision as a solution for presbyopia. However, some people cannot adjust to monovision. You might first consider wearing contact lenses providing monovision or trying it with "trial lenses" in your doctor's office to make sure this approach works for you. CK also provides a type of monovision, but with a fuller range of vision in the corrected eye.

- *Multifocal or accommodating lens implantation*: Your eye's natural lens will be replaced permanently with this procedure. These artificial lenses can produce side effects such as decreased depth perception or night vision problems in the form of halos or glare. Also, you may still need to wear eyeglasses or contact lenses or have a "laser touch-up," because it's possible that the lenses will fall short of restoring a full range of vision.

Warnings about Corrective Eye Surgery

Most eye surgeons will tell you it's unlikely that any vision correction procedure can give you optimal vision for a lifetime. Just as you probably needed to change out eyeglasses and contact lenses in the past, you may need a LASIK enhancement or other surgical correction as you grow older, to maintain good vision.

Also, keep in mind that all vision correction procedures have the usually slight risk of side effects that can range from mild to severe. So be sure you discuss all options and potential risks in detail with your eye surgeon or eye care provider before making any final choices.

The Alternative Approaches

There are several **nutritional supplements** that can improve vision and help keep the lens of your eye healthy. These include:

- *Lutein* (6–11 mg daily) reduces damage from UV sunlight and is an antioxidant. Consumption of 6.9–11.7 mg of lutein through diet has resulted in the lowest risk of developing cataracts.
- *Bilberry with bioflavonoids*, 80 mg (containing 25 percent anthocyanidin content) three times daily.
- *Glutathionine* may protect against UV light; selenium (200 mcg daily) also helps keep glutathionine in its active form. Vitamins B_2 and B_3 are necessary to protect glutathione.
- *Vitamin E* with mixed tocopherols (400 IU daily) may also protect the lens against free radical damage and activates glutathione. "DL" tocopherol products should be avoided.

- *Vitamin C* (1,000 mg daily) is needed to activate vitamin E in the eye.
- *Ginkgo* (120–240 mg daily) increases blood flow to the eye. However, there can be drug-herb interactions with gingko.
- *Grapeseed extract* (150–300 mg per day, containing 95 percent procyanidolic content) may help poor night vision or photophobia (increased sensitivity to bright light).

Skin Rejuvenation

Everyone gets expression lines, thin wrinkles, and sagging skin as they grow older, though to what degree is dependent on your genetics. However, a major reason skin looks older, wrinkled, or contains dark spots is due to sun exposure, referred to as photoaging. If you compare the skin on the outside of the arm with the skin on the underside, you'll notice that the outside, which gets sun exposure, shows far more signs of aging than the unexposed underside surface.

Dr. A's Suggestions:
Make Sure Your Clinician Is Well Trained and Experienced

For major plastic surgery, you can easily determine if a plastic surgeon is board certified, although some are better than others.

For other types of skin rejuvenation, most clinicians are not licensed to do such procedures, including doctors. This is a field that is totally unregulated in most states, and anyone can, without any degree, learn to perform these procedures and convince you to undergo them. Understand that you may get exactly what you pay for, so the cheapest is not necessarily the best.

Be sure to become empowered and check out the credentials of anyone claiming they can rejuvenate you. Ask for references and the names of patients willing to show you their results.

Treatments for Skin Rejuvenation

The Preventive Approaches
Smoking makes skin look older, especially in the facial area, so stopping this habit will certainly improve the health and look of your skin.

Besides sun exposure, UVA and UVB radiation occurs from **tanning beds** as well. They can cause skin damage and accelerate aging skin just like sun exposure (and are often produce more radiation than sunlight), so minimizing such exposure can, again, help prevent your skin from being damaged.

Sunscreen is the most effective preventive action for aging skin. Skin cancers, including melanomas, are on the rise and kill 12,000 people per year, so protect yourself. The following will help:

- You should use *broad-spectrum* sunscreens containing ingredients that protect against both UVA and UVB rays.
- You should use at least a SPF 15, and use 30+ if you are more sensitive to the sun. However, using SPF greater than 50 may only provide minimal additional protection for the cost. *Important Note*: The actual protection can be considerably less than indicated by the SPF on the label because testing of these products utilize large quantities applied to the skin.
- You should apply sunscreen liberally and reapply it after sweating, swimming, or toweling off.
- Reapply *every two hours*; all sunscreens deteriorate within that period of time
- "Waterproof" or "water-resistant" means that the SPF is maintained during eighteen minutes of moderate activity or forty minutes of swimming. This is an average because, depending on the environment and how much is applied, the sunscreen can evaporate more or less quickly.
- Avoid the intense sun between 11:00 a.m. and 3:00 p.m.
- "Spray" sunscreens are easy to use, but much of the spray misses your body. If you use them, apply several times. It is not known whether inhaling the spray is dangerous.

The Conventional Approaches

Prescription medications, primarily vitamin A derivatives tretinoin (Retin-A, Renova) or tazarotene (Avage) are commonly used to treat aging skin. Both cause structural changes in the skin by removing the top skin layers and forming new collagen and blood vessels, which reduces wrinkles, dark spots, and pore size and improves skin tone and smoothness.

Warnings: These drugs are short-lived, and once they are discontinued, the skin will gradually return to the way it was before the drug was started. There is also a possibility that people who use one of these retinoids might have an increased risk of skin cancer if they get excessive exposure to sunlight or sunlamps.

Other than drugs, there are numerous **injections and procedures** that are very successful at reversing the signs of skin aging, at least temporarily.

- *Botox* is given for facial wrinkle lines at rest. Dosage depends on how extensive the wrinkling is as well as how much muscle you have, so men require more than women. Usually two or three areas are done, using two to three injections in each area. Side effects include sagging of eyelids or eyebrows. For this reason, you should also not lie down or have a facial massage for four hours after injection. Results last for three to four months, but duration gets longer the more you undergo the injections, often eventually requiring only twice a year. Cost is $9.95 to $11.95 *per unit*, and each area requires ten to twenty units. **Caution**: Botox does paralyze the muscles, so frowning, smiling, and other facial gestures are often limited or eliminated. **Warning**: Many noncertified people give Botox injections, but they should be avoided due to increased risk of side effects and possible facial distortion. You can check out their credentials through the Botox manufacturer, Allergan.

- *Fillers* are used to fill deeper folds and lines and are often mixed with lidocaine for analgesia and other products to last longer. It usually lasts from six months to one year, although there are longer lasting fillers that can remain for ten years. If done for lip augmentation, physical actions such as sucking through straws, whistling, or smoking uses up the product faster. Costs approximate $500 to $750 for semi permanent and $1,000 for permanent. It is difficult to remove, however, so be sure you want it if it is permanent. **Caution**: Many fillers are actually recycled from old collagen. Always ask your doctor where it was purchased and from what manufacturer. Make sure your doctor uses pharmaceutical-grade silicone as cheaper types can cause harm and even death. There can be side effects such as swelling, inflammation, allergic reactions, facial, lip and eye, palsy, and disfigurement. These usually occur at injection sites away from the nose (the site most commonly used).

- *Fraxel* involves the use of a laser for the purpose of resurfacing the skin. Regular fraxel is done once a month for four months and you achieve 80 percent new skin. Downtime is about a day. An advanced type is fraxel-repair, which achieves 85 to 95 percent new skin, but downtime is about ten days. This type of laser is more powerful and can even perform a nearly complete facelift. It is also useful to remove acne scars, sagging tissues, and cellulite. Cost approximates $5,000.

- *"Permanent" makeup* involves injecting a dye into eyebrows, eyeliner, or lips and may take several sessions. It lasts for three to five years. Costs are $500 to $750.

- *Laser hair removal* is very popular and takes a series of about six sessions. It removes about 80 percent of the hair. The laser destroys the follicle and has replaced electrolysis, which uses electricity and is much more painful.

- *Chemical peels* are commonly done to brighten up aging faces and remove damaged cells by neatly peeling off a layer of skin cells. More than one million people a year undergo chemical peels. There are several acids that can do so, the most common one being trichlorocetic acid (TCA). Although this chemical has come into question as possibly being carcinogenic, research has not proven this conclusively. **Helpful hints**: If you undergo a chemical skin peel, remember that these acids can burn, so make sure your clinician is qualified. There are milder peeling agents, such as glycolic acid, as well as other methods such as dermabrasion and laser resurfacing. Consult with a physician, do your research and check around before deciding.

Plastic surgery is the "gold standard" conventional approach and can provide long term removal of wrinkles, lines, gaps, bags, and so on. Plastic surgery is more time-consuming and much more expensive. Determining whether to undergo the above procedures versus plastic surgery is a matter of degree. If there are many corrections needed or a large area, plastic surgery is more useful; for a few areas or less expense, the above procedures may be advantageous. Costs for plastic surgery are much more expensive than the above, even for the same methods. Some examples include Botox at $200 to $400 an area, collagen injection (filler) at $500 to $1500, facelift at $7,000 to $9,000, and lip augmentation at $600 to $2,000.

Dr. A's Suggestions:
Turning Back the Clock: Not as Much as You May Think

In a 2013 study in *JAMA Facial Plastic Surgery*, volunteers reviewed before and after pictures of patients who had undergone facelifts, brow lifts, and eyelid surgery. Overall, patients looked only three years younger after surgery and had no significant effect on ratings of attractiveness.

Before you plop down thousands of dollars, realize that the benefit you achieve may only be in *your* eyes, not others.

The Alternative Approaches

Most people do not realize that **acupuncture** can be used for cosmetic purposes and may work very well. Cosmetic acupuncture uses even smaller needles than other types of acupuncture and you can actually see the beneficial results after each treatment. It works by increasing blood flow and oxygenation, moisturizing and nourishing the skin, and initiating collagen production. Results include:

- Skin becomes more fair and delicate
- Improvement in facial muscle elasticity
- Reduction and prevention of wrinkles

- Erasing of fine lines and reduction of deeper lines
- Firming of bags
- Reduction of sagging
- Lifting of droopy eyelids
- Minimization of double chins
- Clearing or reduction of age spots

Cosmetic acupuncture involves ten to fifteen treatments but may require occasional maintenance treatments. It usually costs $90 to $120 per treatment, and each session takes about an hour and a half. So, overall, it is much cheaper than conventional means and has minimal to no side effects. Only a small percentage of acupuncturists are trained at cosmetic acupuncture.

Cosmeceuticals: Other than cosmetic acupuncture, there is a huge market for natural, "antiaging" skin care products for aging baby boomers, and these products are often called "cosmeceuticals." They're promoted as being more powerful than regular cosmetics, but not so powerful that they're regulated like drugs. Most are in the form of facial creams or lotions that contain antioxidants and other ingredients and some are taken by mouth. (See sidebar.)

Many Nutritional Products Not Proven Beneficial

There are many different nutrients being tried in cosmeceuticals, but they have not been proven to reduce wrinkles when applied to human skin or taken orally. These include sugar or salt scrubs, sugar cane or fruit extracts, papain, topical vitamin E, vitamin A, beta carotene, papain, papaya, green tea, kineton, aloe gel, CoQ10, acetyl-L-carnitine, resveratrol, grape seed extract, and many others.

Most skin-care products contain a combination of different types of moisturizers. Although dry skin doesn't cause wrinkles, it can make them more pronounced. Using products containing these moisturizers can temporarily puff up the skin with water and reduce wrinkles, but they won't eliminate wrinkled skin altogether.

Occlusive products are the most common moisturizers. They are typically oily or waxy substances that form a layer over the skin and therefore prevent moisture from leaving the skin. These include shea butter, cocoa butter, jojoba, avocado oil, lanolin, emu oil, petrolatum, and mineral oil. Another method of hydrating the skin is to use humectants, which draw water from within the skin to the surface layer. Humectants include glycerin, hyaluronic acid, propylene glycol, lecithin, and many others.

There are also many *nonmoisturizer-type products*. Alpha-hydroxy acids are a common ingredient in scrubs, lotions, and creams used for wrinkles and are commonly used in chemical peels. They are used based on concentration: high concentrations of 50 to 70 percent are only for use in a physician's office; trained cosmetologists use concentrations of 20 to 30 percent for light peeling; low concentrations of less than 10 percent are available in a variety of OTC cosmetic products. These products do seem to be moderately effective for improving the signs of aging skin, including reducing wrinkles. However, they may increase your sensitivity to the sun.

Pyruvic acid is similar to alpha-hydroxy acids but may induce less irritation. Studies show that a 50 percent pyruvic acid chemical peel can smooth skin and decrease wrinkles, but this high concentration is only suitable for application in a physician's office. Lower concentrations are available in cosmetics that are available to consumers, but it's not known if these lower concentrations are effective.

Topical vitamin C appears to reduce wrinkles when used in a 3 percent solution topically after twelve weeks of use. Although vitamin E does not benefit the skin alone, a combination of vitamin E and vitamin C orally may help prevent photoaging. In addition, *green tea* and *grape-seed extract* may help minimize skin damage when exposed to sun or tanning beds.

DHEA is a hormone precursor that appears to increase skin thickness, improve skin hydration, and decrease facial skin pigmentation. It is taken orally, but you should not exceed 50 mg a day. DHEA can induce an increase in hormones, which may be why it works on skin (especially in postmenopausal women), but the 7-keto form may have the same effects, without the increase in hormones. ***Important note***: You should avoid wild yam and soy products labeled as "natural DHEA" because they do not break down into DHEA in the body. Another hormone precursor, DMAE, might have a firming effect on loose skin when used as a topical 3 percent gel, but it is very expensive.

There is some evidence that an antioxidant, *alpha lipoic acid*, in a 5 percent cream daily for twelve weeks, can improve signs of aging skin such as wrinkles and roughness.

Other than these nutrients, which are often contained in OTC lotions and creams, there are some **herbal topicals** that can help make skin look younger. These include herbs such as frankincense, apple-cider vinegar, lavender, witch hazel, chamomile, sea salt, rosehip (contains vitamin C), and even honey. These can be used as washes, masks or to decrease cellulite.

Misleading Claims Common for Skin Products

Manufacturers of beauty products can make claims that are not supported by research or reviewed by the FDA or other government agencies. So you need to be wary if the claims sound too good to be true. Some examples include:

Cosmetics claiming to be organic may be misleading or bogus and may not be any safer or more effective than other products, yet they are usually more expensive. Unless the product contains a USDA or NSF seal, it is not truly organic.

"Hypoallergenic" and "dermatologist tested" are labels that are simply marketing terms and have no official standards. A 2015 study revealed that out of 187 products marketed as hypoallergenic, 89 percent contained at least one chemical known to cause allergic reactions and some contained five or more such chemicals. Most of the allergens were preservatives or fragrances.

There are **homeopathic injections** used to treat wrinkles and help with skin tightening; however, these are only done by specialty trained clinicians.

Body Rejuvenation

Aging not only affects the skin but all the connective tissues, as well as your metabolism. So, it is quite common to have sagging breasts and put on weight in areas where you don't want it. In addition, many people have a tendency to develop cellulite, a skin alteration often described as an "orange peel," "mattress," or "dimpling" appearance on the thighs, buttocks, and sometimes lower abdomen of otherwise healthy women. Again, there are many actions you can take to reverse these effects cosmetically.

Economic Downturn Encourages Cosmetic Changes

You would think that as the economy "sags," fewer people would undergo cosmetic procedures, but that is not the case. In fact, the opposite may be true, and there are other subtle changes as well.

First, more and more older people are seeking cosmetic surgery to look younger so that they can compete better with younger people for jobs. Many older individuals who have lost their jobs are even taking money out of their retirement accounts to do so.

Second, people are shying away from the major surgical procedures and going to the less invasive fillers and chemical peels. The latter do improve appearances, but these procedures are fairly temporary and give more modest improvements.

People who are older most often request facelifts, liposuction, or neck lifts but are postponing some of these procedures in favor of laser procedures or injectables to pump up wrinkles.

Treatments for Body Rejuvenation

The Preventive Approaches

Exercise: The best way to prevent or slow the need for body rejuvenation is exercise. There are many exercises for the face as well as the chest that can slow down aging effects. For the chest, exercises that strengthen and enlarge the pectoralis muscles are beneficial for pulling up the muscles holding the breasts. Exercise, along with diet, is the best way to trim body fat before it becomes a problem.

The Conventional Approaches

Liposuction has been a staple procedure for many years and can remove excess fat from basically any area of the body. This procedure removes large amounts of fat, but it does not tighten the skin, so you may need additional plastic surgery for skin tightening later. You must wear a compression garment or girdle for three weeks to six months afterward, depending on the extent of the procedure.

Cautions: Liposuction can have complications as it is a surgery done under anesthesia, and some deaths have actually occurred. Many of these problems occur if there is too much liposuction done at once or too many areas. Minor complications include superficial irregularities of the skin, collections of fluid under the skin, focal skin death, allergic reactions to drugs, visible or disfiguring scars, discoloration of the skin, fainting during or after surgery, temporary bruising, numbness or nerve injury, and temporary adverse drug reactions. Post-liposuction syncope (fainting) the next morning at home, especially after urinating, is not rare. Costs approximate from $1,500 for one area to $10,000 for five areas.

Important Note:
Fat May Return after Liposuction…To Different Areas

Liposuction can certainly reduce fat, but not for long. A small study published in *Obesity* showed that one year after liposuction, body fat remains the same, but the fat that reaccumulates goes to other areas. For example, liposuctioned thighs remain reduced, but regained fat goes to the upper abdomen.

———

Laser therapy: Another less drastic procedure involves the use of lasers to burn the fat and tighten the skin. There are several types of lasers, all with high wavelengths that produce heat. The laser is placed beneath the skin and heats the fat and skin, which results in dissolving the fat, tightening the skin, and producing collagen. It can be used in any area, including arms, thighs, jowls (neck under the jaw line), abdomen, and so on. The procedure takes between one half to two hours and downtime is two to three days. It does not require anesthesia so has less risks than liposuction. However, in a small percentage of patients, burns can occur. Lasers can also be used in conjunction with traditional liposuction, in order to tighten the skin after fat removal. It is also useful for stretch marks. Cost approximates $3,000 per area, depending on the amount of fat; some abdominal procedures will cost from $5,000 to $12,000.

Endermologie is FDA-approved massage therapy for the temporary reduction of cellulite and involves the use of a high-powered handheld roller and suction device. This method can redistribute the fat but does not get rid of cellulite. It is also costly (average $1,600 for twelve treatments) and may be painful.

Kybella (*deoxycholic acid*) has now been approved by the FDA (2015) for moderate-to-severe chin fat. It is an injection that destroys the cell membranes of fat cells. Patients may receive as many as fifty injections at a time. ***Caution***: injury can occur if not done properly.

Plastic surgery is a common method of body rejuvenation and reshaping. The main procedure for aging women is uplifting the breasts as well as other body parts that are sagging. Some examples of costs are $5,000 to $6,000 for a breast lift and $6,000 to $8,000 for a tummy tuck, so it is much more expensive than other methods.

———

Facts and *Warnings* on Breast Implants

More than three hundred thousand women undergo breast augmentation annually in the United States. Although considered relatively safe, there are some facts that you need to know.

It should be noted that many women have had breast implants at earlier ages, or as a result of reconstruction after mastectomy at older ages. The jury is still out on whether silicone implants may cause other illnesses (most studies have not proven causation), and they are still the most commonly used. You should realize, however, that implants are not "lifetime" devices. Twenty percent of women who receive augmentation and potentially half who receive them for reconstruction will need to have them removed or replaced within ten years.

Contraction of the capsule, implant rupture, wrinkling, asymmetry, scarring, pain, and infection are the most common adverse side effects; and the longer the implants are present, the more likely the complications.

A recent review of post approval studies by the FDA revealed that implants do not appear to cause breast cancer, reproductive problems, or connective tissue disease. However, breast augmentation is associated with higher risk for having a nonlocalized cancer (especially invasive cancer) and for breast cancer death. This is due to missed diagnosis from impaired visualization of breast tissue, insufficient breast compression, and capsular contraction during mammography in women with implants. In such cases, MRI may be recommended but may not be covered by insurance as it is not routine.

The Alternative Approaches

Acupuncture is the primary alternative method that is successful for body rejuvenation. Acupuncture can be used to uplift sagging breasts as well as for other sagging tissues and even tummy tucks. It is also useful for postsurgical or traumatic scars, making them softer, less discolored, tight-feeling, or itchy. It may take ten to fifteen treatments, which can be done two to three times per week and may require intermittent maintenance treatments. Average cost is $100–$125 per session. However, only a small percentage of acupuncturists are trained at body rejuvenation.

The **low level energy laser** *("cold laser or LLEL)* is also excellent for eliminating posttraumatic and postsurgical scars, without any side effects and providing long term resolution. This type of laser does not produce heat like those mentioned above. It appears to break up scar tissue and regenerate new tissue. It usually takes six to eight treatments for definitive changes and can be done three times a week. Cost is approximately $35–$45 per treatment.

There are also other alternative methods that have not been proven effective or, at best, are only temporary. They include:

- *Anticellulite creams* that usually contain amino acids, retinol, caffeine, green tea, and so on, which ostensibly stimulate circulation, decrease water retention, and burn fat.
- *Nutritional supplements* may contain various vitamins or minerals, herbs (like horse chestnut, witch hazel, and hesperidin), fish oil, vinegar, lecithin, and others.

- *Mesotherapy* uses an injection of a combination of drugs with plant extracts, vitamins, homeopathics, and various other substances. There are no standard formulas, so each practitioner uses his or her own concoction; and there can be significant side effects and scarring.
- *Anticellulite spa treatments* usually involve seaweed, aromatherapy, or massage, but they have only temporary results.

Expected Outcome

Most methods for eye, skin, and body rejuvenation are quite successful. However, there are many different approaches, some less expensive than others, some more successful than others, and some longer-lasting than others. The most important issue is to be happy with the finished result, so preparation, research, and choosing the right practitioner are essential.

Depression

What You Need to Know

Depression can occur at any age and can affect anyone. However, as we age, it is even more important to be aware of the risk of depression, which becomes much more common. In fact, up to 35 percent of residents in long-term-care facilities may experience either major depression or clinically significant depressive symptoms. It is reported in 8 to 20 percent of the older population—disproportionately higher in women.

Fast Facts on Depression

- Nearly one out of ten adults in the United States is depressed.
- Depression is most common in the Southwest, with Mississippi having the highest prevalence (14.8 percent) and North Dakota the lowest (4.8 percent).
- Depression is more common among women than men, among blacks and Hispanics than whites, and among middle-aged adults than among younger and older adults.
- Those without health insurance are significantly more likely to be depressed than those with coverage.

Unfortunately, depressive symptoms are commonly not recognized the older we become, because first, depression is *not* a major focus of physicians; and second, depression is frequently intertwined with other aging problems, such as cognitive (brain) impairment, medical illnesses, and functional impairments. Often, depression causes bodily complaints that lead doctors to prescribe more drugs, which often are not necessary and can potentially worsen the depression.

On the other hand, physicians may not just underdiagnose but also overdiagnose depression. In a recent study involving 50,000 cases, it was noted that out of one hundred patients, ten patients with depression will be correctly identified, ten will be missed, and fifteen who are not depressed will be falsely given the diagnosis. Physicians should always search for physical explanations of depressive type symptoms.

It is important to recognize and treat depression because it can worsen diseases of aging such as cancer, asthma, diabetes, and heart disease, and it can even decrease bone density.

Treatments for Depression

The Preventive Approaches

Correctable causes: Depression can be caused by numerous drugs (antihistamines, steroids, antihypertensives, anti-inflammatory agents, tranquilizers or sedatives), marijuana, and environmental toxins (heavy metals, pesticides, herbicides, solvents); so if you are depressed for no specific reason and are taking any medications, check the Physicians' Desk Reference (*PDR*) to see if depression is a side effect of your medication.

Bad habits: In addition, alcohol is a brain depressant, and smoking increases your body's cortisol levels, which can contribute to depression when elevated. Thus, you should curtail these habits as they may make your depression worse.

Diet: Much epidemiological research has shown an association of depression with certain foods, especially refined carbohydrates and trans fats. In fact, it is known that these foods have a potent negative impact on neurotrophins, brain proteins that protect the brain against oxidative stress and promote new brain cell growth. Hence, avoiding these foods and eating more fruits and vegetables (which contain B vitamins and folate) can help fight depression. Omega-3 fatty acids found in freshwater fish (salmon, mackerel, trout, halibut, cod) can also boost your mood.

Exercise helps depression by improving blood flow to the brain, elevating mood, and relieving stress. All types of exercise are beneficial, with aerobic exercise being the best, and can relieve depression substantially faster than medications. In fact, recent studies have shown that the major reason depression increases heart disease risk is due to physical inactivity, not the depression itself.

The Conventional Approaches

Medications are the most common treatment for depression. In fact, three of the top ten medications used in the United States are antidepressants. ***Caution***: Unfortunately, all these drugs can have significant side effects, many of which may be subtle. They most commonly include sleep disturbance, sexual dysfunction, and weight gain; and secondarily, headache, tremor, urinary disturbance, or low blood pressure. In addition, tricyclic antidepressants (see below) have more side effects such as dry mouth, constipation, dizziness, sweating, and blurred vision. Serotonin re-uptake inhibitors (SSRIs) have more nausea, poor appetite, diarrhea, insomnia, agitation and anxiety. If these occur, switching to another antidepressant class that has fewer of these side effects may help.

Important Notes **about Antidepressant Response**

Antidepressant medication *response* is defined as a 50 percent reduction in depressive *symptoms*. This is *not* the same as depression *remission*. Only about one-third of patients achieve full symptom relief after three months of treatment with an initial medication, and only two-thirds achieve full remission, even after trials of three additional medications.

For older people (older than sixty years), antidepressants may help those with a long duration of depression (more than ten years), more so than those who have short-term depression (*American Journal of Psychiatry*, 2013).

Twenty-five percent of patients taking antidepressants will get worse, and if that happens, you need to stop immediately. In general, anxious people and suicidal patients may not do as well on antidepressants.

Of note is that as many as 70 percent of patients fail to continue taking antidepressants, usually because of adverse effects.

In general, prescription antidepressants may be effective in many patients. They include several different classes of drugs:

- SSRIs (fluoxetine [Prozac], sertraline [Zoloft], paroxetine [Paxil], citalopram [Celexa], fluvoxamine [Luvox], Escitalopram [Lexapro])—are the most commonly prescribed antidepressants
- Serotonin-norepinephrine reuptake inhibitors or SNRIs (duloxetine [Cymbalta], Effexor, desvenlafaxine [Pristiq])
- Phenylpiperizine (Serzone)
- Combination SSRI and serotonin-A receptor partial agonist (Viibryd)
- Pyridine (Desyrel)
- Tricyclics/TCA (Elavil [amitriptyline], Pamelor, Sinequan, Anafranil, Doxepin)
- Bupropion (Wellbutrin, Zyban)
- Tetracyclic (Remeron)
- MAO inhibitors (Parnate, Marplan)

Within each of these classes of antidepressants, the drugs are generally equivalent to each other in effectiveness. However, you still may respond differently to different drugs (both in benefits and side effects), whether they are in the same or a different class. So you may have to try several before finding the one that is best for you. There is no overall "best" antidepressant: *The best antidepressant for you is the one that works.*

Sertraline (Zoloft) and duloxetine (Cymbalta) are now generics and are less expensive than prescription antidepressants. In a study published in *Lancet*, Lexapro and Zoloft were the antidepressants that showed the best possible balance between acceptability and benefit. A 2015 study showed that for older patients (>60 years old), Zoloft (sertraline) appears to have the best results with the least side effects. Ziibryd has recently been approved and does not cause the sexual dysfunction or significant weight gain seen with other antidepressants.

Reversing Sexual Dysfunction Caused by Antidepressants

Sexual dysfunction may be a major side effect of antidepressants, occurring in both men and women. Taking gingko biloba (180–240 mg daily) or sildenafil (Viagra), Cialis, or Levitra may reverse this effect and is worth a try. If not, there are other drugs that may be helpful.

A study in November 2013 in *Depression Anxiety* showed that regularly scheduled exercise improves sexual functioning in women. Of note, simply scheduling regular sexual activity improved orgasm, whereas scheduling exercise, especially just before sexual activity, increased desire. However, improvement of sexual function with exercise at least six hours before sex was not statistically significant, but exercise within thirty minutes was.

Warning: SSRI antidepressants have been found to increase the risk of bleeding 50 percent if you are taking blood-thinning medications such as aspirin, warfarin, or clopidogrel (Plavix). The risk is lower but still present even if you are not taking these particular drugs. Taking NSAIDs (including ibuprofen and aspirin) with SSRIs increase bleeding risk six fold! In addition, taking NSAIDs (non-steroidal anti-inflammatory drugs for pain) has also shown an increased risk for not only gastrointestinal bleeding but also brain hemorrhage. This latter effect is more likely in men than women due to differences in metabolism. If you take both, you should be monitored closely for bleeding, especially within the first thirty days of taking them.

Warning: SSRIs Can Increase the Risk of Suicide

SSRIs are the most common antidepressants prescribed and, by reducing depression, can reduce the risk of suicidal behavior. Yet, it is important to know that studies have revealed (and the FDA has added warnings) that this class of antidepressants can ironically increase the risk of suicidal behavior in some people. If you note increased signs of suicidal ideation after starting these medications, you should notify your doctor immediately.

Because a certain antidepressant may not work for you, often another one is prescribed in addition and the two in combination may work better. However, studies show that if two common drugs don't help you, you stand little success (16 percent chance) of a third one helping. Overall, 60 percent of people who have depression gain complete remission by the time they've tried three drugs. Another drug, *Abilify*, is often used to treat depression in adults as an add-on treatment to an antidepressant when an antidepressant alone is not enough. In fact, Abilify is one of the most profitable drugs prescribed in America.

Important Information:
Antidepressant Effectiveness Exaggerated

According to a review of unpublished data, the effectiveness of a dozen popular antidepressants has been exaggerated by selective publication of favorable results. Drug companies often only publish what makes their drugs look beneficial and only tell doctors about those studies. Doctors have no access to the unpublished studies (see chapter 4 under Research for more information). In fact, based on FDA research reviews, antidepressants may only work 40 to 50 percent of the time. According to various studies, Serzone, Zoloft, Remeron, and Wellbutrin are the least effective; Paxil, Prozac, and Lexapro are the most effective.

In the near future, however, a test may be able to help determine what antidepressant will work the best for you. Using an electromyogram (EEG), a test that reveals your brain waves, a certain pattern (called a biomarker) can indicate whether a certain antidepressant is working when performed a week after starting the drug. This test hopefully will be validated soon.

⸻

Important notes: You should see benefit within two weeks of taking an antidepressant (according to a 2006 study in The *Archives of General Psychiatry*), and they should be continued for four to nine months, although some doctors advocate one year of treatment. If one drug doesn't work but has minimal side effects, it should be increased to maximum dose before adding another drug.

Warning: Do not abruptly stop taking any antidepressant. Doing so can cause a wide range of unpleasant side effects. Instead, withdraw the drug slowly (over several weeks), especially if your antidepressant is short-acting (such as Paxil and Luvox). Always consult your doctor before stopping your antidepressant.

⸻

It's More Than the Brain: It's Also the Mind

Most doctors (and patients) think that to treat depression, you need to treat the brain. It has long been surmised that depression is caused by an imbalance of neurotransmitters such as serotonin, dopamine, or norepinephrine. In fact, no studies have actually proven this, and researchers still are not quite sure exactly what causes depression. This may be why antidepressants may not work in many patients; and if they do, it may be because different chemicals can have different effects on the brain.

What you should realize is that there are many different aspects of the brain. Certainly, there are the neurons and nerve pathways that control our bodies and provide learning, memory, and thinking functions, grouped under the heading of "the brain." However, there are also emotions, fantasies, dreams, and unconscious thought, grouped under the heading of "the mind." This latter aspect is in the realm of psychiatry/psychology (see below), and conventional research on the mind has been minimal at best.

The *bottom line* is that drugs alone may not be the answer to depression. If they help, that's great. If they don't, you need to explore other reasons and approaches.

⁂

Although antidepressants are the most *common* conventional treatments for depression, **psychotherapy** is an important conventional step in identifying and addressing the emotional aspects of your depression and providing long-term resolution. Psychotherapy can be equally as or more effective than drugs for treating depression, but it may take several months or longer to observe benefits. ***Important note***: You should realize that although psychotherapy and medications are equally effective, less than half of depressed patients benefit from either one.

Cognitive-behavioral therapy (CBT) has been the main type of psychotherapy for depression, but typically takes an extended period of time, often months or even years. *Psychodynamic psychotherapy* (PP) is a form of in-depth psychology, which is focused on revealing the client's psyche in an effort to alleviate psychic tension. In this way, it is similar to Freudian psychoanalysis. In a 2013 study, remission of depression was seen in 24 percent of CBT patients and 21 percent of PP patients (response rates were 39 percent and 37 percent, respectively).

Interpersonal psychotherapy (IPT) may be superior to the other types in older patients as it is time-limited and focuses on issues more relevant to aging, such as retirement, ceasing to drive, conflicts with children over increasing dependency, or death of a spouse. IPT focuses on present circumstances, not past or early life issues.

Thought field therapy is another type of psychotherapy, which is especially beneficial if traumatic events in the past are causing depression.

Electroconvulsive shock therapy (ECT) is another conventional treatment for depression that is resistant to medications and psychotherapy. This method involves jolting the brain with an electric current to induce a brief seizure, which somehow results in resetting faulty brain connections. ECT was previously used on severe mental illnesses and lost favor over the last few decades, but is making a comeback. In fact, over the past five years, people over the age of sixty-five have accounted for 40 percent of the ECT treatments conducted. This method has an advantage for elderly patients who don't respond well to medications or have major side effects. Because ECT is safer than it was decades ago, there are few side effects, the major one being memory loss (usually short term). *Warning*: Elevations of cardiac troponin, an indication of decreased oxygen to the heart, has been observed in 11.5 percent of patients both before and after ECT, so cardiac evaluation should be done before ECT, especially in older patients.

Transcranial magnetic stimulation (TMS) is another device that has been approved by the FDA for depression. This device uses magnetism, forty minutes every day for four to six weeks, to help depression. Studies from the company show significant relief, but the FDA's Neurological Devices Panel in 2007 concluded that it was not very effective.

The Alternative Approaches

Mind-body methods may determine the underlying reasons for depression and help conquer it long-term. *Interactive imagery (active imagination)*, if available, is perhaps the best psychotherapeutic approach to depression because it works more quickly than most other approaches (including conventional) and adds the benefits of relaxation and meditation. This is a mind-body method in which you mentally interact with images that represent your emotions. It is a powerful method to uncover and deal with subconscious psychological issues you may not be aware of. Unfortunately, there are very few therapists trained in this method. (To obtain references for Interactive Imagery, see Appendix).

Acupuncture is thought to rebalance the neurotransmitters in the brain that are deficient in depression and so may provide long term relief. A 2013 study in *PLoS Medicine* showed benefit of acupuncture in severe depression (other studies show that acupuncture directly stimulates the brain). However, not all styles of acupuncture are beneficial for depression, so be sure to ask the acupuncturist if he or she has experience working with depression. You should notice improvement within six to eight acupuncture treatments but might need additional sessions for maximum benefit.

Along with acupuncture, there are several good **Chinese herbal** antidepressant formulas that are excellent for treating depression. Because these formulas contain a variety of herbs, they are often able to treat forgetfulness, phobias, anxiety, and nervous exhaustion along with depression. *Gui Pi Wan* and *An Shen Bu Xin Dan* are examples. You should notice improvement within three weeks. *An Mian Pian* ("peaceful sleep tablets") can be useful for calming and rest.

Herbal antidepressants can be as effective as conventional drugs but without their side effects. *St. John's wort* (300 mg containing 0.3 percent hypericin three times a day) is the most common, shown in numerous studies to improve mild to moderate depression. It takes from one to three weeks to be effective and is particularly useful for people under the age of fifty. *Cautions*: *Do not take St. John's wort with conventional* *prescription antidepressants*, especially SSRIs, as they all increase serotonin levels, and the combination can cause serotonin syndrome, characterized by some or all of these symptoms: confusion, itching, fast heartbeat, elevated blood pressure, muscle stiffness, restlessness, shaking, nausea, or sweating. If you are on conventional antidepressants and want to change to St. John's wort, you should wean yourself off the conventional drugs first (slowly decrease the amount you take over at least two weeks), and then start St. John's wort. St. John's wort also interferes with a system in the body that metabolizes many conventional drugs, so check with your doctor before starting this herb.

St. John's Wort Linked to Cataracts

New research has shown that there is an increased risk of developing cataracts if you take St. John's wort. This is because a constituent of this herb is photoactive, and the presence of light might damage proteins in the lens of the eye. If you spend significant amount of time in the sun, you should avoid St. John's wort.

Be Careful in Purchasing St. John's Wort Products

In recent testing by ConsumerLab.com, about half of the St. John's wort supplements tested were contaminated with cadmium or lead and/or contained much less active ingredient than claimed. Also be aware that St. John's wort can interfere with the absorption of many conventional medications, so always check with your doctor before taking it.

Gingko biloba (160–240 mg containing 24 percent flavonglycosides per day) may be an effective antidepressant for those of you over the age of fifty. Gingko works by increasing blood and oxygen flow to the brain, but it may take four to eight weeks to be effective.

Fish oil has been demonstrated to be effective even in major depression that hasn't responded to conventional medications. It also has been found to improve the responsiveness when given with conventional antidepressants. Most authorities recommend 1,500 to 3,000 mg daily. *Flaxseed* (1–2 Tbsp daily, fresh only), has also been shown to improve depression. It may take three weeks to notice improvement when taking these omega-3 fatty acids supplements.

The supplement *5-HTP* (100 mg twice daily) is converted to tryptophan, a precursor to serotonin, a brain neurotransmitter that is found to be deficient in many people with depression; it can increase the brain levels of serotonin, thus reducing depressive symptoms. It is equal in effectiveness to most conventional antidepressants, with few side effects. You should observe benefits in two to four weeks. *Warnings*: do not take 5-HTP with conventional antidepressants, due to the possibility of serotonin syndrome. Also, be sure only to use products that are "peak X-free." Peak X is a contaminant that can cause significant side effects and even death. *Helpful Tip*: This supplement can cause abdominal cramping in some people and is best taken by itself (without other medications) with a small piece of fruit.

SAM-e (400 mg daily for mild depression, 800–1,600 for moderate to severe depression) can be an effective antidepressant and has actually been endorsed by the American Psychiatric Association. It affects several brain neurotransmitters and phospholipids that are essential for brain function as well as boosting antioxidants and protecting DNA. It can also improve the effectiveness of the above antidepressants, so it can be added to them if the others are only partially effective. SAM-e starts working in half the time needed for tricyclic antidepressants and does not cause the weight gain or sexual dysfunction seen with other antidepressants. *Important notes*: No studies have compared SAM-e to SSRIs for effectiveness, the top quality products are very expensive ($65 per month), and many SAM-e products contain sub-therapeutic amounts or are poor quality. When used as an injection, this supplement has caused mania in people with bipolar disorder. As with most antidepressants, it may take two to three weeks to have a beneficial effect.

N-acetylcysteine (600–2,400 mg daily) has been shown to be effective in OCD (obsessive-compulsive disorder) in patients who are refractory to antidepressants.

Bright light therapy (using a fluorescent light box for thirty minutes each morning) has long been recognized as beneficial in treating seasonal affective disorder (depression during the winter months) but has now also been shown to be beneficial in non-seasonal major depression.

Your Empowered Patient Plan for Treating Depression

- *Important Note: If your depression is severe, start with steps 1 and 4.*
- *Helpful Tip: I recommend that you continue antidepressant therapy, whether conventional or natural, for four to six months after you are no longer depressed, to reduce the risk of relapse.*

Step #1: Undergo interactive imagery or other psychotherapy for the best chance of long-term relief.
Step #2: Undergo acupuncture if available to also provide long term relief.

*Step #3: **Take SAM-e:*** The best forms are almost as expensive as conventional antidepressants, but they are as or more effective than conventional drugs and have minimal side effects.

*Step #4: **Take a prescription antidepressant:*** The above steps are recommended first because they are less expensive than conventional antidepressants and *may* have fewer side effects.

*Step #5: **Take omega-3 supplements (fish oil or fresh flaxseed)*** alone or with antidepressants to improve mood.

*Step #6: **Try gingko biloba*** if you are over 50 and still have depression, since it can help improve memory as well as depression.

*Step #7: **Take appropriate Chinese herbal remedies:*** If the previous steps have not worked, these may be beneficial. However, some formulas may contain St. John's wort.

*Step #8: **Take St. John's wort or 5-HTP*** if still depressed or if you also have insomnia. If you are taking other medications, check with your doctor to make sure St. John's wort does not interfere with those drugs.

Often, multiple approaches are most effective. Cynthia had moderate depression, as well as some anxiety, for several years. She had taken conventional antidepressants, but they caused her anxiety to worsen, decreased her concentration, and decreased her sexual desire, so she had stopped taking them. I began her on the Chinese herbal formula Gui Pi Wan, which reduced her depression, and also did acupuncture on six occasions, which gave her additional relief. At the same time, I referred her for interactive imagery, which uncovered physical abuse that she had suffered during childhood. After several months of continued psychotherapy, she was able to reduce her herbs and eventually was able to discontinue them.

Expected Outcome

In most cases, depression can be successfully treated. The main keys are diagnosing depression so that it can be treated successfully and finding the treatments that are effective for *you*.

Diabetes

What You Need to Know

After rising steadily from the mid-1990s, the incidence of diabetes has started to drop (from 1.7 million in 2009 to 1.4 million in 2014; *CDC report 2015*). Nevertheless, diabetes is still epidemic in this country. One-third of Americans who have diabetes are not aware that they have the disease, especially African Americans, Hispanics, and Native Americans. Twenty-three percent of people over the age of sixty have diabetes, and it is the seventh leading cause of death. Even if you are aware of having the disease, you may not treat it properly, potentially causing numerous complications.

There are two types of diabetes: type 1, which is genetic, usually occurs in childhood, and in which your pancreas does not make insulin at all; and type 2, which is acquired, has its onset in adulthood and usually is caused by resistance to the insulin your body produces. As type 2 is by far the most common type as we age, this section primarily discusses this type, although some aspects apply to type 1 as well.

Diabetes Is Associated with Increased Incidence of Cancer

A study presented at the annual scientific session of the American Diabetes Association revealed that diabetics have a 25 percent increased risk for developing cancer, a 30 percent greater risk of mortality from any cancer, and a shorter survival time after cancer diagnosis. The risk is highest for liver, pancreatic, and uterine cancers (twofold or more) and less for colorectal, breast, and bladder cancers (1.5-fold). In fact, every 10 mg/dl increase in fasting blood sugar is associated with a 15 percent rise in incidence of pancreatic cancer, according to a 2015 study in *BMJ*. The *bottom line* is that better diabetes care may help prevent the development of cancer in diabetics.

Diabetes is also linked to Barrett's esophagus, a condition caused by long-term acid reflux disease and that predisposes patients to cancer of the esophagus. Patients with insulin resistance and central body fat have a significantly higher risk of Barrett's esophagus as well as esophageal cancer.

Many people who are overweight, eat poorly, and don't exercise may have *prediabetes*, also referred to as glucose intolerance (also called insulin resistance). This means that you develop resistance to insulin, so you can't move glucose (blood sugar) into cells efficiently and utilize it as an efficient body fuel. This can be reversed by exercising and eating better. If you don't, your blood sugar may continue to rise to abnormal levels, and you will develop full-blown diabetes.

Important Information:
Metabolic Syndrome: Risk of Diabetes

People who have metabolic syndrome are at increased risk of developing diabetes and heart disease. This syndrome is characterized by abdominal obesity and insulin resistance (blood-sugar intolerance), which is why it is often called insulin resistance syndrome. Other factors found in the syndrome include lipid abnormalities (high cholesterol, triglycerides), elevated blood pressure and inflammation. About 13 percent of people with metabolic syndrome are normal weight, but most are sedentary.

A 2015 study revealed that 36% of people in the US have metabolic syndrome, with higher prevalence in women and Hispanics. If you have metabolic syndrome, you should receive treatment for all these factors since it can progress to full blown diabetes and increase cardiovascular risk. Of all these, high blood pressure is the most important to control.

At this time, only one in eight people achieve the target goals for glucose, blood pressure (BP), and lipids, despite their importance. The goals are as follows: BP < 130/80, cholesterol < 200 (LDL < 130, best < 100; HDL > 60), and HbA_{1c} <7 (see below).

To *diagnose* diabetes, you measure your blood sugar after an eight-hour fast (100–126 for prediabetes, over 126 for diabetes) or take a glucose tolerance test. Once you have diabetes, most physicians use the HbA_{1c} test to monitor blood sugar, although some now use it to diagnose (prediabetes 5.7 percent to 6.4 percent, diabetes above 6.5 percent). Many experts think the cutoff for diagnosing diabetes should be greater than 7 percent. However, a study in 2010 showed that the HbA_{1c} test varies across assays, and other factors and may not correlate exactly with blood sugar, causing overdiagnosis.

Dr. A's Suggestion
Unnecessary Overtesting for HbA_{1c} Common

Guidelines for diabetics recommend undergoing testing of HbA_{1c} twice a year, but a December 2015 study revealed that 55 percent of people underwent testing three or four times per year and 6 percent received five or more tests. Patients at highest risk for excessive testing were from the Northeast, while those in the Midwest were at lowest risk.

The problem with overtesting is that it leads to additional treatments with antidiabetic drugs or iunsulin that are not needed. This more frequently occurs if several doctors are treating your diabetes, so it is highly recommended to receive your diabetic care from one primary physician.

⁂

A 2014 study (CREDIT study) showed that for every 1 percent increase in HbA_{1c}, there was a 25 percent increased risk of a major cardiovascular event. The risk of cardiovascular death and stroke (36 percent risk) were also increased significantly.

⁂

Self-Monitoring Blood Sugar Levels Often Inconsequential

It has long been standard practice to have diabetic patients measure their own blood sugar levels at home to better control them. In a recent study conducted over a year, patients who monitored their sugar levels did not have any better control of their diabetes than those who did not. In addition, those who monitored their blood sugar had a higher incidence of depression. For these reasons, intermittent blood sugar monitoring (every three to six weeks at your home and every three to six months at the doctor's office) may be just as good for glucose control as daily monitoring.

⁂

Hearing Loss More Common in Diabetics

A recent analysis of 5,100 adults who underwent hearing tests revealed that 21 percent of diabetics had low- or mid-frequency hearing loss versus only 9 percent in nondiabetics. If you are diabetic, you should have your hearing checked and monitored.

⁂

Treatments for Diabetes

The Preventive Approaches
Diabetes self-management education and training (DSMT) is recommended by the American Diabetes Association. It is a covered benefit by most insurers and

can help you become empowered to regulate your diabetes and its treatment better. However, a 2014 *MMWR* report showed that participation ranged from 5 percent (patients on no medication) to 14 percent (patients on insulin), so it is much underused.

Lifestyle interventions can prevent the onset of diabetes for at least a decade. The number one preventive measure is to avoid weight gain and obesity. If you are overweight, simply losing the excess weight may reverse your diabetes or at least lower your blood sugar. In fact, a recent study in the *Archives of Internal Medicine* revealed that just losing weight is more important than what you eat specifically. To prevent or delay the onset of diabetes, you should lose 5 to 10 percent of body weight.

You should also **stop smoking**, which increases the risk of diabetic complications, especially heart attack, stroke, neuropathy, and leg ulcers.

Diet is of tantamount importance in diabetes. Eat a balanced diet that is low in simple carbohydrates and saturated or trans fats and high in whole fruits and non-starchy vegetables. Green leafy vegetables (spinach, kale, lettuce, etc.) are especially preventive of diabetes. Adults who consume certain whole fruits, including apples, grapes, raisins, pears, and blueberries, have a significantly lower risk of type 2 diabetes. Trans-fatty acids, found in commercially baked and deep-fried foods (processed and fast foods), are especially bad, so avoid them.

There are several specific diets that are helpful to follow to prevent worsening of diabetes:

- The *American Diabetes Association (ADA)* diet (go to www.diabetes.org and look under "Nutrition" for further information).
- The *HCF diet*, which means "high-complex-carbohydrate" or "high fiber" diet, can also be beneficial. This diet asks you to follow these daily guidelines in planning your meals: eat 70–75 percent complex carbohydrates, 15–20 percent proteins, and only 5–10 percent unsaturated fats. (It is highly recommended to limit carbohydrates to 55 percent, 20–25 percent for protein, and 20–25 percent for unsaturated fats). The HCF diet is plentiful in grains (bread, cereal, rice, and pasta), starchy vegetables (potatoes, corn, peas), and legumes (dried beans, peas, lentils), and is packed with vitamins, minerals, and fiber. You should consume at least 20 to 35 grams of fiber, but I recommend more if possible as studies have shown that daily consumption of fifty grams of fiber leads to a 10 percent decrease in blood sugar.
- Another diet that also has proven quite effective, as well as more palatable, is the *Mediterranean diet*, which is low in carbohydrates, rich in vegetables, and low in red meat. In a study published in the *Annals of Internal Medicine*, a Mediterranean diet was seen to reduce the need for diabetic medications more than the AHA diet. Another study in a later issue showed that a Mediterranean diet supplemented by extra-virgin olive oil decreased the risk of developing diabetes by 40 percent.

Although the best way to obtain fiber is from food (see Chart 2), you can *supplement fiber* in your diet. Thirty to 50 grams per day of guar, pectin, or oat bran is recommended. As for protein, soy is beneficial for several reasons: First, the protein from soy is the only protein from a plant source that is "complete," meaning that it contains food proteins that provide all the essential amino acids to maintain good health. Second, soy can help control blood-sugar levels. Third, soy can help prevent or reduce complications of diabetes, especially atherosclerosis and nephropathy.

Chart 1
Sources of Water-Soluble Fiber

Legumes (beans)	Oat bran
Psyllium seed husks	Seeds
Most vegetables	Nuts
Pears	Apples

Different carbohydrates can cause variable increases in your blood sugar, and utilizing the *glycemic index* is often recommended. This index tells you how quickly your blood sugar will rise when you eat a particular carbohydrate, and it is suggested that you should eat those foods that have a low glycemic index. Be aware, however, that some low-glycemic foods, such as sausage and ice cream, have high fat, which can contribute to weight gain. ***Important note***: It should be noted that a 2014 study showed for the first time that the glycemic diet has little clinical value and that fine-tuning the index is less important than basic heart-healthy diets. (For a complete listing of glycemic values for all foods, go to www.mendosa.com.)

Nuts, especially pistachios, have been shown to improve blood sugar, insulin levels, and several metabolic risk factors in patients with pre-diabetes. A 2014 study in *Diabetes Care* showed this with patients who consumed two ounces of pistachios daily. I suggest eating one cup of nuts three to four times per week. Walnuts have specifically been found in studies to have a beneficial effect due to the omega-3 content that reduces inflammation in the body.

Adding red wine vinegar (3 tsp) to your salad also can lower your blood sugar after meals by up to 30 percent by slowing digestion. Lemon juice works similarly, so squeeze a fresh lemon into the water you drink.

Several small studies show that eating the broiled stems of one specific prickly pear cactus species, *Opuntia streptacantha*, can reduce blood-glucose levels by 17 to 46 percent. Other species don't seem to have this effect.

Another study showed that eating brown rice in place of white rice might lower the risk for diabetes. Finally, onion and garlic have blood glucose–lowering effects and compete with insulin for liver sites, thus increasing the release of free insulin. I recommend incorporating them into your diet whenever possible. If not following one of the above specific diets, green leafy vegetables are the best food for diabetes prevention.

High dietary magnesium intake is associated with lower fasting insulin concentrations in adults and a reduced risk of developing type 2 diabetes. According to one analysis, a 100 mg/day increase in dietary magnesium intake is associated with a 15 percent risk reduction for developing type 2 diabetes. This is equivalent to the magnesium found in four slices of whole-grain bread, one cup of beans, one-quarter cup of nuts, one-half cup of cooked spinach, or three bananas.

Beware of Artificial Sweeteners Causing Glucose Intolerance

A 2014 study in *Nature* revealed that artificial sweeteners lead to changes in the "good" bacteria in the gut, which can change glucose absorption. In the study, seven healthy volunteers developed glucose intolerance within one week of taking noncaloric sweeteners. Although this has not been fully tested, if your glucose levels or your medication needs to be increased and you consume artificial sweeteners, you should considering not using them.

A recent study revealed that **drinking wine** (150 ml per day) decreased blood sugar, HbA_{1c}, and LDL cholesterol levels. However, realize that alcohol can create a craving for more alcohol and high sugar foods, which would worsen your diabetes. So, it is important to limit your intake to one drink for women and two drinks for men daily.

Don't' Drink Your Calories

A 2015 meta-analysis in *BMJ* confirmed that regular consumption of sugar-sweetened beverages increases the risk of developing diabetes. The increased risk was 18 percent and when adjusted for weight, it was still 13 percent; this means that you don't have to be overweight to have the increased risk. Risk was also increased if consuming artificially sweetened beverages (25 percent; 8% if not overweight).

A Harvard study revealed that for each can of sugary soda consumed daily, there is a 16 percent increase in diabetes risk. In contrast, each cup of daily coffee reduced risk by 6 percent.

Although you can follow the above recommendations by yourself, it may often be difficult for you to plan well-balanced meals, especially if you have a busy schedule. I recommend that you consult with a **licensed dietitian** to help you develop a good diet plan (for referral to a dietitian specializing in diabetes, go to www.eatright.com, the website of the Academy of Nutrition and Dietetics).

Exercise is as important in diabetes as eating healthy. Exercise enhances insulin sensitivity, improves glucose tolerance, reduces serum cholesterol and triglycerides, lowers blood pressure, and helps in weight control. The heart-protective effect of exercise is particularly important.

In general, a combination of aerobic and resistance (weights) exercises have been recommended by most authorities, thirty minutes a day of moderate intensity, five days a week. However, studies differ on the level and amount of activity. One study showed that fewer regular, high-intensity intervals (three days a week with higher intensity) may actually be the best. A 2015 study in the *Annals* showed that more vigorous exercise (five days a week) is associated with better glucose tolerance than low-intensity exercise; in fact, the authors showed that just increasing the incline while walking on a treadmill or walking at a brisker pace attained a higher intensity level and was surprisingly easy to accomplish). A 2013 study in *Diabetes Care* showed that people with prediabetes can control blood sugar better with short bouts of walking after meals than with a single longer daily walk. Another study in the same journal showed that fifteen minutes of exercise after each meal is as effective as once-daily forty-five minutes of exercise.

Exercise must be tailored to your individual needs, especially if you are insulin dependent, as exercise can decrease your blood sugar levels. I recommend that you obtain guidance from your doctor and/or a fitness trainer who has expertise in working with people who have diabetes. You may need to monitor your blood sugar before and after exercise until you establish a standard routine.

Caution: Before starting an exercise program, and especially if you have not exercised before, make sure you obtain a physical examination and exercise tolerance test before beginning vigorous exercise so that you can plan an appropriate program and avoid additional complications. Start slowly with your exercising and build up gradually.

Caution: If you have complications of diabetes, avoid high-impact activities as they can cause further damage to the eyes and kidneys. Also, even small blisters that form on your feet can lead to chronic wounds or infection. Be sure to check your feet and treat any cuts, scrapes, or abrasions (topical antibiotic ointment), and go to your doctor immediately if these do not heal or if they worsen.

Preventing the Progression of Prediabetes

If you have blood sugars that are mildly elevated, you may have prediabetes (otherwise known as insulin resistance or impaired glucose tolerance). This can lead into full-blown diabetes if you don't act. Prediabetics still have increased risks for heart disease. If you do have prediabetes, this is what you should do:

- Undergo annual glucose tolerance test and microalbuminuria (protein in the urine) testing annually.
- Measure fasting blood glucose, HbA_{1c}, and cholesterol every six months.
- Reduce your weight by 5–10 percent.
- Exercise for thirty to sixty minutes five days a week.
- Follow a low-fat, high-fiber diet.
- For high-risk patients (worsening blood sugar or heart disease), start on diabetic treatment (see below).
- Although some studies show that taking various antidiabetic drugs can help prevent progression to diabetes, lifestyle changes are more effective with fewer side effects. In fact, a 2015 study shows that diabetic medications are only effective in the highest-risk patients.

Avoid certain medications: Some over-the-counter remedies contain ingredients that can cause additional problems with blood sugar levels. Aspirin can alter blood-glucose levels if taken in large amounts. Respiratory products containing phenylephrine, ephedrine, or epinephrine can raise blood sugar levels; appetite suppressants containing caffeine can do the same. According to a December 2013 study in *BMJ*, thiazide diuretics used for high blood pressure may result in a higher risk for developing diabetes, but clinical outcomes (including heart disease) may actually be better, so there may be no contraindication to using these drugs (the benefits outweigh the harm).

It is also recognized that statin drugs (for high cholesterol) may increase the risk of developing diabetes by at least 9 percent. Two 2015 studies showed the relative risk was nearly fifty percent higher in statin users. Since high cholesterol is part of the metabolic syndrome, taking statins may be valuable if you have a high risk of developing heart disease but in others, especially pre-diabetics, the risk may be greater than the benefit. So discuss this with your doctor.

You should also be aware that inhaled corticosteroids (for asthma or COPD) have been shown to not only increase the incidence of diabetes but also cause more rapid progression of diabetes. If you have these diseases, talk with your doctor about other alternatives.

Herbs for Other Conditions May Affect Blood Sugar

There are several herbs that can lower blood sugar as a side effect, which can be dangerous if you are unaware of these effects and your blood sugar goes too low (hypoglycemia). These include broom, buchu, dandelion, and juniper. If you take these herbs, monitor your blood sugar more closely.

The Conventional Approaches

Intensive Treatment for Diabetes: Actually Harmful?

Three recent studies have explored whether intensive (strict) control of diabetes is beneficial. One study was halted early because patients lowering their HbA$_{1c}$ to less than 7 percent had higher mortality. Another study revealed that intensive control does not prevent major heart problems.

A study in 2014 showed that diabetes is frequently overtreated in older adults, especially in those who have other medical conditions. Often, such overtreatment leads to hypoglycemia (low blood sugar), which can cause more serious complications.

Please note, however, that evidence suggests that *newly diagnosed* diabetics and young, healthy diabetics may benefit from intense glucose monitoring initially. Overall, experts advise that HbA$_{1c}$ should not be lowered below 7 in older patients with long-standing type 2 diabetes.

In addition, another study showed that intensive treatment of *other* factors associated with diabetes does reduce the risk of heart disease and death. These factors include using statins for cholesterol, ACE inhibitors for blood pressure, and taking aspirin (small doses).

Prescription medication(s) are the primary treatment for diabetes. For mild diabetes or glucose intolerance/insulin resistance (prediabetes), one medication may be adequate.

There are many different types of medications to treat diabetes so it is important to obtain guidance from your doctor or a diabetic specialist (endocrinologist). Depending on your situation, they may recommend one or more of the medications discussed below.

If your liver and kidney tests are normal, *metformin* (Glucophage, Fortamet) is the first most commonly prescribed. It can help prevent progression to type 2 diabetes, but a 2015 study demonstrated that only 4% of prediabetic adults are prescribed this medication. ***Important note***: Some patients cannot tolerate metformin. However, you can take it with a full meal or take the extended-release form instead, which may decrease the side effects. ***Warnings***: Metformin should not be used if you have heart failure. It can also cause Vitamin B_{12} deficiency, which worsens the longer the treatment, and thus your blood levels should be routinely tested. Finally, it increases mortality risk in patients with advanced chronic kidney disease (CDK) and is contraindicated in patients with all stages of CDK.

Dr. A's Suggestions:
Metformin Should Be the First Oral Medication Prescribed

Metformin is commonly the first oral medication prescribed for lowering glucose in type 2 diabetes, but because there are many other oral medications and a lot of pharmaceutical company marketing to promote them, doctors may prescribe another drug first.

Although these other drugs have been approved for first-line use, they should not be started first unless there are contraindications to using metformin. A 2014 study in *JAMA Intern Med* showed that patients given oral drugs other than metformin as first-line therapy are more likely to require additional treatments. In addition, compared with metformin, the other agents did not provide lower risk for cardiovascular events. In fact, sulfonylureas were actually associated with increased risk.

Most patients tolerate metformin, which has been proven to be the best first-line oral medication for type 2 diabetes and thus is recommended. If you find that metformin does not control your blood sugar, then other oral drugs can be added at that time.

If metformin alone does not reduce your HbA$_{1c}$ to normal, another antidiabetic medication is then usually added. There are numerous drugs from several classes that can be added to metformin, and different doctors may prescribe different classes. In general, to help decide which one is best for you, there are several factors that need to be taken into account, including:

- How much reduction in HbA$_{1c}$
- Weight changes (most antidiabetic medications can cause weight gain)
- Reduction in blood lipids (i.e., cholesterol)
- Effects on mortality and cardiovascular events
- Effects on kidneys
- Adverse side effects
- Clinical utility: cost, complexity of use (most of the newer medications may be very expensive and more difficult to dose)

The following are the additional classes of antidiabetic medications that may be added or substituted for metformin. Frequently, some doctors may start you on one of these as initial therapy (see sidebar above).

If your liver and kidney tests are normal and you are *normal weight*, a *sulfonylurea* (Glyburide, Glipizide) may be prescribed. The major side effect is hypoglycemia (blood sugar too low). ***Cautions***: These drugs can interact with trimethoprim (urinary antibiotic), cimetidine (Tagamet, antiulcer), alcohol, and anticoagulants (blood thinners), all of which can increase the chances of hypoglycemia if you take them with sulfonylureas. They can also cause weight gain. You need to know that not all sulfonylureas are the same: glipizide has been proven to be safe in a long-term study.

Important note: If urine testing detects microalbuminuria (too much albumin in the urine), you should take an ACE inhibitor (such as captopril, analapril) along with the sulfonylurea.

If the above medications are not effective or have intolerable side effects, then your doctor may prescribe an *alpha-glucosidase inhibitor* (acarbose, miglitol). These drugs have a high rate of side effects of flatulence, diarrhea, and abdominal cramps, but these effects tend to go away with further use or if the medication is started in a low dose.

Other antidiabetic medications include *thiazolidinediones* (called TZDs for short). These include Actos (pioglitazone) and Avandia (rosiglitazone) as well as combinations of these with other antidiabetic drugs. This class is designed as an "insulin sensitizer" as it improves glucose control while lowering insulin levels. They also may reduce high blood pressure and cholesterol defects associated with insulin resistance. A recent study showed that they are able to slow down the progression of coronary artery disease better than sulfonylureas.

Warning: Taking TZDs for more than a year can increase fracture risk, especially in women, so bone densities should be monitored, and you should avoid taking them if you are prone to falls. They can also cause significant weight gain and swelling in the legs, and a study in 2011 linked them to increased risk of bladder cancer when used for more than twelve months. However, a more recent study in 2015 showed this risk to be minimal but did show a potentially increased risk for pancreatic and prostate cancers.

Five-Year Failure Rate with Diabetic Drugs

Many diabetic drugs may lose their effectiveness within five years or even sooner. A recent study revealed that the percentage of patients with inadequate blood-sugar control at five years was 34 percent with glyburide (a sulfonylurea), 21 percent with metformin, and 34 percent with Avandia.

Several new medications have been developed and are usually used if the above drugs aren't beneficial or along with the above drugs for added benefit. *Dipeptidyl peptidase-4 inhibitors (DPP-4s)*, also commonly called *gliptins*, are one such class. Sitagliptin (Januvia) is the most common, but there are also alogliptin, saxagliptin, and others. These gliptins are safe but reduce $HgbA_{1c}$ only by about 0.3 percent and they do not demonstrate a cardiovascular benefit. In fact, the FDA has backed new safety warnings due to increased risk of heart failure for two of these drugs, saxagliptin (Onglyza) and alogliptin (Nesina). They cost almost $4,000 per year. They are often added to other diabetic drugs, such as metformin, as a second line. A recently approved drug is linagliptin (Tradjenta), which has the same mechanism as Januvia, but it has not been compared to other diabetic drugs. ***Important note***: The FDA is investigating a possible increased risk for heart failure associated with saxigliptin.

Another class of drugs is called *GLP-1 antagonists*. The primary drug in this class, Victoza, appears to be more effective than Januvia, and it can be given once a day. Neither drug, however, improves blood-vessel problems, and Victoza also has an increased risk for pancreatitis and thyroid C-cell tumors. However, Victoza has been demonstrated to help reduce weight in diabetics (25 percent of patients lost more than 10 percent of their body weight over a year). Another GLP-1 agonist newly approved is dulagatide (Trulicity), which can be given by injection once a week. It can be used alone or in combination with other drugs.

Other GLP-1 medications include Byetta and Symli. These are also given by injection under the skin (subcutaneous). A recent study has shown that Byetta given once a week is better than daily injections of insulin glargine (see below) for both blood-sugar control and weight loss; and another study showed it is also superior to Januvia or Actos. In addition, Byetta also helps patients lose weight, whereas insulin can cause weight gain. ***Caution***: Byetta has recently been reported to cause pancreatitis in rare cases.

The latest approved drugs are called *SGLT2 inhibitors* (canagliflozin [Invokana], empagliflozin [Jardiance], and dapagliflozin [Farxigal]), which block the reabsorption of glucose by the kidney. However, the FDA mandated post marketing studies to evaluate various problems, including heart problems, fractures, and bladder cancer. The most common side effects are genital fungal infections and urinary tract infections. ***Warnings***: the FDA in May, 2015 warned that these drugs may cause ketoacidosis occurring within two weeks of taking the drug. (Ketoacidosis lowers the pH of your body and causes very high blood sugars. It requires hospitalization and can be lethal. Symptoms include nausea, vomiting, abdominal pain, fatigue, and difficulty breathing). In November 2015 it also warned that urinary tract infections caused by the drugs could develop into potentially lethal kidney infections.

Many of the above classes of drugs are now being combined together and sold as separate drugs, advertising that the combination is more effective than each drug separately. Although this may be true, these drugs are very expensive and may not have any advantage over less costly diabetic drugs.

Dr. A's Suggestions:
Costs for Diabetic Medications Much Higher Now

Drug costs for diabetics have nearly doubled in just six years, caused by the use of newer, more costly drugs, despite a lack of strong evidence that the new drugs are more beneficial or even safe. This study was published in the *Archives of Internal Medicine*, and an expert panel recommended that doctors should use older, cheaper drugs first.

Insulin is necessary if the above drugs don't control your blood sugar levels. Also, if your blood sugar is above 250, oral medications are usually not effective, and insulin is often started first.

Insulin is injected under the skin (subcutaneously). Some doctors prescribe insulin in combination with oral or other subcutaneous medications, but this is more expensive and usually has no distinct advantage over insulin alone. In fact, a study in the *NEJM* in June 2014 revealed that insulin plus metformin is associated with higher all-cause mortality than sulfonylureas plus metformin.

There are short, intermediate, and long-acting forms of insulin and several different sources (pork, human, RNA). There are also several new forms of insulin, including an inhaled rapid onset form called Afrezza, which allows for faster absorption of insulin. Insulin can cause hypoglycemia and weight gain.

Insulin May Be Better for *New* Diabetics

A recent study compared using intensive insulin treatment (continuous pump infusion or multiple daily injections) against oral medications for newly diagnosed type 2 diabetes. With insulin, control of blood sugar was obtained better and faster; and at one year, half of the patients required no medication, as opposed to only a fourth of those on oral medications.

Because there are so many types of insulin, various combinations can be beneficial. Sliding-scale insulin, in which you measure your blood sugar before every meal and at bedtime and inject short-acting or regular insulin, is burdensome and should be used primarily for initial determination of insulin needs or if hospitalized. The newest combination is using a long-acting insulin at night with a short-acting insulin at mealtimes (called basal-bolus). However, an older approach is using a combination of NPH (intermediate acting) with regular insulin twice daily. This has been shown by studies to still be as beneficial as the basal-bolus approach as well as being much less expensive.

The most recent insulins approved by the FDA are long-lasting drugs; Tresiba is injected once a day but doesn't need to be injected at the same time every day. Ryzodeg 70/30 is a combination long-acting insulin that requires two injections a day. However, most experts state that there is no additional benefit of these insulins over currently existing long-acting insulins and they are expensive.

Aspirin (81 mg is sufficient) is usually recommended daily if you have diabetes, to lower the risk for heart disease. *Caution*: If you take aspirin, you should avoid taking ibuprofen, which blocks the blood-thinning effects of aspirin. If you must take ibuprofen, take the aspirin first and wait at least two hours to take the ibuprofen so that the aspirin has time to exert its beneficial effects. Also, aspirin use can deplete body stores of vitamin C, so replacement by diet or supplementation may be necessary at 600 mg per day. If aspirin irritates your stomach, take a proton pump inhibitor with it.

Finally, **weight-loss (bariatric) surgery** is indicated for grossly obese patients with diabetes. Studies reveal that 75 percent of patients who undergo bariatric surgery see their disease disappear completely. It is not just the weight loss that does this; the surgery also alters the GI tract and apparently affects hormones that, in turn, affect blood sugar. Those with milder disease and the most weight loss fare the best.

There are two basic types of bariatric surgery: placing a band around the stomach (reversible) and rerouting the intestines. The latter seems to improve diabetes faster. However, such surgeries do have complications, including nutritional deficiencies and even death (although rare). The surgery costs $25,000, although some insurance carriers cover the procedure. In the future, doctors are looking at intestines-only surgery, which is simpler and may be more effective, with fewer complications. (See section on weight loss for further discussion of these procedures).

The Alternative Approaches

Be Careful of Claims That Supplements Can Treat or Cure Diabetes

There are many supplements and herbs that may help reduce blood sugar or help prevent or control the side effects of diabetes, but be wary of claims that such products can treat, cure, prevent, or mitigate the disease.

The FDA recently cracked down on fifteen companies that made such claims, finding that most of their products contained ingredients that are unproven and potentially unsafe or contained undeclared pharmaceutical ingredients in unknown quantities.

It is advisable to consult with a naturopathic physician with training in diabetic care before wasting your money on these products.

Certain **nutritional supplements** have been shown to help control and decrease blood sugar and may reduce complications from diabetes. In general, you should obtain the following amounts on a daily basis, from a combination of diet and supplementation:

- Vitamin C, in divided doses of 1,000 mg twice per day
- Vitamin E, 800–1,200 IU
- Vitamin B_{12}, 1,000 mcg
- Vitamin B_6, 100 mg
- Niacin, 1,200–3,000 mg

- Mixed flavonoids, 1,000–2000 mg
- Flaxseed oil, 1 Tbsp, freshly ground
- Zinc, 30 mg

There are two minerals, *magnesium* (700 daily) mg and *chromium* (200 mg twice daily for up to three months) that have received special interest because diabetics are often deficient in these minerals. You should certainly consider supplementation if you are low, but if you have normal levels, it is not known whether or not supplementation will help lower blood sugar.

Low *magnesium* occurs in 25–38 percent of patients and such levels are associated with a more rapid decline in renal function in patients with type 2 diabetes. However, the results of clinical studies using magnesium supplements in patients with type 2 diabetes have been mixed, with some studies showing that magnesium can decrease fasting blood glucose and improve insulin sensitivity and others showing no effect.

Chromium picolinate (200 mcg per day) has been shown to increase insulin sensitivity and binding and can lower blood sugar, primarily if you are deficient in this mineral. Some clinical research shows that patients who take chromium have reduced blood glucose levels, insulin levels, and HbA_{1c}, but much of this research is from small-scale, poor-quality trials, so it is not really known if it is beneficial if your chromium levels are normal. However, a trial run might be worthwhile, especially if you have a poor diet. Unlike magnesium, blood tests for chromium are difficult to obtain. You should see a decrease in blood sugar within three months. **Caution**: Chromium interferes with thyroid drugs and should be taken several hours after taking such drugs.

The antioxidant effects of *selenium* have been thought to be beneficial for both prevention and treatment of diabetes. However, recent studies show that taking selenium alone may significantly *increase* type 2 diabetes over an eight-year period. Fortunately, taking it with vitamin E negated this effect, so if you take it, always take another antioxidant with it. Limit your intake to 200 mcg daily.

A registered dietitian can help you determine whether your diet provides proper amounts of all these nutrients, which is the most effective way to take them. If your diet is poor, then consider supplementation. It may take one to two months to notice any glucose-lowering effects.

There are also several **herbs** that have been noted to decrease and help regulate blood sugar, as well as to make the body's cells more responsive to insulin. They include:

- *Gymnema sylvestre extract*, 200–400 mg daily, appears to increase endogenous insulin production. Initial research shows that taking 200 mg/day of a specific gymnema extract called GS4 seems to cut the required insulin dose in half and lower HbA_{1c} in both type 1 and type 2 diabetes. When GS4 400 mg was taken with conventional hypoglycemic drugs, such as glyburide or tolbutamide, some people were able to reduce the dose or even discontinue their conventional hypoglycemic drug. Whether other Gymnema extracts can do the same is unknown, but it may be worth a try.

- *Banaba extracts* comes from a species of crepe myrtle containing corosolic acid and ellagitannins that seem to have an insulin-like effect and also activate insulin receptors. Initial research shows that type 2 diabetes patients who take a specific banaba extract (Glucosol) for two weeks have an average of 10 percent lower blood glucose levels than patients receiving placebo. Whether other banaba extracts can do the same or if taking it longer is more effective is unknown.
- *Bitter melon*, three to six ounces of fresh juice daily, seems to improve glucose control and decrease HbA_{1c}.
- *Defatted fenugreek powder*, 15–50 g daily, has been found to enhance insulin release and lower glucose levels after eating. This might be due to a bulk laxative effect, slowing carbohydrate absorption from the GI tract.
- *Cinnamon* received a lot of attention when a study from 2004 suggested that taking 1–6 grams (1 tsp = 4.75 grams) could lower fasting blood glucose by 18–29 percent. Another study showed that 1 gram daily could decrease HbA_{1c}. ***Important note***: It should be noted that only one type of cinnamon does this—cassia cinnamon: other types of cinnamon have no significant effect on blood glucose or HbA_{1c}.
- *White mulberry leaf extract* inhibits certain enzymes in the gut, which prevents digestion of carbohydrates, similar to diabetic drugs acarbose (Precose) and miglitol (Glyset). Studies have shown that taking a white mulberry leaf powder, 1 gram three times daily for four weeks, significantly reduced fasting blood glucose by about 27 percent in patients with type 2 diabetes. However, the evidence is considered insufficient at this time to recommend this supplement.
- *Berberine* (500 mg two to three times daily) may lower blood sugar equally as well as metformin and has fewer side effects. It also improves cholesterol ratios. ***Caution***: It should not be used during pregnancy and may enhance blood-thinning effects.

Using these herbs, you should see a decrease in blood sugar within one to two months, and you may be able to take them together, although that could become more expensive than taking conventional medications. If you don't see lowering of blood sugar after that time, they won't be effective. ***Warning***: Minerals, herbs, and supplements may enhance the effects of conventional medications for diabetes and thus drop your blood sugar rapidly. Always monitor your blood sugar closely when first adding a supplement.

Chinese herbs can also affect blood sugar. *Zuo Gui Wan You Gui Yin* in combination with *Zhi Bai Di Huang Wan* may help reduce and regulate blood sugar, as along with reducing symptoms excessive thirst and urination. Another good Chinese herb to decrease blood sugar is from the *Chinese crepe myrtle. Du Huo Ji Sheng Tang* is a kidney tonifier that helps boost energy, retard aging, and increases immunity. You should observe initial benefits from Chinese herbal formulas within three to six weeks (sometimes sooner), but you may need to take them longer, depending on your condition. Consult with a TCM practitioner before taking these formulas.

Panax ginseng (200 mg daily, containing 37 percent ginsenosides) has also been found to help decrease and regulate blood sugar and HbA_{1c}. *American ginseng* (3 g two hours before a meal) can reduce blood sugar after eating. When taking either form of ginseng, make sure that you get the highest levels of ginsenosides.

Acupuncture has been used for centuries to reduce blood sugar, and it can be used in addition to herbs. One of the main acupuncture points is on the middle back, called "pancreas hollow" because it helps control pancreatic function. You should observe improvement within six acupuncture treatments, but you might need additional sessions for maximum benefit.

Yoga is beneficial for diabetes. A recent study revealed that it can reverse the clinical and biochemical changes associated with metabolic syndrome, including lowering blood sugar.

Your Empowered Patient Plan for Treating Diabetes

- **Important note**: *You should have your liver enzymes and creatinine levels tested (reflects kidney function). If they are abnormal, you should consider starting insulin (step 9) and then return to step 1.*
- *If your fasting blood sugar is significantly elevated (greater than 140), or your $HgbA_{1c}$ is greater than 7, start at step 9 and then return to step 1.*

Step #1:   *Exercise and a diet specific for diabetes* should always be followed, no matter what your blood sugar is. These lifestyle changes may be all you need to control your blood sugar, especially if you are a prediabetic or have metabolic syndrome.

Step #2:   *Perform yoga* if you have metabolic syndrome to help prevent the onset of diabetes.

Step #3:   *Take an aspirin* a day to help prevent heart disease unless you have contraindications to its use.

Step #4:   *Make sure you obtain the following preventive exams*: yearly eye, foot, and general exams and blood sugar monitoring every three to four months.

Step #5:   *Take chromium* and *magnesium* if your blood levels are low.

Step #6:   ***Consider metformin*** to prevent further progression if you have mild diabetes (Glucose <140) or are borderline diabetic.

Step #7:   ***Try a strong whole food–based multivitamin along with gymnema sylvestre, bitter melon, defatted fenugreek, banaba, cassia cinnamon and/or American ginseng*** if you are *prediabetic* or *borderline* and/or you don't want to take metformin. You can try each separately or several together in a combination product. If your blood sugar has not decreased, proceed with the next step. These herbs may be preferred over diabetic medications due to fewer side effects and less resistance. However, they may be more costly than metformin if you have insurance.

Step #8:   ***Take the Chinese herbal remedies Zuo Gui Wan You Gui Yin, Zhi Bai Di Huang Wan, and/or Chinese crepe myrtle*** instead of the above herbs if your blood sugar still shows *mild* elevation. If your blood sugar has not decreased after taking these, proceed with the next step.

When Nathan came to see me, his blood sugar was over three hundred, and he was not following a good diet or getting exercise. He was taking two oral diabetic medications. Besides urging him to diet and exercise, I started him on a combination of vitamins, minerals, and herbals to decrease his glucose (steps 6 and 7). After much urging, he finally started an exercise program and the HCF diet. After three months, he started losing weight, and I was able to start reducing the dosage of his medications. He continued taking the vitamins and herbs, and after one year, he was able to discontinue the conventional medications completely.

Step #9:   ***Take a prescription oral medication***: If your blood sugar continues to increase and you are on metformin, take an additional diabetic medication. Because there are so many different drugs and combinations of drugs, not to mention ways to take the drugs, it is important to consult with a diabetes specialist to determine the best drug(s) for you. For recently diagnosed diabetes, you may want to consider short-term intensive insulin therapy before starting oral medications.

Step #10: ***Take insulin*** if your blood sugar is still not controlled on oral medications. As with the oral medications, there are many different types and forms of insulin, so consult with a diabetes specialist.

Step #11: Once again, you can ***try gymnema sylvestre, bitter melon, defatted fenugreek, banaba, cassia cinnamon and/or American ginseng*** if you still have difficulties maintaining a normal blood sugar, if you have side effects of medication, or do not want to take injections. Try one at a time to see if they will decrease your blood sugar and if so, you can decrease the medication dosage. ***Caution***: Be sure to monitor your blood sugar while you are trying these to avoid hypoglycemia. If your blood sugar is well controlled on medications, however, it may be better and less expensive to continue taking them alone.

*Step #12: **Undergo acupuncture*** if you still have problems controlling your blood sugar. If your blood sugar is lowered, you again can decrease the dose of your medication(s).

*Step #13: **Consider undergoing bariatric surgery*** if you are obese.

Expected Outcome

Diabetes is a disease that can be adequately controlled using a combination of preventive, conventional, and/or alternative methods. There is no reason diabetes should interfere with your life or for you to develop complications if you follow the above steps. Diabetes can be prevented at an early stage with weight loss and exercise—or by bariatric surgery if you are obese. If you do suffer from complications, these also can be controlled, as discussed below.

Complications of Diabetes

There are several complications of diabetes that can affect other systems of the body, thus requiring additional treatments. The primary complications are retinopathy (eye), foot problems due to decreased blood supply (primarily infections, ulcers and gangrene), neuropathy (peripheral nerve dysfunction of the lower legs), and heart disease. (For heart disease, see the section on coronary heart disease).

Another complication that is usually unrecognized yet may occur in type 1 diabetes includes *cheiroarthropathy*, which involves thickened skin and limited mobility of hand and finger joints, as well as upper-extremity problems such as frozen shoulder, tendinitis, carpal tunnel, and dupytren's contractures. All of these may be improved or resolved using alternative methods such as acupuncture and low level energy laser (LLEL) (see specific sections on those topics).

Prevention—by strictly maintaining healthy blood-glucose levels—is the best way to avoid complications of diabetes. If complications do occur, however, the following treatments may help with specific conditions.

Treatments for Neuropathy

Neuropathy is a common side effect of diabetes and is thought to be caused by injury to the small blood vessels that supply the nerves of the lower legs and feet. Although the risk increases the more your blood sugar is not controlled, it may occur even with well-controlled diabetes.

The Preventive Approaches

A recent study revealed that long-term *aerobic exercise training* can prevent the onset of neuropathy and improve nerve function in those who already have neuropathy.

The Conventional Approaches

Medications are the primary conventional treatment. The latest guidelines from the American Academy of Neurology recommend the following:

- *Pregabalin* (Lyrica) has level A evidence (the best), but these trials only showed small benefits over placebo. The remaining drugs have level B or C evidence. *Warnings*: Pregabalin does have warnings of causing suicidal tendencies. A recent study from *Neurology* also found that significant neurotoxicity and negative cognitive (thinking) effects occurred with the use of pregabalin, especially when using over 600 mg a day.
- *Anticonvulsants*: Gabapentin (Neurontin), valproate.
- *Antidepressants*: Amitryptiline, venlaxafine, duloxetine. Venlaxafine can be added to gabapentin.
- *Opioids*: Tramadol, oxycodone, morphine, and so on.
- *Skin patches*: Lidoderm, capsaicin.

At present, only pregabalin and duloxetine are FDA-approved for treating diabetic neuropathy. It may take several weeks to observe benefits with any of these medications. ***Important note***: A recent meta-analysis on drugs for diabetic neuropathy revealed that although many of them were statistically superior to placebo, the benefits were minimal, there were few head-to-head comparisons, and most drugs had significant side effects.

Novel Drug May Help Diabetic Neuropathy?

Pentoxifylline (PTX) is a prescription drug approved by the FDA to treat peripheral vascular disease as it improves the flow properties of blood. Those who have diabetes experience accelerated circulatory deficit, which can affect the nerves. In a study on diabetic rats back in 2000, just two weeks of PTX administration improved nerve conduction from 50 percent to 70 percent. However, no studies have been performed on humans.

Electrical devices: Transcutaneous electrostimulation is sometimes successful in relieving some of the pain associated with neuropathy. This device is called a *"rebuilder"* (much like a TENs unit) and is available through a doctor's prescription and can be used at home.

Another electrical device is *H-wave*, which uses different frequencies of electricity than TENS units and also may be effective. These machines are located primarily in California but not in many other areas of the country. However, you can also purchase a home unit.

The Alternative Approaches

Acupuncture is very effective for reducing or even resolving the symptoms of diabetic neuropathy in the majority of patients. You should experience improvement within six acupuncture treatments, but you might need additional sessions for maximum benefit.

The **low level energy laser** ("cold" laser or LLEL) can also significantly reduce symptoms of neuropathy by the apparent healing and regeneration of the damaged nerves. It addresses the underlying cause of the neuropathy and thus can provide long-term relief. It may take between four and eight treatments to obtain benefit and can be used with acupuncture.

There are also various **nutritional supplements** that are beneficial as well. Results may take one to three months to manifest.

- *Alpha-lipoic acid* (ALA), considered a "super-antioxidant," has been used for twenty-five years in Germany to treat diabetic neuropathy and has been demonstrated to decrease numbness and pain in neuropathy after three weeks of treatment, but this is with *intravenous* use. *Oral* alpha-lipoic acid (600–1,200 mg per day) can improve nerve conduction and decrease serum glucose and also has now been shown to provide a significant regression of neuropathic symptoms. You should observe results in one to two months.
- *Gamma-linoleic acid* (GLA) can also improve neuropathy if given long enough to work, often at least a year, although it may be beneficial in several months. Evening primrose oil (480 mg daily) is the most commonly used, but you may want to take borage oil (1 g daily) instead because it is less expensive and contains a greater percentage of GLA.
- *Acetyl-L-carnitine* ((1,500–3,000 mg daily; for example, 1,000 mg two to three times per day) is known to have neuroprotective properties and has been shown to limit the neuropathy associated with diabetes and provide significant reduction in pain.

- *N-acetylcysteine* (NAC) is a powerful antioxidant and a precursor to glutathione, an intrinsic antioxidant. Animal studies have shown that N-acetylcysteine can inhibit diabetic neuropathy.
- *Vitamin B$_1$* (thiamin) and *benfotiamine* (the fat-soluble form of vitamin B$_1$) have been used to treat diabetic neuropathy.
- *Vitamin B$_6$* inhibits glycosylation of proteins, one of the major risk factors for developing diabetic neuropathy. Diabetes patients with neuropathy have been shown to be deficient in vitamin B$_6$ and to benefit from supplementation. Interestingly, the neuropathy caused by vitamin B$_6$ deficiency is indistinguishable from diabetic neuropathy.
- *Vitamin B$_{12}$* supplementation also may have beneficial effects on diabetic neuropathy. There are several forms of B$_{12}$, and the methylcobalamin form appears to be the most effective form of vitamin B$_{12}$ to protect the nerves.
- *Combination*: A recent study published in *Pain Management* concluded that the under consumption of various micronutrients leads to complications of diabetes. In this study, a combination of several nutrients improved neuropathy significantly, especially the burning pain. These included N-acetylcysteine (1–2 g daily), alpha-lipoic acid, L-carnitine (2 grams twice daily), vitamin C (2,000 mg daily), and selenium (200 mcg daily). Symptoms were reduced in one month but reached maximum effectiveness in three months.

Your Empowered Patient Action Plan for Treating Diabetic Neuropathy

*Step #1: **Undergo acupuncture***: This is your best bet for long term resolution and is the most cost effective.

Step #2: ***Undergo cold laser treatment.*** This device also can provide long-term relief and can be used with acupuncture for greater effectiveness.

Step #3: ***Try H-wave stimulation*** or use the ***Rebuilder*** for long-term relief if acupuncture is not effective. ***Transcutaneous electrostimulation*** may also be tried.

Step #4: ***Take nutritional supplements***: Try any of the above supplements alone or in combination, but give them several months to see if they're effective. They may be more effective than medications, with fewer side effects.

Step #5: ***Take a prescription medication***: Pregabalin, low-dose prescription tricyclic antidepressant, or gabapentin may help some patients if the above steps have not helped. However, if you have no benefit within six weeks, these are unlikely to benefit you.

Step #6: ***Consider the use of Pentoxifylline (PTX)*** under the guidance of a doctor if nothing else has helped.

Treatments for Retinopathy

Diabetic retinopathy is a complication of diabetes that results from damage to the blood vessels of the light-sensitive tissue at the back of the eye (retina). At first, diabetic retinopathy may cause no symptoms or only mild vision problems. Eventually, however, diabetic retinopathy can result in blindness.

Diabetic retinopathy can develop in anyone who has type 1 or type 2 diabetes. It affects up to 80 percent of all patients who have had diabetes for ten years or more. The longer you have diabetes, and the less controlled your blood sugar is, the more likely you are to develop diabetic retinopathy.

The Preventive Approaches

Research indicates that at least 90 percent of new retinopathy cases could be reduced if there was proper, vigilant treatment and monitoring of the eyes. It is important to receive yearly eye exams if you have diabetes.

Diet: Carotenoids and antioxidants that can improve vision and help prevent vision loss are high in certain food sources like carrots, butternut squash, raspberries, and blueberries.

The Conventional Approaches

Photocoagulation will be necessary if your retinopathy is severe. This procedure uses high-energy laser to seal leaky blood vessels.

Medications: ACE inhibitors (lisinopril, enalapril…those ending in "pril") and angiotensin-receptor blockers (ARBs; losartan, candasartan…those ending in "sartan"), primarily used to control blood pressure, have been shown to reduce the development of retinopathy in type 1 diabetes and may promote regression of the condition in type 2 diabetes.

Injections: The FDA has now approved two types of injectable medication for diabetic macular edema (swelling); ranibizumab (Lucentis) and afibercept (Eylea), which have been found to produce significant improvement in retinopathy severity compared to laser-based treatment. *Caution*: There can be serious side effects involved with these injections, including eye pain, cataracts, infection and retinal detachment.

The Alternative Approaches

Nutritional supplements containing bilberry (160 mg extract twice daily) may be very helpful if your retinopathy is mild. There are several products that combine bilberry with mixed carotenoids, which may be more effective than bilberry alone. Lutein and zinc may also be beneficial. These supplements protect the eye through their antioxidant effects. You should notice better vision within one to two months.

Your Empowered Patient Action Plan for Treating Diabetic Retinopathy

Step #1: Take bilberry, lutein, and mixed carotenoids if you have mild disease to prevent progression or with severe disease to improve vision and further halt progression.

Step #2: Take ACE inhibitors or ARBs if progression continues, but discontinue if no benefit is observed.

Step #3: Receive photocoagulation if your retinopathy progresses.

Treatments for Nephropathy (Kidney Disease)

Nephropathy means damage to the kidneys, especially the small blood vessels that supply the glomeruli, the structures that filter waste from the blood; high blood sugar from diabetes can destroy these structures. Not everyone with diabetes will develop kidney damage, but it may cause kidney failure in some diabetic patients if not detected and treated early.

Certain factors may increase the risk of developing diabetic nephropathy, including high blood pressure, high cholesterol, or if you smoke. Also, Native Americans, African Americans, and Hispanics (especially Mexican Americans) have a higher risk.

The Preventive Approaches

Diet and nutrient balance can manage nephropathy in the early stages. I highly recommend consultation with a registered dietitian first to help you understand and plan what you need to eat for optimum kidney health, since an imbalance of protein, lipids, sodium, vitamins, minerals, and fluids can make kidney function worse. Adding soy products to your diet may provide needed protein as well as improving kidney function.

Important Information:
Avoid B Vitamins in Nephropathy

B vitamins are often given to decrease homocysteine, an amino acid that is elevated in kidney disease and can cause blood vessel and heart problems and thus may reduce kidney and vascular (blood vessel) complications of diabetes. However, a recent study showed that B vitamins can make kidney function *worse* in diabetics with nephropathy and does not reduce the vascular complications.

The Conventional Approaches

Medications: If your urine tests show that you have proteinuria (excessive protein in your urine), an *ACE inhibitor* (lisinopril, enalapril...those ending in "pril") or an angiotensin receptor blocker (*ARB*, such as losartan, candasartan...those ending in "sartan") is usually prescribed as they supposedly reduce the risk of kidney failure. However, a recent study in the *NEJM* showed that treatment with these drugs did not *prevent* the development of nephropathy. Another drug, *aliskiren* (Tekturna), reduces proteinuria by 20 percent, but it is not yet known if it can reduce kidney failure or heart problems. ***Important Note***: Some people may have the side effect of cough from ACE inhibitors. If you get a cough, take low-dose ibuprofen (200–600 mg per day), which can block the cough in many patients.

Dialysis is required for severe nephropathy to take over the filtering functions of the damaged kidneys. Dialysis requires the creation of an arteriovenous fistula (surgical attachment of a vein to an artery, usually in the forearm) and then weekly or more frequent sessions in which your blood is cleaned of toxins through a dialysis machine. Because this process leaches many important nutrients from your system along with the toxins, your doctor will have these nutrients replaced in the dialysis solution.

The Alternative Approaches

Nutritional supplements and Chinese herbs may be beneficial in stages 3 and 4 of chronic kidney disease, as detailed below.

- *Flaxseed* (1 Tbsp per day, freshly ground) promotes kidney function, due to its effects in preventing artery disease and correcting defects in fatty-acid metabolism seen in people with diabetes. Because of these effects, it may also help prevent heart disease. However, avoid taking the oil or capsules as they deteriorate very quickly.
- *Astragalus* can increase kidney flow, protects the kidney and addresses erythropoietin deficiency.
- *Baking soda* can slow the progression to end-stage renal disease and improve glomerular filtration rate (GFR).
- *Cordyceps sinensis* (Chinese herb) helps protect renal tube damage.
- *Curcumin* can improve kidney function.
- *Melatonin* may reduce oxidative stress, decrease protein in the urine and increases GFR.
- *Omega-3 fatty acids* (fish oil) may improve survival and reduce protein in the urine.

Your Empowered Patient Action Plan for Treating Nephropathy

- **Important note:** *Have your urine checked for microalbuminuria every three to six months. This is the most sensitive test to detect early kidney problems. If abnormal, you should have your creatinine and twenty-four-hour protein and creatinine clearance checked every year.*
- *For further information, see section on Chronic Kidney Disease (CKD)*

Step #1: Make dietary changes to support kidney health to prevent progression of kidney damage. Consult with a registered dietician.

Step #2: Take prescription ACE inhibitors or ARBs to reduce the risk of kidney failure.

Step #3: Take flaxseed (freshly ground) and/or other *nutritional supplements* to promote kidney function.

Step #4: Receive dialysis if your kidneys fail.

Treatments for Diabetic Foot Problems

Diabetes can damage both blood vessels and nerves in the feet. I have already described the treatments for the nerve damage (neuropathy) above, but such a condition can cause your feet to be numb, making it easier to damage without you being aware of it. Along with poor blood flow, such damage can lead to numerous complications, including infections, ulcers and even gangrene (cell death).

The Preventive Approaches

Good foot care and avoiding injury are the best means of preventing foot ulcers. If you do injure your feet, see your regular or diabetes doctor immediately. You should avoid footwear that is constricting.

The Conventional Approaches

Appropriate conventional **wound care** is necessary if an ulcer starts forming. This may include *wound debridement* (removing any dead tissue), appropriate *antibiotics*, and/or *hyperbaric oxygen* treatment. You will likely need *surgery* (amputation) if the ulcer progresses into gangrene, which is caused by the tissue dying and turning black.

A pharmaceutical gel, **becaplermin** (Regranex), has been used to treat ulcers that are not healing, but it has recently been linked to increasing the risk for cancer if used frequently.

The Alternative Approaches

Low level energy lasers ("cold" laser or *LLELs*) are very effective for healing diabetic ulcers by stimulating the damaged cells to heal more quickly and increasing blood flow to the foot. It can also help prevent the development of dry gangrene (non-infectious). You should observe results within one to two weeks.

Acupuncture can also be effective to stimulate blood flow and tissue healing. You should see improvement within six acupuncture treatments, but might need additional sessions for maximum benefits. Acupuncture can be used with the cold laser for faster results.

Your Empowered Patient Action Plan for Treating Diabetic Foot Problems

Step #1: Use good foot care to prevent foot problems in the first place.

Step #2: Receive conventional wound care initially to prevent progression, but add the next steps at the same time to accelerate healing.

Step #3: Undergo low-energy laser treatment: This should accelerate the healing of the ulcer and improve blood circulation.

Step #4: Undergo acupuncture: This can be also done with the above steps for faster and more effective results.

Ethel had diabetes most of her life, and at age seventy-six, she developed dry gangrene (noninfectious disease of tissue from lack of circulation) in several of her toes. Her doctor told her she would need them amputated, but she wanted to do anything to avoid amputation as it would make her wheelchair-bound. I started treating her with LLEL, and after eight treatments, her circulation improved significantly, and most of the gangrenous tissue sloughed off, leaving normal tissue. She did not require amputation.

End-of-Life Care

What You Need to Know

As we approach the end of life, there are special considerations that occur regarding medical care. In many instances, we are not well prepared to deal with these issues, which can cause significant chaos and pain.

End-of-life care used to be considered primarily for cancer patients, but in fact it includes many other terminal illnesses as well as frail individuals, who also can experience more falls, functional impairment, and hospitalization.

Important Information:
Nonbeneficial Treatments Provided to Many Intensive-Care Patients

Critical care doctors at UCLA reviewed the care and outcomes of critically ill patients over a three-month period and found that 11 percent definitely received futile treatment. They suspected another 8.6 percent also received nonbeneficial care. This was borne out by the fact that 68 percent died during hospitalization, and survivors were left in severely compromised health and often dependent on life support.

The doctors' conclusions were based on perceptions that the burdens to the patients, their families, and their care providers definitely outweighed the benefits. Other reasons were that treatment could never reach the patient's goals, death was imminent, and the patient could never survive outside an ICU. Costs amounted to $2.6 million over that three month period.

UCLA is certainly not the only hospital where this occurs; it happens in all hospitals. Just because we have great technology that can prolong survival doesn't mean that you won't suffer and receive needless care. Doctors usually know if you or a loved one fit into this category. Such patients are usually sicker, older, or transferred from nursing homes or long-term-care hospitals. Communication of costs and benefits is the key, but the parties involved are usually reluctant to have that type of discussion.

The key phrase for end of life is *palliative care*, which refers to any form of medical care or treatment that concentrates on reducing the severity of disease symptoms rather than on halting or delaying progression of the disease itself or providing a cure. The goal is to prevent and relieve suffering and to improve quality of life for people facing serious, complex illness.

Caregivers: A Difficult But Often Rewarding Task

Caregivers are essential to take care of patients who are chronically ill or disabled. Caregiving can be very stressful, though, and many studies have found that caregivers' health and well-being can be affected adversely.

However, other studies have shown no adverse health effects and indicate that it may even help people live longer. In a study published in the *American*

Journal of Epidemiology, caregivers had an 18 percent lower mortality rate than noncaregivers. This was especially true when taking care of an elderly parent and when there were low levels of need.

Understandably, when the patient is capable and does express gratitude, caregivers have greater self-esteem and recognition by others.

As death looms, there are a few conditions that commonly occur. Treating these conditions will vastly facilitate a dignified passing and improved quality of life until that event occurs. The major issues include depression, dyspnea (difficulty breathing), and pain. In fact, it has been well documented that there is a high prevalence of pain during the last two years of life, and especially the last few months. Other complications may include loss of strength, fatigue, and weight loss.

Avoid Medical Tests and Procedures at End of Life

Too often, all sorts of medical procedures as well as screenings (PSA, mammograms, colonoscopy, heart, cholesterol) are done that may not benefit us and are done just because they are available. Such procedures are not only expensive but can also cause more pain and discomfort than we already have and lead to further tests and treatments that are unnecessary. If you or a loved one do not have long to live or are frail, avoid these tests.

Treatments for End of Life

The Preventive Approaches

It may seem strange to include prevention with end-of-life care, but this means that you and your family should prepare for end of life as much as possible before major issues occur and cause unnecessary chaos.

Communication is the most important aspect for being prepared. To make appropriate decisions, you must be able to find out important information from your medical providers. This includes understanding the prognosis of what may happen, what complications may occur, and how long the disease may last. *This must be given without false hope.* As the disease progresses, it is important for your medical provider to reassess treatment effectiveness and discuss the values, goals, and preferences of you, the patient, and the family. Everyone is different. Some people want to know about their disease and take an active role; some don't want to be told. It is important that such feelings (from both you and your family) be communicated with your provider.

Medicare to Reimburse Counseling for End-of-Life Care

Medicare has announced that it will reimburse doctors to counsel patients about end-of-life care. This service includes early counseling for patients to decide the type of care they prefer both before an illness progresses and during treatment. The rule will go into effect January 1, 2016.

Medicare currently covers this counseling only when patients first enroll, a time when they may not need or want end-of-life counseling. This is an important decision because previously, many doctors would not provide counseling because of the time involved without receiving reimbursement. This should now change and is to your advantage.

Advanced directives: It is also important to make decisions regarding who will care for you and where the care will be provided—hospital, nursing facility, or home with family. Do you need a visiting nurse, and if so, for how long? A nursing home or assisted care facility? Hospice? These types of issues, along with the financial aspects, should be decided as soon as possible. These are called advanced directives, and they can also include decisions such as management of dementia, tube feeding, discontinuation of chemotherapy for cancer, and whether to deactivate implantable devices to keep the heart beating in end-stage heart failure.

The Conventional Approaches
Many procedures are done to try to save individuals, despite the fact that they may not help, are expensive, and can cause additional problems. But there are some conventional treatments that are beneficial to maintain quality of life (QOL).

Medications are the mainstay for most of the complications. For managing pain, acetaminophen, NSAIDs, and narcotics are the most common. *Caution*: NSAIDs can cause GI, kidney, and cardiac problems and should be used with caution. To avoid GI toxicity, they should be used with a proton pump inhibitor such as Nexium, Prilosec, or Prevacid. Naproxen is the preferred NSAID for older people due to decreased risk of heart problems.

Other medications can provide relief for various conditions, as follows:

- *For fibromyalgia or neuropathic (nerve) pain*, serotonin-norepinephrine reuptake inhibitors (SNRIs), gabapentin, or pregabalin are used, but the latter two can cause drowsiness.
- *For bone pain*, bisphosphonates (alendronate [Fosamax], risedronate [Actonel], ibandronate [Boniva], and so on) may be helpful.
- *For managing dyspnea*, narcotics and oxygen may be valuable.
- *For depression*, tricyclic antidepressants and SSRI antidepressants may be beneficial, as well as counseling.
- *For spasticity/spasm*, Baclofen may be useful (muscle relaxants are often ineffective).

Hospice is a very important end-of-life aspect. Hospice is a special concept of care designed to provide comfort and support to patients and their families when a life-limiting illness no longer responds to cure-oriented treatments. The goal of hospice is to improve the quality of a patient's last days by offering comfort and dignity. It addresses all symptoms of a disease, with a special emphasis on controlling a patient's pain and discomfort, and deals with the emotional, social, and spiritual impact of the disease on the patient and the patient's family and friends.

Hospice is less expensive than a hospital and is covered by Medicare and insurers. To qualify for hospice, two doctors must certify that a patient has no more than six months to live, although patients can be recertified every sixty days and continue to receive care. You should realize, however, that there are for-profit and not-for-profit hospices, the former of which may try to lengthen the amount of hospice care unnecessarily.

Predicting Life Expectancy Inexact

Although doctors may predict that a patient has less than six months to live, many of these predictions end up being inaccurate. Studies show that the closer to death predicted, the more inaccurate the actual event. In fact, doctors who predict death in one to thirty days overestimate the length of life by an average of 69 percent. Predicting greater than 180 days is much more accurate.

Finally, many hospitals now have **ethics consulting teams** to help determine end-of-life issues, such as helping care for dying patients, mediating among family members who disagree on life support and other issues, and helping people with terminal illness make informed decisions. Pursue these programs if they are available.

The Alternative Approaches

There are several alternative methods that can treat end-of-life conditions less expensively and more effectively, especially as compared to drugs.

Relaxation and meditation are very beneficial because stress and anxiety are major reactions to end-of-life problems. They can be done anywhere, at any time, and have little to no cost (usually just the purchase price if you buy meditation CDs: see Appendix for information). Meditation is also excellent for increasing spiritual and emotional awareness, for both the patient and family.

Qigong and tai chi are Chinese exercises that have been proven beneficial for maintaining QOL; increasing strength and endurance; and decreasing pain, depression, and falls. There are many different types of qigong exercises, but several are easy to do and can be done sitting or lying down, so even frail people can do them. Qigong should be done under the directive care of someone who has been appropriately trained, or it could make symptoms worse.

Acupuncture is very effective for the three most common end-of-life conditions (depression, dyspnea, and pain). For these conditions, acupuncture can work very quickly, usually within two to six treatments, and it is also long-lasting. It also can be used regardless of the age or condition of the patient.

A **Chinese herbal formula** called *Jin Gui Shen Qi Wan* (means "pills for restoring vital energy") may help rejuvenate and improve adrenal function.

Homeopathy remedies may be very beneficial and are easy to take, especially for people who cannot swallow. Homeopathy remedies (potencies of 6c or 12c; three pellets underneath tongue every two hours) include:

- *Eupatorium perfoliatum*—used for bone pain.
- *Antimonium tartaricum*—weakened state and end-stage disease, rattling noise during respiration.
- *Carbo vegetabilis*—difficult breathing, must sit up and desires to be fanned.
- *Rhus toxicodendron*—used for joint pain, restless sleep, constant shifting, and inability to find a comfortable position.

Your Empowered Patient Action Plan for End-of-Life Care

Step #1: ***Communicate*** your needs and questions thoroughly with your medical provider. Have advanced directives in place

Step #2: ***Make plans*** for care and finances.

Step #3: **Utilize an ethical consulting team** if your hospital has one.

Step #4: **Use hospice** if there is less than six months to live.

Step #5: **Meditate regularly** to reduce stress and improve quality of life.

Step #6: **Use acupuncture** to control pain, dyspnea, anxiety, or depression.

Step #7: **Use homeopathy** to control QOL symptoms if the above steps are not beneficial.

Step #8: **Use narcotics and oxygen** to control dyspnea if acupuncture is not helpful.

Step #9: **Use medications to control other symptoms** if the above have not been beneficial; NSAIDs or narcotics to control general pain, bisphosphonates to control bone pain, and SSRI or tricyclic antidepressants for depression.

Step #10: **Perform qigong/tai chi**, if able, to improve endurance and balance.

Expected Outcome

The end of life should be a peaceful, restful time. Suffering is not necessary and can be avoided by communicating with your practitioner and using the above steps.

Fatigue and Chronic Fatigue Syndrome (CFS or SEID)

What You Need to Know

Fatigue is a very common problem as we age and can be caused by a myriad of reasons, both physical and mental. To resolve fatigue, therefore, it is important to find the underlying factor(s) first and address those, although sometimes a reason is not evident.

There is a difference between fatigue and weakness. Fatigue is a feeling of tiredness, exhaustion, or lack of energy. Weakness is a lack of physical or muscle strength, often caused by specific diseases, such as hypothyroidism or muscle and nerve diseases.

The most common causes of fatigue are chronic medical conditions, which demand a lot of the body's energy. Some examples include anemia, cancer, diabetes, depression, insomnia (sleep apnea), and hypothyroidism. Even so, there are treatments that can improve fatigue no matter what disease you may have. Stress is also a major cause of fatigue because it may adversely affect the adrenal gland, which produces cortisol and precursors of sex hormones. (Many practitioners refer to this as "adrenal fatigue").

One specific disease in which fatigue is the primary problem is chronic fatigue syndrome (CFS), characterized by extreme fatigue that doesn't improve with rest and actually may worsen with activity. It can also involve unrefreshing sleep and cognitive (thinking) impairment. Studies show that CFS can often follow infections.

Muscle aches, low-grade fever, and swollen lymph nodes can accompany CFS, and it is often observed with fibromyalgia. ***Important note***: The Institute of Medicine renamed this syndrome *systemic exertion intolerance disease, or SEID*, in February 2015. However, in this section I will still use the term CFS until the new name becomes better established.

Beware of Fatigue That Doesn't Improve With Rest

We all encounter fatigue in our daily activities, whether from stress, hard work or activities. When normal, fatigue should resolve after a period of rest.

However, if you rest and you still have fatigue, that may be a symptom of an underlying disease, including cancer. This is especially true if you have involuntary weight loss as well. In such cases, you should see your doctor for an exam and possible testing.

Treatments for Fatigue

The Preventive Approaches
Correctable Causes: Many medications can cause fatigue, and stopping their use may resolve the problem. Antihistamines, cough and cold remedies, beta blockers (for heart disease or blood pressure), some pain relievers, and antidepressants are the most common offenders, but many others can cause fatigue as well.

Sleep: Getting an inadequate amount of sleep is a primary cause of fatigue. As we get older especially, it becomes harder to get uninterrupted sleep, and you sleep less soundly and awaken earlier. (See section on *Insomnia* to address this problem.)

Exercise: Inactivity and being out of shape certainly contributes to fatigue, but even if you have various diseases causing fatigue, exercise can help reduce it. Exercise at least thirty minutes daily, and just walking can improve your overall energy. Especially with CFS, it is difficult to get motivated to exercise, but once you start, you will realize the benefit.

Diet: Not eating properly or drinking enough fluids can cause fatigue because your body needs the fuel to perform functions. Fruits and vegetables are the best because of their high antioxidant content, but protein is important as well. Consult a registered dietitian for recommendations.

Ingesting too much caffeine or simple sugars—from coffee, tea, soft drinks, energy drinks, or candy—can have a rebound effect and make you fatigued.

The Conventional Approaches

Medications: There are no specific conventional treatments for fatigue, and most often medications are used to simply address various related symptoms such as depression, pain, anxiety, or allergy-like symptoms. Some physicians use steroids and amphetamines to bolster energy, especially if you have specific chronic conditions such as cancer, but these drugs have many side effects and should be avoided in the long term. Provigil and Nuvigil, usually used for narcolepsy, are often prescribed for fatigue as well.

For CFS, there are many drugs being used and investigated. Some of these drugs include fludrocortisone, atenolol, and midodrine. Some investigative drugs include methylphenidate (Ritalin, Concerta; used most commonly for ADD), immune globulins, and interferon (which can have serious side effects however).

Psychotherapy: In small trials, patients have benefited from cognitive-behavioral therapy (focused on overcoming the fear of activity).

Graded exercise therapy (focused on gradually improving exercise tolerance) has also been found to be helpful. Another method called **adaptive pacing therapy** (focused on optimizing expenditure of limited energy) has been found to be inferior to the other two therapies.

The Alternative Approaches

Acupuncture is the best overall alternative treatment for fatigue, and several studies have found it to be beneficial in CFS. You should observe benefits within six to eight treatments, although more may be necessary for maximum benefit; and maintenance treatments also may be necessary.

Chinese herbs that can help fatigue depend on which Chinese "syndrome" you may have (there are at least seven different syndromes that can cause fatigue). A general formula is *Zuo Gui Wan/You Gui Yin*, but *Si Jun Zi Tang* and *Ba Zhen Tang* are used for particular syndromes. *Bu Zhong Yo Qi Wan* is useful for restoring energy that is depleted. Proper tongue and pulse diagnosis is necessary to determine which formula will benefit you. *Ginseng* (panax, containing 37.5 percent gensenosides) has long been used in China to increase vitality and is quite beneficial for fatigue. It usually works within one to two weeks, if not sooner. A recent published study showed data to support the benefit of *American ginseng* (2,000 mg daily) over an eight-week period to improve cancer-related fatigue.

There are many **herbs and supplements** that function as adaptogens (maximizing the body's ability to resist stress) and as tonics (enabling the body to reserve and sustain vital energy throughout the day while promoting sound, restful sleep at night). All of these can be beneficial for fatigue, especially adrenal fatigue. Some of these include:

- *D-ribose* (also known as ribose) is a form of sugar that is an essential energy source for your cells. Some research has found that natural D-ribose supplements (5 g three times a day) may significantly improve the symptoms of CFS, with particular benefit in study participants' energy levels and overall well-being.

- *Nicotinamide adenine dinucleotide (NADH)* is a naturally occurring molecule formed from vitamin B_3 (niacin) that plays an essential role in cellular energy production. A recent small study showed that 31 percent of people with fatigue taking 1 mg per day responded favorably to NADH.

- *Vitamin B_{12} and/or B vitamin complex* are often given for fatigue and can help, especially if you are deficient. B_{12} may need to be given by injection or sublingually if you do not absorb it in your GI tract (you can test B12 levels in your blood to find out if you are absorbing it orally).

- *L-carnitine* (2 g daily; for cancer patients, 3–4 g daily) is responsible for transporting long-chain fatty acids into mitochondria, the energy-producing centers of cells and allows these fatty acids to be converted into energy. Some studies have found that carnitine levels in the body are decreased in people with CFS, and one study found L-carnitine to improve CFS in twelve out of eighteen parameters. *Warning*: A rare side effect that has been reported with L-carnitine use is seizures in people with or without preexisting seizure disorders.

- *Coenzyme Q10* is a compound found naturally in the mitochondria, the energy-producing center of our cells, and is involved in the production of ATP, the main energy source of body cells. CoQ10 (30–120 mg daily) is also an antioxidant and has been found in small surveys to benefit approximately 70 percent of people with CFS. It can be expensive, however.

All these supplements have the potential to improve energy. You can try each separately to see their effects, which may take four to six weeks. However, you can also combine several together.

Relaxation/meditation and/or **restorative exercises**, such as QiGong or Yoga, are very helpful in increasing energy. Although it may be difficult to be motivated to perform exercises due to fatigue, once you begin it becomes much easier and more beneficial.

Ayurvedic herb: Numerous studies have found that the Indian herb *Ashwagandha* (500 mg daily, standardized to contain 5 percent withanolides) is very effective in decreasing stress, increasing mental activity, invigorating the body, and functioning as an antioxidant.

For those who have depression, anxiety, or psychological factors that may be contributing to fatigue, **interactive imagery** (active imagination) is an excellent means of finding out the cause and treating the fatigue. (See sections on "Depression" and "Anxiety" for further information.)

Your Empowered Patient Action Plan for Treating Fatigue

Step #1: Rule out other medical conditions and medications as a cause of fatigue. Since these may be common causes of fatigue, successfully treating them may resolve the fatigue.

Step #2: Undergo acupuncture to resolve fatigue long term. This is the best and most cost-effective method for treating fatigue and CFS.

Step #3: Take Chinese herbal formulas or ginseng to temporarily increase energy and protect against stress if the above steps have not helped.

Step #4: Take Ashwaganda, d-Ribose L-carnitine, and/ or CoQ10 to invigorate the body and decrease fatigue.

Step #5: Undergo interactive imagery to discover reasons for your fatigue and to treat it effectively, especially if psychological issues may be causing the condition.

Step #6: Undergo cognitive-behavioral therapy whether or not psychological issues may be a factor in your fatigue and the above steps have not helped or you cannot find a practitioner for step 5.

Step #7: Try graded exercise therapy if you are still having fatigue.

Step #8: Try other supplements and/or vitamins listed above if the above steps have not improved your condition. They can also be used with the above steps.

Expected Outcome

It may be difficult to find a cause for fatigue, which makes it more difficult to treat. However, there are many alternative methods that are beneficial in resolving or at least reducing fatigue, even if caused by other medical conditions or unknown reasons.

Fractures

What You Need to Know

Injuries can occur from numerous sources; and surprisingly, even minor objects can cause injuries, the most common being beds and bedding, household containers, sofas, and footwear. Certainly injuries can occur at any age but as we get older, many of us still think we can do activities we've always been able to do.

Injury occurring at an older age is much different than one occurring when we are younger. Much like skin, soft tissues, blood vessels, and bones also become weaker as we age. Because our tissues degenerate over time, we not only suffer more serious consequences of injuries but also take much longer to heal.

Falls Common as We Age

The primary cause of fractures in the elderly is falling, and almost one-third of community-dwelling elderly people fall each year, with 10 percent sustaining a significant injury. Falls are responsible for 95 percent of all hip fractures in the elderly.

There are many reasons for falls, including over sedation with drugs, , weakness, impaired balance or gait, other blood pressure problems, poor eyesight and hearing (including wearing multifocal glasses), neurological problems, arthritis, sarcopenia (age-related loss of muscle mass), environmental hazards such as slippery floors or uneven ground, orthostatic hypotension (becoming faint when you first stand up, especially from blood pressure medications during the first two months of use) as well as delayed orthostatic hypotension (which can occur several minutes after standing and may be an early manifestation of Parkinson's). Another common reason for falls is walking barefoot or wearing just socks or slippers.

As we age, falls tend to occur sideways or backward, which is in a direction opposite of how younger individuals fall.

Dr. A's Suggestions:
Use Your Alarm!

A recent study showed that elderly people who fell and had access to an alarm system did not use the alarm in 80 percent of cases. Using the alarm is a must because prolonged time on the floor after falling is associated with greater injury and hospitalization.

People who are hospitalized more have a significantly increased risk of all types of fractures. In addition, certain diseases, especially osteoporosis and cancer that has spread to the bones, increase the risk for fractures.

Fractures can occur in any bone in the body, but the most frequent fractures are of bones in the extremities and of the ribs. Fractures are most common in young adults who are adventurous in nature, and in the older population as bones become fragile. The most common fractures as we age are the hip and spine, many of which are a result of osteoporosis.

Although most fractures heal within 6 weeks, hip fractures in older people can be quite significant as 25 percent of older people with such fractures die within one year,

9 percent within thirty days. The cause of mortality following a hip fracture is often due to blood clots, pneumonia, or infection. By getting up and out of bed as soon as possible after hip fracture, the risk of complications is diminished. Unfortunately, only about 25 percent of patients who sustain a broken hip return to their preinjury level of activity.

The majority of patients who sustain a hip fracture will require prolonged specialized care, such as a long-term nursing or rehabilitation facility. About one year after a patient sustains a broken hip, mortality rates return to normal, but a patient who previously sustained a hip fracture is at higher risk of breaking his or her hip again.

X-Rays May Not Be Accurate in Detecting Fractures of the Hips or Pelvis

A recent study revealed that x-rays of the hip and pelvis may miss recent fractures. Furthermore, in many cases when an x-ray ostensibly finds a fracture, there may not be one. MRIs are better at determining fractures but are not indicated in most cases. They should be used when a chance exists that they will change the way you are treated.

Treatments for Fractures

The Preventive Approaches
Correctable causes: Obviously, avoiding injuries and falls is the best way to prevent fractures. Any of the above described medical problems should be addressed and environmental issues modified. You should especially be aware of any prescription drugs that may be causing stumbling, orthostatic hypotension (dizziness when standing quickly), or balance problems. The CDC describes fourteen effective fall-prevention strategies in a new publication, *Preventing Falls: What Works* (http://www.cdc.gov/ncipc/PreventingFalls/).

Beware of Some Drugs Increasing Fracture Risk

In a study published by *CMAJ*, it was noted that two diabetic drugs, rosiglitazone (Avandia) and pioglitazone (Actos), raised the risk for fractures, so they should be avoided if you are a diabetic who is at higher risk for fractures.

In addition, a recent study in *BMJ* revealed that elderly patients are more sensitive to thyroid replacement and do not need as much as younger people; too much thyroid replacement increases fracture risk in such patients and should be monitored more closely.

One unusual cause of falls is decreased blood pressure after eating, which happens to many elderly patients. If that should occur, increased water intake before eating or eating six smaller meals a day rather than three large ones can help prevent this.

Dr. A's Suggestions:
Single-Lens Glasses Lower Risk for Falls

Many active older people wear multifocal glasses (bifocals, trifocals, progressive lenses), no matter what activity they are doing. However, these glasses impair distance perception and raise risk for falls. If you are active and wear multifocal lenses, wear single-lens glasses when you are walking.

Vitamin D$_3$ (800–1,000 mg daily) is an important preventive vitamin to take if your blood levels are below normal. This vitamin has been proven very effective in preventing falls in the elderly, and a majority of older people are deficient in this vitamin. A recent study from the *Annals of Internal Medicine* revealed that low blood levels of vitamin D are definitely associated with increased risk of hip fractures in postmenopausal women. ***Important Note***: The established "normal" blood levels for vitamin D are considered to be 20 ng/ml; however, most naturopaths recommend at least 30-50 ng/ml.

Smoking retards bone healing and may prevent healing altogether, so eliminating this factor can help fractures heal better.

Diet: If you're over sixty-five, a study from Harvard showed that the lower your protein intake, the greater the increased risk for fractures (40–80 percent). However, if you have kidney disease, too much protein can be harmful, so check with a dietician.

The Conventional Approaches
Depending on the fracture site, which bones are involved, and how badly they are fractured, there are different conventional methods.

Casting the arm or leg may be adequate for simple fractures. In some instances, a removable brace may be sufficient. In such cases, the bone usually takes about six weeks to heal.

Surgery may be necessary for more complex fractures or in patients with healing problems. In the limbs, this usually involves using a plate and screws to anchor the bone so that it can heal properly, although sometimes an external fixator device may be necessary. After a specific amount of time and evidence of healing, the screws and/ or plate can be removed.

With ***hip fractures***, surgery can range from simple pinning of the hip to total hip replacement. ***Helpful tips***: An important factor after hip surgery is to begin walking as soon as possible to avoid complications of pneumonia and blood clots. You should be given a blood thinner prophylactically after undergoing hip surgery, usually low-molecular-weight heparin (LMWH).

Dr. A's Suggestions:
Preventing Death from Hip Fractures

In a recent study, two preventable risk factors were noted in patients under-going hip fracture surgery. The first was a delay in surgery of more than four days: The faster surgery is performed the better. In the study, surgery was more likely to be performed within that time frame if the patient was admitted from Sunday through Wednesday, but not on Thursday or Friday. Secondly, those undergoing general anesthesia had a higher death rate, so local anesthesia is recommended if at all possible.

With ***spine fractures*** (also called compression fractures), two procedures, *vertebroplasty* or *balloon kyphoplasty*, are commonly done. Vertebroplasty involves injecting a cement-like substance into the fracture. Kyphoplasty also injects cement but after a balloon is inflated to restore the vertebra's normal height.

No direct studies have compared vertebroplasty (VP) to kyphoplasty (KP) or to nonsurgical techniques. Single studies show that KP is ten to twenty times more expensive than VP and requires anesthesia and overnight hospitalization, but KP is apparently more successful at relieving pain (90 percent vs. 70 percent) and restoring vertebral height (thus preventing "hunching"). There is a possibility of the cement leaking with VP but not so much with KP. ***Important note***: No studies have compared KP to placebo, but several studies have shown that VP is no better than placebo and shouldn't be considered even with recent-onset or severe pain.

There is some thinking that the earlier the surgery is performed, the better the results but again, this has not yet been determined by research. It is known, however, that KP does help relieve pain in cancer patients with metastatic spine disease.

Bisphosphonate drugs (Actonel, Boniva, and Fosamax, and especially Reclast) have been used to prevent subsequent fractures in patients with osteoporosis. However, two well-designed studies revealed that these drugs may not prevent recurrent fractures in older individuals who have underlying factors other than low bone density. In addition, a study presented at the American Academy of Orthopedic Surgeons in 2015 showed that in elderly women with wrist fractures, biphosphonates would reduce hip fractures by about 25% but at a cost of more than $200,000 per prevented fracture. In addition, biphosphonates alone could cause 20,000 more atypical fractures. ***Important Note***: They should be taken at least four hours away from calcium-containing supplements due to absorption issues.

Bone stimulators are sometimes used if the bone does not heal well or as predicted. These stimulators usually involve ultrasound and electrical stimulation, the latter either being applied directly to the bone (invasive) or outside the limb. Such stimulators must be used for three to six months to be effective. During that time, you cannot place weight on the area of bone fracture.

The Alternative Approaches

There are several alternative methods that can accelerate bone healing and are useful in fractures, especially those that don't heal well.

The first is **infrasound** or low-frequency sound (8–14 Hz), which appears to accelerate bone growth by 40 percent. The advantage of infrasound is that it can penetrate casting material, and it has no side effects. Treatment is beneficial over a few weeks.

The **low level energy laser** or *LLEL* (cold laser) is also effective in accelerating bone healing but must be applied directly to the surface, so it cannot be used if your limb is casted (a brace can be removed for treatment with the laser). It is especially useful for spine fractures. You should obtain initial benefit within four to eight treatments (see chapter 4 for more details on cold laser therapy).

Acupuncture is useful in enhancing bone healing, apparently by increasing blood flow to the area, although there may be other mechanisms involved.

Along with acupuncture, several **Chinese herbal formulas** can be beneficial for accelerating healing. These formulas typically include different herbs, depending on the site of the break. For instance, *Mu Gui* and *Niu Xi* are commonly added to formulas for the treatment of fractures in the lower extremities, whereas herbs such as *Chuan Xiong* and *Sang Zhi* are often used to guide the effects of other herbs to the upper extremities. One of the major formulas for bone healing is *Jie Gu Er Halo Fang* ("bone-knitting formula"). *Zhen GU Shui* topical liniment is useful for bone pain.

Strontium (340 mg active strontium, ranelate form, twice daily) is a supplement that is especially beneficial for protecting bones from re-fracture This element provides strength to bones but also helps reduce bone loss from aging and makes new bone (see section on Osteoporosis for more information). Bisphosphonates (see above) reduce bone loss but do not make new bone or strengthen bone like strontium does.

Several **vitamins** may also be of benefit for healing fractures. These include buffered *vitamin C* (500 mg twice daily), *Vitamin D₃* (800–1,000 mg daily) or a combination of *calcium and magnesium* (however, be careful if you have kidney disease when taking this combination). is an important preventive action to take.

A **homeopathic** remedy, Symphytum, is used for fractures and can reduce pain by helping to promote healing of the bone.

Your Empowered Patient Action Plan for Treating Fractures

Step #1: **Cast or Brace the limb** if it is a simple, nondisplaced fracture.

Step #2: **Undergo surgery** for complex limb fractures and hip fractures and **kyphoplasty** for compression fractures of the spine if indicated or if cancer has caused the fracture. Avoid vertebroplasty.

Step #3: **Check your vitamin D levels** and supplement if they are low.

Step #4: **Use infrasound** with either of the above Steps to accelerate healing.

Step #5: **Use LLEL** (cold laser) treatment for nonhealing fractures that have removable casts or braces, to accelerate healing and reduce pain.

Step #6: **Take Chinese herbal formulas** to enhance bone healing along with the above steps.

Step #7: **Take various vitamins** to help accelerate fracture healing.

Step #8: **Take the homeopathic remedy** Symphorum to reduce pain and promote healing.

Step #9: **Undergo acupuncture** if your fracture is still not healing.

Step #10: **Use a bone stimulator** to accelerate healing if the above steps have not helped.

Step #11: **Take strontium** to reduce the risk of recurrent fractures, especially if you have osteoporosis.

Step #12: **Take bisphosphonates** to reduce the risk of recurrent fractures.

Expected Outcome

Most fractures should heal within six weeks, although those requiring surgery may take longer. If your fracture does not heal properly, the use of alternative methods can accelerate healing quicker than conventional means.

Gastroesophageal Reflux Disease (GERD, *Acid Reflux, Heartburn*)

What You Need to Know

GERD (commonly referred to as acid reflux) is a condition primarily caused by a weakness in the muscular valve between the stomach and esophagus (the lower esophageal sphincter, or LES), resulting in stomach acid leaking into and irritating the esophagus. There are two types, nonerosive and erosive; erosive involves inflammation of the esophagus and can eat away the lining.

Heartburn is a *symptom* of GERD, which can occur intermittently or frequently. It is often caused by overeating, but other factors include obesity, cigarette smoking, and consuming certain foods (see "Diet" below), which causes increased pressure on the stomach from the abdomen or directly weakens the LES. Occasionally, heartburn can be a sign of a hiatal hernia (out pouching of the esophagus above the LES).

GERD can cause strictures, Barrett's esophagus (a precancerous change in cell structure), esophageal cancer, irritation and scarring of the vocal cords, and a variety of lung problems, including asthma, cough, and bronchitis (usually due to aspiration into the lungs of refluxed liquids or abnormal stimulation of esophageal nerves). The symptoms of GERD can also imitate those of a heart attack. *Warning*: You should obtain a heart evaluation if you have any chest pain, especially if you have symptoms of shortness of breath, dizziness, pain in the jaw, or pain that is not relieved by antacids.

Endoscopy Overused

Endoscopic examination (EGD) involves placing a scope into your esophagus and stomach to evaluate symptoms. Studies reveal that about 50 percent of patients with reflux symptoms have no objective findings on endoscopy. In addition, the patients who do not have findings may still receive drugs anyway.

Endoscopies are overused by both PCPs (who don't provide optimal medical treatment before referral) and gastroenterologists. However, clear guidelines have now been established for when endoscopy should be done, and you should insist that your doctor follow them. These include:

- "Alarm" symptoms, such as difficulty swallowing, bleeding, unexplained vomiting, unexplained weight loss, or anemia.
- Persistent GERD symptoms despite twice-daily use of medications over four to eight weeks.
- Severe erosive esophagitis (inflammation of the esophagus) after a two-month course of medication, to assess healing.
- A history of esophageal stricture (narrowing) with continued symptoms.
- Established Barrett's esophagus (EGD every three to five years).
- Men over fifty years old with chronic GERD symptoms (persisting longer than five years) and additional risk factors (nighttime symptoms, hiatal hernia, increased BMI, intra-abdominal fat distribution and tobacco use).

Treatments for GERD

The Preventive Approaches

For many people, GERD symptoms worsen when they go to bed. To relieve nighttime symptoms, **elevate the head of your bed**. Do this by elevating the *frame* of the bed (as with blocks) rather than by sleeping with cushions or more pillows, which have a tendency to shift while you sleep. Also, sleep on your *left side*, which reduces the backup of food and acid.

Cigarette **smoking** relaxes the LES, so stopping this habit can help. In addition, numerous **medications** can cause heartburn as a side effect, especially aspirin, NSAIDs, and some antibiotics. Changing to a different medication may relieve the symptoms and prevent the need for additional measures. If you have GERD and are taking medications, check the *PDR* to see if your medication can cause these symptoms, or consult your pharmacist.

Diet: Weight loss (if you are overweight or have gained weight) is recommended and may reverse reflux. Foods that cause relaxation of the LES include acidic foods and caffeine, such as tomatoes, citrus fruits, garlic, onions, chocolate, coffee, alcohol, and peppermint. Foods high in fats and oils also may also cause increased heartburn. However, this does not mean that these foods will cause heartburn, but the only way to know is to eliminate them from your diet and then reintroduce them. Avoid them if they cause symptoms. You might also try small frequent meals and avoid eating a few hours before going to bed or lying flat.

The Conventional Approaches

Medications are the primary conventional treatment for GERD and are effective in most patients.

Antacids are often taken for immediate relief and for mild symptoms. However, taking antacids regularly or long-term may cause other medical problems such as kidney stones or aluminum toxicity.

The primary drugs for GERD are *proton pump inhibitors* or PPIs (generically end in "prazole: there are many brands, including omeprazole [Prilosec], lansoprazole [Prevacid], esomeprazole [Nexium], dexlansoprazole [Dexilant], pantoprazole [Protonix] and rabeprazole [Aciphex]). PPIs are very effective in controlling the symptoms of GERD and can promote healing in areas damaged by exposure to stomach acid, but they may not cure the problem, and they can be very expensive. However, Prilosec, Prevacid and Nexium are now available OTC, both under their trade names and generic names (store-brand), both of which are less expensive than the prescription variety. *Helpful Tips*: Store-brand generics are often just as effective as trade name OTC drugs but are less expensive. Try them first. These drugs should be taken thirty to sixty minutes before the first meal of the day.

———

Important Information:
PPIs Can Increase Risk of Other Medical Problems

It is recognized that taking PPIs can increase the risk of several other medical problems, including pneumonia, *C. difficile* infections, bacterial infections of the abdomen in patients with cirrhosis, electrolyte disturbances, lung and intestinal infections in hospital patients, and nutritional deficiencies (the absorption of many medications and vitamins can be decreased when using these drugs, especially calcium, iron, and magnesium). They also increase the risk of spine, forearm, wrist, and total fractures. A 2016 observational study showed that they are associated with a 20-50 percent increased risk for developing chronic kidney disease.

These side effects primarily occur with long-term use. Experts recommend that you monitor kidney function and magnesium levels if you take PPIs, or switch to H_2 acid blockers when feasible (see below), and not use PPIs for vague complaints of "heartburn".

Important Information:
PPIs Overprescribed

It should be noted that many doctors worry that people self-prescribing OTC PPIs won't get proper medical attention. Yet, even when prescribed by doctors, PPIs are often overused, taken for too long, or taken at too high a dosage or for the wrong condition. A 2012 study in *J Hosp Med* showed that PPIs are overprescribed in 73 percent of hospitalized patients, and many of them are never taken off the drugs after hospitalization. Taking them inappropriately can lead to the other medical problems, as listed in the sidebar above.

If you don't need them, why take them? In a recent editorial in the *Archives of Internal Medicine*, it was concluded that "for most patients, the adverse effects of PPIs outweigh the benefits." But that's only if used inappropriately. So, become empowered, and question your doctor.

Helpful tips: After you take PPIs for at least eight weeks, if your symptoms are eliminated, you may be able to reduce the dose or stop taking them. If symptoms recur, you can restart them for a few more weeks. If your symptoms then continue, you may need to take them long-term, but take the lowest dose necessary to relieve your symptoms. Even with long-term use, you may want to discontinue them after a few months or year to see if the symptoms return. Some people only need them intermittently. PPIs are considered safe during pregnancy.

Dr. A's Suggestions:
Monitor B_{12} Levels if on PPIs

With prolonged use of PPIs in older people, B_{12} levels decrease due to interference with absorption. A *JAMA* study in 2013 showed that using these drugs for more than two years increases the risk for B_{12} deficiency, especially if taking more than 1.5 pills daily.

Just taking the RDA recommended amounts of B_{12} *does not* prevent this decline. If you are on PPIs for extended periods, have your B_{12} blood level checked to make sure it has not declined, and increase your supplementation if low. Cranberry juice increases the absorption of B_{12}.

Caution: There is controversy in regard to using PPIs with clopidogrel (Plavix) (a blood thinner used in heart disease and stroke) as some studies show that they interfere with each other. However, the latest studies refute this. If concerned, consider using an H_2 (see below).

Older drugs that can still be useful for GERD include **H_2 acid blockers** (generally end in "tidine", such as ranitidine [Zantac], famotidine [Pepcid], cimetidine [Tagamet]). These drugs are available OTC and are much less expensive, although they may not be as effective as PPIs. *Caution*: because they work by blocking acid production, they also can cause decreased absorption of other medications—and especially fat-soluble vitamins (vitamins A, D, E, and K), as well as vitamin B_{12}. (If your B_{12} blood level is low, take cranberry juice, which increases the absorption of B_{12}). H_2 blockers can be added to PPIs if nighttime symptoms persist on PPIs alone.

PPIs Vs H_2 blockers: Both of these drug types can work in GERD, but there are pros and cons, as follows:

- H_2 blockers are less expensive
- H_2 blockers work faster than PPIs
- PPIs last longer than H_2 blockers
- PPIs are stronger than H_2 blockers
- You may need to take H_2 blockers twice daily to control symptoms. If so, once daily PPIs may be more cost-effective.

Important Information:
Watch for Rebound Symptoms if Discontinuing GERD Drugs

Some people develop symptoms of hyperacidity if they stop taking PPIs (and possibly H_2 blockers) after taking them for two months or more. This occurs more frequently in patients who take them unnecessarily or for unclear indications. Antacids are the best remedy until the rebound effect is diminished.

Important note: **Sucralfate**, which "coats" the stomach, is sometimes prescribed for GERD but is not indicated except in pregnancy.

If Drugs Are Not Beneficial, Think of Another Diagnosis

Patients for whom GERD drugs don't work may have another, more rare, disease called eosinifilic esophagitis, or EE, which is actually an allergy to food or pollen. Most of these patients describe GERD symptoms refractive to drugs, as well as swallowing difficulties or food caught in their esophagus. If you have these symptoms, see an allergist and gastroenterologist. (You will need a biopsy of the esophagus to prove the disease.)

Surgery may be performed if drugs are not beneficial. A minimally invasive procedure is available in some areas to relieve persistent GERD; called the *Stretta* procedure, it uses high-frequency radio waves to tighten the LES, thus reducing reflux. After this procedure, many people are able to stop taking their acid-blocking medications.

Radiofrequency ablation (RFA) is another surgery that is beneficial for Barrett's esophagus. In a 2014 study in *JAMA*, 74 percent of patients resolved signs of Barrett's, and none progressed to cancer.

If all else has failed, endoscopic surgery called *fundoplication* (using a scope rather than opening the chest) may be necessary to repair the LES if symptoms are severe and do not respond to other treatments. It is most commonly done if you have a large hiatal hernia. This surgery has about 90 percent success rate, but only in the hands of very experienced surgeons. It is expensive, costing up to $10,000.

Helpful tip: *Medical versus surgical treatment*: In comparison between surgery and medical therapy, up to 60 percent of people who undergo surgery still have to take antireflux medications within a year, and most have to take such medications within ten years. In general, it is more effective initially than low-dose PPIs but not high dose.

A study published in *JAMA* in May 2011 compared laparoscopic surgery to PPI use and showed the following after five years:

- Estimated remission (control of symptoms) was 92 percent with PPI and 85 percent with surgery.
- Acid regurgitation was worse with PPI, while dysphagia (difficulty swallowing), bloating, and flatulence were worse with surgery.
- Serious adverse events occurred in 25 percent of patients in each group.

An editorialist concluded that "Given the...potential risks for surgical intervention, long term medical therapy seems to be a resounding best choice for patients who are willing to remain on acid reduction medication."

Important note: Surgery is a consideration for *chronic* GERD, but it is not recommended if you have not responded to PPIs.

Other procedures. There are two other procedures that may be beneficial for GERD and only involve minimal surgical intervention. One approach is the use of *electrical stimulation therapy (EST) of the LES*. Electrodes are placed via laparoscopy into the LES and then the device is implanted in the abdominal wall. An industry-sponsored study (which has some limitations) showed that 77 percent of patients reported either normalization or at least a 50 percent reduction in PPI use. At 12 months after the implant of the device, there was a statistically significant improvement in patients' scores on a scale measuring health-related quality of life for patients with GERD.

The second procedure is the implantation of a *magnetic sphincter augmentation device* in which patients were fitted with bracelet-like magnetic beads that circled their LES and closed, using magnetic attraction, to aid the sphincter in resisting abnormal opening and subsequent reflux. The beads opened with food transport or increased pressure associated with burping or vomiting. An industry-sponsored study (also with some limitations) showed that normalization of acid regurgitation or a 50% or greater reduction in exposure at 1 year was achieved in 64% of patients. A reduction of 50% or more in the use of proton-pump inhibitors occurred in 93% of patients, and there was improvement of 50% or more in quality-of-life scores in 92%. The most frequent adverse event was dysphagia (difficulty swallowing, in 68% of patients postoperatively, in 11% at 1 year, and in 4% at 3 years). However, a third of these patients also underwent fundoplication of their hiatal hernia at the same time.

The Alternative Approaches

Stress is a major factor that causes and worsens heartburn, so **meditation** and **qigong** are both valuable adjuncts to reduce stress.

There are several **home remedies** that have been used successfully to combat symptoms. The two best remedies are raw honey (1 tsp daily) and apple-cider vinegar (1–2 tsp daily; use the best brands). Another remedy commonly used by nurses is drinking a half glass of milk with a half glass of 7-Up. *Caution* with use of raw honey in diabetics, as this may raise blood-glucose levels.

There are several **nutritional supplements** that can be very beneficial in GERD:

- *Digestive enzymes* can help break down food if you have improper digestion. There are many products that contain digestive enzymes, and they should contain some or all of the following: protease, papain, amylase, lipase, bromelain, cellulase, and lactase.
- *Probiotics* are also very useful for many people with GERD, and you can safely take them long-term. You should start to feel better in two to six weeks when using digestive enzymes and probiotics. (See chapter 2 for detailed discussion of probiotics.)
- *Ginger* is another herb that can provide immediate relief. You can take ginger by drinking the tea three times a day (do not exceed 4 g per day), taking 2 ml of tincture daily, taking 250 mg tablets three times a day, or in extracts standardized to 20 percent gingiol and shogoal, 100–200 mg four times a day.
- *Licorice* (deglycyrrhizinated form [DGL], one or two 380 mg chewable tablets before meals) can be taken alone or with ginger. Licorice has antispasmodic, anti-inflammatory, and soothing properties. *Caution*: If you have hypertension, licorice may raise blood pressure. The DGL form of licorice is preferred and does not affect blood pressure.
- *Aloe Vera Juice* may also be effective for controlling GERD. Aloe Vera powder can be added to juice, smoothies or milkshakes. *Caution*: Make sure it is produced for internal use and safe to drink.

There are several **Chinese herbal formulas** that can reduce the symptoms of heartburn and strengthen the LES. *Liu Jun Zi San, Kang Ning Wan, Ping Wei San,* and *Yue Ju Wan* can all be helpful. You should feel better within three weeks, but you may need to take them longer for complete relief.

Acupuncture may also help with long-term reduction of symptoms and also can strengthen the LES. You should notice improvement within six acupuncture treatments but might need additional sessions for maximum benefits.

Several **homeopathic remedies** are useful for specific situations. These include *nux vomica* after eating spicy foods, *carbo vegetabilis* after eating rich foods, and *arsenicum album* for burning pain. These remedies are used in a dosage of 6c, taken every fifteen minutes up to three times. The series can be repeated once, if needed. You should consult a qualified homeopathist for guidance on which remedies will be most beneficial and for proper dosages. You should notice improvement within one to two months.

Your Empowered Patient Action Plan for Treating GERD

Step #1: **Elevate the head of your bed** (using blocks) for mild or occasional reflux symptoms.

Step #2: **Diminish or eliminate foods** that trigger symptoms of GERD.

Step #3: **Try home remedies** (honey or apple-cider vinegar) if you have mild symptoms.

Step #4: **Take ginger, licorice, or antacids for immediate relief** if symptoms occur occasionally.

Step #5: **Try aloe vera juice** or add the powder to other liquids first for long term relief.

Step #6: **Take probiotics and digestive enzymes** if the above steps are not helpful. These (and Steps 3 or 4) are the easiest and least expensive remedies and may benefit other systems of the body as well.

Step #7: **Take the Chinese herbal remedies Kang Ning Wan, Ping Wei San, or Yue Ju Wan** to control symptoms if the above steps aren't helpful.

Step #8: **Undergo acupuncture** along with Step #7 for long term benefit.

Step #9: **Take an OTC H2 blocker medication** or **PPI medication** if you still have symptoms. The decision on which type to take depends on your preference (see above comparison).

Step #10: **Take an appropriate homeopathic remedy** if you still have symptoms.

Step #11: **Consider undergoing a Stretta procedure** to correct anatomical problems causing your GERD if the above steps have not been beneficial.

Step #12: **Consider implantation of an electrical device or magnetic beads** if your symptoms continue or you have symptomatic regurgitation.

Step #13: **Undergo major surgery** as a last resort.

Candice got heartburn every time she ate and at night when she tried to sleep. She tried several PPIs, but neither completely reduced her symptoms. I started her on probiotics and aloe vera juice, which brought about nearly immediate relief of most of her discomfort. I added a Chinese herbal formula and started her on acupuncture to correct her underlying syndromes (stagnant Liver Qi with Damp Heat). After seven acupuncture sessions, Candace had only an occasional episode of heartburn every month or so. She takes her probiotics to make sure her digestion stays normal and takes aloe vera juice whenever she does have an episode of heartburn.

Expected Outcome

GERD can be a difficult condition to overcome, but it can be controlled or even eliminated in most people by using the above steps.

Glaucoma

What You Need to Know

Glaucoma is a group of eye conditions that damage the optic nerve, which is vital to good vision. This damage is often caused by an abnormally high pressure in your eye. The most common forms are primary open-angle glaucoma, caused by increased pressure within the eye (increased intraocular pressure), and low-tension (normal pressure) glaucoma. The higher your intraocular pressures are, the greater the rate of vision loss. Glaucoma can be caused by cataracts, uveitis (inner eye inflammation), eye tumor, injury, or diabetes.

About a fourth of those who have glaucoma don't know it, because they may not be aware of the initial symptoms. This is worrisome because glaucoma is one of the leading causes of blindness. The older you are, the greater your risk, so always have your eyes checked, especially with the following symptoms:

- Peripheral vision loss
- Difficulty moving from a bright room to a darker room
- Difficulty judging steps and curbs
- Headaches
- Need for new glasses
- Tearing
- Aching or throbbing pain
- Visual field abnormalities (blurred vision and loss of peripheral vision)

Treatments for Chronic Glaucoma

The Preventive Approaches

Diet is the primary preventive method for glaucoma. Vitamin C and omega-3 fatty acids are very important in reducing intraocular pressure and improving glaucoma. Fresh fruits and vegetables and cold-water fish (such as herring, salmon, halibut, mackerel, and tuna) are the best sources.

The Conventional Approaches

Medications are the mainstay of conventional treatment. These include *beta blockers*, *carbonic anhydrase inhibitors*, or *pilocarpine*, all of which decrease intraocular pressure. Because these medications all have different side effects and may interfere with other medications, your ophthalmologist should prescribe the specific drug or combination of drugs that is most appropriate for you. These medications do not protect against loss of peripheral vision, but they do decrease the pressure in your eyes and prevent the other complications and dangers of glaucoma.

Warning: NSAIDs, both OTC (such as ibuprofen and Aleve) and prescription (such as naproxen [Naprosyn], meloxicam [Mobic], piroxicam [Feldene], oxaprozin [Daypro], nabumatone [Relafen], ketoprofen [Orudis], diclofenac [Cataflam], and diclofenac/misoprostol [Arthrotec]) may interfere with some of these medications, so you should inform your doctor if you are on NSAIDs.

Surgery: If you have loss of peripheral (side) vision, you may need surgery to preserve your vision. Either *surgical trabeculectomy* or *laser trabeculoplasty* (or both) can be done to protect further visual loss and decrease intraocular pressure. Again, you will need to consult with an ophthalmologist (eye specialist) to determine which procedure is the best for you.

The Alternative Approaches
There are several **nutritional supplements** that can improve vision and decrease intraocular pressure. These include:

- *Vitamin C*, minimum of 2,000 mg daily
- *Magnesium*, 200–400 mg daily
- *Flaxseed*, 1 Tbsp daily, *fresh ground* only (capsules and oil lose their potency quickly)
- *Bilberry with bioflavonoids*, 80 mg (containing 25 percent anthocyanidin content) three times daily
- *Lutein*, 6 mg daily
- *Chromium*, 200–400 mcg

Gingko biloba (240 mg daily) has a mild effect on decreasing intraocular pressure. *Caution*: Gingko may have drug-herb interactions with antihypertensives, antidiabetics, anticonvulsants, anticoagulants, and more.

Infrasound works by increasing the local circulation of blood and lymph and may decrease intraocular pressure in many patients. It may take six to ten treatments to see improvement, but there are no side effects. Numerous chiropractors, naturopathic physicians, acupuncturists, and a few doctors use infrasound.

Acupuncture can reduce intraocular pressure and improve vision. Both body and ear acupuncture are commonly used. You should notice improved vision within six to ten acupuncture treatments but might need additional sessions for maximum benefits. Not all acupuncturists are trained in eye diseases, so make sure yours has experience.

Chinese herbal formulas such as *Qi Ju Di Huang Wan* (for Kidney Yin Deficiency) or *Jen Gui Shen Qi Wan* can be helpful. Consult a TCM practitioner for diagnosis.

Marijuana has been demonstrated to lower intraocular pressure and can be prescribed in states where it is legal to do so. This treatment usually is reserved for people who don't respond to other treatments or have side effects from the medications.

Your Empowered Patient Action Plan for Treating Glaucoma

- *Warning: Acute glaucoma is an emergency, and you should go to an emergency room if you have any of these symptoms: nausea and vomiting, seeing rainbow halos around objects (especially lights), and dilated pupils.*
- *For chronic glaucoma, if your peripheral vision is poor (you can't see things on each side of you, only straight ahead), go to step 7 and then restart at step 1.*

Step #1: Use conventional prescription medications to control your symptoms and reduce intraocular pressure while the other steps have time to work.

Step #2: Receive infrasonic treatment to provide long-term reduction of intraocular pressure. If successful, you may be able to reduce or discontinue the medications in step 1.

Step #3: Undergo acupuncture to provide long-term reduction of intraocular pressure if the above steps have not helped. Again, if it helps, you can reduce or eliminate the medications in step 1.

Step #4: Take bilberry with bioflavonoids, lutein, vitamin c, flaxseed (freshly ground), and/or chromium to improve your vision and decrease intraocular pressure. These can be taken with any of the above steps.

Step #5: Take gingko biloba if your intraocular pressure is still high.

Step #6: Use marijuana if legal to do so in your state and your ocular pressure is still elevated.

Step #7: Undergo surgery for loss of peripheral vision or uncontrolled high intraocular pressure.

Expected Outcome

Most patients with glaucoma should be able to obtain normal intraocular pressure and prevent blindness. The main factor is to detect glaucoma before as early as possible.

Headaches (Tension, Migraine, Cluster, Occipital, Cervicogenic)

What You Need to Know

Headaches refer to any type of pain in the head and can be caused by a variety of factors. There are numerous types of headaches, each one having a different cause and, therefore, a different treatment, although some of the same treatments can be beneficial for several different types. The major types of headaches include:

- *Tension headaches*, the most frequent type, are caused by muscle contractions that pinch nerves or blood vessels. Muscle tension headaches are very common and are usually caused by stress, eyestrain, poor posture, or nighttime grinding of teeth.
- *Migraine headaches* appear to have genetic and environmental causes. They also may be caused by changes in the brainstem or imbalance in brain chemicals such as serotonin. About half of those who have migraine headaches have a family history of migraines. Migraines can be triggered by many factors, including various foods, wind, excessive caffeine, emotional upheaval, sex, cold foods, hormonal fluctuations (called menstrual migraines), exercise, or changes in altitude.
- *Cluster headaches* are similar to migraines (vascular) but occur in clusters, occurring several times in a short period of time and then disappearing, sometimes for months. They usually involve red, watery eyes and nasal congestion. It is unknown what causes cluster headaches, but they may be triggered by certain foods, alcohol, or smoking.
- *"Chronic daily headache"* is a diagnosis to describe headaches that occur at least 50 percent of the time and may occur every day, 24-7. Most of the time, chronic daily headache is a type of migraine or tension headache—or a combination of the two.
- *Cervicogenic headaches* originate from the neck (cervico = neck), usually caused by arthritis or trauma (such as whiplash). The headache starts in the neck but can spread to the top and sides of the head.
- *Occipital headaches* are caused by compression, trauma, or inflammation of the occipital nerve in the back part of the skull, and they can radiate to the eyes.

The different types of headaches can occur together, or one type can precipitate the development of another type. The most common combination involves muscle tension and migraine headaches. Migraines are usually longer-lasting than tension headaches, but the latter can last for days at a time and be chronic as well.

Important Information:
Diagnosing Headaches: Imaging Overused

A research letter published in 2014 in *JAMA Internal Medicine* revealed that neuroimaging (imaging of the head) occurred in roughly 10 percent of office visits for headache, costing nearly $1 billion per year. This was based on data evaluating over fifty million visits for headache between 2007 and 2010. Either MRI or CT was ordered in 12 percent of all headache visits and 10 percent of migraine visits.

Guidelines on evaluating headache recommend against routine imaging for headache complaints. Talk to your doctor about the need for imaging and realize that you may be receiving unnecessary testing.

⸎

Important Note: Numerous conventional medications have the potential to cause headaches or make them worse as a side effect, so it is important to rule out medications as a cause before adding additional medications to treat the headaches. If you have headaches and are on a medication, you can check the *PDR* to see if that medication can cause headaches, or consult with your pharmacist.

Treatments for *Tension* Headaches

The Preventive Approaches

Relaxation and **stress reduction** are essential in the treatment as stress is the major cause and precipitating event for tension headaches.

The Conventional Approaches

Medications are the primary conventional approach for tension headaches. For mild, intermittent muscle tension headaches, *acetaminophen* (Tylenol) or *ibuprofen* can relieve your headache within twenty to forty-five minutes. If these don't seem to be strong enough, medications containing *butalbital* (such as Fiorcet) are often prescribed.

For chronic, recurrent tension headaches, *amitriptyline* (Elavil) is often used. This is a mild antidepressant that affects the pain center in the brain. However, this medication may take at least three weeks for you to observe a beneficial effect.

Botulinum toxin (Botox) injections have been noted to help reduce the frequency of tension headaches. One to four injections are given at three-month intervals and are applied at several different muscle groups, depending on the location of your headache. It is thought that Botox may work by being injected into acupuncture points.

Cognitive/behavioral ("talk") therapy may be beneficial if underlying psychological issues or stress issues are causing or continuing your tension headaches.

The Alternative Approaches

Meditation is one of the best treatments for tension headaches and should be done fifteen to thirty minutes every day. To begin meditation, you can undergo progressive relaxation of your muscles, which can itself relieve the tension.

Massage or acupressure can also relieve acute headaches by applying pressure directly on the trigger points or tense muscles, usually around the neck, forehead, and temples. Applying pressure on the acupuncture point LI-4 often quickly relieves headaches. This point is located in the web between the thumb and index finger and is usually quite tender. Apply firm pressure on this point and massage it for several minutes.

Chinese herbal formulas are very beneficial and can work better than conventional medications and have few side effects. *Ding Xin Wan* is useful if you have general anxiety and stress, but *Chai Hu Mu Li Long Gu Tan* may be the best for relieving tension. *Yan Hu Suo Wan* can be used for short term pain, tension, and spasms. These formulas work quickly and can be taken as needed for headaches.

Acupuncture is also very effective for reducing the frequency or eliminating tension headaches, and can be used with the above herbs. It can also address underlying causes of the tension headache, such as anxiety. You should notice improvement within six acupuncture treatments, but you might need additional sessions for maximum benefit.

If there is anxiety or underlying emotional problems causing the continuation of tension headaches, **interactive imagery** (active imagination) is the fastest psychotherapy method to find and correct these issues. This is a mind-body method in which you mentally interact with images that represent your emotions and/or headache. It is a powerful method to uncover and deal with subconscious psychological issues you may not be aware of. (See chapter 4 for detailed discussion.) *Guided imagery* may also be very effective.

Magnesium (250–400 mg three times a day), and *5-HTP* (100 mg three times daily) supplements can prevent muscle tension headaches in many people, but may take one to two months to observe beneficial results. They are more effective when used together.

Manual therapy may resolve tension headaches that are caused by structural (misalignment) problems with the neck, face, temporomandibular joint TMJ, or skull. Chiropractic manipulation can be effective in relieving muscle tension caused by neck problems, and you should observe relief within four to six treatments. Don't continue these treatments unless your headaches are becoming less frequent and less severe with continued chiropractic treatment. For misalignment of the face, skull, or TMJ, osteopathic manipulation may be more effective. You should obtain relief within three to six treatments.

Biofeedback has been used for decades and, for some people, can be an effective treatment for reducing the frequency and severity of muscle tension headaches when other treatments have failed.

Your Empowered Patient Action Plan for Treating Tension Headaches

Step #1:   *Meditate with progressive relaxation* fifteen to thirty minutes a day to prevent tension headaches. It can also be helpful to decrease or resolve the headache while you are having it.

Step #2:   *Use massage and acupressure for occasional headaches*: Expect resolution within five to thirty minutes.

Step #3:   *Take acetaminophen for occasional headaches*: This should relieve the headache within thirty minutes.

Step #4:   *Take the Chinese herbal remedies Ding Xin Wan or Chai Hu Mu Li Long Gu Tang* for short-term relief if you are still having tension headaches, especially if they are caused by stress. Take as needed every day.

Step #5:   *Undergo interactive imagery or other psychotherapy* if you still have headaches, whether or not underlying psychological or emotional issues are present. This method can provide long lasting relief and decrease reoccurrences.

Step #6:   *Undergo acupuncture,* which is an effective treatment for long-term relief.

Step #7:   *Undergo an osteopathic or chiropractic evaluation* to find underlying structural causes for your headaches if they are still reoccurring. If present, undergo manual therapy.

Step #8:   *Undergo biofeedback* for short- or long-term relief if you still get headaches.

Step #9:   *Take a low-dose prescription tricyclic antidepressant* for chronic tension headaches if none of the above steps have worked.

Step #10: *Try Botox injections* for three to four months of relief if the above steps have not helped.

Expected Outcome

Tension headaches are sometimes difficult to resolve completely, but at the least, they can be controlled well enough with several methods so as to not interfere with your quality of life.

Treatments for *Migraine* Headaches

Migraines Linked to Brain Infarcts

A recent study revealed that migraine headaches occurring in midlife that are accompanied by visual auras (seeing "lights") predicts an increased risk of having brain infarcts in later life. Approximately 4 percent of men and 8 percent of women experience auras with their migraines. People who have other symptoms of migraine do not have an increased risk of later life brain infarcts.

The Preventive Approaches

A recent study showed that **vitamin D** deficiency is common in patients with chronic migraines. Whether taking vitamin D will reverse migraines is not known, but because this vitamin has been found preventive for many medical conditions, it is important to make sure your levels are normal (should be at least 30 ng/ml).

Diet: Food may play a role in migraines and cluster headaches. Food allergy testing and elimination diets may be helpful in determining which foods play a part. Certain foods, including chocolate, cheese, beer, and wine, can also trigger migraine attacks and should be avoided if they do.

Avoid other triggers: An important method of preventing migraines is to avoid factors that trigger their occurrence. Besides the above foods, these include stressful events, bright lights, flying, and changes in barometric pressure.

The Conventional Approaches

Medications are the primary treatment for migraines in conventional medicine. If migraines are mild, *NSAIDs* (such as naproxen [Naprosyn], meloxicam [Mobic], piroxicam [Feldene], oxaprozin [Daypro], nabumatone [Relafen], ketoprofen [Orudis], diclofenac [Cataflam], celocoxib (Celebrex] and diclofenac/misoprostol [Arthrotec]) or a *combination of aspirin, acetaminophen, and caffeine* (which are the "migraine formulas" of Advil, Motrin, or Excedrin) may give you relief until the migraine passes. *Caution*: In July, 2015, the FDA started requiring NSAIDs to carry a warning of increased risk of heart attacks, stroke and heart failure. This is especially evident when taken long term, at higher doses, or by people with pre-existing heart disease. The risks can increase as early as the first weeks of NSAID use. However, ibuprofen and naproxen do not appear to increase the risk, so are the safest and preferred NSAIDs.

If you cannot take medications because of gastrointestinal symptoms caused by your migraine, you can try a new form of *aspirin* called "oral dispersible," which is taken without water and is absorbed in your mouth.

If these medications do not help, or you have more severe migraines, *triptans* are the drugs of choice. Basically, all the triptans can be equally beneficial. When one triptan fails, another one may work, so you may have to try several to see which one is the best for you. Here is some comparative information on the various triptans, based on various studies:

- *Sumatriptan* (Imitrex) was the first and is still the most common triptan used by doctors, but the others can be just as beneficial or more so. Imitrex is available in nasal spray and injectable, in addition to oral. It has also now just been released as a patch for those who can't take pills due to nausea. *Sumatriptan* is less effective when aura is present
- *Zolmitriptan* (Zomig) has the same effectiveness as sumatriptan. It is given through a nasal spray and works faster than the pill forms.
- *Rizatriptan* (Maxalt) can be dissolved on the tongue and can alleviate migraines within thirty minutes. It has better effectiveness than sumatriptan and is the most consistently effective of all the triptans.
- *Almotriptan* (Axert) and naratriptan (Amerge) have fewer side effects than sumatriptan but may be less effective.
- *Frovatriptan* (Frova) lasts the longest (twenty-six hours versus five hours for the others), and is recommended for menstrual migraines.
- *Eletriptan* (Relpax) is more effective than sumatriptan at higher dosages (80 mg), but has more side effects.
- Recently, the FDA has approved *Treximet*, a drug that combines naproxen (anti-inflammatory) with sumatriptan. This combination appears to provide relief faster and last longer than either medication alone.

Caution When Taking Triptans with Antidepressants

People who take a triptan for migraines and are also on an SSRI antidepressant (such as Prozac, Zoloft, Paxil, Celexa, Effexor, or Luvox) are at risk for serotonin syndrome, caused by the buildup of too much serotonin, a brain neurotransmitter. An estimated seven hundred thousand people are at risk for this syndrome. The syndrome causes various symptoms including restlessness, loss of coordination, hypertension, hallucinations, fast heartbeat, fever, sweating, nausea and vomiting, overactive reflexes, coma, and even death.

There are some **older medications** that can be used if the triptans don't work. This includes ergotamine-containing medications (both oral and nasal spray), such as *ergotamine tartrate* and *DHE*. Usually, these drugs work better if you have warning signs that the migraine is going to happen or you are in the early stages of migraine. There are more restrictions on using these drugs because they cause blood vessels to contract.

Narcotic injections such as *Stadol* or *Demerol* may be necessary if the above drugs don't work. These narcotics can "break" the migraine, but you will probably have side effects of drowsiness and be unable to return to normal activity for several hours or even several days. In addition, you may still need a repeat injection if the headache is not completely resolved.

Injections of **botulinum toxin (Botox)** have been noted to help reduce the frequency of migraine headaches. One to four injections are given at three-month intervals and are applied at several different muscle groups, depending on the location of your headache. This treatment is very costly and has only minimal benefit.

Cefaly is the first *device* to prevent migraine headaches approved by the FDA in 2014. It is an electrical device worn in a headband for twenty minutes per day. In studies, about half the patients were satisfied with the device, finding fewer days with migraines per month and not having to take as much migraine medication. However, it did not reduce the intensity of the headaches that occurred.

For prevention or decrease of recurrent migraines:

Other **medications** may be helpful. *Beta-blockers* (propranolol or timolol) or the ACE inhibitor *lisinopril* (Prinivil, Zestril) are approved to reduce migraine severity and frequency. If these drugs are not effective, *amitryptiline*, *divalproex sodium* (Depakote), or *gabapentin* (Neurontin) are the next conventional medications to try. A newer medication, *Topamax*, has shown equal effectiveness but is much more expensive and has been shown to have no advantage over the others. SSRI antidepressants have been used for migraine prevention but are less effective than the above drugs. Each medication may have different results and different side effects for each person, so you may need to try several to find the one that is most effective for you, with the least side effects. It may take several weeks to see improvement.

The Alternative Approaches

Acupuncture is by far the best method for stopping migraines as well as resolving them long term. In an acute migraine attack, most symptoms may be relieved within fifteen to thirty minutes. With continued acupuncture, the severity and frequency of migraine attacks may be reduced and even eliminated. In fact, a 2015 study showed that acupuncture is as effective as drugs in prophylaxis of migraine (50 percent reduction in headache days per month) and half the drug group dropped out due to side effects (none in the acupuncture group). ***Important Note****:* There may be several different underlying syndromes causing migraines, so proper Chinese diagnosis (pulse and tongue) must be made.

There are also numerous **Chinese herbal** combinations that may help reduce migraine severity and frequency. *Chai Hu Mu Li Long Gu Tang, Long Dan Xie Gan Wan, Tian Ma Gou Teng Yin Wan,* or *Qiang Huo Sheng Shi Tang,* may all help. An advantage of Chinese herbs over conventional medications and supplements is that once your migraines are under control, you can reduce or discontinue them. You should notice overall decrease in migraines within three weeks, but you may need to take the formulas longer for complete relief.

There are several **homeopathic remedies** (12c or 30c potency) that may be helpful. They are best taken at onset of headache; if unrelieved, you may take a second dose thirty minutes later:

- *Bryonia* is used for left-sided headaches, averse to slight movement.
- *Glonoinum* used for pulsating and bursting headaches; worse from the sun.
- *Natrum muriaticum* for migraine headaches worse with light, sun, reading.

For prevention or decrease of recurrent migraines:
Nutritional supplements can be beneficial. *Riboflavin* (vitamin B$_2$, 400 mg per day), *magnesium* (250–400 mg), *vitamin B$_6$* (100 mg daily), *5-HTP* (50–100 mg three times daily), and the herb *feverfew* (freeze-dried leaf at 50–125 mg per day, standardized to contain 0.2 percent parthenolide) have all been found effective in studies, either alone or in combination. The combination product Migra-Lieve contains feverfew with riboflavin and magnesium, which may give you adequate relief. *CoQ10* (120 mg daily) may also help prevent migraines and can be taken alone or with the other supplements. You should see improvement within one to two months.

If food allergies are a possible cause of your migraines, the ***Nambudripad Allergy Elimination Treatment***, or NAET, combines acupuncture, kinesiology, chiropractic, herbs, and nutrition to desensitize you to foods to which you are allergic. It may take several months to notice improvement, depending on how many allergens are sensitizing you.

Your Empowered Patient Action Plan to *Stop* an Acute Migraine Attack

Step #1: Undergo acupuncture, which is the fastest way of relieving migraines.
Step #2: Take an NSAID if the migraine is mild and acupuncture is not available.
Step #3: Take a prescription triptan medication if the above steps haven't worked.
Step #4 Take an ergotamine medication if the above steps don't help.
Step #5: Receive a narcotic injection if the migraine is still not relieved.

When Paul came to me, he had a long history of migraine headaches. These would occur once or twice a month and would be very severe, often accompanied by nausea and vomiting and lasting for hours or even days. He had taken many different types of medication that helped reduce the symptoms, but he would still feel badly for several days. During one of these attacks, he came to the clinic. Lights and sounds caused his headache to worsen, and he looked ashen. I performed acupuncture, and within twenty minutes, most of his pain was gone. An hour later, he was able to return to work.

Your Empowered Patient Action Plan to *Prevent* or *Resolve* Chronic Migraines

Step #1: ***Avoid the trigger factors*** mentioned above under "Prevention."

Step #2: ***Undergo regular acupuncture treatments*** to achieve long term prevention and resolution.

Step #3: ***Take an appropriate prescription triptan*** to stop migraines that the above steps don't relieve.

Step #4: ***Use the NAET*** if you suspect food allergies may be causing or initiating your migraines.

Step #5: ***Try homeopathic remedies*** to resolve an acute migraine if the above steps have not worked.

Step #6: ***Take an appropriate prescription medication*** (beta-blocker, ACE inhibitor, or other) to prevent migraines if the above steps have not eliminated them.

Step #7: ***Try the Cefaly device*** to decrease the number of migraines.

Step #8: ***Take riboflavin, magnesium, vitamin B_6, 5-HTP, CoQ10, and/or feverfew*** to prevent reoccurrence.

Step #9: ***Take the Chinese herbal remedies Chai Hu Mu Li Long Gu Tang, Long Dan Xie Gan Wan, Tian Ma Gou Teng Yin Wan, or Qiang Huo Sheng Shi Tang*** for preventive relief if the above treatments have not helped.

Step #10: ***Take Botox injections*** to obtain relief for three to four months if you still have migraines.

Step #11: ***Take combinations of medications***: If the above recommended treatment steps are still not effective, try the following in various combinations: aspirin, multiple NSAIDs, gabapentin (Neurontin), verapamil, other beta-blockers, and the herb feverfew. Again, each medication may have different effects for each person, so you may need to try several to find the one that is most effective for you, with the least side effects.

Joan is a thirty-eight-year-old patient of mine who suffered from migraines for over twenty years, occurring at least twice a week and lasting for hours and sometimes days. She had been tried on numerous medications, which would help dull her headaches but did not diminish the frequency or severity of the attacks. She underwent eight acupuncture treatments along with taking the Chinese herbal formula Chai Hu Mu Li Long Gu Tang. She has not had any more migraines in six years.

Expected Outcome

Migraine headaches are certainly controllable in most people using conventional approaches, but alternative methods can often resolve and prevent them long-term.

Treatments for *Cluster* Headaches

The Preventive Approaches

Food may play a role in cluster headaches. Food-allergy testing and elimination diets may be helpful in determining which foods play a part. Certain foods, including chocolate, cheese, beer, and wine, can also trigger cluster attacks and should be avoided if they do.

The Conventional Approaches

Oxygen inhalation during an acute attack is effective and safe and is the first conventional treatment for cluster headaches. Your doctor needs to prescribe this treatment, which involves breathing oxygen through a face mask at a rate of seven to eight liters per minute for ten to fifteen minutes, in a sitting position.

NSAIDs, especially Naproxen, can be effective if the headache lasts more than forty-five minutes. However, many cluster headaches do not last that long, so you must take it as soon as you have a headache.

Triptan medications (Imitrex, Maxalt, Relpax, Axert, Amerge, and Zomig) are often given for cluster headaches. Basically, all the triptans can be equally beneficial. When one triptan fails, another one may work, so you may have to try several to see which one is the best for you. See under *Migraine Headaches* above for comparisons of the various triptans.

Beware Taking Triptans with Antidepressants

People who take a triptan for migraines and are also on an SSRI antidepressant (such as Prozac, Zoloft, Paxil, Celexa, Effexor, or Luvox) are at risk for serotonin syndrome, caused by the buildup of too much serotonin, a brain neurotransmitter. An estimated seven hundred thousand people are at risk for this syndrome. The syndrome causes various symptoms including restlessness, loss of coordination, hypertension, hallucinations, fast heartbeat, fever, sweating, nausea and vomiting, overactive reflexes, coma, and even death.

Other prescription medications may help for acute attacks if triptans don't. These include DHE 45, Ergotamine, Lidocaine, or methylphenidate. Other medications are used for prevention but you'll need to take them long-term. These include:

- A *combination* of *verapamil* (240 mg/day) and *prednisone* (60–80 mg/day), but use the prednisone for only seven to fourteen days.
- *Methysergide* (2 mg three times a day).
- *Lithium* or *valproic acid* (Depakene) or both together.

There are also some **surgical procedures** that can relieve cluster headaches when all other treatment approaches fail, but there may be serious risks. *Glycerol injection* is the least risky. Surgery should be a treatment of last resort.

The Alternative Approaches

Acupuncture is the best alternative method for both stopping and preventing cluster headaches. However, there may be several different underlying syndromes causing migraines, so proper Chinese diagnosis (pulse and tongue) must be made.

There are also several **nutritional supplements** and herbs that are commonly taken for cluster headaches. For an acute attack, *melatonin* (10 mg) sometimes can abort the attack.

For ***preventing*** cluster headaches, a *combination* of magnesium (250–400 mg), vitamin B_6 (100 mg daily), and 5-HTP (50–100 mg three times daily) may be effective. Magnesium prevents over excitability of nerve cells and maintains the tone of blood vessels, vitamin B_6 helps prevent histamine release (which can trigger headaches), and 5-HTP increases brain neurotransmitters, especially serotonin. It may take one to two months to notice improvement.

Foods and food allergies may trigger cluster headaches. The **NAET** combines acupuncture, kinesiology, chiropractic, herbs, and nutrition to desensitize you to foods you are allergic to. It may take several months to experience improvement, depending on how many allergens are sensitizing you.

Your Empowered Patient Action Plan To *Treat* Acute Cluster Headaches

Step #1: Undergo acupuncture for immediate relief.

Step #2: Receive oxygen inhalation treatment for immediate relief if you are not able to undergo acupuncture.

Step #3: Take melatonin if the above steps are not helpful.

Step #4: Take an NSAID (Naproxen) if symptoms last for more than forty-five minutes and the above steps haven't helped.

Step #5: Take a prescription triptan medication for acute relief if the above steps are ineffective.

Step #6: Take other prescription medications for short-term relief if the above steps don't work.

Your Empowered Patient Action Plan to *Prevent* Cluster Headaches

Step #1: Undergo acupuncture for long term resolution or at least decreased frequency and severity.

Step #2: Take combination magnesium, vitamin B$_6$, and 5-HTP if acupuncture is not effective.

Step #3: Use the NAET if the above steps have not worked and/or food allergies are suspected as a cause of your cluster headaches.

Step #4: Undergo surgery as a last resort.

Expected Outcome

As with migraine headaches, cluster headaches can be well controlled by conventional approaches in most people, but alternative methods may be able to resolve or prevent them completely.

Treatment of Occipital Headaches

Because occipital headaches are caused by injury to a nerve, see section on neuralgia.

Treatment of Cervicogenic Headaches

Because cervicogenic headaches are due to abnormalities with the neck, see section on neck and back problems.

Hearing Loss

What You Need to Know

One condition that occurs to many people as we age is hearing loss. Hearing loss can occur sooner due to noise exposures (sensorineural loss), but there is also age-related hearing loss, called presbycusis, which begins around age fifty. Hearing loss can also be caused by an abnormal growth of bone of the middle ear (called otosclerosis). By sixty-five, one in three people will have hearing loss.

Unfortunately, fewer than one in five people say that their doctor has ever asked them about their hearing or tested them, and few people bring it up themselves. It is important to treat it early because if you wait too long, you may be accustomed to not hearing and find it harder to adjust to a hearing aid.

Sudden sensorineural hearing loss (SSHL), or sudden deafness, occurs as an unexplained, rapid loss of hearing—usually in one ear—either at once or over several days. Some people may hear a "pop" before they lose hearing. Many people may think that it is due to ear wax, sinus infection, or another common condition but delay in treatment can decrease the effectiveness of treatment. Only 15-20 percent of people with SSHL have a cause that can be identified but it still is important to seek immediate care. However, about half of people with SSHL will spontaneously recover their hearing usually within one to two weeks.

Warning:
Sudden Hearing Loss May Lead to Stroke

A recent study published in *Stroke* revealed that sudden hearing loss significantly elevates the risk for stroke. If you have sudden hearing loss, you should undergo a complete neurological and ear examination.

Treatments for Hearing Loss

The Preventive Approaches

The best prevention for hearing loss is to **avoid loud noises**. Although age-related hearing loss is not caused by loud noises, such noises can accelerate and increase the hearing loss and at an earlier age.

A recent study on age-related hearing found that eating at least two servings of **fish** a week decreases the risk of hearing loss by 42 percent, and the higher the intake, the lower the risk.

The Conventional Approaches

Hearing aids are the primary treatment for hearing loss. Hearing aids vary greatly in type, quality, and expense; so you should be careful what you choose. Depending on your needs, you may require extended frequency ranges or one that limits background noises. The most advanced hearing aids use a microchip and can adjust to different background sound levels, and others can be programmed to tailor adjustments, but these are the most expensive. Hearing aids range from $600 per ear to $2,500 or more.

There are three basic types of hearing aids: over the ear or behind the ear (visible), in the ear canal but still visible, and deep in the ear canal and not visible. In general, the larger and more visible the hearing aid, the better you hear.

No hearing aid will fully restore your hearing, but you should notice an improvement quickly. As many hearing aids are very small, make sure you can fit them into place easily.

There are also **assistive listening devices** that can direct more sound to your hearing aid and can be used in situations with increased background noise. There are also amplifying devices to attach to telephones.

In many cases **surgery** is an option for treatment of otosclerosis. In an operation called a *stapedectomy*, a surgeon bypasses the diseased bone with a prosthetic device that allows sound waves to be passed to the inner ear. For severe or total hearing loss, *a cochlear implant* is a safe electronic device that is implanted beneath the skin and into the inner ear. Once the outer skin has healed, an external device is placed on the skin over the implanted device and turned on.

The Alternative Approaches

If the hearing loss is not profound and has existed for a short period of time, **acupuncture** may be helpful to reduce the loss or prevent further deterioration. It also may be helpful if hearing loss (or deafness) is caused by drugs, trauma, or infections. You should obtain some initial benefit within six to eight treatments, although many more may be necessary for optimum benefit.

A **Chinese herbal formula**, *Huan Shao Dan Wan* may be useful along with acupuncture.

Taking **fish oil supplements** may help reduce the rate of hearing loss. *Important notes*: Although regular fish oil can benefit hearing, you should take *at least* 1,500 mg daily to obtain benefits. Many studies were done using 3,000–4,000 mg.

Your Empowered Patient Action Plan for Treating Hearing Loss

- **Warning:** *Sudden hearing loss is considered an emergency. You should be examined and treated as soon as possible by an otolaryngologist (ENT doctor).*

Step #1: Avoid loud noises, which will make hearing loss worse. Use earphones or cuffs if exposed to loud noises.

Step #2: Undergo acupuncture if your hearing loss is mild and has been present for only a short time (less than a year).

Step #3: Obtain a hearing aid. Research the types of hearing aids first. Then be sure to price-shop and make sure you get a thirty-day trial period with a money-back guarantee. Ask about service charges, returns, upgrades, repairs, and training or assistance.

Step #4: Consider surgery for specific treatable causes or severe hearing loss.

Expected Outcome

Hearing loss is difficult to resolve or reverse once it is present, although if diagnosed early, alternative methods may help. Otherwise, hearing aids can at least provide improved hearing.

Heart Disease: Angina and Heart Attacks (Myocardial Infarction or MI)

What You Need to Know

Heart disease is a general term that encompasses several types of heart problems, the primary ones being angina, heart attacks (MI or myocardial infarction), coronary artery disease (CAD), and congestive heart failure (CHF). Other heart problems include arrhythmias (abnormal heart beat), valvular disease (disease of the valves between heart chambers), and cardiomyopathy (disease of the heart muscle). *This section will focus on angina and heart attacks.* (See below for separate sections on other heart conditions)

Heart Attack Facts

- About every 26 seconds, an American will have a heart-related (coronary) event.

- About once every minute, someone will die from a coronary event.
- About 40 percent of people who have a heart attack in a given year will die from it.
- More than 83 percent of people who die of coronary artery disease are age 65 or older.
- Within 6 years of a recognized heart attack:
    - About 22 percent of men and 46 percent of women will be disabled with heart failure
    - 18 percent of men and 35 percent of women will have another heart attack.
    - 8 percent of men and 11 percent of women will have a stroke.
    - 7 percent of men and 6 percent of women will experience sudden death.

Angina is chest pain caused by the heart tissue not getting enough oxygen (called ischemia), usually due to clogged heart arteries (atherosclerosis). The most common type of angina is called *stable angina*, characterized by chest pain only upon exertion. Also known as "effort" angina, the typical presentation is that of chest discomfort and associated symptoms precipitated by some activity (running, walking, etc.) with minimal or nonexistent symptoms at rest. Symptoms typically abate several minutes following cessation of precipitating activities and resume when activity resumes.

Unstable angina, also referred to as "crescendo angina," has at least one of these three features:

- Occurs at rest (or with minimal exertion), usually lasting longer than ten minutes.
- Is severe and of new onset (i.e., within the prior four to six weeks).
- Occurs with a crescendo pattern (i.e., distinctly more severe, prolonged, or frequent than previously).

Studies show that 64 percent of all unstable anginas occur between 10:00 p.m. and 8:00 a.m., when patients are at rest.

Important Information
Sudden Cardiac Arrest May be Preventable in Many People

Sudden cardiac arrest (SCA) is a leading cause of death in the United States, claiming an estimated 325,000 lives each year (1,000 people a day or one person every two minutes)

Unfortunately, almost 95 percent of victims of cardiac arrest die before they reach a hospital or other source of emergency help because death usually occurs within minutes.

SCA is not the same as a heart attack; during a heart attack, the heart usually doesn't suddenly stop beating. SCA, however, may happen after or during recovery from a heart attack and people who have heart disease are at higher risk for SCA. However, SCA can happen in people who appear healthy and have no known heart disease or other risk factors for SCA (commonly from an arrhythmia…a disturbance in the rhythm of the heartbeat).

It has been shown that immediate use of an automated external defibrillator (AED) can prevent a significant number of deaths from SCA (30 to 45 percent survival rate). However, only 3.7 percent of people with SCA are treated with an AED.

Another sobering fact is that half of the people who have SCA had warning signs in the 4 weeks prior to the event, according to a December, 2015 study in *Ann Intern Med*. In addition, 90 percent had symptoms recur in the 24 hours before the arrest. Symptoms were primarily chest pain (mostly in men) or shortness of breath (mostly in women). Only 19 percent of those with symptoms called emergency medical services before cardiac arrest and those people were five times more likely to survive.

The *bottom line* is that you need to recognize the symptoms of angina and arrhythmias and go to an emergency room immediately. If you do, you may be able to prevent a heart attack or sudden death.

A more rare form of angina is called *Prinzmetal*, or variant angina. It occurs mostly in women and is caused by spasm of the heart arteries rather than blockage.

Angina itself causes no permanent damage, but it is a sign that the heart is diseased. Not treating the angina and underlying heart disease can lead to heart attack and death.

Heart attacks have traditionally been diagnosed based on EKG and CPK enzymes, the latter which usually rise from heart cells that are dying. However, it is recognized that many people will have normal EKG results and misleading or delayed CPK results. The best way to diagnose a heart attack is by obtaining *Troponin* levels in the blood.

With Heart Disease, Women May Differ from Men

Heart disease in women may present much differently than in men. To start, it is well recognized that the risk of postmenopausal women to have heart disease quickly catches up to the risk in men. It is also recognized that women may not receive as appropriate heart care as men.

One reason for this appears to be that women suffer from atypical symptoms, including shortness of breath, left *and* right arm pain, dizziness, abdominal pain, and back pain. All of these symptoms may be caused by other problems, so they can be missed.

Women also commonly have "invisible" heart blockages. They are twice as likely as men to have normal results or less than 50 percent of blockage on angiogram tests (dye test that shows blockages in the heart arteries) despite having had a heart attack. Women are also more likely to have misleading EKG or CPK results than men.

More heart attacks occur in winter, which is a time you should be more aware of any heart symptoms. This occurs throughout the United States, even in warmer climate zones. In addition, a heart attack during the winter is more likely to be fatal than at any other time of the year. Heart attack risk is also greater between the hours of 6:00 a.m. and noon.

Heart Test May Not Be Necessary

A frequently ordered test for coronary artery disease is the CT angiogram, which combines infusion of dye into the heart arteries along with a CT scan. Many doctors contend that it has no proven value in most patients. Although this test provides impressive pictures, studies show that it does not alter patient care or improve outcomes. The bottom line is that there are less expensive tests, which are more useful and do not expose patients to relatively high amounts of radiation.

In recent years, several discoveries have contributed to more knowledge about heart disease. First, it has been thought that heart disease is a result of atherosclerosis—clogging or hardening of the arteries. However, it is now recognized that low grade inflammation may also be a major factor. This is important because treatments that only decrease artery clogging may not prevent or improve all heart disease.

The good news is that the rate of heart attacks dropped by 24 percent between 1999 and 2008, and the death rate from heart attack has been cut in half since 1980. This is due primarily to preventive measures and improved treatments, including those now addressing low grade inflammation.

Silent Heart Attacks May Occur During Surgery

In a recent study published in the *Annals of Internal Medicine*, 5 percent of patients undergoing noncardiac surgery who had or were at risk for atherosclerosis suffered heart attacks after surgery. Two-thirds of these patients had no symptoms of ischemia (such as angina).

This is important because these patients are at increased risk for another cardiac event or death within thirty days. Thus, surgeons should order Troponin levels on all surgery patients who have or are at risk for atherosclerosis. Become empowered and make sure you ask for this test if you are at elevated risk.

Treatments for Angina/Heart Attacks

The Preventive Approaches
There are several **tests for inflammation**, homocysteine and C-reactive protein (CRP) being the most common, and they can indicate a higher risk of heart attack. Many drugs and alternative supplements (B vitamins, folate) are known to decrease these so-called "markers," but so far, studies have shown that lowering them does not decrease the risk of heart disease.

Psychological aspects: Hostility, anger or depression can increase CRP, so dealing appropriately with these emotions can reduce the risk of heart disease.

Check Your Vitamin D Levels

A recent study in the *Archives of Internal Medicine* demonstrated that low levels of vitamin D in men are associated with double the risk for heart attacks. Vitamin D has beneficial effects on heart muscle cell growth, blood vessel calcification, inflammation, and blood pressure. Check your vitamin D level (plasma 25-hydroxyvitamin D) to make sure you have a normal level.

———— ⁕ ————

Genomics is adding to our knowledge of how to prevent heart disease. Recently, a genetic variant, called KIF6, has been linked to an increased risk of heart attack as well as a person's chances of reducing that risk by taking statins (for lowering cholesterol). KIF6 is present in 60 percent of the population; it can be measured for about $200, although insurance does not cover the test.

Smoking is a major cause of angina and heart disease and should be discontinued. The heart arteries cannot heal if you continue smoking. Also avoid **excessive coffee drinking**, which can worsen angina. If you have **high cholesterol**, you must reduce it to normal to stop clogging your heart arteries (see section on cholesterol for guidelines).

———— ⁕ ————

Aspirin Does Not Prevent Initial Adverse Cardiac Events

Many doctors prescribe aspirin if you don't have heart disease but are at risk for cardiac events such as angina or heart attacks (such as smoking, family history, etc.) to prevent these from occurring (called *primary* prevention). However, recent studies in *JAMA* show that aspirin may not prevent such cardiac events and is not necessary and, in fact, is used inappropriately in a significant number of patients. Primary prevention is now advised only for people who have a moderate-to-high ten-year risk of developing heart disease (see section on Cholesterol for discussion on measuring risk).

———— ⁕ ————

Poor **diet** is another major cause of angina and heart disease. You need to increase dietary fiber (eat more veggies: every 7-gram increase in daily dietary fiber significantly lowers risk of heart disease) and eat at least two meals of fish per week (cold-water fish such as mackerel, salmon, halibut, tuna, herring, or cod) to help reduce or prevent cholesterol buildup in the heart arteries. Oats and barley have been shown to reduce the risk of heart disease, and high nut consumption has been found to decrease mortality from heart disease.

Avoid, or at least limit, saturated fats, foods high in cholesterol, and animal proteins, all of which increase cholesterol buildup in the heart arteries as well as causing inflammation. Processed meat (cured, salted, fermented, or smoked) is especially bad and doubles the risk of all-cause death, but nonprocessed red meat appears to have minimal effects if not eaten every day and not in high amounts (6 oz or less per day or less than 18 oz per week). Recent guidelines include deriving 5–6 percent of calories from saturated fat but eliminating the percentage of calories from trans fats.

Several *diet plans* have been documented to be beneficial for preventing and reducing heart disease. These include the *DASH* (also good for hypertension), the *USDA Food Pattern*, and the *AHA* diet. According to a 2014 review in the *American Journal of Medicine*, the *Mediterranean* diet has proven to reduce cardiovascular events to a degree greater than low-fat diets and equal to or greater than the benefit of taking statin drugs.

Do Calcium Supplements Cause Increase in Heart-Attack Risk?

A few recent studies have shown that calcium supplements (most often taken for osteoporosis) may raise the risk for heart attacks in healthy older women. Based on data from a *BMJ* study, treating one thousand people with calcium supplements for five years would prevent only twenty-six fractures but would cause an additional fourteen heart attacks. However, it should be noted that there were significant limitations and possible errors in this study, and many experts disagree with these findings. However, another study showed that high calcium intake (1,400 mg) is associated with earlier death in women. Yet another study showed that high supplemental calcium increases the risk for heart death in men.

If you eat a diet rich in low-fat dairy products, you may not need any calcium supplementation. Otherwise, a total of 1,000–1,200 mg daily (as much from diet as possible) appears more than adequate. In addition, adding vitamin D_3 to the calcium appears to help negate heart-related effects.

Alcohol: drinking one glass of wine daily with meals may be beneficial to help prevent heart disease. Red wine is the best choice because it contains antioxidants called polyphenols, but beer, white wine, cocktails, and grape juice can also provide benefit (if imbibed moderately…see chapter 2). Trying to "catch up" by binge drinking actually increases the risk of heart attack.

Moderate Drinking May Be Better than
Abstinence in Heart Attack Patients

A study presented at an American College of Cardiology annual meeting revealed that moderate drinkers who quit after a heart attack have worse long-term outcomes than those who continue mild to moderate drinking.

※

Drinking *pomegranate juice* (240 ml daily for three months) appears to decrease stress-induced myocardial ischemia (lack of oxygen delivery to heart muscle) in patients with coronary heart disease. The average improvement is about 17 percent with pomegranate juice compared with an 18 percent *worsening* of myocardial perfusion in patients treated with placebo. However, it is not known whether drinking pomegranate juice (and thus its effects on perfusion) translates to reducing the risk of a myocardial infarction or other cardiovascular outcomes.

※

Cold Beverages May Be Bad for the Heart

Most people have a cold drink after meals, but this may not be good if you have heart disease. The cold beverage can solidify the oily stuff that you consume and slow down digestion. It then reacts with acid in the stomach, breaks down, and is absorbed faster, which then becomes fat in the body. The Chinese and Japanese drink hot tea with their meals, which appears to lower the risk of heart attack.

※

Exercise is important because it helps you improve the ability of your cells to use oxygen efficiently, which reduces symptoms. Unfortunately, studies reveal that most people with heart disease are less likely to comply with physical activity recommendations. If you truly want to live longer and healthier, exercise is a must. ***Helpful tip***: Before starting an exercise program, however, you should undergo an exercise tolerance test (ETT) to determine your safe exercise level. Based on the ETT results, your doctor can advise you on a carefully graded, progressive aerobic exercise program.

Finally, good **oral hygiene** (i.e., brushing your teeth) is an important preventive. A recent study in the *British Medical Journal* found that poor oral hygiene is associated with higher risks for cardiovascular events such as angina, heart attacks, and arrhythmias.

Sex Helps Prevent Heart Attacks

Studies reveal that men who have the highest frequency of orgasm have half the death rate. In addition, men who have sex three or more times a week reduce their risk of stroke or heart attack by half. Whether the same effect occurs with women is not known (and has not been studied).

The Conventional Approaches For Unstable Angina

Initially, certain **medications** are given to thin the blood, followed by a test to determine if you have clogged arteries and how severe they are (angiography/cardiac catheterization). The medications may include *beta-blockers* to rest the heart, or drugs to thin the blood and prevent clotting, such as *aspirin, clopidogrel* (Plavix), *low molecular weight heparin* (LMWH) or a *glycoprotein IIb/IIIa inhibitor.*

Depending on how severe your condition is, an **invasive procedure/surgery** is often done for unstable angina or an acute heart attack, as most frequently there is an obstructing clot in a heart artery that needs to be removed immediately to prevent further damage. There are three procedures that can be done for unstable angina or an acute heart attack. The first two are classified as "percutaneous coronary intervention *(PCI),*" in which a catheter is threaded through a leg artery into a clogged heart (coronary) artery to open it, and the other is *coronary artery bypass grafting (CABG),* which involves major surgery to open the chest and bypass clogged arteries with veins taken from the legs.

Patients' Understanding of PCI Differ from Physicians' Understanding

A recent study from the *Annals of Internal Medicine* showed that patients undergoing PCI overestimate its benefits. Even with informed consent, patients were over four times as likely as physicians to believe that PCI would prevent heart attacks and almost five times as likely to believe that it would prevent a fatal attack. Fully 88 percent of patients believed that PCI lowers risk for heart attack compared to 17 percent of cardiologists, and 82 percent felt it would decrease the risk of death compared to 15 percent of cardiologists.

Studies show that PCI reduces symptoms but does not affect mortality or risk of heart attack. It is important for your doctor to tell you not only the risks involved with the procedure but also the anticipated benefits. Of course, it helps if your cardiologist knows the true statistics as well.

PCI: *Angioplasty* (short for *PTCA*, percutaneous transluminal coronary angioplasty) was the first PCI and involves using a balloon that is inflated inside the artery. It should be done within twelve hours from onset of symptoms, although it may still be helpful up to three days later. It appears to not help at all after three days and should not be done in such patients.

Important note: Unfortunately, arteries cleaned out by angioplasty may re-clog (called restenosis) in over half the patients. If this occurs, another angio-plasty is usually attempted. Restenosis may occur after several months to a year. To prevent restenosis, patients should take a combination of aspirin and a thi-enopyridine drug (clopidogrel [Plavix] or prasugrel [Effient]). It is unknown how long you should take this combination, with most doctors recommending about nine months. **Important note**: Many people think they are resistant to aspirin, but in actuality, most of these people are taking enteric-coated aspirin, which pro-tects the stomach but does not have as much blood-thinning effect as noncoated aspirin.

The second PCI procedure is *stenting*, which places a small device into the artery that holds the artery walls open to increase blood flow. Additional external radiation is often used with this procedure to activate substances in the catheter/stent to prevent recurrences of the blockage. The restenosis rate for stents ranges widely, from 11 per-cent to 46 percent, but it is less than with angioplasty.

Four factors increase the risk of restenosis:

- Age over sixty-three years
- Female sex
- Lesion length greater than 12 mm
- Type C lesion (the most complex).

The restenosis rate is nearly four times greater for long, complex lesions treated by multiple stent implantations as compared with simple lesions. As with angioplasty, to prevent restenosis, patients should take a combination of aspirin and a thienopyridine drug after stenting (see above). **Important note**: African American recipients of stents have a twofold increased risk of stents reclogging than do other ethnic groups; this is thought to be due to genetic factors.

Stent Comparison: Which is Best?

There are two types of stents: bare metal (BMS) and drug eluting (DES), the latter of which was designed to decrease occurrences of reclogging (restenosis) of the artery. The DES is the primary one used, although 80 percent of its use is for off-label conditions, as confirmed by studies.

Initial studies showed DES to decrease reclogging of arteries compared to BMS, but later studies showed that reclogging does occur more often in DES after thirty days. Following this study, the use dropped significantly, but it still leads the other PCI procedures. This is an area that is very controversial, with some experts saying that the risks outweigh the benefits. The latest research shows that DES has a lower risk for needing another procedure and lower risk of death than BMS.

The most important factor to prevent reclogging is to take aspirin and a thienopyridine drug (clopidogrel [Plavix] or prasugrel [Effient]) after the procedure. Many of the failures of DES are because patients stop taking these drugs. In addition, one study shows that it may be dangerous to suddenly stop these drugs, due to an increased risk of rebound coronary events such as heart attack. Be sure to discuss this with your cardiologist.

Helpful tip: During PCI, clot material can break off and imbed further in the artery, which compromises blood flow. This can be improved by using an aspiration catheter, with studies showing almost a twofold decrease in cardiac-related death or nonfatal repeat heart attack. Unfortunately, many centers do not have these catheters. Become empowered and make sure your doctor uses one.

Hospitals Not Using New Drugs before PCI

A study reported from Duke University revealed that doctors are not using the latest, potentially life-saving heart drugs in nearly two-thirds of patients presenting to the emergency room. These drugs (called glycoprotein [GP] llb/llla inbitors; Eptifibatide, Integrilin) are used if there are certain findings in patients having acute coronary syndromes at high risk of death or a nonfatal myocardial infarction and those patients are to undergo PCI. These drugs can decrease death rates by 50 percent if used within twenty-four hours of admission.

Coronary artery bypass grafting (CABG): Studies have shown that CABG may be slightly better than PTCA to reduce symptoms, but only in the hands of a skilled surgeon. With coronary disease in more than two arteries (multivessel disease) and in the sickest heart patients (three clogged arteries or clog in the left main artery), CABG has been found to be superior, causing fewer deaths and heart attacks. CABG has also been found to be superior to PCI in survival benefits in patients over sixty-five and in diabetics.

Important note: A large study in 2012 confirmed other studies that taking statin drugs (see section on "Cholesterol") prior to surgery lowers the risk for acute kidney injury from cardiac surgery.

Important note: Atrial fibrillation (AF), a cardiac arrhythmia (see section on arrhythmias), occurs relatively often after cardiac surgery and can cause complications. Most doctors prescribe beta blockers (metoprolol) to prevent AF, but many doctors are using a newer drug, amiodarone. This drug is equally effective but more expensive, and so far it shows no advantage over metoprolol.

Warning: Trasydol, a drug commonly used in bypass surgery to control bleeding, has been found to have increased risks of kidney failure, heart attack, and stroke in comparison to similar drugs.

Comparison of PCI Vs CABG

Two advantages with CABG include a lower incidence of needing to repeat the procedure and the need for taking two antiplatelet drugs, as with stents. A more recent study from the *NEJM* showed that CABG offers a slight advantage over drug-eluting stents (DES) in terms of improving quality of life after one year. Finally, a 2014 study showed that quality of life was better after CABG than medical treatment. On the negative side, CABG has a slightly higher risk of stroke and longer recuperation times.

The choice from the three procedures depends on the skills and experience of your cardiologist/cardiac surgeon, the condition of your heart arteries, and other medical conditions that you may have. *Important Note*: Even though these procedures will reduce your symptoms, they alone may not prolong life.

— ∞ —

Important Information:
Cognitive Decline Associated with Heart Procedures and Medical Treatment

Several studies have revealed that cognitive functioning (thinking, intellectual functions) is affected by both bypass surgery and PCI interventions. In general, the incidence of cognitive decline is 53 percent of people at discharge,

36 percent at six weeks, 24 percent at six months, and 42 percent at five years. However, the benefits may outweigh the risks if angina is unstable or you are having a heart attack.

A recent study showed that it is not just surgery that can cause cognitive decline; patients who were treated with various heart drugs also showed cognitive decline, and there was no significant difference between using heart drugs versus surgery.

Treatments After Stabilization of Angina

Once your angina is stabilized with these procedures, other **medications** are usually prescribed. *Aspirin* reduces the risk of heart attack and death in unstable angina by blocking platelets—the blood cells that cause clotting. If you are not already taking it, your doctor will probably recommend it after your angina is stabilized, whether you undergo interventions or not. You should take no more than 325 mg per day, as increased doses can cause harm and provide no additional benefit (*81 mg is often a sufficient dose*). **Important note**: Many people think they are resistant to aspirin, but in actuality, most of these people are taking enteric-coated aspirin, which protects the stomach but does not have as much blood-thinning effect as noncoated aspirin (also see sidebar below for additional reasons).

Aspirin Resistance: Real or Not?

In patients with coronary artery disease, aspirin has been found to reduce the rate of death due to all causes by about 18 percent and the rate of vascular problems (heart/blood vessels) by 25–30 percent. Some patients, however, are thought to have aspirin resistance, in which aspirin does not have the anti-platelet effect to prevent clots. People who are nonresponsive to aspirin have a fourfold increased risk of adverse coronary events. However, a recent study revealed that 90 percent of patients who are unresponsive to aspirin have simply not taken their aspirin on a regular basis. You can find out if you are truly aspirin resistant by undergoing arachidonic acid testing.

Cautions: Ibuprofen blocks the blood-thinning effects of aspirin, so try not to take it if you are taking aspirin. If you must take ibuprofen, take the aspirin first and wait at least an hour to take the ibuprofen, and take the lowest ibuprofen dose you can.

Aspirin can decrease body stores of vitamin C, so you should take 600 mg by diet or supplementation. In addition, aspirin can cause stomach irritation and bleeding in some people. Taking OTC PPIs/H$_2$ blockers is recommended (see section on GERD).

If you are sensitive or allergic to aspirin, your doctor may recommend the prescription drug *ticlopidine* instead for the same effect.

In addition to aspirin, most studies show that taking *clopidogrel* (Plavix) with aspirin provides more heart protection in patients with *acute* coronary syndromes.

Warning: Avoid NSAIDs after Heart Attack

A study published in *Circulation* in May 2011 demonstrated that taking NSAIDs (including naproxen [Naprosyn], meloxicam [Mobic], piroxicam [Feldene], oxaprozin [Daypro], nabumatone [Relafen], ketoprofen [Orudis], diclofenac [Cataflam], diclofenac/misoprostol [Arthrotec] or celocoxib [Celebrex] after heart attack increases the risk for death and recurrent heart attacks.

The AHA had recommended low-dose, short-term use of NSAIDs as being safe, but this study shows that taking NSAIDs for even brief periods increases the risk. Diclofenac (Feldene) was associated with the greatest risk, and naproxen was the least problematic.

It is not known how long after having a heart attack you should avoid NSAIDs.

Cardiac rehabilitation is a must for all patients who have a first heart attack because it raises a person's chances of surviving at least three years after a heart attack by more than 50 percent. Unfortunately, referrals and follow-through rates are often very low, so it's important to discuss rehab with your physician and obtain a referral.

Heart Attack Patients Not Receiving Appropriate Rehab

A study conducted at the Mayo Clinic revealed that nearly half of heart attack victims do not participate in cardiac rehabilitation. Women are 55 percent less likely than men to undergo rehab. Only about 32 percent of men and women over the age of seventy participate, compared with 66 percent of sixty- to sixty-nine-year-olds and 81 percent of those younger than sixty.

Some reasons include lack of referral from a doctor, access to rehab, or financial reasons.

⎯⎯⎯⎯∞⎯⎯⎯⎯

The Conventional Approaches For Stable Angina

Medications are considered the primary treatment for stable angina. You should definitely take aspirin (81 mg daily), but there is no additional advantage in taking clopidogrel unless you have a stent. Depending on your symptoms, other drugs may be prescribed as follows:

- *Nitrates*, such as nitroglycerin tablets under the tongue (sublingual) or spray, are usually effective for anginal symptoms that occur occasionally. Oral or transdermal (skin patches) nitrates can be used more long-term, but resistance can occur and decrease their effectiveness. This problem may be reversed by taking vitamin E (200 IU three times daily) so that you can continue using these forms of medication.
- *Beta-blockers* (such as propranolol, atenolol, metoprolol, or nadolol) or *calcium channel blockers* (such as dihydropyridine, diphenylalklylamine, or benzothiazepine) can provide long-term relief or prevention of your symptoms for chronic angina (angina that occurs frequently).

These drug types may be used together, depending on the severity and frequency of the angina. The particular formulation and dosage should be determined with your physician.

These drugs should be beneficial in reducing or preventing anginal symptoms very quickly (usually within a few days). Beta-blockers can also help prevent heart attacks, so they serve two good purposes. ***Important note***: In some men, beta-blockers can cause blood cholesterol to drop to low levels that can be harmful (less than 160 mg/dl). If this occurs, you should take chromium picolinate, 200 mcg three times per day, to reverse this side effect.

⎯⎯⎯⎯∞⎯⎯⎯⎯

Dr. A's Suggestions:
Surgery versus Medical Treatment for *Stable* Angina: Which Is Preferred?

In our procedure-oriented reimbursement system, if you have stable coronary artery disease detected, it often results in testing and procedures including coronary angiograpy (dye test), angioplasty, stenting, and/or CABG. However, these interventions have been shown not to prolong life or prevent future heart attacks. Nevertheless, Americans undergo one million angioplasties and more than 350,000 CABG procedures every year.

Two studies, one in *JAMA* and another in *Lancet*, reveal that many doctors perform PCI without appropriate evaluation. Thus, patients may not benefit. For this reason, you should insist on undergoing stress testing before PCI if you are not symptomatic (stable), to make sure it will be beneficial.

A recent study called Clinical Outcomes Utilizing Revascularization and Aggressive Drug Evaluation (COURAGE) revealed that stable angina can be successfully managed with aggressive medical therapy, permitting a delay in invasive procedures and without causing any increased death rates. For most of those who have not had a heart attack and have chronic stable angina, medical management should be the preferred conventional approach.

The Alternative Approaches
Nutritional Supplements: Studies have shown that *following angioplasty*, B vitamins and fish oil reduce the risk of the artery reclogging, as follows.

- *Fish oil*, 1,500–3,000 mg daily
- *Folic acid*, 1 mg daily
- *Vitamin B₁₂*, 400 mcg daily
- *Vitamin B₆*, 10 mg daily

Warning: However, antioxidant vitamins, C, E and beta carotene *should not be taken*, because they interfere with the artery repair process following angioplasty.

Most of you who have unstable angina may have already taken nitroglycerin to reduce your symptoms. Adding *N-acetylcysteine* (600 mg three times daily) to transdermal nitroglycerin has been found to be very beneficial in stabilizing angina in many people. However, headaches can occur with nitroglycerin and can become even more severe with the addition of N-acetylcysteine.

Other nutritional supplements that can be beneficial for angina include *L-carnitine* (500 mg three times daily) and/or *coenzyme Q10* (150–300 mg daily) *in combination with prescription drug therapies*. These supplements allow the heart to utilize oxygen more efficiently. It may take several weeks to notice improvement. If your symptoms are improved with these supplements, you may then be able to reduce the dosages of your prescription medications; however, *consult* with your doctor before doing so. CoQ10 has been shown to help prevent complications (especially arrhythmias) if you are having heart surgery (120 mg daily starting a week before your surgery).

Warning: Avoid Arginine

L-arginine (3 g three times a day) is another supplement that augments nitric oxide in the blood (thus helping open your arteries) and has been used for angina. However, a study at John's Hopkins revealed that arginine supplements given to heart-attack patients dramatically increased deaths. It should be avoided.

If spasm of the heart blood vessels (Prinzmetal angina) causes your symptoms, *magnesium* (200–400 mg three times daily) can be of benefit.

Meditation and relaxation reduce the factors that accelerate atherosclerosis, including stress; emotions such as anger, anxiety, and frustration; and certain personality types. Studies reveal that stress, especially from job strain, is associated with recurrent cardiac events such as heart attacks and angina, most likely caused by biologic factors. In addition, panic attacks increase the risk of heart attack in women. Along with exercise and diet, meditation has been proven to actually reverse coronary artery disease.

Homeopathic remedies, such as nux vomica or arsenicum album, can sometimes relieve angina that fails to respond to other measures. You should consult a qualified homeopathist for guidance on which remedies will be most beneficial and for proper dosages. Benefits should be observed in one to two months.

Chelation: Many alternative practitioners believe that various metals accumulate in our bodies and cause atherosclerosis and angina. They recommend intravenous chelation, a process in which a specific substance (called EDTA) is injected into your bloodstream and binds to these metals and helps the body dispose of them. Chelation has been controversial lately; an NIH trial investigating chelation for heart disease actually showed it to be beneficial compared to placebo, especially in patients who had a heart attack in the front portion of the heart (anterior) and in diabetics. It is, however, very expensive ($2,500–$4,000) and is not covered by insurance.

Less expensively, you can use some herbs taken orally that can chelate. Although no good studies have been done on these herbs, they are generally not harmful, so they are worth a try. Malic acid (800–1,200 mg daily) is particularly useful for removing aluminum from the body. Cilantro is excellent for cleaning all heavy metals out of the blood (see recipe in sidebar below).

Cilantro Chelation Recipe

Use the following recipe: Blend one cup of fresh cilantro with six tablespoons of olive oil until the cilantro is completely chopped. Add one clove of garlic, half a cup of nuts (cashews or almonds are the best), and two tablespoons of lemon juice. Blend these into a paste (which will be lumpy), adding hot water if necessary. Take two to three teaspoons per day for two to three weeks, every few months. If you make large amounts, you can freeze it for later use. You should see benefits within two to three weeks.

—⚬⚬⚬—

Your Empowered Patient Action Plan for Treating *Unstable* Angina/Heart Attacks

- *Warning: Unstable angina is considered an emergency, and you should go to an emergency room immediately*.

Step #1: **Take beta-blockers and blood thinners** to prevent further progression and symptoms.

Step #2: **Undergo procedures** to unclog coronary arteries if not controlled by medications or if you have had a heart attack. Make sure you understand the pros and cons of PCI (Percutaneous Cardiac Intervention) versus CABG (Coronary Artery Bypass Grafting) before proceeding. If undergoing PCI, further understand the pros and cons of bare metal stents (BMS) versus drug-eluting stents (DES) Vs angioplasty.

Step #2a: **Take CoQ10 before heart surgery** to reduce complications

Step #3: **Take B-vitamins and fish oil** after any procedures to prevent reclotting. **Avoid** antioxidant vitamins.

Step #4: Always **undergo cardiac rehabilitation** after a heart attack.

Step #5: **Take aspirin and clopidogrel (Plavix)** after the procedure to prevent reclotting, especially if you have a stent. Consider taking an H_2 blocker or PPI if taking aspirin to prevent stomach bleeding or irritation.

Your Empowered Patient Action Plan for Treating *Stable* Angina

Step #1: **Take aspirin, 81 mg daily** to help prevent future cardiovascular problems. Consider taking a proton pump inhibitor or H_2 blocker with the aspirin to prevent bleeding or stomach irritation.

Step #2: **Take other appropriate prescription medications** (nitrates, beta blockers, and/or calcium channel blockers) to stabilize your heart and control your angina symptoms, per your doctor.

Step #3: ***Change to a cardiac diet*** like DASH or the Mediterranean diet or one that is lower in saturated fat, cholesterol and animal protein

Step #4: ***Exercise***, even walking, is a must. Make sure you undergo an exercise tolerance test before beginning any vigorous exercise.

Step #5: ***Meditate regularly*** to slow the progression of atherosclerosis caused by stress.

Step #6: ***Take L-carnitine and coenzyme Q10*** to improve your heart function once your symptoms are stabilized.

Step #7: ***Take magnesium*** for Prinzmetal Angina.

Step #8: ***Take malic acid or cilantro*** for prevention or recurrence of angina.

Step #9: ***Consider chelation*** if your angina continues, even if controlled by medications.

*Step #10: **Add homeopathic remedies*** for continued angina.

Joe, a sixty-four-year-old mechanic, would get chest pain whenever he performed strenuous activities such as mowing his lawn or his favorite hobby, woodworking. He was taking both a beta–blocker and a calcium channel blocker, which controlled his angina until he did something strenuous. When the angina occurred, nitroglycerin and rest relieved the pain, but he wanted to be able to perform his activities without having to stop all the time. I placed him on a good cardiac diet, L-carnitine, and CoQ10. After one month he was able to start walking up to five miles on a regular basis and do his woodworking without having to take nitroglycerin. After two months he was able to discontinue the calcium channel blocker, but he did continue taking the beta-blocker, primarily to prevent heart attacks in the future.

Expected Outcome

Angina is a warning that must be heeded. The most important action is to obtain timely and appropriate treatment, especially if it is unstable, which can prevent further complications and prolong life. Even if you have had a heart attack, using the above steps can slow or even reverse the underlying condition, providing a longer and improved quality of life.

Heart Disease: Arrhythmias

What You Should Know

Arrhythmias (abnormal heartbeat or rhythm) can occur commonly with angina, coronary artery disease, or heart failure and often require different types of treatment. The four most important types of arrhythmia that are encountered are discussed below.

Atrial fibrillation (AF) arises from the small chambers of the heart. Almost 5 percent of people older than sixty-nine years and 8 percent of those older than eighty years have this problem. Thus, the prevalence of AF increases with advancing age. While patients can be asymptomatic, many experience a wide variety of symptoms, including palpitations, shortness of breath, fatigue, or dizziness. It can also increase the risk for serious conditions such as angina, congestive heart failure (CHF), stroke, and transient ischemic attacks (TIAs).

Atrial Fibrillation Deadlier in Women Than in Men

A 2016 meta-analysis of 30 studies published in the *BMJ* revealed that atrial fibrillation poses a higher risk for side effects, complications and death in women than in men. The higher risk includes all-cause deaths, heart deaths, strokes, cardiac events (such as heart attacks) and heart failure.

The most serious danger of AF is embolism (blood clot causing stroke), which is associated with a 1.5- to 1.9-fold higher risk of death. Overall, approximately 15–25 percent of all strokes in the United States (seventy-five thousand per year) can be attributed to AF. There are different forms of AF: 46 percent of AF patients have the permanent type, 25 percent have paroxysmal (comes and goes), 22 percent have persistent, and 5 percent have occasional.

Atrial Fibrillation Undertreated

Recent studies have shown that atrial fibrillation is commonly undertreated, which results in an increase in strokes and death. There are international guidelines for treatment of atrial fibrillation, and it is important to make sure you are treated appropriately.

Supraventricular Tachycardia **(SVT):** This category refers to fast heartbeats of 150–250 per minute, also originating from the atria (small chambers of the heart), but without an irregular heartbeat like AF. These include *sinus tachycardia* and *junctional tachycardia*. Stress, exercise, or emotion can precipitate SVT. They can last a few minutes or as long as one or two days, sometimes continuing until treated. The rapid beating of the heart during SVT can make the heart a less-effective pump, decreasing cardiac output and blood pressure and causing symptoms of pounding heart, shortness of breath, chest pain, and rapid breathing.

Ventricular arrhythmias arise from the large chambers of the heart and can be very dangerous, causing fast heartbeat (tachycardia) and sudden death. It can manifest either as ventricular tachycardia (heart beats very fast) or ventricular fibrillation (no contractions of the heart muscle occurs), the latter of which is responsible for 75–85 percent of sudden deaths in persons with heart problems.

Bradycardia means slow heartbeat. When you have bradycardia, either your heart's natural pacemaker isn't working properly, or passage of the electrical signal is disrupted elsewhere in the electrical system, causing an abnormally slow heart rhythm. Aging-related damage to the heart muscle, as well as loss of the cells responsible for transmitting electrical signals, can contribute to bradycardia.

Treatments for Arrhythmias

The Preventive Approaches

Change habits: The best way to prevent arrhythmias is to prevent heart disease. However, if you have heart disease with arrhythmias, there are factors that can make them worse, primarily caffeine and alcohol. Even moderate alcohol intake is associated with AF (increases risk 10–20 percent), according to a 2014 study in the *Journal of the American College of Cardiology*. Continued smoking can also worsen arrhythmias.

Beware of certain medication effects: Many common medications for heart disease and high blood pressure are designed to slow the heart rate to help it beat more efficiently. But sometimes your medications may need to be adjusted if your heart rate is too slow. These medications include beta blockers, calcium channel blockers, and even anti-arrhythmic drugs. Recently, a study revealed that bisphosphonates taken for osteoporosis (especially alendronate—Fosamax) can increase the risk of AF.

Dehydration is a common cause of sinus tachycardias, and can easily be corrected by **drinking more fluids**.

Control other medical conditions: According to the 2011 ARIC study, over half the cases of AF could be prevented by modifying risk factors including high blood pressure, obesity and smoking. In addition, obstructive sleep apnea (OSA) can be a causal factor for atrial fibrillation and treating OSA will reduce its occurrence.

The Conventional Approaches

For emergencies: For any arrhythmia that is causing significant symptoms (chest pain, shortness of breath, fainting, etc.), you should go to the emergency room. Usually, intravenous medications are prescribed to control rate and irregular heartbeats (rhythm), or electrical cardioversion is performed (electrical pads placed on the chest producing electrical shocks). For severe bradycardia, a temporary pacemaker may be placed.

For arrhythmias that are persistent but are not causing significant, life-threatening symptoms, treatments depend on the kind of arrhythmia.

For AF/flutter, it should be noted that a primary result of AF causing symptoms is a fast heartbeat. A goal of treatment is to *reduce the heart rate* to 80 beats per minute, which is considered strict control. A recent study, however, shows that a heart rate of up to 110 has the same outcomes as strict control. Many patients, however, may have a normal heart rate (under 100) and no symptoms but still have the abnormal rhythm (heart beats irregularly). Even this can lead to complications (primarily stroke), so another goal is to *control the rhythm* (decreasing the number of abnormal beats), which is now considered more efficacious than rate control. Rate and/or rhythm control are accomplished with various medications.

Atrial Fibrillation (AF) Facts

- Control of AF is achieved in just 59 percent of patients.
- Even if controlled, 56 percent of patients will still have at least one symptom.
- Controlling the *rate* is the most popular but least effective treatment strategy. Seventy-one percent of people ultimately fail to achieve rate control. *Rhythm* control is superior.
- Most people with AF have other diseases, including hypertension, high cholesterol, and other types of heart disease. All of these need to be treated.
- Guideline adherence is suboptimal. Twenty-five percent of people on medication (amiodarone) do not qualify for that drug. Forty-seven percent of patients who should be on blood thinners are not, and 46 percent who should not be on blood thinners are.

Cardioversion is often necessary for atrial fibrillation, meaning that the heart beat is "converted" to a normal beat. Cardioversion can be accomplished either by use of drugs (control rate) or by electrical shocks (control rhythm). Outcomes of death, stroke, and worsening heart failure do not differ between the two treatments. Using shocks is faster but requires sedation and more hospitalizations. Medical conversion is usually accomplished using the drug amiodarone (Cardarone). ***Warning***: If you take the cholesterol drugs simvastatin Vytorin or Zocor, amiodarone increases the risk of a severe muscle side effect (called rhabdomyolysis).

Radiofrequency ablation (destruction) of some heart nerves that cause this arrhythmia is indicated if medical conversion does not return the heart rhythm to normal or if you have recurrent AF with symptoms. Ablation is a fairly low-risk procedure that uses a catheter inside the heart to deliver radio frequency energy to locate and destroy the abnormal electrical pathways. Ablation is primarily considered if this arrhythmia interferes with your quality of life. Studies show that the single-procedure success rate is about 57 percent when patients are not on anti-arrhythmic drugs and 72 percent when they are. If a single procedure doesn't work (50 percent of patients), it may be repeated. For multiple ablation procedures, the success rates are 71 percent and 77 percent, respectively. Younger patients may benefit from first-line therapy using ablation. ***Caution***: Major complications occur in 4.9 percent of patients who undergo RF ablation; overall mortality is 0.7 percent.

Medications: AF that cannot be or is not converted to normal rhythm usually requires a blood thinner to prevent blood clots that can cause stroke. *Aspirin* (with or without *clopidogrel* [Plavix]) or *warfarin* (Coumadin) have been the most common medications, and the choice depends on a rating system called the CHADS$_2$ score, which predicts the risk of having a stroke. ***Warning:*** Using aspirin and clopidogrel (Plavix) for heart disease *along with* warfarin significantly raises the risk for serious and sometimes fatal bleeding, and most of the time, all three medications should not be used together.

Warfarin requires frequent dose adjustments, and many different types of foods and medications (especially antibiotics) can interfere with its absorption. Therefore, frequent monitoring with a specific blood test (INR) is necessary. ***Warning***s: If you are on warfarin and take a statin (for cholesterol), you can also have a higher risk of gastrointestinal bleeding. Pravastatin has *not* been associated with increased risk and is the preferred statin in these situations. You should avoid the supplement quercetin, which can decrease the effect of warfarin.

Four relatively new medications (called *Factor Xa inhibitors*)—dabigatran (Pradaxa), rivaroxaban (Xarelto), apixaban (Eliquis) and the newest, edoxaban (Savaysa)—have been found to be superior in outcome to Coumadin and are fixed doses, so they do not require blood monitoring or dose adjustments. A December 2013 meta-analysis published in *Lancet* showed that these drugs seem to offer clear advantages over warfarin in effectiveness, safety, and convenience. Their downside was that they had no known antidote for their blood-thinning effects, but studies show this is not a great concern, and there is now an antidote for dabigatran that has been approved by the FDA (idarucizumab [Praxbind]). ***Cautions***: A 2014 study in *JAMA Intern Med* showed that dabigatran has a higher incidence of major bleeding and GI bleeding, so it should be prescribed with caution. Additional 2014 data indicate that these medications can cause increased GI bleeding, primarily in patients older than sixty-five. The FDA will be performing a new assessment of dabigatran due to persistent concerns about its safety, but not on the other two same-class medications. It should not be used if you have GERD (acid reflux).

Warning: An older medication used for atrial fibrillation in almost one-third of patients is *digoxin* (digitalis). However, several studies have found that use of digoxin increases the likelihood of heart failure, diabetes and persistent atrial fibrillation, as well as higher mortality. It should only be used as a last-line agent, if at all.

Important note: AF occurs relatively often after cardiac surgery and can cause complications. Most doctors prescribe *beta-blockers* (metoprolol) to prevent AF, but many doctors are using a newer drug, *amiodarone*. This drug is equally effective but more expensive; and so far it shows no advantage over metoprolol.

An investigational device called "*the Watchman*" is a closure device to prevent clots, and studies have shown it to be equal to or superior to taking warfarin. It has not yet been approved by the FDA due to initial safety and effectiveness concerns, but the latest studies show these factors to have improved.

For SVT, a number of **physical maneuvers** can often stop the fast heart rate immediately (these also are called vagal maneuvers because they stimulate the vagus nerve, which can slow the heart). The *Valsalva* maneuver should be the first vagal maneuver tried, although it's only effective in less than 20 percent of patients. It is carried out by asking patients to hold their breath and try to exhale forcibly, as if straining during a bowel movement, or by getting them to hold their noses and blow out against it. There are many other vagal maneuvers, including holding one's breath for a few seconds, coughing, plunging the face into cold water, drinking a glass of ice-cold water, and standing on one's head. If necessary, the act of defecation can sometimes halt an episode, again through vagal stimulation. Urination has also been found to work, especially if there has been a delay in voiding. *Helpful Tips*: A good way to use a Valsalva maneuver is to blow into a 10-ml syringe until the plunger just moves. A 2015 study showed that if you follow the maneuver by laying down via reclining the head of your bed and then having someone raise one of your legs to 45 degrees, it returns your rhythm to normal 43 percent of the time.

If vagal maneuvers are not effective, **adenosine**, an ultra-short-acting drug, may be effective.

Carotid sinus massage, carried out by firmly pressing the bulb at the top of *one* of the carotid arteries in the neck, is effective but is often not recommended due to risks of stroke in those with plaque in the carotid arteries.

If you are unstable or other treatments have not been effective, **electrical cardioversion** may be used and is almost always effective. If the tachycardia continues to recur, **radiofrequency ablation** has been shown to be around 90 percent effective.

Once the acute episode has been terminated, ongoing treatment may be indicated to prevent a recurrence of the arrhythmia. Patients who have a single isolated episode, or infrequent and minimally symptomatic episodes usually do not warrant any treatment except observation.

Patients who have more frequent or disabling symptoms from their episodes generally warrant some form of preventive therapy. A variety of **drugs** including diltiazem, verapamil, or metoprolol may be used, usually with good effect. Some SVTs may respond to other anti-arrhythmic drugs such as sotalol or amiodarone.

**For bradycardia** there are no particular long term medications that are prescribed (_atropine_ is often given for short term reversal if you have adverse symptoms). Implanting a **pacemaker** is the primary treatment, especially if symptoms such as fainting occur. A pacemaker is a wallet-sized device with wires and electrodes attached. The electrodes are threaded through your veins and into your heart. The pacemaker device is implanted under your collarbone and generates electrical impulses through the electrodes to regulate your heartbeat.

There are many different types of pacemakers, and many patients receive pacemakers that have "bells and whistles" that they don't need. Depending on your condition, your doctor may recommend a dual-chamber pacemaker. Whereas a traditional pacemaker only stimulates the ventricles (or, less commonly, the atria), a dual-chamber device has electrodes in both the atria and the ventricles. Some pacemakers even have three leads, one for the right atrium and one for each ventricle (biventricular pacemaker). Biventricular pacemakers are most commonly used in individuals who have heart failure.

Dr. A's Suggestions
Be Cautious Using Smartphones with Implanted Medical Devices

It is being recognized that smartphones can interfere with the signals from electronic devices, including pacemakers, defibrillators and other implanted devices. For example, a pacemaker may stop working or a defibrillator may produce an unnecessary shock.

If you have an implanted medical device, you should keep the smartphone at least 7 inches away from the device. Especially with cardiac devices, don't keep your smartphone in your pocket. Furthermore, when in use, hold the phone to the ear farthest from the device.

For Ventricular Arrhythmias
There are several types of ventricular arrhythmias, some benign and some life-threatening. The latter, including ventricular tachycardia or fibrillation, are emergencies, which will not be discussed here.

Occasionally, *premature ventricular complexes* (isolated abnormal beats, called PVCs) can be seen on EKG in patients without heart disease and is more an annoyance than a medical risk; and treatment is not commonly required. In fact, anti-arrhythmic drug therapy in such patients may increase, rather than decrease, the risk of dying. It is important to review medications, determine whether stimulants are being used, and correct electrolyte abnormalities.

Patients with established heart disease and premature ventricular complexes, however, have a higher likelihood of developing ventricular tachycardia or fibrillation and might need to be treated. Undergoing an ETT (treadmill) test or other cardiac tests can help determine if you need treatment.

Medications: If patients with multiple premature ventricular complexes have severe, disabling symptoms, *beta-blockers* (such as metoprolol or atenolol) are the safest initial choice. Referral to a cardiologist is indicated if beta-blocker therapy is not effective. In this situation, the next agents to be tried are usually class I anti-arrhythmic drugs, such as flecainide (Tambocor) or amiodarone (Cordarone), although radiofrequency ablation of an ectopic focus may also be an appropriate treatment.

Defibrillator implantation is beneficial in older patients with heart failure who have ventricular arrhythmias and thus a high risk of sudden death. However, it is controversial whether to use such devices in elderly people. On the negative side, they are expensive ($44,000 plus $8,000 yearly), they can have complications (6.9 percent), and, as one gets older, the survival benefit is almost nil. A recent 2008 study revealed that just receiving the shocks can increase mortality; 20–30 percent of people get inappropriate shocks, which doubles all-cause mortality. But even the 30–60 percent of people who receive appropriate shocks have a tripling of all-cause mortality. On the plus side, if you are otherwise healthy, over the age of seventy, have an ejection fraction (percent of blood pumped out by the heart) of less than 30 percent, and have a stage 3 heart failure classification, there can be up to 50 percent reduction in total mortality. After all, if you have an arrhythmia that can kill you, the shock can be lifesaving.

Cautions: Defibrillators should not be implanted in people who have a lot of other medical conditions or have a life expectancy of no more than six months to a year. They also do not decrease mortality if implanted after a heart attack. You should also be aware that taking fish oil is contraindicated with implantable defibrillators.

The Alternative Approaches

There are not very many alternative methods that are beneficial for arrhythmias. **Magnesium** (200–400 mg three times per day) is very important in stabilizing the heart's electrical system and can be beneficial for several different types of benign (non-life-threatening) arrhythmias.

A recent study at the University of Kansas in April 2011 showed that practicing **yoga** can significantly reduce irregular heart beat episodes as well as improve anxiety and depression in patients with paroxysmal atrial fibrillation.

The only other method that can be helpful is **acupuncture**. A particular point on the back (at the level of the fifth thoracic vertebra) is beneficial for bradycardia and several in the hand can be helpful for irregular heart beat and bradycardia. You should see benefits within six to eight treatments.

Your Empowered Patient Action Plan for Treating *Atrial/Supraventricular Arrhythmias*

- *Warning: If you have severe symptoms such as palpitations/fluttering of your heart, shortness of breath, and/or chest pain, you should go to the emergency room.*

Step #1: Only for supraventricular tachycardia, try the physical maneuvers (described above) first.

Step #2: Use the appropriate conventional medications to try to get your heartbeat/ rhythm under control.

Step #3. Undergo electrical cardioversion if the above medications have not controlled your arrhythmia and you continue to have recurrent tachycardia.

Step #4: Take a Factor Xa inhibitor long term to prevent stroke if you continue to have atrial fibrillation, even with a normal heart rate.

Step #5: Practice yoga to help reduce episodes of irregular heartbeat.

Step #6: Undergo acupuncture to see if it will control your irregular heartbeat.

Step #7: Undergo radiofrequency ablation if the above steps have not been effective and if the benefits outweigh the possible side effects.

Step #8: Take appropriate anti-arrhythmic medications once your supraventricular tachycardia is controlled to prevent recurrence.

Your Empowered Patient Action Plan for Treating *Bradycardia*

Step #1: Undergo acupuncture to speed up your heart rate if your slow rate is not life-threatening or symptomatic.

Step #2: Take magnesium with or without the acupuncture.

Step #3: Undergo pacemaker implantation for symptomatic bradycardia or if the above steps are ineffective.

Your Empowered Patient Action Plan for Treating *Ventricular Arrhythmias*

- *Warning: If you have severe symptoms such as palpitations/fluttering of your heart, shortness of breath, and/or chest pain, you should go to the emergency room.*

*Step #1: **Take beta blockers*** to decrease abnormal beats and/or rhythm.

*Step #2: **Take other antiarrhythmic medications*** under a cardiologist's supervision if the beta blockers are not effective.

*Step #3: **Consider taking magnesium*** if the arrhythmia is not life-threatening, especially if the above steps are not totally effective.

*Step #4: **Consider implantation of an ICD device*** for dangerous ventricular arrhythmias, if appropriate for your age and medical conditions.

Expected Outcome

If you don't have heart disease, most arrhythmias are benign; and unless symptomatic, these may not need treatment. If you do have heart disease, however, there are many appropriate treatments that can both control the arrhythmias and heart rate and prevent sudden death or other complications.

Heart Disease: Congestive Heart Failure

What You Need to Know

When the heart has been damaged from heart attacks, high blood pressure, or coronary artery disease, the muscle tissue may not receive enough oxygen, and it weakens. The heart may start failing and is unable to pump blood out into the body. As fluid cannot get out of the heart fast enough, it backs up into the lungs, causing congestion, which is why it is called *congestive* heart failure (CHF).

—⁂—

Heart Failure Patients Overestimate Their Life Expectancy

A recent report in *JAMA* revealed that most heart failure patients predict a life expectancy of thirteen years, when actual measurements indicate a ten-year survival.

—⁂—

One older test to determine heart function is how much blood your heart is pumping with each beat, called an ejection fraction. Normal ejection fraction is over 55 percent: below 40 percent requires treatment. Although chest x-rays are commonly used for diagnosing heart failure, lung ultrasound has been shown to be more accurate.

A blood test called BNP (B-type natriuretic peptide) has been important for diagnosing CHF more quickly. Patients with CHF are clinically misdiagnosed 50–75 percent of the time because its main symptom, shortness of breath, can be caused by lung problems as well and often it is difficult to find the source. A normal BNP level is about 98 percent accurate in ruling out the diagnosis, freeing doctors to hunt for other conditions that may be causing shortness of breath or fluid retention. BNP values of 1,000–4,000 usually indicate CHF: lung conditions have BNPs less than 100. BNP is also very helpful in determining the outlook for patients with CHF; in general, the higher the level, the worse the CHF (greater than 4,000 is especially worrisome). Finally, BNP is very helpful in guiding the treatment of CHF because it will decrease if treatment is successful.

Symptoms of Heart Failure Often Not Addressed

Patients with heart failure often have severe symptoms of dyspnea (shortness of breath) and fatigue, but they also may have less typical symptoms, including anxiety, depression, and pain. According to a research letter published in a 2015 *JAMA Internal Medicine*, hospitalized patients often had no symptom improvement after discharge; nearly 60 percent showed no improvement in fatigue and 40 percent had no improvement in anxiety, dyspnea or pain.

Most participants in the study were unfamiliar with quality of life (also called palliative care) to reduce symptoms, but two-thirds were interested in receiving it once the concept was explained. The *bottom line* is that these symptoms can be treated successfully by both conventional and alternative approaches, but you may have to become empowered and make sure these symptoms are addressed.

Treatments for Congestive Heart Failure

The Preventive Approaches
Correctable causes: The best ways to prevent heart failure are the same as preventing coronary artery disease, including eating a *proper diet*, *getting exercise*, and *stopping smoking* (see next section on *Coronary Artery Disease* for more detailed explanation). Alcoholism can cause heart failure as well.

Important Information:
Avoid the Use of NSAIDs in Heart Failure

Current guidelines recommend avoiding NSAIDs (nonsteroidal anti-inflammatory drugs, including naproxen [Naprosyn], meloxicam [Mobic], piroxicam [Feldene], oxaprozin [Daypro], nabumatone [Relafen], ketoprofen [Orudis], diclofenac [Cataflam], or diclofenac/misoprostol [Arthrotec] or celocoxib [Celebrex]) because they can make heart failure worse as well as interfere with the action of proper medications. Nevertheless, one-third of heart failure patients are receiving NSAIDs, which means that physicians are unaware of the recommendations.

In addition, there are several **medical conditions** that can predispose people to heart failure, so controlling them is important. They include high blood pressure, diabetes, thyroid disease, and anemia.

A recent study revealed that 20–30 percent of heart failure patients are **iron deficient**. If so, giving intravenous iron improves heart function and symptoms (oral iron supplementation has not been studied but also may be of benefit). This effect occurs whether you are anemic or not. Always have your doctor check your iron levels if you have heart failure. *Caution*: Harm can be caused by having too much iron, so you need to be closely monitored if you are not iron deficient and receive iron.

Sleep Apnea Increases Risk of Heart Failure

Sleep apnea is a condition that cause lower oxygen levels while sleeping. Men with severe obstructive sleep apnea are 58 percent more likely to develop new congestive heart failure over eight years. It is present in about 33 percent of patients who have congestive heart failure and can make it worse; this is not found in women, for unknown reasons.

It is hypothesized that the lack of oxygen from sleep apnea sets the body into a type of panic, raising blood pressure and thus stressing the heart. If you have heart failure, you should be tested in a sleep lab and, if results are abnormal, use a breathing device at night called a CPAP machine.

If you have stable heart failure, you may need to monitor and **restrict your intake of salt** (sodium) **and fluids**. Retention of fluid can be detected early by noting a change in weight. You should weigh yourself three times a week in the morning after waking, after you go to the bathroom but before you eat anything. If your weight suddenly rises, that means you may be retaining fluid, and you should contact your doctor. Catching this early can avoid hospitalization. *Important note*: If hospitalized, however, most doctors routinely restrict salt and free fluid in patients with *decompensated* heart failure. A 2014 study in *JAMA Internal Medicine*, however, showed this to be ineffective.

Soda Linked to Heart Failure

A long-term Swedish study has demonstrated that people who drink soda daily may be at higher risk for heart failure. This observational study revealed that subjects who drank more than two sweetened drinks daily had a 23 percent greater risk of developing heart failure.

Besides the diet suggestions in the following section on heart disease, you should **avoid processed meats**, including bacon, ham, and salami. A study in *Circulation: Heart Failure* linked moderate intake of these meats (2.5 ounces daily) to a 28 percent increased risk of heart failure.

Chocolate Consumption Lowers Risk for Heart Failure

A study in *Circulation* showed that women who eat chocolate moderately have a 30 percent reduced risk of developing heart failure. Moderate consumption was defined as one to three servings a week and higher intake did not appear to have a protective effect. Beware that in the United States, most chocolate consumed contains less cocoa than that consumed in this study. Dark chocolate is the preferred form.

Beetroot Juice May be Beneficial for Heart Failure

It is recognized that nitrates are the active ingredient in beet juice. Nitrates are converted to nitric oxide, which has beneficial effects on blood pressure and heart health, comparable to the benefits of aerobic exercise.

In an interesting study in *Circulation: Heart Failure*, researchers showed that drinking beet juice increased the power in the heart muscles by 13 percent, and this occurred just two hours after drinking the juice.

If you don't like beets, nitrates are also plentiful in spinach and other leafy vegetables, including arugula and celery.

Exercise is important for heart failure patients although some doctors are hesitant to prescribe it due to the patient's shortness of breath, which makes physical exertion difficult. However, exercise has been shown to be beneficial although you should start slowly and obtain some guidance from a trained exercise therapist.

30 Minutes of Exercise Daily May Not Be Enough to Ward Off Heart Disease

It has long been recommended that adults get 30 minutes of moderate intensity exercise daily to promote good heart health. However, a 2015 study demonstrates that the more exercise you get, the less the risk of heart disease.

In the study, people who exercised 30 minutes a day had modest reductions in the risk for heart failure. Doubling the standard 30 minutes resulted in a 20 percent lower risk and those who exercised four times as much registered a 35 percent drop.

The Conventional Approaches

Medications are the primary treatment for heart failure, and there are several that can be beneficial, depending on your particular condition and other conditions. Drugs from different classes may be combined in some people for better effectiveness. These include:

- *Diuretics*, which remove excess fluid that builds up in your lungs and lower extremities. There are several types used, ranging from HCTZ (very mild) to Lasix (very strong). Another type of diuretic (spironolactone) inhibits a hormone (aldosterone) that is deleterious to the heart and has been shown to decrease heart disease–related deaths in those with moderate to severe heart failure. Eplerenone, another aldosterone inhibitor, has also been shown advantageous; however, it is more expensive, and no studies have compared it to spironolactone. ***Warning***: Taking diuretics can lower your potassium level, so you may need to supplement. Spironolactone, however, is a diuretic that does not lower potassium, although it is not as strong as Lasix.

- *ACE inhibitors* (ACEI [end in "pril," such as captopril, lisinopril or enalapril]), which dilate blood vessels and make it easier for the heart to pump blood. They improve symptoms and exercise tolerance and can prolong survival. An uncommon side effect is coughing.
  - ***Caution***: Taking NSAIDs for arthritis can blunt the effects of ACE inhibitors. If you are on both types of drugs, be sure to monitor your blood pressure closely.
- *ARBs* (Angiotensin Receptor Blockers [end in "sartan"]) may lower all-cause mortality in patients with heart failure but are not considered superior to ACEIs and provide no added benefit if given with ACEI. A study in *JAMA* showed that the ARB candesartan (Atacand) had better survival advantage than losartan (Cozaar).
- *Beta-blockers* block the high levels of adrenaline often seen in heart failure. Metoprolol, carvedilol, and bisoprolol are the most common. This class of drugs had traditionally been considered contraindicated in CHF, but more recent studies showed that they improve mortality rates in people being treated with the above medications. They are useful in CHF patients who are stable, who do not have shortness of breath at rest, and who have no other contraindications to the use of these agents.
- *Ivabadrine (Corlanor)* is a drug approved in 2015 for stable patients with heart failure on maximal doses of beta blockers. It reduces the risk for hospitalization from worsening heart failure.
- *Digoxin* strengthens the heart muscle to improve the symptoms of heart failure and is used for mild to moderate CHF. It is one of the original drugs used for heart failure and is derived from the herb foxglove, which has actually been used for centuries for CHF.
- *Sacubitril/valsartan (Entresto)* is a combination drug just approved in 2015 by the FDA under a fast-track application. This drug was found to reduce the rate of heart death and heart-failure related hospitalization compared to an ACE inhibitor. However, it will cost roughly $4500 per year.

There are two **implantable devices** that may be of benefit if your heart continues to fail. The first is called *cardiac resynchronization therapy (CRT)*, which is indicated for mild-to-moderate heart failure in some patients. This device provides electrical pacing of both ventricles (the large chambers of the heart) and has been shown to decrease cardiac events and death.

The second is called a *ventricular assist device (VAD)*, which can keep your heart functioning while waiting for a heart transplant. A VAD is a mechanical pump that helps a weak heart pump blood. VADs were originally intended for short-term use but can be used for long-term in patients who cannot undergo transplant. Interestingly, because this advice allows the heart to rest, the hearts of a few patients may return to normal or near normal function, and the devices may be removed without the need for further surgery. The main pitfall with VADs is that they require battery replacement every three to four hours.

Heart transplant is the last resort for a failing heart, performed in numerous medical centers throughout the country. To be considered, you have to be less than sixty-nine years old, stop smoking and drinking alcohol (forever), not have arterial disease in your arms or legs or have cancer, and have insurance coverage. You must be unresponsive to other treatment, and your other vital organs must be in good shape. Donor hearts last six hours outside the body, so surgery must be done quickly. There is a 70 percent survival rate for heart transplantation. After heart transplant, you must be on drugs to suppress your immune system and follow a healthy lifestyle.

Cardiac rehabilitation therapy can improve heart patients' quality of life and reduce the risk of hospitalization, according to a 2015 study. Unfortunately, the study points out that 90 percent of heart failure patients are not referred to such programs after hospitalization.

Dr. A's Suggestions:
Many Hospitals Fail Follow-Up with Heart Failure Patients

All patients hospitalized with heart failure should receive five actions when discharged from the hospital, which significantly reduces death rate and rehospitalization. The four actions are:

- Measurement of left heart function,
- Prescription for an ACE inhibitor,
- Smoking cessation counseling as indicated
- Issuance of a complete set of patient discharge instructions.
- Referral to a cardiac rehabilitation program.

You need to make sure you receive these actions.

—∞—

The Alternative Approaches

There are several **nutritional supplements** that may be very beneficial for heart failure:

- *Hawthorn* (Craetageus) is an herb that dilates coronary arteries and thus may improve oxygen flow to the heart. It may be used if you have angina along with NYHA (New York Heart Association) stage 1 or 2 heart failure, in which you are comfortable at rest but ordinary physical activity results in fatigue, palpitation, breathing problems, or angina. However, if used with other conventional heart medications, hawthorn can possibly either increase the effect or interfere with these medications; so check with your doctor before taking it. Dosage is 100–250 mg of extract containing 1.8 percent vitexin-4'rhamnoside or 10 percent procyanidin content, three times a day. The solid extract is the best form to take of this herb.

- *Coenzyme Q10* (150–200 mg daily) added to conventional treatments has been shown in some studies to improve quality of life, decrease hospitalization rates, and decrease symptoms of heart failure such as dyspnea, peripheral edema, enlarged liver, and insomnia in patients with stage 3–4 heart failure. Heart failure patients with low blood levels of CoQ10 are known to have higher death rates.

- *Fish oil* supplements were noted in a 2008 study to work slightly better than cholesterol-lowering drugs in patients with heart failure. Another study in November 2010 showed that taking five grams of omega-3s for one month followed by two grams daily for eleven months substantially improved chronic heart failure. ***Important notes***: There are problems with fish oil that you need to be aware of. Many fish oils deteriorate very rapidly (three months); so by the time you buy them, they may already be partially deteriorated. Another alternative is krill oil, which is stable, contains two natural antioxidants, and has few to no side effects. However, some krill oil products differ in their combinations with other ingredients, so check the label.

  - ***Warning***: Regular fish oil in high doses may decrease HDL cholesterol (the good cholesterol) in some people. If you take fish oil and your HDL is reduced to below normal, you can take vitamin E with mixed tocopherols and tocotrienols (200 IU daily) and garlic (4,000 mg daily) or niacin (1–3 g daily) to raise HDL. Niacin may cause flushing, but there are nonflushing products. It also can be prescribed, but the prescription form is much more expensive and does not have any advantage over OTC forms.

- *L-carnitine* (300 mg three times daily) increases energy production in heart tissue and can be used with hawthorn.
- *L-arginine* (2–5 g three times daily) improves circulation and quality of life. **Caution**: L-arginine should be avoided if you have asthma.
- *Khella* (100 mg of powdered extract containing 12 percent khellin three times daily) dilates the coronary blood vessels and can be helpful with heart failure and angina.
- *Creatine* (20 g per day for five to ten days) is helpful to increase your strength and endurance.

Acupuncture decreases overstimulation of the heart, helping improve heart failure, as noted in a 2014 study done at John's Hopkins. Acupuncture is also excellent at reducing symptoms such as dyspnea, fatigue, anxiety and pain. Always seek evaluation and treatment from a practitioner certified in acupuncture. You should notice improvement within six acupuncture treatments, but you might need additional sessions for maximum benefit.

Daily sauna therapy, consisting of fifteen minutes lying supine (on your back) in a 60-degree centigrade (140-degree Fahrenheit) dry sauna, followed by thirty minutes of lying under blankets at room temperature, can reduce irregular heartbeat, fatigue, shortness of breath, insomnia, and other symptoms of congestive heart failure. It only takes two weeks to see the benefits.

Your Empowered Patient Action Plan for Treating Heart Failure

Step #1: Modify your lifestyle (proper diet, exercise, stop smoking) to prevent heart failure or decrease your symptoms if you already have it.

Step #2: Take prescription medications to stabilize your heart failure, as per your doctor's recommendations.

Step #3: Take fish oil supplements along with the medications in the above step to improve your symptoms and condition,

Step #4: Undergo acupuncture for long term benefit of both heart failure and its symptoms. If your symptoms improve, you may be able to decrease or discontinue the drugs in Step #2.

Step #5: Use a dry sauna daily to decrease irregular heart rhythms and numerous symptoms of CHF.

Step #6: Take CoQ10 and/or hawthorn to improve cardiac function and reduce symptoms. As with acupuncture, if your condition improves, you may be able to decrease or discontinue the medications in step 2.

Joe had high cholesterol and high blood pressure and suffered two heart attacks in the past ten years. He took medications to lower his blood pressure and cholesterol and took one aspirin daily, as well as beta-blockers. He was prescribed a balanced diet but did not follow it very well. He developed congestive heart failure, with swelling in his ankles and difficulty breathing. He started taking diuretics and digoxin, which helped but did not eliminate his symptoms. The amount of blood he was pumping from his heart (called ejection fraction) was only 25 percent of normal. I started him on CoQ10, L-carnitine, hawthorn, and krill oil and he underwent several acupuncture treatments. After three months, his ejection fraction had risen to 45 percent, his swelling and shortness of breath improved considerably, and he was able to discontinue the digoxin.

Step #7: ***Undergo sleep apnea evaluation****.* If positive, obtain proper treatment to avoid developing or worsening CHF.

Step #8: ***Try additional herbs and supplements*** (L-carnitine, L-arginine) if symptoms continue despite the above steps.

Step #9: ***Take the herb khella*** for heart failure with angina.

Step #10: ***Undergo cardiac resynchronization*** if your heart continues to fail.

Step #11: ***Receive a VAD*** to rest the heart and keep it pumping until heart transplant is available if you continue to deteriorate despite the above steps.

Step #12: ***Undergo a heart transplant*** as a last resort, if you qualify.

Expected Outcome

Heart failure has an expected life expectancy of ten years, but with proper treatment and the use of alternative methods, life expectancy and quality of life can both be increased.

Heart Disease: Coronary Artery Disease (CAD)

What You Need to Know

Heart disease is a term that encompasses several types of heart problems, the primary ones being angina (and heart attacks), coronary artery disease (CAD), and congestive heart failure (CHF). Other heart problems include arrhythmias (abnormal heart beat), valvular disease (disease of the valves between heart chambers), and cardiomyopathy (disease of the heart muscle).

Previous sections in this book discuss treatments for some of the above conditions including *symptomatic* heart disease (angina), but many people have underlying, chronic heart disease (coronary artery disease—CAD) *with no or minimal symptoms.* This condition will be discussed in this section.

Heart disease is the number one killer of Americans and is the most expensive medical condition to treat, about $76 billion yearly. Most heart attacks are a direct and eventual result of coronary artery disease (disease of the arteries supplying oxygen to the heart muscle), which in turn is usually due to atherosclerosis, a condition in which an artery wall thickens as the result of a buildup of fatty materials such as cholesterol.

Important note: It is well recognized that the risk of postmenopausal women to have heart disease quickly catches up to the risk in men. It is also recognized that women may not receive as appropriate heart care as men. One reason for this appears to be that women suffer from nontypical symptoms and have "invisible" heart blockages (see section on *Angina/Heart Attack* for more information).

In recent years, several discoveries have contributed to more knowledge about heart disease. First, it has been thought that heart disease is a result of atherosclerosis—clogging or hardening of the arteries. However, it is now recognized that low grade inflammation may also be a major factor. This is important because treatments that only decrease artery clogging may not prevent or benefit all heart disease.

—❦—

Heart Test May Not Be Necessary

A frequently ordered test for coronary artery disease is the CT angiogram, which combines infusion of dye into the heart arteries along with a CT scan. Many doctors contend that it has no proven value in most patients. Although this test provides impressive pictures, studies show that it does not alter patient care or improve outcomes. The bottom line is that there are less expensive tests, which are more useful and do not expose patients to relatively high amounts of radiation.

—❦—

A good test for detecting coronary artery disease is a heart coronary artery calcium test (CAC…this is not the same test as described in the sidebar above). A CAC can indicate how much calcium is detected in your arteries and can predict mortality at 15 years, according to a 2015 study. If you have a score of 0, you have a very low risk of a heart event. Mortality (from all causes) ranged from 3 percent among patients with CAC scores of 0 to roughly 28 percent with scores of greater than 1000. Since CT scans do produce radiation, you should find a site that uses protocols that deliver the lowest radiation possible (approximately 1 mSv).

Treatments for Coronary Artery Disease

The Preventive Approaches

There are several **tests for inflammation**, homocysteine and C-reactive protein (CRP) being the most common, which can indicate higher risk for CAD. Many drugs and alternative supplements (B vitamins, folate) are known to decrease these so-called "markers," but so far, studies have shown that just lowering them does not apparently decrease the risk of CAD.

Psychological factors: Hostility, anger, or depression can increase the risk of heart disease, so dealing appropriately with these emotions may reduce the risk.

Genomics is adding to our knowledge of heart disease. Recently, a genetic variant, called KIF6, has been linked to an increased risk of heart attack as well as a person's chances of reducing that risk by taking statins (for lowering cholesterol). KIF6 is present in 60 percent of the population. KIF6 can be measured for about $200, but insurance does not cover the test.

Controlling medical conditions including diabetes, hypertension and high cholesterol will decrease the risk of CAD and prevent its progression (see those specific sections for treatment recommendations).

One of the major causes of CAD is **smoking**, including secondhand inhalation. As soon as you *quit smoking*, the disease can stop progressing. Women who quit smoking have a 21 percent lower risk of death from CAD.

Caution: If you are a woman who is past menopause, and you already have CAD, be very cautious about taking synthetic HRT or synthetic estrogen. Recent studies show an increased chance of death, heart attack, or unstable angina when taking estrogen, especially the first few years. Although this risk decreases with long-term use, it is doubtful that synthetic estrogen has any long-term benefits for women who already have heart disease. (See the section on menopause for alternate recommendations for treating menopausal symptoms).

Important Information:
Taking Aspirin for Primary Prevention
of Heart Disease and Stroke

All health organizations recommend aspirin (81 mg) if you already have atherosclerosis. This is called *secondary prevention* and can save tens of thousands of lives.

Some of these organizations also recommend aspirin for *primary* prevention (preventing stroke or heart attack in those not having atherosclerosis).

However, several studies have shown that aspirin is not beneficial for primary prevention. The caveat is that these studies used low doses (81–167 mg), and it may be that higher doses do protect you. A registry analysis showed that 10 percent of heart patients are inappropriately prescribed aspirin (80 percent were women). Be aware though that aspirin can cause ulcers and bleeding, especially in older individuals on blood thinners.

Until studies are conducted using high-dose aspirin, you do not need to take it if you don't have cardiovascular disease or if your ten-year risk of having a heart event is less than 6 percent.

⸻

Eating habits and **nutrition** are major factors in causing, preventing, and reversing CAD. High fat content, processed and fried foods, fast foods, and high-cholesterol foods all worsen the atherosclerotic process. Even minor improvements in diet can help a great deal. Increasing your fiber is recommended for decreasing the risk of CAD, especially if you are a woman. Eating five to nine servings of fruits and vegetables daily can increase your fiber intake and also provide other ingredients that protect the heart, such as antioxidants. Every seven-gram increase in daily dietary fiber significantly lowers risk of heart disease.

Green leafy vegetables and vitamin-C rich fruits and vegetables are especially protective against CAD and its progression. One meal per week of cold-water fish (mackerel, tuna, herring, salmon, cod, trout, or halibut) can reduce the risk of heart attack by half, by increasing HDL (the "good" cholesterol) and decreasing LDL (the "bad" cholesterol). Barley and oats decrease the risk of developing and worsening heart disease, and high consumption of nuts have been found to decrease mortality from heart disease.

Avoid, or at least limit, saturated fats, foods high in cholesterol, and animal proteins, all of which increase cholesterol buildup in the heart arteries as well as causing inflammation. Processed meat (cured, salted, fermented, or smoked) is especially bad and doubles the risk of all-cause death, but nonprocessed red meat has minimal effects if not eaten every day—and not in high amounts (6 oz or less at one time or less than 18 oz per week). Recent guidelines include deriving 5–6 percent of calories from saturated fat but eliminating the percentage of calories from trans-fat.

⸻

Six Foods That Protect Your Heart

- *Almonds*: a handful a day lowers LDL cholesterol by 5 percent. Other nuts can do the same.

- *Cold-water fish*: Four servings a week (4 oz) can lower CAD risk by 14 percent. However, above that amount may raise blood mercury levels.
- *Garlic*: A daily dose (one fresh clove, opened, or 600–900 mg in dried capsule form) can reduce CAD risk by 25 percent.
- *Produce*: 5 to 9 servings of fruits and vegetables daily can cut heart risk by 25–40 percent.
- *Wine*: A daily glass decreases CAD risk by a third.
- *Dark Chocolate*: 1.6 oz a day can reduce high blood pressure that leads to heart disease.

Chocolate Can Be Healthy for the Heart

A recent study in the *Journal of Internal Medicine* showed that chocolate consumption decreased mortality related to the heart. Risk was 44 percent lower for weekly chocolate eaters and 66 percent for those who ate chocolate two or more times a week. If you eat chocolate, just don't overdo it (obesity is a risk factor) and eat *dark* chocolate (60–70 percent cocoa); a good guide is to eat about one ounce a day.

Several **heart diets** have been documented to be beneficial for preventing and reducing heart disease. These include the *DASH* (also good for hypertension), the *USDA Food Pattern*, and the *AHA* diets. The *low-fat diet* designed by Dean Ornish, MD, has been proven to actually reverse heart disease. According to a 2014 review in the *American Journal of Medicine*, the *Mediterranean* diet has proven to reduce cardiovascular events to a degree greater than low fat diets and equal to or greater than the benefit of taking statin drugs.

Low blood levels of vitamin D are associated with increased heart disease risk, so supplementation may be beneficial (you can measure your 25-dihydroxyvitamin D levels in a blood test).

Drinking one to two glasses of ***wine*** daily (5 oz) has been shown to help prevent the development of atherosclerosis (causing CAD) due to its antioxidant and anti-inflammatory properties. Red wine is the best choice because it contains resveratrol and antioxidants called polyphenols, but beer, white wine, cocktails and grape juice can also provide benefit (if imbibed moderately…see Chapter 2). To help avoid weight gain from drinking alcoholic beverages, drink them during meals.

Drinking **black or green tea** has also been shown to help prevent CAD as well as heart attacks, because of its antioxidants, anti-inflammatories, and blood-thinning ingredients. A recent study showed that eating lots of **dairy products**, such as milk, yogurt, cheese, or ice cream, may reduce the risk of CAD, even when the dairy products are high fat (although low fat is the better choice).

Drinking **pomegranate juice** (240 ml daily for three months) seems to decrease stress-induced myocardial ischemia (lack of oxygen delivery to heart muscle) in patients with coronary artery disease. The average improvement in myocardial perfusion is about 17 percent with pomegranate juice compared with an 18 percent *worsening* of myocardial perfusion in patients treated with placebo; however, it is not known if drinking pomegranate juice can prevent or reduce the risk of a myocardial infarction or other cardiovascular outcomes.

A Soda a Day Raises Heart Disease Risk

A study published in March 2012 revealed that sugary drinks increase the risk of heart disease. Even one soda a day was associated with a 20 percent increase in risk. However, *diet* soda was not associated with increased risk, although other studies have shown it to be associated with weight gain and metabolic diseases (such as diabetes), which can lead to heart disease.

Exercise is essential in preventing and reversing CAD. Aerobic exercise is the primary form necessary to do so. I support the AHA guidelines, which include a minimum of thirty to sixty minutes of moderate intensity activity, three to four times a week, supplemented by an increase in daily lifestyle activities, such as gardening, walking the stairs, or doing household chores. However, if you have not exercised before, have your doctor order an exercise tolerance test (ETT) to evaluate your heart condition and help you plan a graded exercise program.

Lifestyle Factors Can Prevent Most Coronary Artery Disease in Women

A 2015 study revealed that a healthy lifestyle might prevent coronary artery disease in nearly 75 percent of women. In this study, 92 percent of women who had six healthy lifestyle habits were less likely to develop heart disease. The six healthy lifestyle habits were as follows:

- Not smoking
- Greater than 2.5 hours weekly of physical activity
- Healthy diet
- Normal body-mass index
- Average less than or equal to one alcoholic drink per day
- Less than seven hours weekly of watching television

If you are not able to accomplish all six, the more of them you attain, the less the risk of developing heart disease.

The **mind-body connection** is also important for prevention of heart disease. A study published in *Circulation* showed that women who were optimists had significantly lower rates of heart disease. Those who had cynical hostility had higher rates. So, a sunny disposition is to your advantage.

The Conventional Approaches

An **aspirin** a day is the most important drug in slowing the progression of atherosclerosis because of both its blood thinning and anti-inflammatory effects. Take no more than 325 mg per day (81 mg is usually sufficient to thin the blood). ***Important note***: Many people think they are resistant to aspirin, but in actuality, most of these people are taking enteric-coated aspirin, which protects the stomach but does not have as much blood-thinning effect as noncoated aspirin (also see sidebar below for additional reasons).

Aspirin Resistance: Real or Not?

In patients with coronary artery disease, aspirin has been found to reduce the rate of death due to all causes by about 18 percent and the rate of vascular problems (heart/blood vessels) by 25–30 percent. Some patients, however, are thought to have aspirin resistance, in which aspirin does not have the antiplatelet effect to prevent clots. People who are nonresponsive to aspirin have a fourfold increased risk of adverse coronary events. However, a recent study revealed that 90 percent of patients who are unresponsive to aspirin have simply not taken their aspirin on a regular basis. You can find out if you are truly aspirin resistant by undergoing arachidonic acid testing.

Caution: Be aware that ibuprofen blocks the blood-thinning effects of aspirin. If you must take ibuprofen, take the aspirin first and wait at least two hours to take the ibuprofen so that the aspirin has time to exert its beneficial effects. Take the lowest dose of ibuprofen necessary. Aspirin use can deplete body stores of vitamin C, so make sure you get 600 mg a day through diet or by taking a supplement. It also can cause stomach irritation and bleeding in some people. OTC PPIs (such as Prilosec, Prevacid or Nexium) can protect the stomach if this occurs.

Warning: If you don't have heart disease, aspirin is not indicated. It may cause more harm (bleeding) than good and hasn't been shown to decrease deaths from heart attacks or strokes.

Other than aspirin, there are no particular medications to treat coronary artery disease if you do not have symptoms. Instead, you should take medications to control medical conditions that can cause CAD and to prevent the progression of atherosclerosis, such as diabetes, hypertension or high cholesterol (see those sections for specific recommendations).

Warning: Do Not Undergo Heart Procedures before Optimal Medical Treatment in Stable CAD

If you have unstable angina or a heart attack, you may need a procedure done called percutaneous coronary intervention (PCI) (see section above "*Heart Disease: Angina and Heart Attack*"). However, in *stable* coronary artery disease, a study done in 2007 called COURAGE determined that PCI had no advantage over optimal medical therapy (beta-blocker, statin, and aspirin) as an initial strategy to treat conditions predisposing to heart disease.

However, that is not what is occurring; despite stenting being shown to be ineffective and unnecessary in stable heart disease, it is significantly overused. A study published by *JAMA* in March 2011 revealed that only 45 percent of patients were receiving optimal medical therapy at the time of PCI. In addition, only 65 percent of patients were receiving optimal medical therapy *after* undergoing PCI. To make matters worse, there was no change in the use of medical therapy after the study was released

The *bottom line* is that optimal medical therapy is less expensive, less invasive, has fewer side effects, and is just as effective or more effective than PCI if you have stable disease. So don't be convinced to rush into a procedure you don't really need.

The Alternative Approaches

Several **nutritional supplements** may help prevent the progression of atherosclerosis and its complications.

Flaxseed (1 Tbsp. daily) is a plant omega-3 that helps prevent deposition of fats into the arteries. Use only freshly ground because encapsulated or oil forms deteriorate very quickly.

Fish oil has been found to significantly lower risk for cardiac death by 20 percent and sudden cardiac death (probably from arrhythmia) by 26 percent. Omega-3s from fish oil are more potent than from plants. ***Important notes***: There are problems with fish oil that you need to be aware of. Although regular fish oil can decrease cholesterol levels and protect the heart, you must take *at least* 1,500 mg daily to obtain benefits. Most studies have been done using 3,000–4,000 mg. Many fish oils also deteriorate very rapidly (three months); so by the time you buy them, they may already be partially deteriorated. Krill oil may be more potent and stable and contains two natural antioxidants and has few to no side effects. However, krill oil products differ in their concentrations of omega-3s and combinations with other ingredients, so check the label. Decrease in cholesterol levels will take about two months when taking krill oil.

Caution: Regular fish oil in high doses may decrease HDL cholesterol (the good cholesterol) in some people. If you take fish oil, and your HDL is reduced to below normal, take vitamin E (200 IU daily) and garlic (4,000 mg daily) or niacin (1–3 g daily) to raise HDL. Niacin may cause flushing, but there are nonflushing products. It also can be prescribed, but the prescription form is much more expensive and does not have any advantage over OTC forms.

Studies reveal that stress, especially from job strain, is associated with recurrent cardiac events, most likely caused by biologic factors. In addition, panic attacks increase the risk of coronary artery disease in women. **Meditation** and **relaxation** reduce the factors that accelerate atherosclerosis, including stress and emotions such as anger, anxiety, frustration, and certain personality types. Along with exercise and diet, meditation has been proven to actually reverse coronary artery disease.

Intravenous **chelation** is another alternative method that has been used to lower cholesterol and prevent heart disease. Chelation has recently been controversial. An NIH trial investigating chelation for heart disease actually showed it to be beneficial compared to placebo, especially in patients who had a heart attack in the front portion of the heart (anterior) and in diabetics. This type of chelation is very expensive, costing around $4,000.

Oral Chelation Recipe

An easier and simpler way of reducing your cholesterol (and helping clean your arteries) may be by using an oral, herbal chelation recipe. Blend one cup of fresh cilantro with six tablespoons of olive oil until the cilantro is completely chopped. Then add one clove of garlic, half a cup of nuts (cashews or almonds are best), and two tablespoons of lemon juice. Blend these into a paste (which will be lumpy), adding hot water if necessary. Take one to three teaspoons per day. If you make large amounts, you can freeze it for later use.

Your Empowered Patient Action Plan for Treating Chronic (stable) Coronary Artery Disease

Step #1: Aerobic exercise and a heart-healthy diet are a must for preventing and treating coronary artery disease or improving the condition if you already have it, along with a healthy water intake of at least eight glasses of purified water daily.

Step #2: Stop smoking and consider drinking a glass of wine daily, tea and/or pomegranate juice.

Step #3: Take an aspirin a day **(81 mg)** to prevent the progression of atherosclerosis and the risk of heart attack.

Step #4: Control other medical conditions that can lead to CAD to prevent its progression

Step #5: Take fish oil or ground flaxseed to prevent heart attack and progression of coronary artery disease and complications of coronary artery disease. Take vitamin E with mixed tocopherols and tocotrienols and garlic or niacin if you need to raise HDL due to lowering by fish oil.

Step #6: Meditate daily to reduce stress.

Step #7: Take cilantro as oral chelation to help decrease atherosclerosis buildup.

Step #8: Consider *IV chelation* if you still have progressive CAD.

Expected Outcome

Heart disease is the number one killer of Americans, but in fact, it can be slowed and even reversed using the above steps. In fact, deaths from heart disease have steadily decreased over the past two decades, but this can be lowered even more.

Hypertension (High Blood Pressure or HBP)

What You Need to Know

Blood pressure is a measurement of the pressure blood exerts against the walls of your arteries. There are two numbers that are important: The *systolic* (top) number is the peak force of the blood against the artery wall when the heart contracts. The *diastolic* (bottom) number is the force of blood against the artery wall as the heart is filling.

Quick Facts on High Blood Pressure*

- 82% of Americans with hypertension are aware of it.
- 76% of those aware are taking medications for it.
- 52% of hypertensive adults do not have their condition under control, despite the fact that 90% have a regular source of care.
- Of those with *uncontrolled* hypertension, 40% are not aware of their condition; 16% are aware but not receiving medication.

*CDC, 2013

For years, the diastolic measurement was considered the most important blood pressure measurement, but we now recognize that the systolic component may be as important as the diastolic. Elevation of either or both can cause heart, kidney, and brain damage; strokes; dementia; heart attacks and heart failure; kidney failure; vision problems; and death. One in three Americans has hypertension, and it accounts for one in six adult deaths annually. Elevated systolic pressure is strongly linked to intracerebral hemorrhage (causing stroke), subarachnoid hemorrhage (back of brain), and stable angina. Diastolic blood pressure is a less powerful predictor of the above but is a strong predictor of aortic aneurysm.

The levels of high blood pressure (in mm/Hg) are:

- Borderline: 120–140/90–94
- Mild: 140–160/95–104

- Moderate: 140–180/105–114
- Severe: 160+/115+

Hypertension Can Be Worse in African Americans

Many studies have noted that African Americans have greater risk for hypertension, can have more complications, and may require more intense treatment. Recently, the International Society on Hypertension in Blacks updated their recommendations for blood pressure control:

- Lifestyle modification should begin at BP > 115/75
- Target BP is < 135/85 rather than 140/90 (in Caucasians)
- If the patient has heart or kidney disease, target BP < 130/80.

"White-Coat" and "Masked" Hypertension: Not Benign

Often, your blood pressure will be falsely elevated in the doctor's office or in the emergency room, called "white-coat hypertension." It is thought that this may be due to anxiety, even if you don't feel anxious. Most doctors don't treat this type of hypertension, but recent studies indicate that such hypertension can increase the risk of future heart problems in nearly 10 percent of patients. Monitoring should be more frequent in such patients.

Opposite to white-coat hypertension, blood pressure readings may be normal in a doctor's office yet abnormal at home, called "masked hypertension." Blood pressure can also be episodic, varying at any time. All of these can cause higher mortality and should be treated.

In such cases, ambulatory monitoring should be done in addition to office and home monitoring (see below). With this device, you can measure blood pressure during day-to-day activities and while asleep, providing a more accurate determination of BP.

Measuring blood pressure: Most heart and hypertension associations recommend the use of home monitoring for more accuracy. However, ambulatory readings are more accurate and have been recommended by the USPSTF as the reference standard for confirming a diagnosis of hypertension. If taking your home blood pressure, you should note the following:

- The most reliable devices are validated by a manufacturer-sponsored educational trust and have electrically inflated cuffs (automatic), oscillometric detection, and memory. All of these should be described on the box. (A list of validated devices is available at www.dableducational.org.)
- *Important note*: Since home units use sound to determine BP, you should take readings in a quiet room with minimal noise.
- You should take readings after resting for five minutes and take at least two to three readings each time for better accuracy (the latter readings are the most accurate).
- You should take readings at least twice daily, each morning and each evening, for seven days before determining need for medication or for change in medication. For long-term follow-up, it should be performed for one week every three months.
- A study published in *BMJ* in 2011 revealed that taking multiple readings while at rest while using an automated blood pressure monitor is more accurate than manual monitoring, especially in measuring systolic blood pressure. Manual monitoring shows blood pressure to be higher than with automated measuring and can lead to unnecessary treatment.

Measuring Blood Pressure: *Helpful Tips*

You might notice that some doctors take blood pressure using your bare arm and others on a sleeved arm. A recent study showed that either way can give accurate readings. In patients who cannot use their arms to measure blood pressure (mainly breast cancer patients or those with blood clots), blood pressure can be measured in the leg, with readings being about 90 percent of the arm results.

Many kiosks allow you to check your blood pressure at pharmacies, grocery stores, gyms or other public places. Beware that these are not "one-size-fits-all," so different kiosks can yield different results. If a cuff is too small or too large, it will also give you inaccurate results.

Controlling hypertension is one of the easiest and most significant ways to prevent heart disease, stroke, circulation problems, and death. For each 10 mm decrease in systolic blood pressure, heart disease risk decreases by 30 percent and stroke by 40 percent. Untreated hypertension is certain to lead to other health problems and possibly even death.

Treatment Guidelines for BP: Controversial

There have been several guidelines issued regarding hypertension, many from medical associations (AHA, American College of Cardiology) and others from a committee called the JNC (Joint National Committee on Prevention, Detection, Evaluation, and Treatment of High Blood Pressure). Many of the guideline recommendations are similar, but some are not, and some are controversial.

The JNC-7 recommended that prehypertension should be treated, which would create forty-five million more patients for blood pressure drugs. Prehypertension is a systolic pressure from 120 to 139 millimeters of mercury (mm Hg) and/or a diastolic pressure from 80 to 89 mm Hg.

Numerous researchers not affiliated with drug companies, as well as the editor of the *American Journal of Hypertension*, flatly stated that such a recommendation "is garbage" and other recommendations made by the committee were "utter nonsense." They stated that many experts were excluded in the process of generating the guidelines and urged doctors to not take the guidelines seriously.

The JNC-8 featured some more unusual twists. Basically, its guidelines were to be endorsed by the above associations, but those arrangements fell through, so the report was issued anyway. Then a minority report was issued, disagreeing with the majority report. The main report recommended increasing the target systolic pressure to 150 for sixty to seventy-nine-year-olds, which is still controversial.

Complicating matters is a recent *Cochrane Review* in summer 2012 that found that benefits of treating patients with even mildly elevated blood pressure (140–159/90–99) and who are free of heart disease are unclear.

In general, prehypertension commonly becomes hypertension in many people, but it can be prevented by making lifestyle changes. Most experts think that, at this time, there is not sufficient evidence to warrant taking blood pressure medications for these measurements. On the other side of the spectrum, most authorities still recommend a target systolic blood pressure of 140. The bottom line is that you should consult with your doctor, especially if you have other medical conditions.

Treatments for Hypertension

The Preventive Approaches

Smoking is a key contributor to high blood pressure; if you smoke, it will be more difficult to control your blood pressure without medication.

Screen for Diabetes If You Have Hypertension

The USP-STF recommends that all people with blood pressure above 135/80 should be screened for type 2 (adult onset) diabetes due to a significantly increased risk.

Changes in lifestyle (diet and exercise) can prevent or control blood pressure in 80 percent of people who have borderline to moderate hypertension. In fact, if you are overweight, losing weight can significantly lower your blood pressure as well as help prevent heart disease from hypertension.

Diet: The *DASH* diet (Dietary Approaches to Stop Hypertension) is specifically designed to reduce blood pressure. This diet emphasizes fruits, vegetables, low-fat dairy, and includes whole grains, poultry, fish, and nuts. (For a copy of the DASH die, go to www.nhlbi.nih.gov/health/public/heart/hbp/dash/). If you don't follow this diet, any of the following dietary recommendations will still be helpful. *Warning*: Women with hypertension *should not* eat a very-low-fat diet (less than 10 percent saturated fat) as this can increase a type of hemorrhagic stroke.

Forget the Salt

One important part of the diet is *salt*, and Americans use an average of sixteen times the recommended amount. Most hypertensive people are salt-sensitive, especially in hypertension resistant to most drugs and especially in postmenopausal women.

Studies reveal that simply reducing salt intake may lower blood pressure, although only a small amount in some people. This is especially true in postmenopausal women, who can lower blood pressure up to 16 mm by limiting their intake of salt to one teaspoon a day.

It is also important to read food labels as there are many processed foods that also contain salt, including cereals and other snacks. Salt is often used to enhance sweetness in various foods. Preparing foods from their natural sources will minimize the additional salt and preservatives used to increase shelf life.

In addition, a 2013 study in *BMJ* revealed that many medications contain sodium, some at high levels. If you have hypertension, you should ask about any medications that you take to make sure that they are in non-sodium forms. This especially includes effervescent, soluble or dispersible tablets.

You should reduce the salt content of the food you eat to 2300 mg per day (although the American Heart Association recommends a cap of 1500 mg, a 2013 report from the Institute of Medicine found insufficient evidence to support the lower figure).

Low fat dairy products have been shown to reduce hypertension risk by 16 percent via the natural calcium in such products. A Japanese study revealed that drinking sour milk can significantly decrease both systolic and diastolic blood pressure.

Increase your *vegetable* intake (three cups per day) and decrease your animal meats (less than 4–6 oz daily). Using extra-virgin olive oil can lower your blood pressure after six months. Certain foods can help lower blood pressure, including celery, garlic, onions, nuts and seeds, cold-water fish (mackerel, cod, trout, shark, salmon, tuna, herring, or halibut), and legumes. Whole grains alone have been noted to decrease blood pressure about six points. Tomatoes and tomato products are also beneficial in lowering blood pressure due to their lycopene content, and eating them with oil (especially olive) increases this effect. A berry eaten in Asia (which tastes like cranberries), called *autumn olives*, has up to eighteen times the amount of lycopene found in tomatoes. Foods with high vitamin C content (primarily fruits) are also beneficial for reducing high blood pressure. A 2015 study showed that eating blueberries or blueberry powder over eight weeks reduced blood pressure by 7mm systolic and 5mm diastolic, as well as reducing arterial stiffness.

Beet juice, which contains inorganic nitrates was shown to lower blood pressure 7.7 mm systolic and 2.4 mm diastolic in a 2015 study (250 ml of beet juice daily). Such consumption was also associated with improved blood-vessel function.

Sugar: Worse Than Salt for Hypertension?

It is not just salt that may increase blood pressure, but another white substance that people overeat...sugar. Sugar can increase blood pressure by excess consumption and weight gain, as well as causing fluid retention. The worse culprit is sugar-sweetened beverages.

Reducing your intake of sugary drinks will decrease your blood pressure, even if drinking just one less sugar-sweetened beverage a day. A study in England in 2011 showed that for each serving of a sugar-sweetened beverage consumed per day, blood pressure increased by 1.6/0.8 mm (systolic/diastolic). The authors recommended drinking less than three twelve-ounce cans per week.

It was also noted that these associations were strongest among people with higher sodium excretion, which correlates to salt intake (see above).

One glass of **wine** a day may be beneficial: Red may be the best, but white wine is also beneficial. Other alcoholic drinks, such as beer and cocktails, can also be beneficial, if taken in moderate amounts.

Moderate **exercise** can reduce blood pressure by an average of 7 mm. I recommend primarily aerobic exercise, but resistance exercise can safely be done at 30–60 percent of maximum heart rate. Be aware, however, that resistance exercise can initially increase blood pressure, but this phenomenon goes away as you continue the exercise program. Interestingly, some small studies purport to show that using hand (grip) exercises for twelve minutes, three to five times a week, can reduce blood pressure up to 15 mm. The standard routine is to squeeze a device using 30 percent of your maximum strength in two minute intervals.

Be sure to undergo a thorough physical exam from your doctor before beginning an aggressive exercise program, especially if you have not exercised previously or for more than a year.

Exercise Pattern Can Help Decrease Prehypertension

A study published in *Medicine and Science in Sports & Exercise* showed that if you have mildly elevated blood pressure, breaking up your exercise workouts into shorter sessions during the day can be more beneficial than one long session. This was defined as walking briskly three times a day for ten minutes each versus one time for thirty minutes.

The Conventional Approaches

Important Note:
Doctors Not Treating Hypertension According to Guidelines

Multiple studies have shown that physicians are not providing treatment for hypertension consistent with published guidelines. Certainly, the guidelines may be controversial in certain aspects (see above), but they are beneficial for standard care. In particular, physicians are less aggressive about treating older patients, who are most likely to have the condition and who do benefit from therapy. They are also less likely to treat isolated systolic hypertension. A recent study showed that few patients have their medications adjusted at visits where blood pressure is still elevated. For this reason, you should be empowered and make sure you get treated in such instances.

Medications are the primary conventional treatment for hypertension. There are numerous and varied medications for high blood pressure available. Your blood pressure should be lowered within a few days to a week when taking these medications. Other health conditions, age, gender, race, and other medical conditions may dictate the choice of antihypertensive medications appropriate for you, among the following:

- *Diuretics* (such as thiazide diuretic or chlorthalidone) are the least expensive and are very effective. If you take a diuretic, your potassium excretion through the urine is increased (and your blood potassium level may drop), so you should check your potassium and supplement if necessary (10–20 meq per day) and eat more vegetables that contain potassium (primarily vegetables). However, another type of diuretic, called a potassium-sparing diuretic (aldosterone antagonists), such as spironolactone, triamterene, and ameloride, does not decrease potassium (however, they may cause an *increase* in potassium levels with certain other medications or conditions). A 2015 study showed that spironolactone was the most effective add on drug for hypertension that is resistant to other medications.

Important notes

- Older men who take loop diuretics (Lasix, bumex, demadex), commonly prescribed for heart failure and hypertension, are at higher risk for bone loss. If you take such drugs, undergo a bone density test for osteoporosis.

- People who take thiazide diuretics (especially Diuril) are at mild increased risk of developing diabetes. However, studies show that even if you do take them, risk for heart disease, stroke, kidney disease and all-cause mortality are not elevated and may, in fact, be less (so benefit is greater than potential harm).
- A 2014 study in the *Journal of the American Geriatric Society* showed that electrolyte disturbances or decline in kidney function are fairly frequent in older patients taking diuretics especially in the first nine months. These need to be monitored.

- *ACEIs* (angiotensin-converting enzyme inhibitors, such as captopril, lisinopril, or enalapril) may be considered next, to replace or combine with diuretics. ACE inhibitors are also commonly used as a first choice in diabetics with protein in their urine or used with diuretics in patients with congestive heart failure. Cough is sometimes a side effect of ACE inhibitors but may be reduced by taking ibuprofen.
  - *Caution*: Taking NSAIDs for arthritis can blunt the effects of ACE inhibitors. If you are on both types of drugs, be sure to monitor your blood pressure closely.
- *ARBs* (angiotensin receptor blockers) are similar in effectiveness to ACE inhibitors and can help prevent kidney failure in diabetes and hypertension. In comparisons of ARBs, irbesartan (Avapro) and candesartan (Atacand) have demonstrated superior blood pressure lowering as compared with losartan (Cozaar). Irbesartan also has shown better blood pressure reduction than valsartan (Diovan). Atacand can be obtained as a generic.

Important Information:
Older Patients Beware of Antibiotic Interaction with ACEIs or ARBs

A 2014 study in *BMJ* revealed that older patients who are taking ACE inhibitors, ARBs, or spironolactone have excess risk of sudden death if also taking trimethoprim/sulfamethoxazole (Bactrim, Septra), a common antibiotic. The risk approximates to three out of one thousand patients. A possible reason is that all these drugs increase potassium level, which can cause heart arrhythmias at elevated levels.

Although the risk is small, it is a good idea to have your potassium levels checked if you are on a combination of these drugs.

—⟨∞⟩—

- *Calcium channel blockers*, such as nifedipine, verapamil, or diltiazem, are effective but can also cause chronic eczematous rash. They are usually used if the above have not controlled your blood pressure. ***Warning***: several small studies have suggested an association between calcium channel blockers and excess risk for breast cancer. This is not yet definitive, but if you are at high risk, you should take other medications first.
- *Beta-blockers*: These drugs were commonly used as first-line therapy but have now lost favor, especially in older people with systolic hypertension. However, they can be used after heart attacks and if you have an arrhythmia. ***Cautions***: In some people, beta-blockers can sometimes reduce blood cholesterol levels to harmfully low levels. This can be reversed by taking chromium picolinate, 200 mcg three times per day. ***Important Note***: Beta-blockers may *raise* blood pressure in some African Americans.
- *Central α–antagonists* (such as clonidine or methyldopa) may be the last choice. However, clonidine is excellent at quickly reducing blood pressure if the levels are dangerously high. ***Important note***: Clonidine should not be used with a beta-blocker as it can cause a decrease in heart rate and a rebound in high blood pressure if it is stopped abruptly.

—⟨∞⟩—

Blood Pressure *Variability* for Medications Linked to Stroke Risk

If you go for doctor visits and your systolic (upper number) blood pressure changes each time, you are at higher risk for stroke. If that should occur, certain classes of blood pressure medication are better to take; these include calcium channel blockers and nonloop diuretics.

—⟨∞⟩—

Dr. A's Suggestions: Some Antihypertensives Can Make Blood Pressure Worse: Have Your Renin Level Checked

Beware that there can be substantial differences in response to different antihypertensive drugs depending on race and age. For example, beta-blockers can raise blood pressure in some African Americans.

One key to outcome is your renin level. Renin is a kidney enzyme that regulates fluid in the body and thus can play a significant role in regulating blood pressure. According to two recent studies, patients with low renin have elevated blood pressure because of excess fluid volume and those with high renin have hypertension with low fluid volume. Low renin patients with excess volume respond best with diuretics, and those with high rennin respond best to beta-blockers, ACE inhibitors, and ARBs.

You should realize that most doctors do not order renin tests and do not base their treatment on such results, so you may have to request it. Also be aware that some blood-pressure medications combine two drugs; if one is for high renin and the other for low renin, there could be a negating effect.

Most doctors will prescribe one antihypertensive and then add other antihypertensives if your pressure is still not controlled, which is very common. However, a recent study published in *Lancet* showed that starting therapy with a two-drug combination may work better than starting with just one drug. Nevertheless, some combinations don't work as well as others. ***Important Note:*** It is common for doctors to combine ACE inhibitors with ARBs, but several studies show that they are not as effective as using either class in combination with aldosterone antagonists. ***Important Note***: If blood pressure does not decrease with a medication, some doctors will start adding another drug rather than increasing the first drug(s) to maximum dosage. I have examined patients who are taking three or four drugs but none of which are at maximum dose; this is not advised unless side effects occur with the higher dosages.

Dr. A's Suggestions:
Take Blood Pressure Medications at Night

A recent review of twenty-one studies revealed that blood pressure is better controlled and there is less risk of heart attack and stroke if the medication(s) are taken at night.

It is also recognized that elevated nighttime blood pressure is predictive of new-onset type 2 diabetes but two 2015 studies showed that taking your medication at night reduces diabetes risk.

Important notes: An important reason patients do not continue taking blood-pressure medications is the side effects, many of which can be very subtle, such as just "not feeling right," but also involving problems with thinking and libido. They can also cause dizziness and subsequent falls, especially within the first two months after starting them (2014, *JAMA Internal Medicine*). However, there are many types of blood pressure medications, and you should ask your doctor to change yours rather than simply not taking the medications.

Adherence to Blood Pressure Drugs a Problem

One of the main reasons blood pressure may not be not controlled is lack of compliance. A recent study of compliance revealed that at one year, nearly half the patients had stopped taking medications altogether. On any given day, about 10 percent of scheduled doses were missed. Nearly half the patients took drug "holidays" lasting at least three days and this was more common during summer and weekends. Taking medications in the morning seemed to be easier to comply with than in the evening.

As uncontrolled blood pressure can cause serious complications and early death, you should make sure you take it as prescribed. If side effects occur, ask your doctor for a different type.

The Alternative Approaches

Most **mind-body techniques**, including biofeedback, meditation, progressive muscle relaxation, and hypnosis, can reduce high blood pressure by relaxing the blood-vessel walls and offsetting the effects of stimulant substances in the body such as adrenalin and cortisol.

Biofeedback (which teaches you how to relax and lower blood pressure using your mind) is most effective for borderline to mild hypertension.

Yoga has been shown to help lower blood pressure by reducing stress, and I recommend it if your blood pressure goes up when you are anxious. A study in *The European Journal of Preventive Cardiology* analyzed thirty-seven studies that showed yoga modestly improving blood pressure, cholesterol, and body weight. Systolic blood pressure decreased by 10 mm and diastolic by 6 mm. Consult a qualified yoga instructor for guidance on which postures are the best and how to perform them correctly. It may take up to several months to see results with yoga.

Storytelling Can Lower Blood Pressure

A study published in the *Annals of Internal Medicine* in 2011 showed that culturally appropriate storytelling may lower blood pressure as much as medication. In the study, black patients described their experiences with high blood pressure on DVDs, offering lessons about how to interact with physicians and how to achieve better medication adherence, diet, and exercise. Patients with controlled hypertension did not benefit, but those with *uncontrolled* hypertension lowered their blood pressures by 15 mm systolic and 3 mm diastolic.

Interactive imagery or other forms of **psychotherapy** have been successful at reducing blood pressure in some people by helping to release repressed emotions and stress/anxiety reduction that may be underlying the condition. Interactive imagery is a mind-body method in which you mentally interact with images that represent your emotions. It is a powerful method to uncover and deal with subconscious psychological issues you may not be aware of.

Qigong and **tai chi** have both been shown in studies to reduce blood pressure 8–10 mm over a course of twelve weeks.

A **Chinese herbal formula** called Jian Ya Ping Pian can be used in mild cases only, but is best used for prehypertension.

There are several **nutritional supplements** that can lower your blood pressure if it is borderline or mild. You can take these alone or together. You should observe lowering of your blood pressure within one to two months of using these nutrients. There are products that combine many of these together in the same compound. These include the following:

- *Lycopene*, an antioxidant found in tomatoes and tomato products can reduce blood pressure by 7–9 mm in mildly hypertensive patients. This effect can be obtained by taking lycopene extracts containing at least 15 mg of lycopene. (Lyc-O-Mato is the product used in the study.)
- *Stevioside* (750–1,500 mg daily) appears to reduce systolic blood pressure by 6–14 mm. The effect can begin within one week.
- *Flaxseed* (1 Tbsp per day, freshly ground only) or *fish oil* (1,500–3,000 mg daily) may be very effective in reducing mildly elevated blood pressure, as well as helping prevent complications of cardiovascular disease. A 2013 study in *Hypertension* showed that 30 g of milled flaxseed could decrease systolic blood pressure by 10 mm and diastolic BP by 7 mm. (***Caution***: This high dose may be associated with loose stool and/or diarrhea and may interact with antihypertensives or blood thinners.) ***Important notes***: There are problems with fish

oil that you need to be aware of. Although regular fish oil can decrease blood pressure and protect the heart, you must take *at least* 1,500 mg daily to obtain benefits. Many studies were done using 3,000–4,000 mg. Many fish oils also deteriorate very rapidly (three months); so by the time you buy them, they may already be partially deteriorated. For this reason, I recommend krill oil, which is more stable, contains two natural antioxidants, and has few to no side effects. However, some krill oil products differ in their combinations with other ingredients, so check the label.

- *Coenzyme Q10* (30–75 mg per day for mild, 120–150 mg per day for moderate high blood pressure) may reduce hypertension through its effects on dilating blood vessels. It can lower systolic blood pressure up to 11–17 mm and diastolic 8–10 mm. Hypertension also tends to deplete your body's supply of this nutrient.
- *Garlic* (containing 4,000 mg allicin daily) has been reported to lower blood pressure up to 20–30 mg systolic and 10–20 mg diastolic, but this effect varies greatly among patients.
- *Hawthorn* (100–250 mg, containing 10 percent procyanidins, three times daily) can also reduce high blood pressure in much the same way as CoQ10 does. **Caution**: If used with other conventional heart medications, hawthorn can possibly heighten the effect or interfere with successful treatment, so check with your doctor before taking it. It can also increase the risk of stroke.
- *Olive leaf* (containing 20 percent Olueropein, twice daily) has also been found to help lower blood pressure.
- *Hibiscus tea*, three cups a day for six weeks, has been shown in a recent study to lower blood pressure about 7.2 mm.
- *Cocoa flavanols* (215–500 mg per day) can decrease systolic blood pressure by 5 mm and diastolic by 3 mm.
- *Probiotics* may help reduce blood pressure, but only modestly (2–3 mm reduction).
- *Calcium* (800 mg per day) and magnesium (800 mg per day) have both been found to be effective in reducing blood pressure in many patients. Try one at a time for one month to see if each is effective, although they can be taken together. **Caution**: Recent studies have implied that taking supplemental calcium may increase the risk of heart disease. (See section on *Osteoporosis* for more information).

Acupuncture has been used quite successfully to reduce blood pressure, primarily borderline to mild, but only if you've had it a short time. Otherwise, the results may only be temporary. There are at least five possible underlying causes for hypertension in Chinese medicine, so acupuncture points will vary. Always seek evaluation and treatment from a practitioner certified in acupuncture. You should notice improvement within six acupuncture treatments, but you might need additional sessions for maximum benefits. However, the longer you have been on antihypertensive medication, the less the likelihood that acupuncture will help lower your blood pressure.

Your Empowered Patient Action Plan for Treating Hypertension

- *Important Note: For moderate to severe hypertension, start with steps 5 and 1; then return to step 2.*

Step #1: Make lifestyle modifications by adopting the DASH or Mediterranean diet and exercising to prevent hypertension or lower blood pressure if high.

Step #2: Practice qigong/tai chi to reduce mildly elevated blood pressure. It may take two to three months to observe the maximum effects.

Overweight and a twenty-year smoker, Ted had mildly elevated blood pressure. He did not want to take blood-pressure medications, but he was willing to change his lifestyle to try to control his blood pressure. First, he stopped smoking by using acupuncture and Chinese herbs (see chapter 2). I placed him on the DASH diet, and he began an exercise program, primarily walking (he gradually increased up to four miles per day). He also practiced qigong, although not as regularly as instructed. After several months, he had lost nearly thirty pounds, and his blood pressure returned to normal.

Step #3: Try acupuncture if hypertension has been recently diagnosed and is mild.

Step #4: Try various herbal supplements to reduce blood pressure if it is mild to moderate. These may be preferred over drugs because they have fewer side effects. However, taking one or two medications may be easier and less costly than several herbs.

Controlling blood pressure often requires multiple approaches. Beatrice had hypertension for over fifteen years. Her blood pressure had been controlled on prescription medications, but she didn't like the side effects, so she stopped taking them, which caused her blood pressure to go up. I recommended the DASH diet, and she began exercising. I prescribed both magnesium, flaxseed oil, and a lycopene supplement. These efforts brought Beatrice's blood pressure to mildly elevated.

I then recommended qigong, which further reduced her blood pressure, but it was still borderline high. At that point, I prescribed a mild diuretic, which did not have any side effects and brought her blood pressure back to normal.

⸺

Step #5: ***Take prescription antihypertensive medications*** to control your blood pressure if the above measures have not been effective or if your blood pressure is moderate or greater.

Step #6: ***Undergo interactive imagery or other forms of psychotherapy*** to reduce blood pressure further if stress induces or increases your blood pressure. If blood pressure is lowered, you may be able to decrease the dose or discontinue the medications in step 5 and the herbs in step 4.

Step #7: ***Practice appropriate yoga postures*** to maintain blood pressure.

Step #8: ***Practice biofeedback*** to reduce blood pressure further if still elevated.

Expected Outcome

The most common reason for failure to control blood pressure is non-compliance or not knowing that you have hypertension. It is essential that blood pressure be controlled; treatment reduces the risk of stroke by 35–40 percent, heart attacks by 25 percent, and heart failure by 50 percent.

Incontinence/Overactive Bladder

What You Need to Know

Incontinence is the involuntary loss of urine. There are three main types:

- **Stress incontinence**, caused by weakness of the muscles surrounding the opening of the urethra (the tube from the bladder), in which a cough, sneeze, or laughter can cause leakage.
- **Urge incontinence**, due to uncontrolled contractions of the bladder, is when leakage occurs as soon as the bladder is full.
- **Overflow incontinence**, caused by decreased sensation of the bladder, causes unexpected, sudden leakage.

Although incontinence occurs eight times more often in women (most often due to childbirth or aging), it can also occur in men, usually secondary to prostate problems or treatment of prostate cancer (radiation, surgery).

Overactive bladder (OAB) is a symptom *complex* that is characterized by urinary urgency, with or without associated urinary incontinence. Urgency, the hallmark of OAB, is defined as the sudden compelling desire to urinate, a sensation that is difficult to defer. Often, there will also be urinary *frequency*, defined as voiding eight or more times in a twenty-four-hour period, as well as *nocturia*, the need to wake one or more times per night to void.

OAB impacts approximately 34 million Americans. Though OAB is a common condition, it is estimated that < less than 30 percent of patients receive treatment, likely attributed to the reluctance of patients to talk to their healthcare providers about the condition. Overall, about 17 percent of women have OAB. Men tend to develop OAB slightly later in life than women do, and women are more likely to develop urgency incontinence. Thirty-seven to 39 percent of OAB cases remit during a given year, but the majority of patients have symptoms for years.

Treatments for Incontinence and Overactive Bladder

The Preventive Approaches

Correctable causes: Incontinence is a potential side effect of many medications, including diuretics, sedatives, antidepressants, antihistamines, and many forms of synthetic estrogen. If you take any of these medications, check the *PDR*; and if the medication you take can cause incontinence, have your doctor switch you to another one.

Obesity can predispose you to incontinence, and **losing weight** can reduce or reverse it. Even losing a modest amount of weight can make a difference.

Smoking cessation can lower the risk for incontinence.

Voiding at specified times during the day can also help increase bladder tone and train the bladder to function better.

Often, discontinuing **beverages that contain caffeine**, including coffee, tea, and soft drinks, can reduce incontinence.

Exercises Helpful for Incontinence

For women, Kegel exercises (pelvic-floor muscle training) increase the strength and tone of the "pelvic floor" muscles, the ones that control your urine flow. They are indicated primarily for stress incontinence.

To perform Kegel exercises, first find the muscle: stop the flow while you are urinating to feel this muscle; however, do not exercise the muscle during urination. You can also place your finger inside your vagina and squeeze down; the muscle will tighten. Once you learn which muscle it is, you can voluntarily contract and relax this muscle whenever you want. The more you exercise it, the stronger it will become. You can perform these exercises lying down (easiest initially), seated, or standing. Contract the muscles for three seconds and relax for three seconds; repeat ten to twelve times. Gradually work up to ten-second contractions. Don't use other muscles (abdominal, buttock, thigh) during this time, and don't hold your breath.

For urgency incontinence, pelvic floor training is not helpful, but bladder training (e.g. lengthening the time between voids) is recommended. For mixed stress and urgency incontinence, both pelvic floor exercises and bladder training may be beneficial.

There are other, more **specific exercises** to strengthen the pelvic floor muscles besides Kegel exercises, but you must learn these from registered physical therapists specifically trained in these techniques (check with your state physical therapy association). These exercises are especially valuable after childbirth, for preventing stress incontinence.

The Conventional Approaches

A recent study showed that **behavioral therapy** was beneficial for postprostatectomy incontinence. Such therapy consists of pelvic floor muscle training, bladder control strategies, fluid management, and self-monitoring with a bladder diet. ***Important note***: The study found that there was no benefit from biofeedback or pelvic floor electrical stimulation.

Estrogen has been shown to decrease irritative symptoms of incontinence in some women, but it can worsen incontinence in others. If taking HRT, I recommend taking natural estrogen or raloxiphene; the latter is the only synthetic estrogen that does not cause incontinence problems

There are numerous **medications** for treatment of incontinence/OAB. It should be noted, however, that these drugs are *only modestly effective* and can have limiting side effects. They are indicated for urgency incontinence if bladder training hasn't been effective. In men, use of these drugs can sometimes cause acute urinary retention, especially in the first few weeks of treatment. The drugs are listed below:

- *Oxybutynin* (Ditropan) is called an antimuscarinic agent (anticholinergic) and can be effective for both OAB and urge incontinence patients. It is the only one available in generic form in the United States (and thus is the least expensive), but it has the highest rate of side effects, including dry mouth and constipation. It comes in a short-acting pill, long-acting pill, transdermal patch (every three to four days), and gel. It can be obtained OTC at a lower cost.

- *Tolterodine* (Detrol) is another antimuscarinic drug that relaxes the bladder muscles and can also be effective for both OAB and urge incontinence patients. It comes as short-acting and long-acting. It is more expensive than oxybutynin but has the same side effects but occurs less than oxybutynin. (You can obtain the less expensive generic form from Canadian pharmacies online).
- *Trospium* (Sanctura; short-acting and long-acting), solifenacin (Vesicare), and darifenacin (Enablex) (the latter both long acting) all have less research regarding effectiveness and safety than the above drugs. Again, the main side effects are constipation and dry mouth.
- *Tesoferodine* (Toviaz), reduces bladder spasms and has recently been approved for OAB. It is structurally similar to and is actually just a repackaged form of Detrol. Toviaz is much more expensive but may be more effective in patients who lack a specific enzyme that is necessary for Detrol to work. It has the highest success rate in achieving continence compared to oxybutynin and Detrol, but even so, the success rate is only 13 percent.

Cautions: The above drugs have a high discontinuation rate due to the side effects. In fact, the majority of patients stop taking them after a few weeks. They should not be used in patients with narrow angle glaucoma, urinary retention, or impaired stomach emptying.

- *Mirabegron* (Myrbetriq) relaxes the smooth muscle and increases the capacity of the bladder, a different mechanism than the medications above. Approval studies showed almost a 40 percent efficacy.
- *Duloxetine* (Cymbalta), an SSRI antidepressant, has *not been shown* to be beneficial for stress incontinence.

Botox has been approved for urge incontinence in patients with OAB who cannot or do not respond adequately to the above drugs and for urinary incontinence in patients with neurological diseases such as multiple sclerosis or spinal injuries. It helps reduce leakage (from five down to three episodes daily) in 70 percent of women. However, the injection must be repeated every nine months to a year.

Invasive procedures are often done to correct any structural problems. *Collagen injection* can be beneficial for stress incontinence, but it usually breaks down over time. A new injectable, called Durasphere, is as effective as collagen but is longer-lasting. Collagen injections have a 20-30 percent success rate. Some women obtain relieve from using *pessaries* and cone-shaped vaginal weights.

Surgery for incontinence may be necessary to repair weakened or damaged pelvic muscles, called pelvic floor disorders (often the result of pregnancy or childbirth). *Suspension* and *midurethral sling* procedures are the most common and can be done as an outpatient, and are reported to have an 82% success rate. A 2013 study in the *NEJM* showed that outcomes at twelve months were better with surgery than with physiotherapy. *Tension-free vaginal tape* procedures for stress incontinence are performed under local anesthesia, with a reported cure rate of 91%, a 7% improvement rate, and a 2% failure rate and is very safe. In obese patients, *bariatric surgery* can reduce symptoms of incontinence.

Anti-incontinence surgery called *urethropexy* may be done for stress urinary incontinence caused by pelvic organ prolapse (organs "falling down" due to weakening of the muscles holding them). However, a long-term study published in *JAMA* revealed that at seven years, prolapse failure was greater with urethropexy (48 percent compared to 34 percent with no surgery).

Warning: The FDA warned that using mesh in surgery, especially transvaginally, has much higher risk of complications than not using mesh and has no advantage. If mesh is considered, it should be placed through the abdomen, not the vagina.

Nerve stimulation procedures can be done for OAB as well, using small, electrical impulses to control the nerves that signal the need to urinate. It may help with urge incontinence but not for stress incontinence. There are two types: sacral nerve and tibial nerve stimulators. Pacemaker-like devices are implanted under the skin with electrodes to stimulate these nerves. They are not as successful as surgery.

The Alternative Approaches

Acupuncture is very effective in reducing and sometimes resolving all forms of incontinence and overactive bladder long-term by increasing the tone of the bladder muscles and improving bladder sensation. You should notice improvement within six to eight acupuncture treatments, but you might need additional sessions for maximum benefit. Acupuncture can be effective for incontinence caused by prostatectomy.

Yoga was found in a 2014 study to reduce the frequency of incontinence—primarily stress incontinence but not urgency incontinence (OAB). The researchers showed that yoga benefits the pelvic floor muscles as well as the anxiety associated with incontinence. The yoga in the study involved eight postures used in Iyengar (Hatha) yoga.

Biofeedback and **hypnosis** are mind-body methods that have been shown to lead to improved or complete bladder control.

There are several **Chinese herbal formulas** that can be helpful as well. *Zuo Gui Wan/You Gui Yin* can reduce frequent urination, especially at night. *Jin Gui Shen Qi Wan* and *Jin Suo Gu* are "lifting" formulas that, in TCM, take pressure off of organs. *Jing Wan* can help with urge incontinence. You should notice improvement within three weeks, but you may need to take them longer for complete relief.

A **homeopathic remedy**, Equisetum, may help with urging from a full bladder that is unable to fully void.

Marshmallow tea (althea) may reduce bladder irritation.

Your Empowered Patient Action Plan for Treating Incontinence and Overactive Bladder

- *Important note: Injectable devices and artificial slings have not been thoroughly researched and cannot be recommended at this time.*

Step #1: Practice Kegel and pelvic floor exercises to prevent or reduce incontinence problems.

Step #2: Undergo acupuncture to obtain long-term resolution of incontinence or overactive bladder.

Step #3: Practice biofeedback, yoga, and/ or undergo hypnosis to help control overactive bladder if the above steps have not helped.

Step #4: Take the Chinese herbal products Zuo Gui Wan/You Gui Yin or Jin Suo Gu Jing Wan to control incontinence symptoms or overactive bladder if the above medications are not helpful.

Step #5: Take an appropriate prescription medication to control incontinence or overactive bladder symptoms if you still have them. Remember that these drugs have limited effectiveness so don't continue taking them if they have not helped.

Step #6: Undergo surgery if the above steps have not been beneficial. Be sure to obtain a second opinion since there are many different types of procedures.

Step #7: Receive collagen injection treatments if appropriate and the above steps aren't beneficial.

Step #9: Try *nerve stimulators* if none of the above Steps have worked.

Frances had urge incontinence with OAB. Her urologist had placed her on Detrol, but this drug had not controlled her symptoms. I referred her to a physical therapist, who taught Frances various exercises to strengthen her pelvic muscles. I then performed acupuncture. After one month her remaining incontinence had gone away, but when she tried to stop taking the Detrol, she still had intermittent leakage. I prescribed the Chinese herbal formula Jin Suo Gu Jing Wan, continued acupuncture treatments, and had Frances continue her exercises. Her leakage stopped completely, and she was able to discontinue the Chinese herbs and Detrol.

∞

Expected Outcome

Urinary incontinence and overactive bladder are common problems but can potentially be resolved completely by using alternative methods. If not, it may be able to be controlled adequately by medications.

Dangerous Infections (Pneumonia, MRSA, VRE, C. Difficile)

What You Need to Know

There are certain infections that are especially dangerous to people as they age, as immune systems are not as strong, although younger people can get them as well. If you have concurrent chronic conditions, this can further weaken the immune system and thus predispose you to these dangerous agents. It is thus important for you to realize what these infections are and what you should do about them. With infections, the sooner they are recognized and treated, the better your outcome.

The diagnosis of infection as we age becomes more difficult, yet is very important because of the higher incidence of complications and death. Many signs and symptoms of infection that are common in younger adults, particularly fever and leukocytosis (high white blood cell count—the cells that fight infection), occur less frequently or not at all in older adults. While 60 percent of older adults with serious infections *do* develop leukocytosis, its *absence* does not rule out an infectious process. Because frail older adults tend to have poorer body temperature response, elevations in body temperature of 1.1°C (2°F) from their normal baseline temperatures should be considered a high temperature. Fevers higher than 38.3°C (101°F) often indicate severe, life-threatening infections in older adults, and hospitalization should be considered for these patients.

In addition, changes caused by infection in the elderly are subtle, and nonspecific symptoms may be the only indications. Elderly patients with infections commonly present with thinking impairment or a change in mental status; delirium occurs in 50 percent of older adults with infections. Furthermore, anorexia (no appetite), functional decline, falls, weight loss, or a slight increase in breathing rate may be the only signs indicating infection in older patients.

Although most dangerous infections are primarily seen in hospitals and nursing homes, they can also occur at home. So be aware of any subtle changes that may occur.

Below are the most common dangerous infections you need to be aware of.

Pneumonia

Pneumonia and influenza combined are the sixth leading cause of death in the United States, and about 90 percent of these deaths occur in adults sixty-five years old and older. In fact, more than 60 percent of people sixty-five years old and older are admitted to hospitals because of pneumonia.

The diagnosis of pneumonia in older adults is difficult to make as the signs and symptoms can be subtle, so the initiation of antibiotic therapy is often delayed, which may contribute to higher death rates.

Regardless of age, bacterial causes of pneumonia can only be identified in 20–50 percent of patients. In fact, a 2015 study showed that a bacterial cause was found in only 38 percent of cases, with the rest being viruses. For that reason, treatment of pneumonia is initially guesswork and treatment is usually directed toward bacteria that would most likely cause it.

Quality Measurements for Treating Pneumonia

One of the core quality measurements dictated by Medicare was to start treatment for pneumonia within four hours of presentation. Studies have shown, however, that rushing to diagnose pneumonia in this short period leads to inaccuracy in diagnosis and the use of unnecessary antibiotics, which can in turn lead resistance and to other infections, such as *C. difficile* (see below). Other studies show that an eight-hour cap is just as effective and reduces the errors, but the measure has nevertheless been amended only to six hours.

Methicillin-Resistant Staphylococcus Aureus (MRSA)

Methicillin-resistant Staphylococcus aureus (MRSA) presents a major problem for patients, especially those in institutional settings, such as nursing homes. Because of overuse of antibiotics, this bacterium has become very resistant to most antibiotics and therefore is difficult to kill.

Many people are already carriers of MRSA, and those people are at increased risk of MRSA infection. They also have a higher risk of death from MRSA resulting from its resistance to common antibiotics. While MRSA infection is more likely to occur in hospitalized patients than in nursing home residents, poor functional status is associated with being an MRSA carrier. Therefore, nursing homes and other institutional settings must be especially careful to prevent the spread of infection caused by this organism.

Screening for MRSA May Not Be Helpful

Because MRSA is associated with severe complications and death, preventing the infection is a top priority in hospitals. A specific test called PCR screening can detect MRSA within one day, compared to two to three days for conventional testing. However, studies show that despite leading to less use of inappropriate antibiotics, this test does not reduce the spread of MRSA.

Vancomycin-Resistant Enterococcus (VRE)

As with MRSA, VRE presents a major problem in older patients, especially when an outbreak occurs in an institutional setting. Enterococci are the second most common organism in hospital-acquired urinary tract and wound infections. Over the past two decades, enterococci have become more resistant to most of the major antibiotics, increasing death rates to 50 percent. Because of the high level of antibiotic resistance, prevention of outbreaks and spread of VRE is crucial.

Clostridium difficile (C. difficile, C. diff)

C. difficile (commonly called *C. diff*) bacteria are everywhere—in soil, air, water, human and animal feces, and on most surfaces. The bacteria don't create problems until they grow in abnormally large numbers in the intestinal tracts of people taking antibiotics or other antimicrobial drugs. Then, *C. difficile* can cause symptoms ranging from diarrhea to life-threatening inflammations of the colon.

C. Difficile Can Be Deadly

A report from the CDC in 2013 showed that more than two million people contract drug-resistant infections, and twenty-three thousand die, primarily in the hospital. *C difficile* is the main culprit, killing fourteen thousand people, accounting for over half of all deaths from drug-resistant infections. The incidence of *C difficile* infections is increasing steadily.

The reason *C. difficile* occurs starts with common bacteria, which play a key role in suppressing the growth of harmful organisms. When you take an antibiotic to treat an infection, it often destroys these beneficial bacteria along with the bacteria that may be causing the illness. Without enough *healthy* bacteria, potentially harmful bacteria such as *C. difficile* can quickly grow out of control.

Dr. A's Suggestions:
PPIs May Increase Risk of *C. Difficile*

Several recent studies have shown that taking PPIs (e.g., Nexium, Prilosec, Prevacid and others) for acid reflux may increase the risk for developing *C. difficile* in the hospital. Often, these drugs are given to hospitalized patients who don't really need them. Avoid them if possible.

Once it takes hold, *C. difficile* can produce two virulent toxins that attack the lining of the intestine. The toxins destroy cells and produce pseudomembranes, telltale patches of inflammatory cells and decaying cellular debris on the interior surface of the colon.

Almost any antibiotic can cause harmful bacteria to proliferate in the intestine, but clindamycin, fluoroquinolones, and cephalosporins are most often implicated in *C. difficile* infections. The use of such broad-spectrum drugs that target a wide range of bacteria and the taking of antibiotics for a prolonged period increase the chance of infection. (That's why taking a drug like Cipro for urinary infections or upper respiratory infections should not be first line). Other antimicrobials (including antiviral and antifungal drugs), PPIs for acid reflux (see sidebar above), and chemotherapy medications can also lead to an increased risk of infection with *C. difficile*.

Health experts are especially alarmed by the emergence of new, aggressive strains of *C. difficile* that produce far more deadly toxins than ordinary strains do. The new strains are more resistant to treatment with certain medications and are increasingly showing up in people who haven't been in the hospital or taken antibiotics. In fact, it is occurring more frequently in outpatients and in people who don't have the common risk factors. It's not clear why or how these low-risk people become infected.

Another major problem is that the major test for *C difficile* is unreliable, and 20 percent of patients that have the infection test negative. If not treated, such patients have many more complications.

Treatments for Dangerous Infections

The Preventive Approaches

Most of the infectious diseases discussed in this section are preventable. Most pneumonias are caused by a bacteria called pneumococcus and a pneumococcal vaccine called *Prevnar 13* (PCV13) protects against 13 types of pneumococcal bacteria, decreasing the risk by 75 percent in healthy persons sixty-five years old or older. In nursing home residents, the vaccine is 50 to 60 percent effective in preventing bacteria in the blood and 80 percent effective in preventing death from pneumonia. An additional vaccine called PPSV23 has shown to further increase immunity from this bacteria and should be given one year after receiving the PCV13. ***Important Note***: a *lower* immune response may be observed if PPSV23 is given before PCV13.

Hand washing, isolation of infected patients, and proper handling of bodily secretions are essential to prevent the spread of MRSA and VRE. The most common areas where these bacteria originate from are the nose and throat. Skin contamination from persons already colonized in these areas may also be a source for MRSA infection.

Attempts to identify the original infected person (source case) must be made by swabbing the noses and throats of patients and staff near to the outbreak and treating those found to have MRSA or VRE infections. Staff and patients who are carriers should be isolated, and some authorities recommend treatment with topical mupirocin (Bactroban), which is applied twice daily for two weeks to the nose or other areas of skin (e.g., wounds) to reduce spread. Colonization recurs in about half of treated subjects.

The Conventional Approaches

Medications: Antibiotics are the primary treatment for these infections, although other treatments may be given as adjuncts or as first line therapy.

Antibiotic Dosing Requirements Different If Obese

Most antibiotics are given based on a fixed dose, even though they should be calculated on body-mass index. An example is vancomycin, which a recent study finds is under dosed in more than 70 percent of patients. A study in the journal *Pharmacotherapy* showed that very obese people taking short courses of drugs, especially antibiotics, may be getting as little as half the level of medication they need.

Underdosing leads to worsened outcomes as well as increased antibiotic resistance. If you are obese, make sure your doctor prescribes antibiotics based on your weight. Also know that vancomycin levels should be checked by your doctor from a blood test after the third dose.

Other studies have shown that overweight people receiving injections in the buttocks may not be receiving proper dosage because the needles are too short to reach the desired blood vessels to be absorbed. The result is, of course, less response and more resistance. Again, be sure to question your doctor regarding the need for increased dosage if you are overweight.

For MRSA, active infection is usually treated IV with the powerful antibiotic *vancomycin*. However, two new drugs (*dalbavancin, oritavancin*) that are long-acting and require only a once-weekly dose have now been approved by the FDA and have fewer side effects than vancomycin. *Caution*: Older adults may require decreased dosage adjustment based on renal function. Other regimens include vancomycin plus gentamicin (Garamycin) or rifampin (Rifadin).
Some people may be carriers of MRSA, which can grow (colonize) in the nose. *Mupirocin nasal* spray alone offers 93 percent effectiveness initially, but at 90-days post-treatment, effectiveness drops to 61 percent. More often, *multiple antibiotics* must be given together to eradicate the MRSA; the regimens include various combinations of mupirocin, rifampin, doxycycline and trimethoprim-sulfamethoxazole. These combinations can produce an 88 percent eradication rate at one year.

For VRE, vancomycin is also the most frequently used drug to treat infections. Of course, other potent antibiotics are required if the bacteria is resistant to vancomycin.

For C. difficile antibiotics are also given—but different ones, of course, than the ones that may have caused it. Doctors usually prescribe oral *metronidazole* or IV *vancomycin*. These antibiotics eradicate *C. difficile*, allowing normal bacteria to flourish again in the intestine. Both antibiotics kill only the active form of *C. difficile*, not the tough, long-lived spores it produces. Because the spores may persist in the body after treatment, the infection can return, requiring a second or even a third round of antibiotics. Some people have repeat bouts of *C. difficile* for years. Another antibiotic, *tigecycline*, has been shown effective in those resistant to the above antibiotics; and another recently approved antibiotic, *Dificid* (fidamoxin), is also more effective in preventing recurrences. Both, however, are very expensive.

A recent anecdotal report showed that a combination of an antibiotic staggered and tapered over six weeks along with the fermented dairy drink *Kefir* (which is a probiotic and available in supermarkets) had an excellent success rate against C diff.

Fecal microbiota transplant (FMT) is a procedure that has become the treatment of choice for recurrent *C. difficile*, when available. FMT involves restoration of the colonic flora (bacteria) by introducing healthy bacterial flora through infusion of stool, obtained from a healthy human donor. There are several modes of delivery, including enema or duodenal infusion through the upper GI tract, and both have lower cure rates than using colonoscopy for the infusion. This therapy, however, is not widely available.

For people with severe pain, organ failure (of the colon), or inflammation of the lining of the abdominal wall caused by C. difficile, **surgery** to remove the diseased portion of the bowel may be the only option to resolve the condition.

For community-acquired pneumonia (*CAP*) (not acquired in the hospital), *antibiotics* are the treatment of choice, but not the ones that may commonly be recommended. Guidelines recommend the combination use of beta-lactam (drugs ending in "cillin", "cephem," or "penem" with a macrolide (drugs ending in "mycin") or flouroquinolone monotherapy (drugs ending in "quin"). A 2015 study, however, reveals that these broad spectrum drugs (that destroy many types of bacteria) are no better than using a macrolide antibiotic alone.

Steroids have been demonstrated to confer benefits in people with CAP, especially those with severe pneumonia. Two 2015 studies showed that steroids are valuable in hospitalized patients with CAP due to their effect at reducing the body's inflammatory response.

The Alternative Approaches

Dangerous infections should be treated by conventional means, but alternative methods can assist in healing and recovering from these infections.

Probiotics, meaning "for life," are "live bacteria" in the form of dietary supplements that help restore a healthy balance to the intestinal tract. A natural yeast called Saccharomyces boulardii has proved effective in treating *C. difficile* infections in conjunction with antibiotics as well as significantly decreasing the incidence of recurrent *C. difficile* infections.

Other alternative therapies such as **acupuncture** can be very useful during the recovery phase, helping the body to rebalance after the illness and contributing to the prevention of recurrences.

In addition, **Chinese herbal formulas** can speed up recovery. *Zuo Gui Wan/You Gui Wan* strengthens the immune system and speeds recovery from illness. *Don Chai Xia Cao* strengthens the lungs, boosts the immune system, and strengthens resistance to disease, so it is especially beneficial after pneumonia. For energy, *panax ginseng* is very beneficial and also strengthens the immune system.

Your Empowered Patient Action Plan for Treating Dangerous Infections

*Step #1: **Be sure to maintain good hygiene*** at all times, especially hand washing, whether you have an infection yourself or are around people who have one.

*Step #2: **Obtain proper vaccines*** to prevent bacterial infection if you are over the age of sixty five.

*Step #3: **Take appropriate antibiotics*** to kill whichever bacteria are causing your illness. Take only antibiotics that are indicated for your infection (question your doctor). For CAP, consider adding steroid to the treatment regimen.

*Step #4: **Take probiotics*** (Saccharomyces or a "broad-spectrum" probiotic) to assist recovery and prevent recurrence of *C. difficile* infection.

*Step #5: **Undergo fecal microbiota transplant*** for recurrent C difficile infection.

*Step #6: **Take Chinese herbs or use acupuncture*** to accelerate healing and strengthen the immune system after the infection treatment is initiated through the above steps.

*Step #7: **Undergo surgery*** for organ failure, severe pain, or abdominal inflammation.

Expected Outcome

Dangerous infections are just that: dangerous. They have the potential for serious complications and death. With appropriate preventive measures, and judicious use of specific antibiotics and other treatments, such infections can be cured, but timely diagnosis is of utmost importance for success of treatment.

Insomnia (and Sleep Apnea)

What You Need to Know

Sleep is a very important aspect of health, and insomnia can lead to many health problems, including mental and cognitive dysfunction (memory, concentration), depression of your immune system, increased risk for heart disease, high blood pressure, diabetes, stroke, psychological problems, and even weight gain. A recent study revealed that chronic insomnia triples the risk of death. It also hampers recovery from major illness or injury. Surveys show that almost one-third of adults seeing their PCPs suffer from insomnia.

Dr. A's Suggestions:
Segmented Sleep: Not Insomnia

As we get older, we require as much sleep as when we were young, but we may not sleep as soundly or for as long a duration. Thirty-four percent of people report waking up several times at night. Many people fall asleep easily but wake up in the middle of the night.

This may not be abnormal and may be a common sleep pattern. In fact, many languages have names for "first sleep" and "second sleep." If this occurs, reading a book, having sex, or just talking to someone for a half hour can help you fall asleep again.

Sleep problems can vary significantly. They can be transient or long-lasting; you may have trouble falling asleep, staying asleep, or both. You may fall asleep easily but wake up and be unable to fall back asleep. You may have intermittent sleep problems. Whatever your pattern, lack of sleep can make you feel tired and impair your thinking and working, in addition to the physical and mental problems mentioned above.

How much sleep do you need? Basically, when you feel refreshed and alert the next day, you've had adequate sleep. It varies from person to person, but on average, seven to nine hours is recommended for the best health. Thirty-nine percent of Americans do not obtain this amount of sleep. Of those who do obtain adequate sleep, 74 percent still may experience sleep *problems* that affect the quality of their sleep.

Consider Sleep Apnea

Ten percent of people have a disorder called obstructive sleep apnea*, a condition in which your airway is obstructed at night, resulting in periods when you don't breathe fully (apnea or hypopnea) and your oxygen level decreases. With this condition, you can stop breathing for a period of ten seconds to a minute, and this can occur multiple times per night. Sleep apnea can prevent you from getting a full night's sleep or restful sleep and can cause excessive daytime sleepiness. Many people who have sleep apnea may snore, but not everyone who snores has sleep apnea.

Sleep apnea alone has been linked to heart attacks, strokes, hypertension, diabetes, depression, and many other diseases. In 2012, a study showed that cancer patients with untreated sleep apnea have up to a fivefold increase in the risk of death.

A major cause of sleep apnea is being overweight, but even normal-weight people can have it. If you snore, wake up gasping for air, have twitching/jerking at night, have excessive daytime sleepiness, don't feel you are obtaining "restful" sleep, or someone has witnessed you not breathing for short periods of time while asleep, you should see a sleep specialist and be evaluated for sleep apnea.

Also note that polysomnography (sleep study in a lab) is the gold standard for diagnosing sleep apnea. An alternative is a portable monitor ("home" study), but a 2014 study showed that these do not measure all the relevant parameters and cannot distinguish between types of sleep apnea. Nevertheless, many insurance companies will only reimburse the home study but if it is abnormal, a formal sleep study will still be necessary.

Note: There are other causes of sleep apnea, but *obstructive* sleep apnea is by far the most frequent. Polysomnography will diagnose all types of sleep apnea.

Treatments for Insomnia

The Preventive Approaches

Psychological factors, especially anxiety, tension, and depression, are often the cause of insomnia; so these need to be addressed if you have them (see sections on *Depression* or *Anxiety* for further treatment recommendations).

Physical conditions can also cause insomnia, so they need to be properly addressed and controlled. These include pain, heartburn, breathing disorders, hot flashes, diabetes, acid reflux, ulcers, Parkinson's disease, kidney disease, restless legs syndrome, hyperthyroidism, stress, excessive caffeine, irregular sleeping patterns (naps), alcohol, and drugs.

Many **medications** that commonly cause insomnia include alcohol, beta-blockers, caffeine, some antidepressants, decongestants (some cold, asthma, and allergy medications), drugs for digestive disorders, and thyroid medications. If you are on any of these drugs, consult your doctor about changing to another drug that may not cause insomnia or whether taking them at a different time will avert the insomnia.

Diet: Carbohydrates at dinner can drop blood sugar, making insomnia worse. You should eat a combination of protein, fat, and fiber. If eating fish, you should increase your fat; and if you eat beef or chicken, you can have a little starch but not much. You want to avoid a heavy meal before sleep but there are certain snacks that have been research supported to help improve your ability to fall asleep and stay asleep, as noted in the chart below.

Bedtime Snacks That May Help Promote Better Sleep

Hummus and Veggies   Cherry and Pistachio Rice Pudding
Rice   Popcorn; spiced or parmesan cheese
Ham and Cheese   Cherries or Tart Cherry Juice
Banana Smoothie   Sweet potato fries
Walnuts, Almonds or Brazil nuts   Crackers and peanut butter
Ginger Tea With Dried Dates   Banana with nuts
Kale chips   Applesauce with Cinnamon and Raisins
Cereal and milk   Yogurt with Berries
Whole Grain Toast with Almond Butter
Oatmeal with Bananas and Almond Butter

Moderate exercise, both aerobic and resistance, can help you sleep better, but timing is important. A recent study showed that women who take a brisk, half-hour morning walk improved their ability to fall asleep by 70 percent. Afternoon exercise also helps sleep, but exercise within three hours of sleep can cause more insomnia.

There are several other **lifestyle suggestions** that may help you sleep better, which include:

- Start slowing down an hour before bed.
- Limit the time you spend in bed not sleeping or for sex
- Avoid watching TV or using electronic devices (computers, smart phones, ebooks, and so on). These emit blue wavelength light, which can cause more insomnia than other artificial light.
  - Red or green light is the best to use before bed.
- If you want light, use 40 watt bulbs. Higher wattage stimulates the pineal gland, which keeps you awake.
- Don't substitute a nap for a good night's sleep. If you nap, limit it to between half an hour and an hour.
- Limit your intake of caffeine-containing foods and beverages; don't drink coffee after 2:00 p.m.

- Limit alcohol, which can help you fall asleep but can cause you to wake up in the middle of the night.
- Think warmth, such as keeping your extremities warm with socks or mittens.
- Don't smoke for at least two hours before bedtime.
- Face your alarm clock away from the bed.
- Even small light sources, such as LED alarm clocks, can prevent sleep; the darker the better.
- Maintain a regular sleep schedule seven days a week. Set a regular time to go to bed and get up, even on weekends.
- Use a jasmine scent (potpourri or a single spritz)

Dr. A's Suggestions:
Do Expensive Beds and Mattresses Help?

You might be familiar with ads on television, radio, and in magazines that advertise mattresses and sleeping "systems" that can help you sleep at night. Most of these cost $1,500 or more. There have been no studies that show these beds and mattresses help you sleep, and many people actually sleep better on mats on the floor. If you do buy an expensive sleep system or mattress, be sure you can return it within thirty days if it doesn't help.

Snoring: New Approach May Be Beneficial

Oropharyngeal exercises strengthen the muscles of the throat and have been used in sleep apnea (see below). Researchers in Brazil tested whether snoring also could be decreased by doing these exercises (done for 8 minutes three times a day). The results of their 2015 study in *Chest* revealed that both the number of snores per hour and a composite measure of loudness of snoring decreased by about 50 percent in those practicing the oropharyngeal exercises. They can be taught to you by a speech therapist.

The Conventional Approaches
A **sleep medicine specialist** is highly recommended if you suffer from chronic insomnia or if intermittent insomnia interferes with your quality of life or daily functioning.

Since insomnia may be the result of a variety of causes and every person may respond differently to various therapies, such a specialist can both diagnose and treat insomnia more appropriately and more successfully, saving you time and money in the long term.

Medications are the primary conventional treatment for insomnia. Several prescription medications may be effective, including *benzodiazepines* (Halcion, Valium, Dalmane), but because they do not metabolize as quickly as we age, they can make you drowsy the next day.

Nonbenzodiazepine sleeping pills (called "Z" *drugs*) like zolpidem (Ambien), eszopiclone (Lunesta), and rozerem (Sonata) are better tolerated and don't often cause hangover. Rozerem works by mimicking the actions of melatonin. These have become very popular in the past few years and are the most commonly prescribed sleep aids. However, zolpidem and eszoplicone should be used only when you expect to sleep for eight hours. Rozerem has a shorter duration of action (four hours) and can be taken if you wake up in the middle of the night. These drugs are expensive, but zolpidem and eszoplicone can be purchased as a generic. A newer drug, zolpidem tartrate (Intermezzo), is the first one to be approved for those waking in the middle of the night and having trouble falling back to sleep. It is expensive (two to three dollars per pill), and you should not take it only if you have less than four hours of sleep time left.

Warning: In 2007, the FDA issued risk warnings regarding Z drugs. These include sleep-driving, sleep-eating (including binge eating), and making phone calls without realizing it. In fact, the recommended dose of zolpidem was reduced from 10 mg to 5 mg as a result of this problem. Allergic reactions and facial swelling can also occur. It can also impair balance and thinking if you awake during the night. It is advised that you should hide your car keys or unplug the phone if you do this.

Z Drugs May Help, but Effect Is Small

Z drugs such as Ambien, Sonata, and Lunesta are the most common drugs used for insomnia. In a recent meta-analysis, however, these drugs were associated with only slight improvements in sleep latency (how much time it takes to fall asleep).

Compared to placebo, Z drugs decreased the amount of time to fall asleep by an average of twenty-two minutes. The subjective time (the person's perception) of falling asleep was only seven minutes. Larger doses were associated with greater improvements but also greater side effects, such as drowsiness. Furthermore, the placebo response accounted for about half of the drug response; so often, psychological aspects are involved.

A drug approved in August 2014 is *suvorexant* (Belsomra), which works differently than the above drugs by altering the signals of neurotransmitters responsible for regulating the sleep-wake cycle. In the studies, however, total sleep time was improved only by eleven to twenty-two minutes. **Caution**: This is a class IV controlled substance, and next-morning drowsiness and activities while still asleep are common, so start at the lowest dose.

Some doctors prescribe *sedating antidepressants*, and some patients do respond to these. The most common are trazadone and doxepin. Remeron is an antidepressant that appears to reduce insomnia as well. Rozerem is another sleep medication that works by mimicking the actions of melatonin (see "Alternative Treatments" below).

Another common and inexpensive drug is *diphenhydramine* (Benadryl), which is commonly used for allergies. Its major side effect, however, is drowsiness; so many older people sleep well without after-effects. Dosage is usually 25 to 50 mg at bedtime. Seroquel, an antipsychotic drug, has been used off-label as a low dose (25 mg) for insomnia and can work quite well.

Warning: All insomnia drugs in the long term can cause abnormal sleep patterns and dependence. It is not advised to take prescription sleep medications for more than fourteen days at a time, although it is commonly done.

Important Information:
Sleeping Pills Associated with Increased Risk of Death

A February 2012 study in the journal *BMJ Open* revealed that people who take sleeping pills are four times more likely to die than those who don't take them. The pills also raise the risk for certain cancers, including esophageal, lymphoma, lung, colon, and prostate. Other cancers were not increased. Those who took up to 18 doses per year were 3.6 times more likely to die, between 18 and 132 doses more than four times, and over 132 doses five times the risk. This was an observational study and cause and effect cannot be determined.

However, another 2014 study in *BMJ* showed that Z drugs and benzodiazepines were associated with increased risk for death and were dose-dependent (the higher the dose, the higher the risk). It is better to try other methods first or at least take sleeping pills only when you really need them.

Cognitive/behavioral therapy may be helpful whether or not psychological issues underlie your insomnia. This type of therapy attempts to change your behavior as well as altering the way you think. A study in 2011 published in the *Archives of Internal Medicine* showed that just two hours of counseling by a nurse without specialized sleep training helped 55 percent of patients resolve their insomnia. The intervention focused on four goals:

1) Reducing amount of time in bed
2) Getting up at the same time every day
3) Going to bed only when sleepy
4) Staying in bed only when asleep.

For sleep apnea

Most patients are placed on a **CPAP** machine, which is attached to a mask or nasal tube. Some patients do not respond to CPAP and need other types of machines, either BiPaP or ASV (Adapto-Servo-Ventilation). In addition, some people cannot tolerate the full face masks, but there are numerous types, as well as nasal masks and nasal pillows that may work.

If you can't tolerate these machines, there is alternative equipment that can be helpful, although not as effective. There are numerous devices designed to pull the tongue and jaw forward, but most are unreliable and also not well tolerated for the most part. The **Mandibular Advancement Device** is probably the best tolerated and works almost as well as CPAP.

The FDA approved a **neurostimulator implant** in 2014 in patients with moderate to severe sleep apnea (greater than 20 apnea episodes per hour) who cannot tolerate CPAP. This implant, called Inspire Upper Airway Stimulator, contracts upper airway muscles to pull the base of the tongue forward. Side effects include tongue weakness, dry mouth, pain, and numbness. In the approval study, more than half of all patients experienced at least a 50% reduction in apnea episodes and also experienced at least a 25% reduction in oxygen desaturation index.

A new technique developed in Brazil involves **oropharyngeal exercises**, taught by speech therapists, which can lead to better objective and subjective outcomes in sleep apnea. A 2009 study showed that these exercises may reduce sleep apnea episodes up to 50 percent.

Finally, **surgery** can be done for sleep apnea if there is significant obstruction, but outcomes are generally poor. There are several types of surgery, so be sure to evaluate the types and their published outcomes.

The Alternative Approaches

A recent study showed that **listening to soft music** can help older people sleep better, so it's worth a try.

Because stress and tension are major factors in insomnia, **meditation** and **imagery** are very beneficial, whether done during the waking hours or at bedtime. I recommend listening to a meditation tape specifically designed for sleep when you go to bed.

Interactive imagery (active imagination) is very beneficial and may take only a few sessions to correct the problem if psychological issues are the cause of your insomnia. Interactive imagery is a mind-body method in which you mentally interact with images that represent your emotions. It is a powerful method to uncover and deal with subconscious psychological issues you may not be aware of (see chapter 4 for more information).

Tai chi and **qigong** are also very useful for combating insomnia. A recent study from UCLA showed that older people with moderate sleep complaints reported better sleep and daytime functioning (less drowsiness) after twenty-five weeks (six months) of tai chi.

There are several **nutritional supplements** that may be quite beneficial for insomnia:

- *Valerian* (up to 400 mg per night) may be effective for both insomnia and anxiety that is keeping you up or waking you at night, or if you have lots of thoughts on your mind. ***Caution***: May cause vivid dreams in some people.
- *5-HTP* (100–300 mg per night) can also help if you have depression that is keeping you awake, or if you have anxiety with your depression.
- *Melatonin* is effective for insomnia primarily when body melatonin levels are low. It affects circadian rhythms (sleep/wake cycle) and promotes drowsiness. Quick-release melatonin can help you fall asleep faster, and slow release may benefit those who wake up after a few hours of sleep. ***Important note***: Effective dosages vary widely and are specific to each person. Too much or too little can cause more insomnia or simply not work. Start with 0.5 mg daily for a few days and then increase every few days by 0.5 mg. When you find the "right dose for you," you'll know, because it'll work very well.
- *GABA* is often decreased in people with insomnia, and some of the above medications work by improving GABA binding in the brain. However, it cannot get into the brain as a compound and thus is probably ineffective. However, one form, Kavinace, appears to get into the brain. ***Caution***: Start slowly and work up to an ideal dose as it can make you sleepy in the morning if you take too much.

- *Ashwaghanda*, up to 1 gram, is an ayurvedic herb that is used as a tonic but also may help sleep in some people.
- Many alternative products contain a *combination of herbs*. A study in 2011 showed that a combination of melatonin (5 mg), zinc (11.25 mg), and magnesium (225 mg) was safe and effective for not only insomnia but also QOL and depression.
- *Calcium/magnesium* can help with relaxation of muscles and help with inducing sleep.
- You can combine any of these herbs with *Passiflora* (passionflower; 6–8 ml of the tincture, tea, or capsules). Other common herbs found in formulas include chamomile, skullcap, lemon balm, and hops, all of which have relaxing effects.
- ***Caution***: If you use supplements for other conditions, make sure they are not excitatory compounds, which can cause insomnia. Examples include phosphatidylcholine, ginseng, and B vitamins.

Chinese herbal formulas containing Schizandra fruit can be very effective as well. Formulations that can be helpful include *Ding Xin Wan and Chai Hu Mu Li Long Gu Tang. An Mian Pien* ("peaceful sleep tablets") works like OTC sleep aids but can be used long-term in certain syndromes. You should notice improvement within three days to a week, but you may need to take them longer for complete benefit.

Certain styles of **acupuncture** can address both the insomnia and underlying factors. At my clinic, we developed a specific protocol of acupuncture that can also significantly reduce sleep apnea symptoms as well as insomnia. There are auricular (ear points) that are specific for insomnia, and tacks placed in these insomnia points can be very effective.

Sleep restriction therapy may help some people. The idea is to shorten your sleep time initially to about five hours and then gradually go to bed earlier and sleep later. A study at Duke University showed that this reduced wakefulness at night by more than half.

Foot soaking may help many people. Soak your feet in water as hot as you can stand; then put socks on and go immediately to bed.

Essential oils in a diffuser can also help with sleep. There are many different oils that may be beneficial, and many companies have combinations. However, make sure you get a diffuser that is not loud! Jasmine appears to be one of the most beneficial for sleep.

There are several **apps** that you can find on the Internet and download to your cellphone that may help you fall asleep.

Dr. A's Suggestion
Counting Sleep: Does It Work?

The old method of **counting sheep actually** has been shown to worsen insomnia in many people, so avoid it. However, studies have shown that many people can get to sleep more easily by reciting in your mind favorite song lyrics or the plot of a favorite book.

Your Empowered Patient Action Plan for
Treating Insomnia and Sleep Apnea.

Step #1: *Undergo sleep studies* if you have the symptoms of sleep apnea listed above. If abnormal, use CPAP or other machines to treat the condition.

Step #2: *Use lifestyle changes* to improve sleep patterns naturally. This is your best course—and the least expensive.

Step #3: *Play soft music and/or use meditation/imagery CDs or apps* to help you sleep.

Step #4: *Undergo interactive imagery or cognitive therapy* if underlying psychological issues (anxiety/depression) may be causing your insomnia.

Step #5: *Practice qigong/tai chi* to help you sleep better and improve daytime functioning.

Step #6: *Undergo acupuncture* for long term benefit if you still have insomnia.

Edna had trouble falling asleep at night. She had tried various herbal remedies as well as prescription drugs, but they were either not effective or made her too drowsy the next day. I placed ear seeds in the two insomnia points in her ear, which remained in her ear for two weeks. She reported no problem falling or staying asleep during that time and only had occasional insomnia when the seeds eventually fell out.

Step #7: *Take Chinese herbal remedies* if you still have insomnia.

Step #8: *Take valerian or 5-HTP, with or without passionflower,* if the above steps have still not helped.

Step #9: ***Take melatonin*** if you are still having trouble sleeping. Start with a low dose and increase every few days until it is beneficial. Combine it with zinc and magnesium if the melatonin alone is not effective.

Step #10: ***Take prescription sleep-aid medications*** if nothing else has helped. Start with OTC or generics first. I prefer the previous steps first because these drugs may have side effects and can cause dependency.

Step #11: ***Consult with a sleep specialist*** if the above steps have not been effective, especially if your insomnia continues to interfere with your daily functioning.

Expected Outcome

Insomnia can be a significant problem at all ages. By investigating the underlying causes and using the above methods, however, most people can conquer their insomnia.

Irritable Bowel Syndrome (IBS)

What You Need to Know

Irritable bowel syndrome is a disorder affecting the intestines, in which peristalsis (wavelike movements that move food) becomes irregular and uncoordinated. It is the most common of all digestive disorders. Studies show that IBS involves dysfunction of feedback loops and chemical substances in both the intestines and the brain.

Psychological factors can cause or complicate IBS in a significant number of cases and must be addressed as well.

Food sensitivities (not allergies) may also play a role in some patients with IBS. One study of two hundred patients found that roughly half of them were sensitive to one or more foods. Other studies have demonstrated that approximately one-third of people with IBS are sensitive to certain foods. The most common problematic foods include dairy and grains. Because most people with IBS suffer from food sensitivities rather than true allergies, many allergy tests may be inconclusive.

Treatments for IBS

The Preventive Approaches

Diet: As food sensitivities may affect your symptoms, a one-week elimination diet may be necessary to determine which foods may be causative factors. It's important for patients with IBS to keep a food diary to record the elimination diet. Dairy products are often the cause of IBS symptoms; so eliminate them for a week or two to see if that has any effect. Some patients with diarrhea-prominent IBS can respond to a gluten-free diet.

Although only helping a minority of patients, increasing soluble dietary fiber may help control the symptoms of IBS, so increase intake of fruits and vegetables. Foods high in refined sugar and fats also can contribute to IBS, and you should avoid or decrease them.

In a randomized trial, IBS symptoms improved with a diet *low* in short-chain carbohydrates known as FODMAPs (fermentable, oligo-, di-, monosaccharides, and polyols), which include fructose, lactose, and polyol sweeteners. In fact, a 2014 study in *Gastroenterology* showed that FODMAPs deficiency may be a cause of IBS.

Exercising at an aerobic pace for twenty to thirty minutes has been shown to help reduce symptoms.

The Conventional Approaches

Medications are the primary treatment from conventional medicine but are highly ineffective in most cases. Drugs such as *hyocyamine* (Levsin) or *dicyclomine* (Bentyl) are the most common and may offer temporary relief at best.

For IBS with diarrhea, loperamide (Imodium) is often prescribed for symptomatic relief. Another drug called *alosetron* (Lotronex) was found to be effective for IBS, but due to several deaths and adverse gastrointestinal side effects, it was withdrawn from the market by the FDA. *Caution*: It has now been reapproved for IBS with severe diarrhea, but only under strict regulations, and it can only be prescribed by approved physicians.

More recently, a drug-company study published in the *NEJM* showed that an antibiotic, *rifaximin*, ameliorates diarrheal symptoms of IBS after a two-week course in 41 percent of patients (but only 10 percent more than placebo). It may increase bacterial resistance, and long-term safety and efficacy are unknown.

For IBS with constipation, linoclotide (Linzess) has been shown to be better than placebo. *Tegaserod* (Zelnorm) is a medication for women with IBS who have constipation, but it only helps a small percentage and also has a large array of side effects. *Caution*: It was also taken off the market and then restored with warnings of increased risk for heart attack, stroke, and angina. It also has numerous potential side effects.

A newly approved drug for IBS with constipation is *lubiprostone* (Amitiza), which was previously used only for non-IBS constipation and works by drawing more fluid into the colon. However, this drug is approved only for women and not for men or children. It also has many side effects, including nausea, heartburn, and breathing problems, and may not work in the majority of patients.

Buspar, an antianxiety medication, can also be helpful for some people if anxiety increases symptoms.

The Alternative Approaches

Acupuncture is one of the best treatments for IBS as it may eliminate the symptoms of IBS for long periods of time—or even permanently. You should notice improvement within six acupuncture treatments but might need additional sessions for maximum benefit.

Several **Chinese herbal formulas** are excellent for controlling IBS symptoms—much better than drugs. I recommend the formula *Bo He Wan*, but there are several others that are beneficial, such as *Mu Xiang Shun Qi Wan*. *Shi Jun Zi Tang* and *Ba Zhen Tang* are beneficial, depending on your particular Chinese diagnostic syndrome. You should usually notice improvement within a few days or up to a week.

Hypnosis or ***Interactive imagery*** (*active imagination*) may be effective if your IBS has an underlying psychological component that needs to be unearthed and resolved. However, even in patients without psychological factors, these methods can help. The mechanism of action for hypnosis is unknown, but some studies report a 96 percent success rate in reducing or resolving IBS symptoms in as few as one or two sessions.

Interactive imagery is a mind-body method in which you mentally interact with images that represent your emotions. It is a powerful method to uncover and deal with subconscious psychological issues you may not be aware of. Often, it only takes a few sessions for resolution of IBS (see chapter 4 for detailed discussion).

A 2014 published in the *American Journal of Gastroenterology* revealed that an eight-week course in **mindfulness meditation**-based stress reduction significantly reduced the severity of IBS as measured six and twelve months later.

Probiotics and **digestive enzymes** are also commonly utilized. A 2014 study showed that certain probiotics can improve symptoms in 68 percent of patients. Probiotics consist of live cultures of organisms (the "good" bacteria) that help digest and excrete food properly (see chapter 2 for an in-depth discussion). There are many different species. In the above study, *Bifidobacterium lactis*, *Lactobacillus rhamnosus*, and *Streptococcus thermophiles* were the beneficial ones. *B. infantis* was found to be beneficial in another study.

Yogurt, although it contains some beneficial microorganisms, is not a good substitute for probiotics, although several OTC yogurt products (e.g., Dan Active, Activia, Align) have been shown to help some women with IBS constipation. You should notice improvement within one to three weeks. You may have increased gas or bloating initially and should reduce your dosage if this occurs.

The dysfunction of your colon may be caused or made worse because of toxins, chemicals, and old fecal matter that have been retained. **Detoxification** of the colon, using herbal supplements to remove these substances and soothe your colon, is commonly prescribed by CAM providers. Such products should contain some or all of the following: apple pectin, slippery elm bark, marshmallow root, licorice root, fennel seed, activated willow charcoal, and montmorillonite clay.

There are also several **supplements and herbs** that may help control IBS symptoms. *Enteric-coated peppermint* oil (0.2–0.4 ml twice a day or one to two capsules three times daily for three weeks) or *flaxseed* (1 Tbsp daily, freshly ground), can help bulk up your stool and reduce diarrhea. There is also a *five-herb formula* consisting of chamomile flower, peppermint leaf, caraway fruit, licorice root, and lemon balm leaves. (This formula is a modification of *Iberogast*, an herbal preparation now available in health food stores.) You should notice improvement within one to three months using these herbs.

The **NAET** may be of help if food sensitivities are a cause of your symptoms. It combines acupuncture, kinesiology, chiropractic, herbs, and nutrition to desensitize you to foods. It may take several months for its effectiveness to be observed, depending on how many allergens are sensitizing you (see Chapter 4 for more information).

There are also **homeopathic remedies**, such as *mercurius vivus* and *nux vomica*, which can help control symptoms. You should consult a qualified homeopathist for guidance on which remedies will be most beneficial and for proper dosages. You should notice improvement within one to two months.

Your Empowered Patient Action Guide for Treating IBS

Step #1: Take the Chinese herbal remedies Bo He Wan or Mu Xiang Shun Qi Wan to temporarily control your symptoms while undergoing the following steps.

Step #2: Undergo hypnosis, which may be the best treatment for resolving IBS.

Step #3: Undergo acupuncture to resolve your IBS long-term if hypnosis is not effective.

Step #4: Undergo interactive imagery if the above steps have not been beneficial.

Step #5: Detoxify your colon and then take probiotics to regulate your intestines as well as control symptoms of diarrhea or constipation.

Step #6: Undergo the NAET if the above steps have not been effective and/or you have detected food sensitivities after undergoing an elimination diet.

Step #7: Take enteric-coated peppermint oil, flaxseed, or five-herb formula if you still have symptoms.

Step #8: Try homeopathy is the above steps have not been effective.

Step #9: Take conventional medications to control symptoms if nothing else has worked. This is the last step due to the side effects and poor effectiveness for most people.

Suzanne is a thirty-four-year-old patient of mine who had had irritable bowel syndrome since fourth grade. She always had to be near a bathroom due to sudden cramping and diarrhea. Over the years, doctors had tried her on various conventional medications, but none ever worked very well. I started her on the Chinese herbal formula Bo He Wan, which eliminated most of her symptoms. However, every time she tried to discontinue the Chinese herbs, her symptoms would reoccur. At that point I began acupuncture and also interactive imagery. The imagery revealed that in fourth grade, another student stayed home a lot because of sickness (nausea and vomiting), and Suzanne began doing the same. Her parents also divorced, which caused many repressed negative feelings, which all came out during the imagery sessions. Within two months, her symptoms went away completely and have not returned.

<hr />

Expected Outcome

Most people should be able to resolve IBS long-term using the alternative methods listed, or at least control symptoms enough to have a good quality of life.

Chronic Kidney Disease (CKD)

What You Need to Know

The kidneys filter the blood and dispose of wastes and excess fluid as urine. The kidneys have many functions, including regulating the "acid-base" balance of the body and electrolytes such as sodium and potassium.

Beginning in our midforties, most of us experience a decline in kidney function, although they continue to function adequately under ordinary circumstances. Blood flow to the kidneys decreases by as much as 10 percent per decade and can be decreased by nearly half that of younger people in those who are age eighty or older. As we age, the kidneys lose one-quarter to one-third of their mass as both the number and size of nephrons (filtering units) decreases. By age eighty, the total number falls by 30–40 percent, and another 30 percent may become sclerotic (scarred) and nonfunctional. These changes reduce the rate at which the blood is filtered by the kidneys.

In addition, the regulation of hormones that respond to dehydration and the ability to conserve salt can decline with age. These changes make older adults particularly vulnerable to dehydration. As a result of these physiologic changes, the kidneys become less efficient in concentrating urine and eliminating solutes from the blood stream.

<hr />

Dr. A's Suggestions:
CKD Often Overdiagnosed in Older People

The definition of CKD is based on a test called estimated glomerular filtration rate (eGFR), which basically measures the amount of fluid going through your kidneys. Using this method, 14 percent of Americans meet criteria for CKD, defined as an eGFR under 60 ml/min.

This definition does not account for age. In an article from *BMJ*, the authors noted that most people meeting that criteria are over the age of sixty-five, yet those eGFRs may be considered normal for that age. The harm is that people are often aggressively treated, especially for their blood pressure, unnecessarily.

Make sure to ask your doctor what a normal eGFR is *for your age*: if you have no other risk factors for kidney disease, treatment may not be necessary.

For the most part, kidney function is well preserved during aging, although it may be slower. Most changes do not cause significant problems, but they do leave the kidney vulnerable to illness or medications that can depress kidney function and lead to acute or chronic kidney failure. Because CKD may have no symptoms until it is severe, it is important to identify kidney problems at their earliest stages to avoid complications.

At present, 1 out of every 7 adults is affected by CKD and mortality has doubled in the past 20 years. As the population of the U.S. ages, it is predicted that almost half of individuals 30 to 64 years old may likely be affected. So it is important to check kidney function so disease can be prevented or treated appropriately at an early stage.

Be Cautious With Certain Medical Compounds for Testing If You Have CKD

Before you undergo colonoscopy, you may be prescribed sodium phosphate to clean out your colon. This compound has been found to decrease kidney function and should be avoided, even if your kidney function is only minimally impaired.

When undergoing certain tests, such as CT and MRI, contrast material (especially gadolinium) may be injected to improve the diagnosis. Older iodine preps as well as gadolinium may cause further damage to diseased kidneys. This may be prevented by taking N-acetylcysteine prior to the test, but you may need to undergo the test without contrast or undergo a different test.

It is also important to realize that CKD can cause many other conditions, including anemia, osteoporosis, hypertension, increased blood phosphate, elevated lipids, and premature heart disease. Thus, it is important to have CKD diagnosed (using simple blood and urine tests), yet fully one-third of all people with CKD are not diagnosed by their doctors. In fact, a study in *JAMA* revealed that 5.5 percent of women and 11.6 percent of men are not aware of having moderately severe CKD.

Beware of Drug Dosages as You Age

Medication dosages often need to be reduced in the elderly because the reduction in kidney function can affect clearance of some drugs and lead to toxicity or adverse effects. Drugs that are toxic to the kidneys should be used cautiously in older adults.

Beware of Lowering Blood Pressure Too Much in CKD

Optimal blood pressure control is very important in CKD. Generally, doctors try to decrease both systolic and diastolic pressures (the upper and lower numbers), but a 2013 study in the *NEJM* showed that lowering the diastolic below 70 mm increased death significantly.

You should aim for a blood pressure of 130–140/80–90, which shows the lowest mortality rate in this study (see below under "Conventional Treatments").

Treatments for CKD

The Preventive Approaches
Correctable causes: Diabetes and hypertension are responsible for the bulk of CDK, accounting for one-half and one-quarter respectively. For this reason, it is important to control those conditions if you have them (See sections on *Hypertension* and *Diabetes*). It is recommended to keep your blood pressure at or below 130/80 mm Hg if you have kidney disease. It is often useful to monitor blood pressure at home using an automated monitor.

You should also **stop smoking** because smoking can cause narrowing of your kidney arteries and increases the risk of CKD. Being overweight can also be a factor in CKD, so **losing weight** is important.

Several **medications** can be toxic to the kidneys and may need to be avoided or given in adjusted doses. These include some OTC medications, such as:

- Certain *analgesics* such as aspirin; NSAIDs such as ibuprofen.
- Fleets or phosphosoda *enemas* because of their high phosphorus content.
- *Laxatives* and *antacids* containing magnesium and aluminum, such as milk of magnesia and Mylanta.
- *Ulcer medications*: H2-receptor antagonists cimetidine (Tagamet) and ranitidine (Zantac). Decrease dosage with kidney disease.
- *Decongestants* like pseudoephedrine (Sudafed), especially if you have high blood pressure.
- *Metformin* (for diabetes) is contraindicated in CDK due to an increased risk of lactic acidosis. It increases mortality in those with advanced CDK.
- *Alka Seltzer*, as this contains a lot of salt.
- *Herbal medications*: many may be hazardous to kidneys, and you should check with a certified herbalist.
- *Proton Pump Inhibitors (PPI's)* have been shown in a 2016 observational study to increase the risk for developing chronic kidney disease by 20-50 percent.

Diet: There are several important dietary rules you can follow to help slow the progression of your kidney disease and decrease the likelihood of complications. However, this can be quite complex and must be individualized, generally with the help of your health care provider and a registered dietitian. The following are general dietary guidelines:

- *Protein restriction*: Decreasing protein intake may slow the progression of CKD. A dietitian can help you determine the appropriate amount of protein for you.
- *Salt restriction*: Limit to 4–6 grams per day to avoid fluid retention and help control high blood pressure.
- *Fluid intake*: Excessive water intake does not help prevent CKD. In fact, your doctor may recommend restriction of water intake. At the same time, you don't want to get dehydrated, either (see chapter 2 on regulating water intake).
- *Potassium restriction*: This is necessary in advanced CKD because the kidneys are unable to remove potassium. High levels of potassium can cause abnormal heart rhythms. Examples of foods high in potassium include bananas, oranges, nuts, and potatoes.
- *Phosphorus restriction*: Decreasing phosphorus intake is recommended to protect bones. Eggs, beans, cola drinks, and dairy products are examples of foods high in phosphorus.

- *Vegetarian protein sources* are better than meat sources.
- *Alkali supplementation*: Because CKD patients have a tendency to retain increased acid, sources of alkali can be helpful, primarily fruits and vegetables. However, again you should be careful of elevated potassium blood levels.

The Conventional Approaches

Medications are the main conventional treatment for CKD. I already mentioned that you should control diabetes and hypertension, which slows progression of chronic kidney disease. Blood pressure medications known as *angiotensin converting enzyme inhibitors (ACEi)* with *calcium channel blockers* have the most benefit in CKD. If you have albumin in your urine, blood pressure should be at or lower than 130/80; with no albumin, it should be at or lower than 140/90. *Important note*: Combination of ACE inhibitors *with* ARBs (another class of blood pressure medication) is not recommended, although ARBs alone can be beneficial (see section on *Hypertension* for further information).

If you have fluid retention (swelling in your ankles especially), *diuretics* remove excess water from the body. However, these drugs are not suitable for all patients, and you should check with your doctor. *Caution*: They can also decrease your potassium levels.

Some patients with CKD develop elevated phosphate levels in their blood, which is associated with increased death from heart problems. It is usually treated or prevented with medications called *phosphate binders*. There are two forms: calcium-based and non-calcium-based binders. A recent meta-analysis showed that those who receive non-calcium-based binders have a 22 percent lower risk for death than calcium-based.

If you have anemia, *erythropoiesis stimulating agents* (ESAs) may be used, replacing the deficiency of erythropoietin, which is normally produced by healthy kidneys and promotes the production of red blood cells. Often, patients treated with such drugs must take iron by mouth or sometimes even intravenously. *Warning*: ESAs can significantly increase the risk of cardiovascular events and death when given above a hemoglobin level of 11 g/dl. The smallest dose needed to avoid transfusions should be used.

Acidosis—too much acid—may develop with kidney disease, which in turn can cause breakdown of proteins, inflammation, and bone disease. If the acidosis is significant, *sodium bicarbonate* (baking soda) may correct the problem

Dialysis is instituted if kidney function continues to deteriorate and the kidneys fail. If you don't have significant symptoms, dialysis is usually instituted when the GFR (glomerular filtration rate) falls to the range of 5–7 ml/min; if you have symptoms, it may need to be instituted earlier.

Dialysis is a method of removing toxic substances (impurities or wastes) from the blood when the kidneys are unable to do so. It can be performed using several different methods. Peritoneal dialysis is done through the abdomen and can be done at home, but it must be done every day. Hemodialysis works by circulating the blood through special filters outside the body. Blood is diverted from an access point in the body to a dialysis machine where the blood flows across a filter, along with solutions that help remove toxins. The chemical imbalances and impurities of the blood are corrected, and the blood is then returned to the body. Typically, most patients undergo hemodialysis for three sessions every week. Each session lasts three to four hours.

Delayed Initiation of Dialysis Better

There has been a trend toward early initiation of dialysis for patients with chronic renal failure, based on a specific eGFR (the rate at which your kidneys circulate blood) cutoff. A study published in *CMAJ* in 2011 revealed that starting dialysis with eGFRs greater than 10.5 ml/min increased mortality and should not be used in patients without symptoms.

It should also be noted that the rates of dialysis in the very elderly (over eighty) has steadily increased in the last ten years, despite the fact that the survival rate is only about 54 percent. Before instituting dialysis, estimates of survival and expected QOL should be considered.

If all else fails, **kidney transplant surgery** can be done and generally requires four to seven days in the hospital. All transplant recipients require lifelong immunosuppressant medications to prevent their bodies from rejecting the new kidney. Immunosuppressant medications require careful monitoring of blood levels and increase the risk of infection as well as some types of cancer. Transplants are successful in the majority of patients, but some transplant kidneys can be rejected. A recent study revealed that overall rejection occurs more often from female *donors*, and transplants of male kidneys into females have an increased risk for failure. However, female *recipients* from both sexes have fewer failures.

Beware of Vitamin D

Because CKD causes bone loss, vitamin D compounds are routinely prescribed by doctors for CKD patients. However, a recent study in the *Annals of Internal Medicine* reveals that it is costly, provides no proven benefit, and has the potential to be harmful.

The Alternative Approaches

Acupuncture is the best CAM method for CKD, but it is most effective if used early in the course. Acupuncture can address several complications of kidney disease, including high blood pressure, swelling, and increased protein leakage. You should observe benefits within six to eight treatments, although maintenance treatments are usually required.

A **Chinese herbal formula** called *Jin Gui Shen Qi Wan* is used frequently in kidney disease. *Cordyceps sinensis*, another Chinese herb, may improve anemia but should be used within a formula.

There are several **nutritional supplements** that also may be of benefit. These include:

- *Astragalus* (Chinese) increases kidney blood flow and can protect the kidney from further damage, but it is usually used within a formula.
- *Baking soda* can slow progression to end-stage kidney disease and improve the eGFR.
- *Curcumin* may improve kidney function.
- *Melatonin* can decrease protein in the urine and increase eGFR, as well as having beneficial effects on blood pressure.
- *Omega-3 fatty acids* (fish oil) can reduce protein in the urine and improves survival in CKD.
- *Buchu tea, dandelion, cranberry, uva ursi,* and *hydrangea* are diuretics, and these may be useful to prevent urinary tract infections.

Supplements to Avoid in CKD

Alfalfa	Aloe	Bayberry	Blue cohosh
Broom	Buckthorn	Capsicum	Cascara
Coltsfoot	Dandelion	Ginger	Ginseng
Horse chestnut	Horsetail	Licorice	Mate
Nettle	Noni juice	Rhubarb	Senna

Your Empowered Patient Action Plan for Treating Chronic Kidney Disease

Step #1: Prevention is the best treatment. Be sure to control all concurrent diseases, especially diabetes and high blood pressure and avoid medications that may worsen CKD.

Step #2: Follow the dietary rules explained above. This will help slow the progression of CKD. Be sure to consult with a registered dietician.

Step #3: Take appropriate medications as needed for complications.

Step #4: Undergo a trial of acupuncture to slow the progression of the condition. If this helps, you may be able to decrease or discontinue the medications in step 3.

Step #5: Take Chinese herbal formulas if you still have decreasing kidney function.

Step #6: Take nutritional supplements if the above steps are not helping. You can take them *with* the above steps as well.

Step #7: Undergo dialysis to take over kidney function if your CKD is severe. Hemodialysis is the most common type.

Step #8: Undergo kidney transplant for total kidney failure. If successful, dialysis will no longer be required.

Expected Outcome

Kidney disease is a silent killer, and the most important issue is to detect and treat it early—and treat other conditions that can cause it. If caught early, kidney function can be maintained, and you can avoid serious complications. However, if you are older, make sure you are not incorrectly diagnosed.

Macular Degeneration (AMD)

What You Need to Know

Age-related macular degeneration (called AMD, atrophic macular degeneration) is scarring of the macula, a small area at the back of the eye that is necessary for focused, straight-ahead vision such as reading, watching TV, driving, and sewing. There are two types: exudative ("wet") and atrophic ("dry"), the latter being the most common.

AMD is a result of the free-radical damage and decreased blood and oxygen supply to the eye that occurs with aging. It is slowly progressive, taking about five to ten years to cause legal blindness after it begins.

Exudative macular degeneration is responsible for 90 percent of sudden, severe visual loss in people with AMD and is considered an emergency, requiring surgery. This section will primarily discuss the dry AMD.

Treatments for Macular Degeneration

The Preventive Approaches

Correctable causes: The major risk factors for macular degeneration are smoking, atherosclerosis, and high blood pressure, so these conditions must be treated to prevent or slow the progress of AMD. (See sections on *Cholesterol*, *Heart Disease* [chronic], and *Hypertension* for further treatment guidelines if you have these conditions.)

Nutrition designed to reduce atherosclerosis and increase antioxidants will help if this is the cause of your macular degeneration. I recommend increasing the fruits and vegetables you eat, which can lower your risk for macular degeneration and slow down its progression.

Physical activity is very important for preventing macular degeneration, including the "wet" variety. Any physical activity three times per week lessens the risk by 70 percent. Simply walking is adequate.

Warning: A recent study revealed that *aspirin* use may double the risk of wet AMD. If you have increased risk for heart disease complications, the benefits of taking aspirin outweigh the harm (which is small); but for primary prevention of heart disease, aspirin is not beneficial, and you should avoid its use (see section on *Heart disease*).

The Conventional Approaches

Laser photocoagulation is a surgical procedure commonly used for exudative AMD. It decreases the rate of severe visual loss. For dry AMD, **photodynamic treatment** with verteporfin reduces the risk of moderate and severe visual loss and can be used with photocoagulation.

Medications: *Ranibizumab* (Lucentis) significantly improves visual acuity in AMD. However, one dose costs nearly $2,000. Some ophthalmologists are instead using a closely related drug called *bevacizumb* (Avastin) which is used for various types of cancer but is used off-label for AMD and is just as effective as (and much less costly than) ranibizumab ($50 per dose). *Afibercept* (eylea) is another injection recently approved. *Caution*: These injections may cause serious side effects, including eye pain, cataracts, infection, and retinal detachment.

Important notes: For exudative AMD, studies have not shown benefit from external beam radiation, submacular surgery, or subcutaneous interferon α.

The Alternative Approaches

There are many **nutritional supplements** that can improve eye health, vision, and AMD:

- A 2013 study published in *JAMA* showed that a combination of vitamins C and E, beta carotene, and zinc (called the *AREDS formula*) reduced the risk of progression of AMD. Adding lutein plus zeaxanthin, docosahexanoic acid (DHA), or eicosapentanoic acid (EPA) did not add any benefit to this formula. This is the only formula that is substantiated by research studies, although there are other companies making combination products with similar ingredients.

- *Bilberry extract with carotenoids* (40–80 mg per day, containing 25 percent anthocyanidin content) is very effective at halting and even reversing dry macular degeneration. These supplements increase blood flow to the retina and improve visual processes. You should notice improvement within one month.
- *Gingko biloba* (160–240 mg per day, containing 24 percent gingko flavonglycosides) is also very effective in slowing the progression of this condition. Gingko acts similarly to bilberry by increasing blood flow. It may take up to two months to observe benefit from gingko.
- *Zinc* alone, in doses of at least 70 mg per day, can also improve poor vision. Zinc helps reduce symptoms and halts the progression of macular degeneration, especially in combination with vitamin E (800 IU per day). Too much zinc, however, can interfere with copper absorption and immune function.
- *Grapeseed extract* (150–300 mg per day, containing 95 percent procyanidolic content) may help if you are having problems with poor night vision or photophobia (increased sensitivity to bright light). It may take one to two months to notice improvement.

A **Chinese herbal formula** called *Ming Mu Di Huang Wan* may help when eyes are dry.

Your Empowered Patient Action Plan for Treating Atrophic (Dry) AMD

- *Warning: For exudative ("wet") AMD, undergo laser photocoagulation surgery immediately.*
- *For moderate to severe dry AMD, go to Step #6 or #7, and then return to Step #1.*

Step #1: Take the AREDS formula and/or bilberry with carotenoids to prevent or slow down the progression of AMD. These combinations have been shown to be the most effective.

Josh was a sixteen-year-old patient whose uncle and grandfather both had macular degeneration, and which he developed at age fourteen. He was denied a driver's license because he could not pass the eye exam. I started him on a formula containing bilberry and carotenoids. After two months, he was able to pass the eye test and was given his driver's license.

*Step #2: **Take gingko biloba*** to slow the progression of AMD. It can be used with Step #1.

*Step #3: **Take zinc and vitamin E*** to reduce symptoms and halt the progression of AMD. It can be used alone if the above steps have not helped or can be used with the above steps to further improve vision.

*Step #4: **Take fish oil*** (or krill oil) to improve eyesight.

*Step #5: **Take grape-seed extract*** to improve night vision.

*Step #6: **Take bevacizumb (Avastin) or ranibizumab (Lucentis)*** to increase vision if the above steps have not been effective. Use Avastin first if possible as it is less expensive.

*Step #7: **Consider photodynamic treatment*** if you have dry AMD and the previous steps have been ineffective.

Expected Outcome

Most people with atrophic AMD should be able to prevent further deterioration and vision loss and improve their vision by using the above steps.

Memory Loss

What You Need to Know

It is obvious to most of us that, as we age, our brains may not function as well as when we were younger. When you're in your twenties, you begin to lose brain cells a few at a time. Your body also starts to make less of the chemicals your brain cells need in order to work properly. The older you are, the more these changes can affect your memory. Aging may affect memory by changing the way the brain stores information and by making it harder to recall stored information.

Your short-term and remote memories aren't usually affected by aging, but your *recent* memory may be affected. Aging is usually the cause, but many other factors can cause memory problems; these include depression, dementia (severe problems with memory and thinking, such as Alzheimer's disease), side effects of drugs, strokes, head injury, thyroid dysfunction, and alcoholism.

It is important to realize that research has proven that new brain cells can be made even into the late eighties (called neuroplasticity). So, even if brain cells die, they can be regenerated.

Treatments for Memory Loss

The Preventive Approaches

You should rule out **correctable causes** of memory loss. Medications are the primary culprits, especially blood pressure medicines, antidepressants, antihistamines, and even diet pills.

Alcohol use can also affect memory if overused or from binge drinking. However, moderate drinking may improve memory.

A good **diet** with plenty of fruits and vegetables can help prevent memory loss and preserve brain function because they contain powerful antioxidants. In fact, a recent study done in rats showed that blueberries reversed age-related memory declines in elderly rats, and their brains showed greater activation of proteins involved in memory and learning. Proper daily exercise has also been proven to enhance memory and cerebral (brain) blood flow.

Recent studies show that people with vitamin B_{12} deficiency have a six times greater risk of having brain atrophy and cognitive (thinking) impairment. **B_{12} supplementation** may be helpful to prevent such a risk if blood tests show you to be B_{12} deficient.

The Conventional Approaches

To help remember things, there are some actions you can take, including:

- Make lists
- Follow a routine
- Keep a detailed calendar
- Place important items in the same place every time
- Repeat names when you meet new people

More importantly, however, you need to keep your brain active. We actually have "two" brains—the left and right—which perform different functions, so we need to "exercise" both.

As the left brain is more analytical and systematic, we must take actions that enhance these aspects. Any games, puzzles, or activities that require logic, use words and language, or apply math and science can enhance the functioning of the left brain. Working on a project, making detailed lists, planning functions or trips, working crossword puzzles, doing your taxes, and participating in sports that require strategy (even golf) are actions that empower the left brain.

The right brain requires imagination and fantasy, so creative endeavors are important, such as writing, art, or crafts. Trying to decipher symbols such as dreams or contemplating and debating philosophy or religion can also empower the right brain.

Random Line Technique for Improving Right Brain Function

A good example of how to increase right brain power is called the random line technique. On a piece of paper, draw a line randomly but don't consciously guide the pencil or pen...just let it go where it will, up and down and around, until a pattern has developed. Then guide the line back to its starting point. You will see that this has created several spaces, which you can fill in with different colors or shading. This technique has been shown useful for decreasing stress in hospital waiting rooms.

There are also actions you can take to activate *both* sides of the brain. One action is to use one or more of your senses in a way you have not done before. An example is taking a shower or eating with your eyes closed, or communicating with someone using only visual or hand cues rather than talking. Another action is to break a routine in a new way. If you drive somewhere, take a different route, or shop somewhere different, or rearrange your living room.

One of the best ways to enhance brain function and keep the brain "alive" is to do something that you have never done before but always wanted to do. This could be exploring a new hobby, taking up a new sport such as golf or tennis or lawn bowling, traveling more often, learning to paint or sculpt, writing a short story or even a book, and so on. Be creative—the possibilities are endless.

Important note: You should understand, however, that if something becomes too routine, it does not stimulate the brain, and you can lose brain cells. If something you do becomes automatic, it's time for a change.

There are **medications** that can be prescribed to slow degradation of the brain and support mental functioning (see chapter on Alzheimer's/dementia). However, most of these drugs have only minimal effects, yet they have potentially serious side effects, so they are not recommended. The only one that may be effective is *Cerefolin*, which contains high-dose folate.

The Alternative Approaches

There are numerous alternative methods that can help improve memory as well as improve brain function.

Mind-body methods are excellent at helping brain function, with meditation being the easiest but most effective. Even meditating five minutes a day is helpful, but a half hour is the best.

There are several **nutritional supplements** that can be quite beneficial for improving overall brain function. They increase blood flow to the brain and increase production of neurotransmitters. However, they may take up to eight weeks to have an effect. These include:

- *Gingko biloba* (240 mg daily), which is one of the most studied herbs. It may take six to eight weeks to observe benefit.
- *Panax Ginseng* (containing 37.5 percent gensenosides) has been shown to improve abstract thinking, mental arithmetic skills, and reaction times. Panax ginseng alone does not seem to improve memory, but there is some evidence that a combination of panax ginseng and ginkgo leaf extract can improve memory in otherwise healthy people ages thirty-eight to sixty-six years.
- *Omega-3's* from fish oil are important to brain function because a particular omega-3 (DHA) is concentrated in the brain. ***Important notes***: There are problems with fish oil that you need to be aware of. First, you must take *at least* 1,500 mg daily to obtain benefits. Most studies showing benefit for memory were done using 3,000–4,000 mg. Many fish oils also deteriorate very rapidly (three months); so by the time you buy them, they may already be partially deteriorated. Krill oil may be more potent and stable, and it contains two natural antioxidants and has few to no side effects. However, krill oil products differ in their concentrations of omega-3s and combinations with other ingredients, so check the label. Krill oil also has been shown to improve blood circulation in the brain.
- *Huperzine A* (50–200 mg daily) increases brain levels of a neurotransmitter thought to be involved in memory (acetylcholine) and may improve memory through that mechanism.
- *Green tea* helps with mental alertness during the day.
- *Acetyl-L-carnitine* (1,500–2,000 mg daily) seems to improve some measures of cognitive function and memory in elderly people with age-related mental impairment.
- *Phosphatidylcholine* (25 g daily) is the largest reservoir of choline in the body. Choline is a precursor to acetylcholine.

- *Phosphatidylserine* (200–300 mg daily for one to two months, then 100 mg daily) increases levels of several neurotransmitters, including acetylcholine, dopamine, and serotonin.
- *DMAE* (300–200 mg daily) is a precursor to choline as well.
- *7-KETO DHEA* (25–50 mg daily) appears to help memory loss resulting from menopause. ***Important note***: You should avoid wild yam and soy products labeled as "natural DHEA" because they do not break down into DHEA in the body.
- *Curcumin* (1.5 grams twice per day with food) may help with memory loss.

There are also several **Chinese herbal formulas** that can increase blood flow in the brain and improve memory. These include *Dan Shen, Yin Xing Ye, Chuan Xiong*, and *Mao Dong Qing*. An excellent formula for treating deterioration of brain function and loss of memory is *Zuo Gui Wan/You Gui Yin*.

Your Empowered Patient Action Plan for Retarding and Treating Memory Loss

*Step #1: **Maintain a good diet and exercise*** to prevent brain dysfunction.
*Step #2: **Exercise your brain*** as you age to prevent brain deterioration and make new brain cells.
*Step #3: **Take gingko biloba and/or krill oil*** to improve memory and brain function.
*Step #4. **Try Cerefolin*** if the above has not helped.
*Step #5: **Take other herbal supplements***, either alone or in combination, if the above steps have not helped. Of these, Huperzine A and acetyl-L-carnitine may be the best, or a combination of gingko and ginseng.

Expected Outcome
Memory loss is quite common as we age, but does not have to be a major deterrent to quality of life. In fact, by using various lifestyle changes and herbs, memory loss may be "forgotten."

Menopause

What You Need to Know
Symptoms of menopause will usually resolve with time, but it may take several years to do so. Not all women will get menopausal symptoms, but the

majority of American women do, and it can definitely interfere with your quality of life.

Duration of Hot Flashes Depends on When They Begin

The most common side effects of menopause are vasomotor symptoms (VMS), that is, hot flashes and night sweats. A 2015 study showed that the median total VMS duration for all women was 7.4 years. However, this varied with the time VMS started. The women who were premenopausal or early menopausal when they first felt VMS had the longest duration, with a median greater than 11.8 years. The women who were postmenopausal when VMS began had the shortest duration, with a median of 3.4 years.

In Asian countries, very few women have menopausal symptoms, most likely due to a different diet, which is higher in plant estrogens. They also have less obesity: it should be noted that the more body fat you have, the more likely you are to have hot flashes and night sweats during menopause.

Hot Flashes Not the Only Cause of Sleep Disturbance

Many women feel that hot flashes are the cause of sleep disturbance, but other causes are usually more prevalent. In a recent study published in 2007 in *Menopause*, sleep apnea and periodic limb movements (such as restless legs syndrome) were the major predictors of reduced sleep.

Menopause can herald the deterioration of various organ systems, especially the heart, brain, and bones. Many conditions can occur subsequent to this, including depression, heart disease, incontinence, insomnia, and osteoporosis. In fact, a 2014 study showed that women who have hot flashes are at increased risk for osteoporosis. For this reason, there are several steps that women need to take to protect these organ systems, whether they have menopausal symptoms or not (see steps below).

Dr. A's Suggestions:
Menopause Affects Oral Health

After menopause, women become more susceptible to periodontal disease. This is most likely due to estrogen deficiency with resulting bone loss and inflammation. This is best diagnosed early so that treatment can be provided; so see your dentist regularly.

———

Dr. A's Suggestions:
Be Sure to Check Your Cholesterol Levels

Lipids undergo substantial changes from the year before to the year after menopause. It is important to check your lipid levels after you reach menopause to enhance protection against cardiac problems.

———

Warning: If you have vaginal bleeding after you are menopausal, you should seek gynecological care immediately to rule out uterine or cervical cancer. All women who are menopausal and postmenopausal should still have gynecological exams at least every two to three years to check for other pelvic and gynecological diseases that can still occur.

In this section, I will provide a guide for treating menopausal *symptoms*. For postmenopausal *medical conditions*, refer to the sections for those particular conditions.

Treatments for Menopause

The Preventive Approaches

A balanced **diet** can help all the symptoms of menopause, especially eating foods that contain plant estrogens (phytoestrogens), particularly soy and lima beans. Other beneficial foods include nuts and seeds, fennel, celery, and parsley. These foods can increase the levels of estrogen in your body, although they may not be enough to prevent all menopausal symptoms (they contain "weak" estrogens).

A diet low in saturated fat can help prevent postmenopausal heart disease. If you are a postmenopausal woman, you can be especially sensitive to salt, and limiting salt intake to one teaspoon daily can significantly reduce your blood pressure if it is high. Synthetic hormone replacement therapy (HRT; see below) can deplete your body's stores of vitamin B$_6$ and folic acid, which you can replace or supplement by eating more vegetables and fruits or fortified food products.

Caffeine may increase hot flashes and related problems, but it also improves memory and mood, according to a 2104 study from the Mayo Clinic.

Many menopausal women gain weight, especially around the midsection. **Exercise** is the primary method of reducing this particular type of weight gain (diet alone has not been shown to be very effective unless accompanied by exercise). Aerobic exercise can help prevent postmenopausal heart disease (it increases HDL cholesterol) and improve brain function, and resistance (strength training) exercises can help prevent bone loss and make new bone, as well as decreasing LDL cholesterol, total cholesterol, and body fat. Strength training will also increase your metabolism. I recommend at least thirty minutes of strength training and aerobic activity three times per week. Exercise does not decrease vasomotor symptoms (hot flashes) but does improve sleep quality.

The Conventional Approaches

For more than sixty years, **HRT** was the mainstay of treatment for menopausal symptoms, ostensibly preventing chronic conditions that commonly develop after menopause, such as heart disease and osteoporosis. However, the studies done to support this were inadequately designed (see sidebar below), and a landmark study (Women's Health Initiative, WHI) eventually demonstrated that HRT could be more harmful than beneficial.

HRT primarily refers to the use of equine (horse) estrogens in combination with progesterone, which is rarely recommended anymore. Although many doctors have stopped prescribing HRT, they also have stopped using estrogen alone (ERT), which has been shown to be beneficial at relieving many menopausal symptoms with minimal risks (although a 2015 study showed slight increased risk of ovarian cancer).

The Fall of HRT

Beginning in the 1940s, doctors prescribed estrogen to prevent menopausal symptoms and to protect the body from accelerated deterioration. This treatment with estrogen was called estrogen replacement therapy (ERT). It was thought that the lack of estrogen in menopausal women caused all of the symptoms of menopause, as well as the complications of menopause. It was assumed that replacing the lost estrogen would ameliorate the problems that accompany menopause.

However, it was discovered that women who took estrogen over a long period of time had a significant increase in cancer of the uterus. To counteract the harmful effects of taking estrogen alone, progesterone was prescribed in conjunction with estrogen, and this combination treatment was referred to as hormone replacement therapy, or HRT. The progesterone protected the uterus from too much estrogen. The estrogen and progesterone were given in the form of synthetic drugs, derived either from chemical compounds or from animal sources such as horse urine.

For decades, these two hormones were the standard treatment for the symptoms and complications of menopause. Unfortunately, however, the long-term consequences of this treatment were not truly recognized until a landmark study called the Women's Health Initiative (WHI; see below) found that these combination hormones did not, in fact, adequately protect women from the aging process: HRT did not prevent heart disease, osteoporosis, and decreased cognitive functioning in aging women. Furthermore, it caused significant side effects, including increased risk of stroke, gall bladder disease, acid reflux, cataracts, blood clots, and cancer (increased incidence of breast cancer and higher death rate with lung cancer). These potential dangers far outweighed the possible benefits. As a result, millions of women stopped taking HRT.

However, you should realize that these studies were only done on one type of estrogen, that being equine (horse)-derived, along with synthetic progesterone. Other estrogens alone have not been found to have the same dangers, but they can reduce hot flashes. Follow-up studies from the WHI have also shown that after ten years of taking estrogen alone, the treatment neither increases nor decreases the risks for coronary artery disease, deep vein thrombosis, stroke, hip fracture, colorectal cancer, or total mortality.

Nevertheless, many doctors have turned to other treatments to relieve the symptoms of menopause and the deterioration of women's organs from the aging process.

This is the information concluded by the WHI study:

- Avoid the use of equine estrogen with medroxyprogesterone. They do not prevent chronic diseases in postmenopausal women but can cause increased risk of other diseases.
- Estrogen therapy (ERT) alone remains the most effective *conventional* treatment for hot flashes.

- If you use ERT, use it for as short a period of time as possible. It can still increase the risk of breast and ovarian cancer, albeit small.
  - Both current and past users of HRT are at significantly higher cancer risk than never-users, and risk increases with duration of use. Risk declines rapidly after stopping use, falling to that of never-users within three years.
- Even with lower doses of estrogen, however, there is still an increased risk of blood clots, stroke, and heart disease within the first one to four years. The increased risk of heart disease and blood clots begin to appear within year one, and the risk of stroke between years three and four. At ten years, the risk disappears.
- The risk/benefit ratio is most favorable when initiated in younger menopausal women. Those women who begin therapy at ages fifty to fifty-nine and who use it for five years appear to have less risks as well as less mortality (30–40 percent) than those who start after age sixty.
- Use of ERT to prevent osteoporosis is appropriate in selected women at risk for this condition.
- Estrogen's heart protection was thought to occur if started close to the time of menopause but only in women younger than sixty years of age. A 2014 study demonstrated this to not be true.

Certain Women Less Prone to Breast Cancer with HRT

In a study published in the *Journal of the National Cancer Institute*, black women, obese women, and those with less dense breasts have minimal excess risk of breast cancer than whites, Asians, and Hispanics who take HRT. The association between HRT and breast cancer was greatest for underweight or lean women with extremely dense breasts, and the associations were almost nil for obese women with fatty breasts.

If you do take *estrogen*, you should start with the lowest-dose estrogen, which may be able to decrease symptoms without as much of the increased risk of cancer, blood clots, and gallstones seen with higher doses. Estrogen can be prescribed in several forms, including pills, patches, injections, and intravaginal creams, depending on your symptoms. The risk of gall bladder disease, stroke, and blood clots has been found to be lower with estrogen patches (transdermal) than with the oral form, so it may be preferred. One transdermal patch, Vivelle-Dot, can be obtained as a generic.

After four years, the risk for these side effects levels off, but there is still an increased risk for other side effects, such as breast cancer and gallstones. The dangers increase more in the decade after menopause. However, the WHI study noted that after discontinuing estrogen, risks for stroke and blood clots diminish, and there was a reduction in the risk of breast cancer.

Duration of Hot Flashes Same with or without Estrogen

A study in the journal *Menopause* reveals that the mean duration of hot flashes is 5.2 years in women not using hormones and 5.5 years if using hormones. Two-thirds of women experience hot flashes intermittently.

Another study done at the Helsinki University in 2013 showed that HRT helps women who have seven or more moderate to severe hot flashes per day but not those who have less than three daily. In the women with more hot flashes, other symptoms of menopause, including disturbed sleep, impaired memory and concentration, anxiety, exhaustion, irritability, swelling of extremities, and vaginal dryness, were also helped—but not in the women with few hot flashes.

Warning: Combining Alcohol with Estrogen Increases Risk of Breast Cancer

It is already recognized that too much alcohol can slightly increase the risk of breast cancer. A twenty-year Danish study revealed that women who take hormones and averaged a drink a day had a two- to threefold higher risk of breast cancer, and those drinking two drinks a day had a fivefold increase. In women who did not take hormones, alcohol did not increase cancer risk. As hormones themselves increase the risk, alcohol with hormones is even more worrisome.

Raloxiphene is a type of estrogen called a selective estrogen receptor modulator (SERM) that demonstrates no increased risk of cancer or blood clots, and so it is often used in place of other estrogens.

Two drugs that contain **estrogen derived from plants**, instead of animals or synthetic substances, are promoted as an alternative to HRT and ERT. These drugs (Enjuvia, Cenestin) are prescribed to control hot flashes, vaginal dryness, and night sweats. It is not known, however, whether these pills are safer than estrogen made from animal sources. These drugs were created to be available by prescription only, and they had to get FDA approval; so even though they are derived from plants, they are considered a conventional treatment rather than alternative.

Other medications for menopausal symptoms: Because of the problems with synthetic hormones, other drugs have been tried to reduce menopausal symptoms:

- *Zyrtec*, an allergy medication, was noted in one small study to decrease hot flashes by 40 percent after four weeks of therapy.
- *Trazadone* is an antidepressant that is used to help combat insomnia in menopausal women.
- *Clonidine* or *methyldopa*, both blood pressure medications, can decrease the frequency and severity of hot flashes but not eliminate them.
- *Selective serotonin reuptake inhibitors (SSRIs)* are usually used for depression, but have been found to decrease hot flashes in about 50 percent of women. No studies have been done to indicate which SSRI is the most beneficial, and different women react differently to each one. SSRIs (and a few other classes; see section on *Depression*) used for menopausal symptoms include paroxetine (Paxil), fluoxetine (Prozac), bupropion (Wellbutrin), citalopram (Celexa), Escitalopram (Lexapro), and venlafaxine (Effexor). A 2014 *JAMA Internal Medicine* study showed that Effexor and low dose estrogen are similarly effective. Another antidepressant, sertraline (Zoloft), has been found to be ineffective. Low dose paroxetine (7.5 mg) can be obtained OTC at a lower cost.
- For problems with decreased libido (sex drive), *testosterone supplementation* by pill, patch, or injection may help. **Caution**: However, testosterone can have some masculinizing effects. It may also have long-term side effects and an increased risk for breast cancer, so is not recommended by most authorities.
- The FDA has approved *ospemifen* (Osphena) to treat moderate-to-severe dyspareunia (painful intercourse) due to vaginal atrophy during menopause.

Factors Involved with Sexual Dysfunction during Menopause

In a recent study published in the journal *Menopause*, sexual desire declined in late menopause. The most common variable associated with sexual functioning in menopause was the *perceived importance* of sex. Vaginal dryness was associated with vaginal or pelvic pain and with decreased arousal, emotional satisfaction, and physical pleasure. So addressing vaginal dryness can alleviate these problems: estrogen cream or suppositories, using a lubricant for sex, or alternative methods (see below) can be helpful.

—∞—

A newer treatment for vasomotor symptoms in menopause is **stellate ganglion block**, in which an injection is given in a large group of nerves near the spinal column. A 2014 study in *Menopause* showed that such treatment may work for some women, although it provides only short-term relief, mainly in number of occurrences and intensity.

A machine called **EROS** is FDA-approved and has been found effective if you have sexual dysfunction, such as poor lubrication due to menopause. You can use this machine at home, applying gentle suction to the clitoris one minute a day initially and then building up to five minutes a day. As sexual function returns, you can use the device occasionally, as needed. EROS therapy requires a prescription from your doctor. (for more options, see section on *Sexual Dysfunction in Women*).

Finally, **surgery** is also done to control menopausal symptoms, but it is more frequently performed for dysfunctional uterine bleeding and fibroids (if symptomatic).

Hysterectomies are overused in this country, almost four times as much as any other industrialized nation. They do have complications, including doubling the likelihood of urinary incontinence. Other methods can be just as effective as hysterectomy for controlling post-menopausal symptoms. The following are indications for hysterectomy:

- Uterine fibroids that cause pain, bleeding, or other problems
- Uterine prolapse, which is a sliding of the uterus from its normal position into the vaginal canal
- Cancer of the uterus, cervix, or ovaries
- Endometriosis
- Abnormal vaginal bleeding
- Chronic pelvic pain
- Adenomyosis, or a thickening of the uterus

There are three types of hysterectomies:

- In a *supracervical or subtotal (partial) hysterectomy*, a surgeon removes only the upper part of the uterus, keeping the cervix in place. This may have the advantage of increased sexual pleasure.
- A *total hysterectomy* removes the whole uterus and cervix.
- In a *radical hysterectomy*, a surgeon removes the whole uterus, tissue on the sides of the uterus, the cervix, and the top part of the vagina. Radical hysterectomy is generally only done when cancer is present.

There are also different surgical techniques:

- An *abdominal* hysterectomy is an open surgery. This is the most common approach to hysterectomy, accounting for about 65% of all procedures.
- *Vaginal* hysterectomy: The surgeon makes a cut in the vagina and removes the uterus through this incision. The incision is closed, leaving no visible scar.
- *Laparoscopic* hysterectomy: This surgery is done using a laparoscope, which is a tube with a lighted camera, and surgical tools inserted through several small cuts made in the belly or, in the case of a single site laparoscopic procedure, one small cut made in the belly button. The surgeon performs the hysterectomy from outside the body, viewing the operation on a video screen. This can be done through the vagina.
- *Laparoscopic-assisted vaginal* hysterectomy: Using laparoscopic surgical tools, a surgeon removes the uterus through an incision in the vagina.
- *Robot-assisted laparoscopic* hysterectomy: This procedure is similar to a laparoscopic hysterectomy, but the surgeon controls a sophisticated robotic system of surgical tools from outside the body. Advanced technology allows the surgeon to use natural wrist movements and view the hysterectomy on a three-dimensional screen.

The last three are considered *minimally invasive procedures* (MIP). In general, an MIP allows for faster recovery, shorter hospital stays, less pain and scarring, and a lower chance of infection than does an abdominal hysterectomy.

Comparison of MIP procedures: With an MIP, women are generally able to resume their normal activity within an average of three to four weeks, compared to four to six weeks for an abdominal hysterectomy. The costs associated with an MIP are generally lower than the costs associated with open surgery, depending on the instruments used and the time spent in the operating room. There is also less risk of incisional hernias with an MIP. ***Caution***: Robotic procedures, however, can be much more expensive without any clear advantage and there has been some concern that it can spread uterine cancer that is not detected at time of surgery.

Not every woman is a good candidate for a minimally invasive procedure. The presence of scar tissue from previous surgeries, obesity, and health status can all affect whether or not an MIP is advisable. Because there are different types, indications, and techniques for getting a hysterectomy, you should always be empowered and get a second opinion.

Endometrial ablation is another option for bleeding problems. It is not quite as effective as hysterectomy (25 percent require retreatment, mostly women under the age of forty) but has significantly fewer side effects and complications and is much less expensive.

For fibroids, *embolization* to cut off the blood supply and thus shrink the fibroid can be done as an outpatient by interventional radiologists and is just as effective as open surgery for this condition.

Helpful Tip: If undergoing surgery, it is recommended that you avoid removing your ovaries unless you have a predilection for ovarian cancer. Studies show that removing the ovaries along with the uterus can cause an increase in heart disease and deaths from heart disease and stroke.

The Alternative Approaches

Acupuncture is the best treatment for menopausal symptoms, which can reduce symptoms long-term without the need for taking drugs or even herbs. Often, night sweats resolve in three or four sessions and hot flashes in five or six. You might need additional sessions for maximum benefits, or for other symptoms such as libido, vaginal dryness, and mood swings. Acupuncture is also beneficial for other conditions related to menopause, including dysfunctional uterine bleeding and incontinence. Auricular (ear) acupuncture and body acupuncture both may be effective, with ear acupuncture better for increasing libido (there is a point called the *sexual desire* point).

Several **Chinese herbal formulas** are very effective at reducing menopausal symptoms. I recommend the formula *Er Xian Tang*. If hot flashes persist, and there is evidence of Yin deficiency, *Zhi Bai Di Huang Wan* can be added. *Liu Wei Di Huang Wan* can be used for hot flashes and chronic urinary tract infections. You should notice improvement within three weeks but may need to take them longer for complete or ongoing relief.

There are several **Western herbs and supplements** that can be beneficial for menopausal symptoms:

- *Black cohosh* is the best supported by research and helps reduce many menopausal symptoms through its phytoestrogen (plant estrogen) content. Phytoestrogens have been shown in studies to have no adverse effects. A recent study using 40 mg black cohosh daily in women with uterine fibroids for twelve weeks showed not only a decrease in hot flashes but also benefit of decreased volume of the fibroids. The best studied (over ninety studies) standardized natural black cohosh is *Remefemin*.
- *Flaxseed* (1 Tbsp per day freshly ground flax seeds—not capsule or oil) is also very effective for this purpose, and you can take it along with black cohosh.
- *Gamma-oryzanol* (150 mg twice daily), derived from rice bran oil, has been used primarily in Japan for hot flashes but also can lower cholesterol.
- *Soy extract* (250 mg twice daily, standardized to 10 percent isoflavones) can often reduce symptoms. **Caution**: doses greater than 150 mg daily does increase the risk of endometrial hyperplasia (thickening of the lining of your uterus); do not take this if you have fibroids or fibrocystic breast disease.
- *Red clover* (liquid extract, 1:1 in 25 percent alcohol, taken 1.5–3 ml three times a day, or tincture, 1:10 in 45 percent alcohol, 1–2 ml three times a day) contains phytoestrogens as well, but they are weaker than those in black cohosh.

- A *rhubarb extract* (4 mg daily) found in Germany was found to significantly reduce menopausal symptoms.
- Applying *vitamin E oil* helps to hydrate vaginal membranes and counteract vaginal dryness. Also, taking vitamin E with mixed tocopherols can be helpful in minimizing hot flashes.
- *Calendula*, *comfrey*, and/or *St. John's wort* can be made into creams or ointments that reduce vaginal burning, itching, and other symptoms caused by thinning of the vaginal skin. ***Caution***: Avoid the use of comfrey on an open wound area.
- *DHEA* (12.5–50 mg daily; start low and gradually increase if no side effects) has been used to increase energy and well-being, and also may help with cognitive functions such as memory. DHEA breaks down into estrogen and androgens (like testosterone), although doses greater than 50 mg can cause masculinizing effects. DHEA may also help reducing the central fat that occurs during menopause (you need to take 50 mg daily for that effect). ***Caution***: There can be a risk in taking DHEA daily, so it is important to have your hormone levels checked by your PCP. ***Important note***: You should avoid wild yam and soy products labeled as "natural DHEA" because they do not break down into DHEA in the body.

If one of these supplements is not totally effective, you can safely combine many of them together for better results.

There are also so-called **natural ("bioidentical") hormones** available, which are synthesized from plant compounds. *Natural progesterone* is the most prescribed (50–200 mg once daily if in oral form or 20–40 mg daily as a cream, days seven through twenty-seven if you still have periods and every day if menopausal). ***Important notes***: There are some recent studies showing that natural progesterone used with *synthetic* estrogen confers less or even no risk of breast cancer as opposed to using synthetic progesterone.

Natural estrogens (Tri-est or Bi-est, 0.625–2.5 mg daily for the first twenty-one days of your cycle, or every twenty-five days with a five-day rest period if your periods have stopped) are also used, but usually only if you still have symptoms that are not relieved by natural progesterone. ***Caution***: Avoid if you have been diagnosed with or have a strong family history of breast cancer.

Natural testosterone (0.25–2 mg daily) is also available to treat low sex drive, but it can be harmful over the long term (increasing the risk of heart disease).

Natural hormones can be purchased in health food stores or over the Internet, or they can be compounded (mixed together) by a compounding pharmacist trained in these techniques. You should also have your hormone levels tested to help the compounding pharmacist know specifically how to make a product with the best individualized results. You can take natural hormones in several forms, including creams, capsules, troches, and suppositories. Natural testosterone, however, must be prescribed by a doctor.

⁂

"Bioidentical" Hormones: In Controversy

Because of the problems with HRT, many women have turned to so-called bi-oidentical hormones—or natural hormones made from plant compounds. The FDA started cracking down on claims for these compounds, stating that there is no evidence that they are effective or have fewer side effects than synthetic hormones and that they do not prevent postmenopausal diseases, including Alzheimer's. They have tried to prevent pharmacists from compounding natural hormones.

In actuality, these compounds do help control menopausal symptoms in many women. However, it is true that they do not prevent Alzheimer's, and studies have not been done to show whether they have the same side effects and increased risks that synthetic hormones have (there is a current study under-way). In addition, dosing and purity can vary, with a 2011 review finding that 34 percent of product samples tested failed one or more quality tests—90 percent of those due to less of the active ingredient.

What you should know is that most compounding pharmacists are very knowledgeable and provide excellent products, and they can individualize them for you. However, some pharmacists and companies that produce standard products provide poor products that will not benefit you. So, you need to become empowered and make sure you are obtaining quality products.

Finally, the term "bioidentical" has no scientific definition; it is primarily a marketing term.

⁂

Fish oil has been found to significantly lower risk for cardiac disease if you are meno-pausal. It has not been found to be useful to alleviate vasomotor symptoms. Omega-3s from fish oil are more potent than from plants. ***Important notes***: There are problems with fish oil that you need to be aware of. Although regular fish oil can decrease cho-lesterol levels and protect the heart, you must take *at least* 1,500 mg daily to obtain benefits. Many studies were done using 3,000–4,000 mg. Many fish oils also deterio-rate very rapidly (three months); so by the time you buy them, they may already be partially deteriorated. Krill oil may be more potent, more stable and contains two natural antioxidants and has little to no side effects. However, krill oil products differ in their concentrations of omega-3s and combinations with other ingredients, so check the label.

Warning: Regular fish oil in high doses may decrease HDL cholesterol (the good cholesterol) in some people. If you take fish oil, and your HDL is reduced to below normal, take vitamin E with mixed tocopherols and tocotrienols (200 IU daily) and garlic (4,000 mg daily) or niacin (1–3 grams daily) to raise HDL. Niacin may cause flushing, but there are nonflushing products available. It also can be prescribed, but the prescription form is much more expensive and does not have any advantage over OTC forms.

Intravaginal natural estrogen cream can be used for vaginal dryness. The cream should contain primarily estriol, which works the best and has the least risks of all the estrogen forms. If that does not work, micronized progesterone (which is also natural but must be prescribed by a doctor) is helpful in place of the cream form of natural progesterone.

Use It or Lose It: Maintain Lubrication the Natural Way

You may think that you need hormones such as DHEA or testosterone to increase vaginal lubrication and maintain sexual function, but studies have shown that for many people, having sex several times a week will stimulate the vagina, produce natural lubrication, and maintain sexual desire, without the need for supplemental hormones.

Your Empowered Patient Action Plan for Treating Menopausal Symptoms

Step #1:   *Undergo acupuncture* for long-term relief of menopausal symptoms. This is the most cost-effective therapy. Acupuncture is also beneficial for dysfunctional bleeding, but use only after cancer has been ruled out as a cause.

Step #2:   *Take natural progesterone* for control of menopausal symptoms if acupuncture doesn't relieve your symptoms. Be sure to have your hormone levels checked before having it compounded.

Step #3:   ***Take the Chinese herbal remedies Er Xian Tang, Zhi Bai Di Huang Wan, or Gan Mai Da Zao Wan*** if the above steps have not worked.

Step #4: **Take black cohosh, flaxseed oil, gamma-oryzanol, rhubarb extract, red clover,** or a combination of these herbs if you still have menopausal symptoms.

Step #5: **Take natural estrogen** if your hot flashes and night sweats continue. It can be combined with natural progesterone for better results. Use *caution* if you have been diagnosed with breast cancer or have a strong family history of gynecologic cancers.

Step #6: **Take natural testosterone** to improve memory and libido, with caution over the long term (obtain guidance from a doctor, who must prescribe it).

Step #7: **Take DHEA** to improve memory and libido and to help promote weight loss.

Step #8: **Take fish or krill oil** to improve cognitive (memory) function and protect against heart disease and stroke.

Step #9: **Use natural estrogen and/or vitamin E intravaginal creams** for vaginal dryness and/or use lubricants when you have sex.

Step #10: **Take synthetic estrogen** in low dose (transdermal is preferred) or **raloxiphene** if the above steps have not reduced your menopausal symptoms and if you are under the age of sixty. Avoid taking synthetic progesterone.

Step #11: **Undergo embolization** for symptomatic fibroids.

Step #12: **Undergo surgery** only if indicated or if symptoms interfere with your quality of life and cannot be relieved by the previous steps. Be sure to investigate the different types and techniques and obtain a second opinion.

At age fifty-three, Norma had stopped having periods three years earlier. Although her hot flashes had eventually gone away on their own, she now had depression, trouble sleeping, weight gain, decreased sex drive, and vaginal dryness. I started her on an exercise program, acupuncture, and natural progesterone. After three months, the majority of her symptoms were gone, but she still had some vaginal dryness. I suggested that she take natural estrogen as a vaginal cream, along with vitamin E vaginal cream. This addition eliminated her vaginal dryness.

Expected Outcome

Menopause does not need to interfere with quality of life for any woman. Menopausal symptoms can be controlled adequately and most often resolved completely by using the above steps. For diseases of aging that occur after menopause, see sections on *Heart Disease (CAD)* and *Osteoporosis*.

Neuralgia (Trigeminal, Postherpetic)

What You Need to Know
Neuralgia is nerve pain caused by irritation or damage to a nerve. The most common forms include trigeminal neuralgia, which involves a nerve in the face (the trigeminal nerve, or the fifth cranial nerve) and postherpetic neuralgia, which involves nerves primarily in the torso (along rib margins) but can occur anywhere on the body that shingles occurs, including the face, eyes, legs, and arms.

Pressure from a blood vessel or trauma to the face can cause trigeminal neuralgia. Postherpetic neuralgia is caused by the chicken pox virus (herpes zoster), which has remained dormant after having chickenpox until some factor causes it to reappear (such as stress or trauma). The *acute* infection is more commonly known as shingles and neuralgia can occur as a result of damage to the nerve during the infection (see section on shingles for more information and treatment of the infection).

Treatments for Neuralgia

The Preventive Approaches
There is no actual method for preventing neuralgia. However, some forms of neuralgia (shingles especially) can be precipitated by stress, and stress can cause all forms of neuralgia to become worse or more painful. For this reason, **meditation**, interactive imagery, or **psychotherapy** may be useful to address the stress.

Obtaining a **shingles vaccine** over the age of sixty decreases the risk of getting shingles infections and also decreases the risk of recurrence if you have already have had shingles (see section on shingles for discussion of the types of shingles vaccines available).

The Conventional Approaches
Medications are the first choice of treatment in conventional medicine. Carbamazepine (Tegretol, Carbatrol) is the most commonly prescribed, followed by oxcarbazepine. Baclofen is a muscle relaxant that is sometimes used with carbamazepine if not helpful

alone. Other drugs used include lamotrigine (Lamictal), gabapentin (Neurontin), and pregabalin (Lyrica). Occasionally, clonazepam (Klonopin) is used. All of these except Baclofen and Klonopin are primarily antiseizure medications.

Important note: You should understand that all these medications may work initially but lose their effectiveness over the long term. *Warning*: Recently, the FDA warned that antiseizure medications may cause an increased risk of suicidal ideation.

Tricyclic antidepressants (amitriptyline) may help up to two-thirds of patients but must be started within three months to a year, or they won't be effective. Amitriptyline can have severe side effects in the elderly, and other tricyclics (desiprimine, nortriptyline) are preferred.

Botulinum toxin (Botox) has also been used for neuralgias, but there are no good studies, and benefits are variable, ranging from five weeks to six months.

There are also several conventional drug **topical pain solutions** that can give you temporary relief. These include some of the above drugs that have been made into a solution. An intranasal spray containing lidocaine may help trigeminal neuralgia as a branch of that nerve passes near the nose.

Lidocaine patches (Lidoderm) are also commonly prescribed to control pain and can be obtained as generics.

The medications of last resort are **narcotics**, which are only indicated for severe, unrelenting neuralgia that has not responded to any other treatments. They are used only to control your pain but are highly addictive and have many side effects. They vary in potency from hydrocodone to oxycodone to morphine to fentanyl. Your use of these drugs should be monitored by a specialist in pain management.

There are several **injections** that may provide relief, although they are not without side effects:

- *Alcohol injections* may offer temporary pain relief by numbing the areas for weeks or months. Because the pain relief isn't permanent, you may need repeated injections or a different procedure.
- *Glycerol injections* (percutaneous glycerol rhizotomy [PGR]) are another option. After three or four hours, the glycerol damages the nerve and blocks pain signals. Initially, PGR relieves pain in most people. It works in about 85 percent of people, but you can have a recurrence of pain, and many people experience facial numbness or tingling when used in trigeminal neuralgia.

Surgery is another option, especially if drugs do not work or have significant side effects. Surgery is done primarily for trigeminal neuralgia, but *not for postherpetic neuralgia*. The usual goal of surgical procedures is to either damage or destroy the part of the nerve that is the source of your pain. Because the success of these procedures depends on damaging the nerve, numbness of varying degree is a common side effect. These procedures include:

- *Microvascular decompression* (MVD) doesn't damage or destroy part of the trigeminal nerve. Instead, MVD involves relocating or removing blood vessels that are in contact with the nerve and separating the nerve root and blood vessels with a small pad. This is the gold standard among surgical options. However, it is the most invasive of all surgeries (requires opening the skull) but also offers the lowest probability that pain will return. While MVD has a high success rate, it also carries risks. There are small chances of decreased hearing, facial weakness, facial numbness, double vision, and even a stroke or death. The risk of facial numbness is less with MVD than with procedures that involve damaging the trigeminal nerve.
- *Balloon compression* successfully controls pain in most people, at least for a while. Most people undergoing this method experience facial numbness of varying degrees, and more than half experience nerve damage resulting in a temporary or permanent weakness of the muscles used to chew.
- *Electric current*: A procedure called percutaneous stereotactic radiofrequency thermal rhizotomy (*PSRTR*) selectively destroys nerve fibers associated with pain. Numbness is a common side effect of this type of treatment. Although it provides relief in almost all patients (90 percent), you can have sensation loss, weakness, and eye sensitivity, and the pain can return after six months in 20–30 percent of patients.
- *Severing the nerve*: A procedure called partial sensory rhizotomy (*PSR*) involves cutting part of the trigeminal nerve at the base of your brain. This procedure usually is helpful, but almost always causes facial numbness and it's possible for pain to recur. If your doctor doesn't find an artery or vein in contact with the trigeminal nerve, he or she won't be able to perform an MVD (above), and a PSR may be done instead.

Radiation: Gamma-knife radiosurgery (GKR) involves delivering a focused high dose of radiation to the root of the trigeminal nerve. The radiation damages the trigeminal nerve and may reduce or eliminate the pain. Relief isn't immediate, but it gives 70 percent of patients complete relief after one year. However, after five to six years, only 56 percent of patients still have complete or partial relief.

The Alternative Approaches

Acupuncture is the best treatment for all types of neuralgia as it has a high success rate, is noninvasive, and has no side effects. You should notice improvement within six acupuncture treatments (often sooner) but might need additional sessions for maximum benefit. For trigeminal neuralgia, there are auricular (ear) points that can be stimulated. Press tacks (which stay in the ear for up to two weeks) can be placed in these points as well. Because acupuncture addresses the underlying cause, it can provide long-term relief.

Low level energy laser ("cold" laser or *LLEL)* may also be very effective, appearing to reduce inflammation, heal the nerves, and give long-lasting pain relief. These lasers are called "cold" lasers because they do not produce heat like the hot lasers used in surgical procedures. You should notice improvement within two to six treatments (two to three weeks). The laser can be used with acupuncture for better, faster results (see chapter 4 for more detailed discussion). Because LLEL addresses the underlying cause, it can also provide long-term relief.

Chinese herbal formulas can speed up the healing and rebalancing process. With *Qi Ye Lian* (orally), you should observe initial benefits within one to two weeks, but you may need to take it longer for complete relief. Topically, you can use *Bao Zhen Gao*, but this should not be used in inflamed conditions. Another excellent Chinese herb topical is *Zheng Gu Shui*.

Topical pain-relieving creams or lotions can be used for temporary relief. Natural topicals include EMU oil (usually with aloe vera and MSM), long crystal menthol, Biofreeze, capsaicin, Topricin (homeopathic cream), and other herbal combinations. These topicals should give you pain relief in just a few minutes. They don't cure the underlying causes of pain, but they may provide pain relief for two to eight hours or longer and have minimal side effects (skin allergy or sensitivity are the most common).

A **homeopathic remedy**, Hypericum 30c, can be used to help reduce nerve and/ or phantom pain.

Certain **nutritional supplements** that may be beneficial include B_{12} injections, L-lysine (500 mg two to three times daily), B-complex, and/or fish oil.

Your Empowered Patient Action Plan for Treating Neuralgias

Step #1: Apply EMU oil, long crystal menthol, Biofreeze, capsaicin, or prescription compounds to the painful area for temporary relief if the above steps have not helped or with those treatments.

Step #2: Undergo acupuncture for long-term resolution of all types of neuralgia. This is the most cost-effective treatment available and most successful.

Earl had trigeminal neuralgia for several years. He had tried numerous medications and had even undergone surgical intervention, but the pain returned. Because he lived over two hundred miles away, I placed press tacks in the trigeminal acupuncture area of both ears. These completely relieved his pain. He returned on two more occasions (three weeks apart) to have them replaced, but after that his pain went away for good.

Step #3: Receive LLEL treatment if symptoms do not improve or use it with acupuncture if available.

Step #4: Take the Chinese herbal remedy Shoa Yao Gan Cao Tang along with acupuncture.

Step #5: Take non-narcotic prescription medications to help control the pain temporarily if you are still suffering.

Although the sores from a shingles outbreak healed after a few months, Margaret continued to have severe pain in her face and chest (where the outbreaks occurred). She had seen several doctors, who had prescribed Tegretol, Neurontin, and Elavil, none of which helped. The pain was so severe that she felt like it wasn't worth living anymore. Surgery had been recommended and she was considering it but wanted to try alternative methods first. I gave her an herbal topical, which gave her temporary relief for four to six hours. I then gave her the Chinese herbal formula Shoa Yao Gan Cao Tang, and also performed acupuncture, which started working almost immediately. She only needed 5 acupuncture sessions to completely end her pain.

Step #6: Take prescription amitriptyline to help control the pain if the above steps have not helped.

Step #7: Take prescription narcotics if severe pain continues despite the above steps.

Step #8: Undergo surgical intervention as a last resort. The choice is dependent on the skill of the doctor and the various side effects and other risks.

Expected Outcome

Neuralgias can be very severe and difficult to treat. With the use of alternative methods, however, most people may obtain complete resolution without necessitating drugs or surgery.

Neuromas

What You Need to Know

Many people think of a neuroma as a nerve tumor, but in actuality, it is a thickening of the nerve caused by abnormal compression and irritation of the nerve. It is usually located between the third and fourth toes but can occur between other toes and the forefoot as well.

Often, other foot symptoms (primarily pain or numbness) may preceed the development of neuromas because of abnormalities in the structure of your foot. Your foot may be able to compensate for these problems initially but as you get older, the symptoms can become manifest. It is advised that you see a podiatrist or an orthopedist specializing in foot conditions to evaluate and correct any structural abnormalities.

The Preventive Approaches

The primary way to prevent neuromas is to *avoid activities that cause them*. This includes not wearing high-heeled, tight, or ill-fitting shoes or those that have a tapered toe box. High-impact athletics activities, including jogging or any repetitive trauma to your feet, can also cause them.

The Conventional Approaches

Most conservative conventional methods may not work well for neuromas. Some of these include:

- *Padding techniques* that provide support for the arch and can decrease the compression on the nerve may help in some cases.
- *Icing* reduces swelling but does not resolve the neuroma.
- *Orthotics* to support your arch may help but can be very expensive and work only in a minority of people. Often, less expensive OTC orthotics may work just as well as prescription orthotics (although they don't help much, either).

NSAIDs (such as naproxen [Naprosyn], meloxicam [Mobic], piroxicam [Feldene], oxaprozin [Daypro], nabumatone [Relafen], ketoprofen [Orudis], diclofenac [Cataflam], diclofenac/misoprostol [Arthrotec] or celocoxib [Celebrex]) are usually prescribed and can help reduce inflammation but also do not resolve the condition. **Caution**: In July, 2015, the FDA started requiring NSAIDs to carry a warning of increased risk of heart attacks, stroke and heart failure. This is especially evident when taken long term, at higher doses, or by people with pre-existing heart disease. The risks can increase as early as the first weeks of NSAID use. However, ibuprofen and naproxen do not appear to increase the risk, so are the safest and preferred NSAIDs.

Steroid injections are also routinely done but, again, are not very successful.

Usually, **surgery** is done as a last resort. This involves removal of the tissue, including the nerve, and often results in numbness. In addition, studies show that 70 percent of the time, neuromas will return after surgery.

The Alternative Approaches

There are two alternative methods that are quite effective for resolving neuromas long-term, but most people are not aware of them as most podiatrists do not use them.

The first is **low level energy laser** ("cold" laser or *LLEL*), a device that projects "cold" light into the tissue and has been shown to reduce or eliminate scar tissue and overgrowths. It usually takes eight to twelve treatments (see chapter 4 for in-depth discussion). Because LLEL addresses the underlying cause, it can provide long-term relief.

A specific style of **acupuncture**, called Tung style, is also exceptional for neuromas and resolves them completely in most cases, usually taking six to ten sessions. Standard Chinese acupuncture or other styles may help in many cases. Because acupuncture addresses the underlying cause, it can provide long-term relief.

The laser and acupuncture can be used together for faster results, if you can find a practitioner that does both. With these two methods, neuromas usually do not regrow.

Your Empowered Patient Action Plan for Treating Neuromas

Step #1: Avoid wearing ill-fitting footwear if you are predisposed to getting foot pain.

Step #2: Undergo LLEL treatment for long-term resolution. This is the most cost-effective and successful treatment.

Step #3: Undergo acupuncture for long-term resolution. It can be used with step 2 for faster results, if available.

Margaret was a fifty-eight-year-old woman who presented with neuromas in both feet. She had used orthotics, steroid injections, and surgery on one foot, but her pain returned; and she developed numbness due to nerve damage. She did not want surgery on her other foot and elected to try Tung-style acupuncture with LLEL. After each treatment, her neuroma decreased in size; and after seven sessions, her neuroma and pain resolved completely.

Step #4: Undergo padding and/or orthotics to reduce pressure on your toes if the above steps have not helped or to correct anatomical abnormalities.

Step #5: Undergo steroid injection if you still have pain. If one does not work, do not repeat it. If it does work, avoid repetitive injections due to long-term side effects.

Step #6: Undergo surgery as a last resort if the above steps have not helped.

Expected Outcome

Neuromas are most commonly removed by surgery, which may be unsuccessful long-term in many people. With alternative methods, neuromas can be resolved long-term without the need for surgery and without risk for recurrence.

Neuropathy (Peripheral, Chemotherapy-Induced)

What You Need to Know

Peripheral neuropathy is a degeneration of the nerves in your limbs, particularly the feet but sometimes the hands. When it occurs, it usually starts at the toes or fingers and spreads up the lower legs or arms, usually stopping at the level of your knees or elbows. If you have pain above these areas or shooting pain down your arms or legs, it is most likely a different condition.

It is unknown how many patients have peripheral neuropathy, but the incidence increases with advancing age. There are many known causes of neuropathy; B_{12} deficiency and autoimmune diseases can cause neuropathies and need to be addressed to lessen the symptoms. Other causes of neuropathy include alcohol abuse, as a side effect of certain chemotherapy drugs, and as a consequence of diabetes (see section *Complications of Diabetes*).

However, the cause of other neuropathies may not be known (called idiopathic), although it may be caused by environmental toxins. Peripheral neuropathy can be a progressive disease, gradually worsening, and can cause secondary problems with balance and the development of wounds due to numbness.

Treatments for Neuropathy

The Preventive Approaches

The best way to prevent peripheral neuropathy is to **avoid toxins** that may cause neuropathy, including overuse of alcohol. Unfortunately, most toxins that cause neuropathy are unknown, or you may not be aware of exposure.

Correctable causes: Some *medications* can cause neuropathy: These include amiodarone (heart), colchicine (gout), hydralazine (BP), nitrofurantoin (antibiotic), and metronidazole (Flagyl [antibiotic]). *Diseases*, especially diabetes, must be well controlled to help prevent neuropathy.

Eating a healthy **diet** that's rich in fruits, vegetables, whole grains, and lean protein may also help prevent neuropathy or reduce the symptoms. Some vitamins, especially B_{12}, are most important for maintaining nerve function. The best food sources of B vitamins are meats, fish, eggs, low-fat dairy foods, and fortified cereals. If you're a strict vegetarian, fortified cereals are a good source of vitamin B_{12} for you, but you may also want to talk to your doctor about B_{12} supplements. If you are B_{12} deficient (determined by a blood test), you may not be able to absorb B_{12} from your stomach, but other forms are available, including intramuscular injection and sublingual (under the tongue).

As much as possible, avoid repetitive motions, cramped positions, and toxic chemicals, all of which may cause more nerve damage.

The Conventional Approaches

Medications are the principal conventional treatments for neuropathy. *Gabapentin* (Neurontin), *pregabalin* (Lyrica), or *topiramate* (Topamax) are the primary drugs used and may reduce symptoms to acceptable levels, but they also may have intolerable side effects at higher doses (e.g., drowsiness, fatigue, dizziness). In addition, they may only be effective only in about 15 percent of patients. *Warning*: These drugs may cause increased suicidal ideation in some people.

Other medications that may be used for neuropathic pain include low-dose amitriptyline (25–50 mg per day), serotonin-noradrenaline reuptake inhibitors, nortriptyline, ketamine, amantadine, orphenadrine, haloperidol, carbamazepine, valproic acid, phenytoin, mexilitene, baclofen, prazosin, baclofen, and nifidepine. A recent study from *Lancet* showed that the combination of nortrityline and gabapentin decreased pain more than either alone. These drugs can be given orally or by injection or, in some, sublingually (under the tongue), rectally, nasally, and buccally (dissolves in your cheek). Most of these drugs should reduce pain in one to three weeks, if they are beneficial.

Thyroid Drug May Help Neuropathy?

Research done in 2006 showed that Cytomel, a drug used to treat hypothyroidism, is also effective at regenerating damaged peripheral nerves. This has only been tested on animals and not on humans.

Many physicians prescribe **topicals** made from conventional drugs and mixed in a gel that is absorbed into the soft tissues. The topical forms of these drugs usually don't have the side effects that can occur if you take them orally. Drugs that can be made into topical include gabapentin (Neurontin), amitriptyline, baclofen, ketamine, ketoprofen, and others. There is now a pharmaceutical 8 percent capsaicin patch called Qutenza, which can provide pain relief for up to three months; studies show a greater than 30 percent decrease in pain reduction at each week during the three-month period. However, this patch can cause significant burning when applied.

Transcutaneous electrostimulation is sometimes successful in relieving some of the pain associated with neuropathy. This method is performed by registered physical therapists under prescription from your doctor

Other electrical devices include *H-wave* and the *Rebuilder*, which use different frequencies of sound than TENS units and are also more effective. You can purchase a home unit.

The Alternative Approaches

Acupuncture may be the best method for reducing the symptoms of neuropathy, although it may only work in 50 percent of patients with *idiopathic* peripheral neuropathy. However, for diabetic neuropathy or that caused by chemotherapy, the success rate is much greater. If it is beneficial, you should notice improvement within one to eight acupuncture treatments, but you might need additional sessions for maximum benefits. Because acupuncture addresses the underlying cause, it can provide long-term relief.

Low level energy laser ("cold" laser or *LLEL)* has also been found to be as good as acupuncture in reducing or resolving neuropathy caused by diabetes or chemotherapy. It may take two to eight treatments to obtain the maximum benefit and has few to no side effects. Because LLEL addresses the underlying cause, it can provide long-term relief.

Chinese herbal formulas such as *Zuo Gu Shen, Jing San*, and *Xiao Huo Luo Dan Wan* can be used, depending on your pulse/tongue diagnosis.

Infrasound, the use of low-frequency sound, has been found to help reduce symptoms and can be used with acupuncture or LLEL. It can be used in a sweeping motion down the legs and/or over specific acupuncture points. Infrasound works by increasing the local circulation of blood and lymph and the activity of the nervous system to accelerate the healing process. It can not only reduce pain but also decrease spasms and swelling. Numerous chiropractors, naturopaths and acupuncturists and a few doctors use infrasound.

There are a number of **nutritional supplements** that have been shown to interfere with the underlying mechanisms of a variety of forms of neuropathy:

- *Gamma linoleic acid* may help reduce pain in some patients. The best source of GLA is borage oil (1,500 mg daily). It may take two months to observe benefits.
- *Acetyl-L-carnitine* (500–1,000 mg daily) is known to have neuroprotective properties and has been shown to yield significant reductions in pain. Two

studies found that acetyl-L-carnitine can limit the neuropathy associated with some chemotherapy drugs, and other studies have shown indications that it can improve diabetic-induced neuropathy.

- *Alpha lipoic acid* (600–800 mg daily) is a powerful antioxidant that has also been shown to reduce the pain associated with diabetic and chemotherapy-induced neuropathy as and sometimes complete regression of neuropathic symptoms.
- *N-acetylcysteine* is another powerful antioxidant. Animal studies have shown that it can inhibit diabetic neuropathy and protect against neuropathies caused by chemotherapy drugs.
- *Curcumin* has been shown to relieve neuropathy symptoms in a study of inherited peripheral neuropathies. It has also shown promise in animal studies of diabetic neuropathy.
- *Vitamin B$_1$* (thiamin) and *benfotiamine* (the fat-soluble form of vitamin B$_1$) have shown a decrease in pain when combined with vitamin B$_6$ and vitamin B$_{12}$. It also has been used effectively to treat alcoholic and diabetic neuropathies.
- *Vitamin B$_6$* (100 mg two to three times daily) for two months can help decrease symptoms of neuropathy.
- *Vitamin E* with mixed tocopherols and tocotrienols (400 IU daily) has been shown to reduce platinum-induced (chemotherapy) neuropathy (i.e., Cisplatin or carboplatin).

Medical Marijuana and Derivatives May Be Helpful

As of March, 2015, twenty-three states and the District of Columbia had medical marijuana laws in place. These laws allow the use of marijuana for a variety of medical conditions, which vary among the states. However, it is approved in most of these states for treating neuropathic pain and chronic pain, as well as pain and spasticity in multiple sclerosis. There is high-quality research evidence to support this use.

There are some extracts and a spray being used in other countries but they have not been approved in the US. However, marijuana itself is more potent, being comprised of more than 400 compounds, of which 70 are cannabinoids. Cannabinoids appear to be the active compounds and have individual, interactive and entourage effects (entourage means that a compound has an effect only in the presence of other compounds).

Although medical marijuana may be beneficial, you can develop a tolerance requiring higher doses and may also have withdrawal symptoms. It may also interfere with the action of opioid medications for pain, which are commonly prescribed to chronic pain patients. Approximately 1 out of 10 people will develop an addiction to marijuana. It should be avoided in patients with psychoses such as schizophrenia and bipolar disorder. It is usually indicated if you have chronic pain that has not been responsive to other medications or are limited due to intolerable side effects.

There are also natural **topical pain-relieving creams** or lotions that may provide temporary relief. Natural topicals include the Chinese topical Zheng Gu Shui, EMU oil (usually with aloe vera and MSM), long crystal menthol, Biofreeze, capsaicin, Topricin cream (homeopathic), and other herbal combinations. Some topicals may work better than others, so you may have to try several to find the best one. You can also mix several different topicals together for better results. These topicals should provide you with pain relief in just a few minutes. In my clinic, I applied samples to my patients so they'd know if a product worked before purchasing it. Encourage your doctor or practitioner to do the same. They don't cure the underlying problem, but they may provide pain relief for two to eight hours or longer and have minimal side effects (skin allergy or sensitivity are the most common).

Your Empowered Patient Action Plan for Treating Neuropathy

Step #1: Undergo acupuncture for long-term relief. This is the most cost-effective treatment available.

Step #2: Use the LLEL for long-term relief. It can be used alone or with acupuncture for faster results.

Regina had progressive neuropathy for ten years, with constant pain and numbness in both legs that became worse at night. She was taking large doses of neurontin (2,400 mg per day), which helped somewhat but caused fatigue and drowsiness. I started her on acupuncture. She required about twelve treatments but was able to decrease the dose of her neurontin to 300 mg daily. I added cold laser, and after five treatments, her neuropathy was resolved.

Step #3: Use H-wave stimulation or the Rebuilder if the above steps have not helped.

Step #4: Use infrasound for long-term relief. This method can be used with acupuncture and laser for faster results.

*Step #5: **Apply EMU oil, long crystal menthol, Biofreeze, Topricin cream (homeo-pathic), and/or capsaicin** to the painful areas for temporary relief if the above steps have not been beneficial.*

*Step #6: **Take various nutritional supplements,** either alone or in combinations, if the above steps have not reduced your symptoms. Give each one to two months to work before trying another.*

*Step #7: **Apply prescription topical compounds** if you are still suffering from neuro-pathic pain.*

*Step #8: **Try appropriate prescription medications** to control pain if still present.*

Expected Outcome

Peripheral neuropathy of unknown cause is a difficult condition to resolve, but symp-toms can be reduced using the above methods. However, neuropathy caused by che-motherapy and diabetes may respond very well—and quickly—to acupuncture and/or LLEL. Overall, several methods, both conventional and alternative, can significantly reduce symptoms and improve quality of life for all types of neuropathy.

Osteoporosis

What You Need to Know

Osteoporosis is the thinning and weakening of your bones. Osteopenia is sometimes confused with osteoporosis, but it represents only the initial stages of bone loss and may not progress to osteoporosis in many cases.

Dr. A's Suggestions:
Don't Treat Osteopenia

You should understand that although osteopenia does not always progress to osteoporosis, many doctors and the pharmaceutical companies that manufac-ture drugs for osteoporosis recommend taking these drugs at this stage. *Studies show that you do not need these drugs if you have osteopenia, so don't waste your money.*

Women account for 80 percent of the osteoporosis diagnoses, but that means that 20 percent of men will also have this condition, which is often overlooked. Men tend to develop osteoporosis about ten years later than women because they have larger bones, and it comes on more gradually. Caucasian men at sixty years of age have a 29 percent chance of experiencing a fracture during their remaining lifetime, so it is advisable for men as well as women to undergo osteoporosis testing if they have increased risk factors (chart see below).

Factors in Men Increasing Risk of Osteoporosis

Age > 70   Body-mass index < 25 (thin)
Recent weight loss > 10%   Physical inactivity
Corticosteroid use   Testosterone treatment
Previous fragility fracture   Loop diuretic treatment for hypertension

---

When osteoporosis was first thought to be a condition that needed treatment, doctors focused on correcting the amount of bone (*quantity*). More recently, many experts have become more concerned with bone fractures and preventing them by improving the *quality* or strength of the bone. The reason this is important is that treatment is based primarily on a test of bone mineral density (BMD), but this test (DEXA scan) cannot be totally relied upon to prevent fractures. The DEXA scan uses what is called a T-score to determine how thin the bones are; normal should be below negative 1.0 (- 0.1). However, it is known that some people with T-scores greater than negative 3.5 (- 3.5) (severe osteoporosis) will never have a fracture, and others will fracture at a T-score of -1.0. In other words, improving BMD may not reflect the change in bone *quality*.

Even so, most doctors still focus only on quantity of bone and not quality or strength of the bone. As the main goal of treating osteoporosis is to prevent fractures and bone density testing may not always predict the exact risk, it is helpful to use better tools to predict your fracture risk before beginning treatment. There is now a web-based calculator for predicting your ten-year fracture risk, which is more accurate. Women should undergo treatment if their risk is high (greater than 20 percent). To find your risk free of charge, go to: www.apps.sbgh.mb.ca/bmd-web-calculator/calculator.action. You can also use the FRAX (WHO Fracture Risk Assessment Tool): www.shef.ac.uk/FRAX/ and go to "calculation tool." You should especially check your risk if you have some of the factors listed below.

Risk Factors for Bone Fractures*

Increasing age
Any fracture over age fifty-four
White race
Sedentary lifestyle
Current smoking
Treatment for diabetes
Bariatric (weight loss) surgery

Relatively greater height
Relatively lighter weight
Fair to poor self-reported health
Parental hip fracture
Current steroid use
History of falls

It is very important to treat osteoporosis if your fracture risk is high because fractures caused by it, especially in the hip and spine, increase the risk of premature death. This excess risk occurs regardless of location or severity of fracture and can persist for several years after hip fracture.

You should also realize that an abnormal bone density does not necessarily mean you have osteoporosis. There can be other reasons for low bone density, such as gastric bypass, kidney disease, or transplantation. Several clues to another diagnosis include a family history of kidney stones, unexplained anemia, thyroid disease, an unexplained change in blood pressure, frequent loose stools, and disturbances of phosphate or calcium.

Repeat Testing for Bone-Density: How Frequent?

Most doctors repeat bone density screening every year while you are undergoing treatment, but this is not necessary for many women. A recent study in *JW General Medicine* and the *NEJM* showed the following:

- For women with normal bone-density scores (T-score of -1.49 or better), repeat testing in ten to fifteen years appears appropriate.
- Women with T-scores of -1.50 to -1.99 (moderate osteopenia) can be tested every four to five years
- Women with T-scores between -2.00 to -2.49 (advanced osteopenia) should be tested yearly.

Note: Medicare and most insurance companies reimburse for DEXA every two years if medically necessary.

Treatments for Osteoporosis

The Preventive Approaches

Correctible causes: First, you need to look at any *medications* you are taking as many can cause osteoporosis (see chart below). If you are taking these medications and have osteoporosis, you may need to take another medication or use a different method if possible. If you are diabetic, thiazolidinedione (TZD) drugs (Avandia and Actos) increase fracture risk, and other antidiabetic drugs should be considered instead.

Medications That Can Cause Osteoporosis

SSRI antidepressants

Oral anticoagulants (warfarin)

Excessive thyroid medications

Antiretroviral drugs (AIDS)

Proton pump inhibitors (PPIs)

Loop diuretics (water pills like Lasix)

Lupron (given for prostate cancer, endometriosis)

Breast-cancer drugs (aromatase inhibitors)

Antiseizure medications

Steroids

Aluminum containing antacids

Steroid inhalers

Immunosuppressive drugs

Depression May Contribute to Osteoporosis

Antidepressants can cause bone loss, but just being depressed causes certain biochemical reactions in the body that can also cause bone loss. If you are depressed, and especially if you are taking an antidepressant, you may need to check your BMD earlier and more often.

Medications that help: On the other hand, however, certain medications typically prescribed for other diseases can *reduce* bone loss, including thiazide diuretics for swelling or hypertension and statins for high cholesterol. These are preferred medications to take if you have these diseases and have osteoporosis as well.

Poor lifestyle habits, including smoking, excessive alcohol use, excessive caffeine intake, inadequate exercise, and low calcium intake also induce bone loss, so reversing these factors can help prevent osteoporosis.

Diet: Vegetarians have a lower risk of osteoporosis in the later decades of life, so increased intake of vegetables is recommended for helping prevent and treat osteoporosis, especially vitamin K–rich foods such as broccoli, spinach, and other green, leafy vegetables. Dairy products and calcium-fortified juices and cereals are important sources of calcium and vitamin D. For those who are lactose intolerant, almond milk and whole almonds are another great source of calcium. Long-term tea drinkers have been found to have greater bone density than nondrinkers.

Cod-Liver Oil May Weaken Bones

A Norwegian study of middle aged women showed that those who took cod liver oil were twice as likely to have low bone mass as those who didn't. Several studies have corroborated this. The cause is a very high level of vitamin A, which is not found in other fish oil supplements—or in fish, for that matter.

Important Note: Most consumers think that taking *supplemental* calcium and vitamin D will *prevent* fractures, but a recent study revealed that taking these supplements alone does not reduce the risk of bone fractures in healthy, asymptomatic people and is recommended against taking by the USP-STF. In fact, vitamin D as well as calcium do not increase bone-mineral density to any important degree (see "Alternative Approaches" for more information). Again, obtain these minerals from diet if at all possible for prevention purposes.

Important Information
Calcium in Fortified Foods: Are They Worth It?

Many foods and drinks are now fortified with calcium and marketed to improve bone strength. These can vary from soy milk to energy bars. Will these foods supply enough calcium?

In fact, calcium in fortified food acts as a supplement, not like the food. In addition, the amount of calcium in these foods is variable, and some forms of calcium may not be absorbed as well as others. You also need to look at the label to make sure you are not getting too much calcium.

There have been studies on orange juice showing that, when fortified, the calcium does get utilized as much as from milk, but other foods have not been well studied.

Carbonation May Cause Bone Loss

Several studies have demonstrated that women who drink more carbonated drinks increase their risk of osteoporosis. In the Nurse's Health Study, it was found that for each twelve ounces of soda, there was a 14 percent increase in risk fracture. Although it is not known why this occurs, it may be because the sodas simply replace more nutritious drinks that contain beneficial elements such as calcium. Although the American Beverage Association disputes these studies, if you have osteoporosis, it is better to drink healthy drinks in place of carbonated soft drinks.

Weight loss/dieting: If you undergo bariatric weight loss surgery, this can cause malabsorption and secondary bone loss. Postmenopausal women who diet (calorie restriction) may have an increased loss of bone mass. This effect is more pronounced if you are on estrogen and discontinue it. Exercise that results in weight loss, however, has no negative effect on bone mass.

Exercise: One of the most important methods for preventing osteoporosis is exercise. Weight-bearing (resistance) exercises are recommended because they stress the bone, which stimulates new bone formation. I recommend exercises such as walking, running, tennis, stair climbing, and weight lifting. Exercises such as swimming and bicycling are not helpful for osteoporosis, because they do not provide enough stress on the bones. You should exercise for at least thirty minutes on a daily basis.

The Conventional Approaches

Some Doctors Not Following Guidelines for Osteoporosis

A study in *Menopause* (October 2011) revealed that many doctors are not following guidelines for either screening or treating women with osteoporosis. In the study, 41 percent of women who were screened should not have been screened, 35 percent of women who should have been prescribed medications did not receive treatment, and 18 percent of women who did not meet criteria for osteoporosis received therapy anyway.

Screening for osteoporosis should not be initiated until age sixty-five (unless high risk or early menopause), and women should be considered for treatment if they have osteoporosis and are at elevated risk, not if they have osteopenia or are at low risk.

Medications are the mainstay of osteoporosis treatment in conventional medicine. The primary drugs used are called *bisphosphonates* (Alendronate [Fosamax], risedronate [Actonel], ibandronate [Boniva], teriparatide [Forteo], zoledronic acid [Reclast/Zometa]), which help prevent bone loss (antiresorptive therapy). What they *don't* do is make new bone. Studies show that they can reduce fracture risk up to 50 percent. Some bisphosphonates can be taken monthly, and zoledronic acid can be taken intravenously once a year, which has a distinct advantage for those who forget easily. Zoledronic acid can be obtained as a generic. It can also reduce further hip fractures after already having one. Risedronate will become a generic in 2014.

You must remain upright for at least thirty minutes to one hour after taking these medications, or they may not be effective. A study in the *American Journal of Medicine* showed that people are more likely to adhere to weekly or monthly dosing than daily dosing. ***Important note***: A study at Cornell University revealed that bisphosphonates are much more effective if your vitamin D blood levels are above 33 ng/ml.

Zoledronic acid is also indicated for multiple myeloma and metastatic cancer to bone, but some doctors are using it off-label because it needs only two injections a year for osteoporosis. It reduces risk fracture in the hip by 41 percent and in the spine by 77 percent. However, it can cause several side effects and does not have a great advantage over the other medications.

Important Information:
Beware Side Effects and Long-Term Problems of Bisphosphonates

Increasingly, some potentially harmful side effects of bisphosphonates have been noted. First, bisphosphonates may cause severe and sometimes incapacitating *musculoskeletal pain*, which most doctors may not recognize and thus seek other causes. This can develop within days, months, or even years of starting treatment.

In addition, recent studies have shown that alendronate (Fosamax) doubles the risk of atrial fibrillation, a heart arrhythmia, in older women. The other bisphosphonates have not been studied in regard to this condition but may also have this effect.

In long-term users of bisphosphonates (over five years), *atypical fractures* may occur in the leg bones (femur), although this is uncommon.

Another less common side effect is *osteonecrosis* (bone death) of the jaw. This occurs primarily with people taking IV bisphosphonates for cancer (multiple myeloma) but can occur occasionally if taking oral bisphosphonates long-term (1 in 1,700 people). In fact, most dentists will not provide a dental procedure if a patient is on bisphosphonates for more than three years because such procedures may *initiate* osteonecrosis. In such cases, patients should discontinue bisphosphonates three months before oral surgery and restart only after bone healing has occurred.

Many experts are concerned that taking bisphosphonates for more than three to five years may decrease bone strength by suppressing bone turnover. In fact, a recent report published in the *JAMA* revealed that prolonged use of bisphosphonates increase the risk of low-energy fractures of the upper leg bone and hip bone.

In addition, a recent study published in *BMJ* found that bisphosphonates are associated with an increased risk of esophageal cancer. The study found that the increased risk was 30 percent and mainly found in people taking more than ten medications.

Recent guidelines have been issued for determining long-term use of biphosphonates. It is recommended that physicians reassess a woman's fracture risk after 5 years of oral biphosphonates or 3 years of IV therapy, then:

- For women at high risk (low T score, previous fracture history), oral thrapy can be continued for 10 years or IV therapy for 6 years. Fracture risk should be reassessed every 2-3 years.
- For women at low risk after theray, treatment can be stopped, but fracture risk should be reassessed periodically (see above).

Should Not Routinely Receive Biphosphonates

A study presented at the 2015 meeting of the American Academy of Orthopedic Surgeons evaluated whether elderly women who had sustained a wrist fracture should be given biphosphonates to prevent subsequent hip fractures.

Results indicated that taking biphosphonates would reduce hip fractures by 25% but this would cost $200,000 per prevented fracture. In addition, expanded biphosphonate use could cause an additional 20,000 atypical femur (thigh bone) fractures, thus negating any benefits. Recommendations were against using biphosphonates in such cases.

Important Information:
Bisphosphonates Not Beneficial for Other Causes of Fractures

According to various studies, if you are at increased fracture risk due to factors other than low BMD (see risk factors above), bisphosphonates alone will *not* decrease your risk of hip fractures.

Other medications: Another antiresorptive medication is *Evista*, which is a synthetic estrogen that doesn't increase breast cancer risk. It also decreases fracture risk by 50 percent, but only vertebral (spine) fractures, not hip fractures.

Should You Take Estrogen to Prevent Osteoporosis?

For years, doctors have recommended taking estrogen replacement after menopause, one reason being to reduce bone loss. A large study, the WHI, revealed that estrogen does not significantly prevent osteoporosis and its potential harm outweighs its benefits for this disease. Evista is the only estrogen that has been shown to reduce osteoporosis.

If antiresorptive therapy doesn't help or side effects occur (primarily GI upset), most doctors may prescribe *calcitonin-salmon*, which is given through nasal spray. Calcitonin is a hormone made by the thyroid gland that both prevents bone loss and makes new bone. It is commonly used if you have had a fracture because it also helps reduce pain while your fracture is healing. **Caution**: Calcitonin does have a number of side effects, can cause allergic reactions, and is expensive, which is why it is not a first-line treatment. **Warning**: FDA advisors recommend against the use of calcitonin-salmon because the potential cancer risks outweigh the benefits, and questions remain about whether the therapy is effective in reducing fractures.

For women who have had bone fractures from osteoporosis, your doctor may prescribe daily injections of *parathyroid hormone* (PTH, a natural hormone that regulates calcium in the body) to increase bone density and help prevent future fractures. Like the above drugs, PTH decreases fracture risk by 50 percent, even though it increases BMD twice as much as the above medications. It has been shown to reduce the incidence of spine fractures, but not hip fractures. PTH does improve both bone quantity and quality, but is very expensive ($10,000 per year), requires daily injections, and few insurance companies pay for it. After taking PTH for eighteen to twenty months, you must take a bisphosphonate, or you will lose most of the benefits of PTH.

A study published in *JAMA* in February 2011 showed that *nitroglycerin ointment* (15 mg per day) can produce a modest increase in bone mineral density and decrease bone resorption. Nitroglycerin is known to stimulate bone formation and inhibit bone resorption.

Denosumab (Prolia) has now been approved by the FDA for the prevention of fracture in postmenopausal women with osteoporosis and high fracture risk (i.e., have had fracture or failed other treatments.) It is given as an injection twice a year, with a cost of $825 per injection. Adverse effects include pain in muscles and extremities, high cholesterol, and bladder infection. A higher dose version of desonumab (Xgeva) is used for metastatic cancer to the bones and can help slow progression as well as decrease pain.

Important Information
Combination of Drugs Not Necessary

As each type of medication for osteoporosis appears to reduce fracture risk, you might think that combining them would decrease the risk even more, but this is not so. The effects of these drugs are not additive, even though many doctors commonly prescribe several together if your osteoporosis does not respond to a single agent.

In addition, understand that the benefit of treatment using any of these drugs may take eighteen to twenty-four months, so more frequent testing is unnecessary and will just lead to increasing dosages or adding other medications.

Adherence to Taking Osteoporosis Medications Poor

A recent study in *Mayo Clinic Proceedings* demonstrated that one-third to one-half of osteoporosis patients do not take their medication as directed. Nonadherence usually occurs shortly after starting the medication. There may be many reasons for this, including cost and side effects.

A **vibration platform** is a new conventional therapy that uses high-frequency sound waves to increase bone mass. It has not yet been approved.

The Alternative Approaches

The **supplements** calcium (800–1,200 mg daily), magnesium (400–800 mg daily), and vitamin D (800–2,000 mg daily, depending on baseline levels; low-sunlight areas may need to take 1,200 mg daily) have long been recommended to prevent and treat osteoporosis. A recent study published in the *Annals of Internal Medicine* revealed that low blood levels of vitamin D definitely increase the risk of hip fractures, so you should undergo a blood test for vitamin D and supplement if it is below 20–25 ng/ml (many naturopathic physicians think that the optimal range is around 50, and as high as 80 if you have heart disease or cancer: above 100 is dangerous). *Important Note*: As mentioned previously, studies show that vitamin D *alone* does not prevent fractures in healthy people, but does if you have osteoporosis and take it with calcium. That being said, studies have now shown that neither vitamin D nor calcium increases BMD to any degree (see sidebar below).

Cautions: *High-dose* intermittent vitamin D as standard replacement may increase the risk of falls and fractures and other side effects. This includes monthly 50,000 IU, but some doctors prescribe it weekly, which may be indicated if you are very deficient or don't absorb it well. A common dose is 2000 IU to 5000 IU daily. Remember to use the D_3 form, not the D_2 form, and to check blood levels if you take the high dose form (see chapter 2 for details).

Important note: Chelated forms and coral calcium are commonly marketed as superior products, but no scientific proof has supported this contention, and they are much more expensive. They may offer no advantage over cheaper forms of calcium.

Do You Really Need Calcium for Bone Health?

As mentioned above, it has long been standard practice to prescribe calcium to protect your bones from osteoporosis and fracture. But now those recommendations are being placed in doubt, especially in light of some long-term adverse effects from taking supplemental calcium (see sidebar below).

This was confirmed by a 2015 meta-analysis in the *BMJ* showing that augmenting dietary calcium intake or taking supplements results in only small increases in BMD, which are unlikely to translate into clinically meaningful reductions in fracture incidence.

The bottom line is that you should eat a diet with the recommended daily intakes for calcium (and vitamin D), and exercise (non-aerobic) to prevent fractures, but supplementation may not be necessary.

Magnesium is also essential for bone formation, and not taking it with calcium and vitamin D can intensify the risk of heart disease. These products should be taken all together, in a form that is highly absorbable, such as citrate, tricalcium phosphate, or hydroxyapatite. Carbonate forms are probably the most commonly used but are less absorbable. Carbonate and phosphate forms should be taken with meals. However, be aware that supplemental calcium may cause harm in some patients (see sidebar below).

Dr. A's Suggestions:
Caution: Avoid Some Calcium Combinations

Several companies are now producing OTC products that contain calcium with aspirin (Bayer Women's Aspirin is an example). However, you may have to take three or four capsules a day to get the recommended calcium dosage, which then means you receive high doses of aspirin, which can cause GI problems. Taking generic aspirin and calcium separately are just as effective and much cheaper.

Vitamin K is also now being included in many supplements that contain calcium and magnesium to prevent or treat osteoporosis. Although vitamin K is a cofactor in some bone-forming processes, and low vitamin K is associated with reduced bone density and increased fracture risk, research shows conflicting evidence on its benefits for supplementation. In addition, and more importantly, vitamin K can interfere with the effects of blood-thinning medications;

so if you are on warfarin (Coumadin) or heparins, you should avoid taking these supplements or tell your doctor to monitor your blood carefully.

***

Dr. A's Suggestions:
Can Calcium Supplements Cause Increase in Heart-Attack Risk?

Recent studies have shown that calcium *supplements* may hasten atherosclerosis and death in patients with kidney failure and moderately raise the risk for cardiovascular events (primarily heart attacks) in healthy older women. A more recent study in *BMJ* showed that supplementation in women increases all-cause and heart-related mortality, and in another study in *JAMA Internal Medicine*, supplements raised the risk of heart disease in men but not women.

Many authorities state that calcium supplements have only marginal-to-modest benefits on bone density and fracture risk to begin with, so the negative effects on the heart may outweigh the benefits for osteoporosis. Based on data from a *BMJ* study, treating one thousand people with calcium supplements for five years would prevent only twenty-six fractures but would cause an additional fourteen heart attacks. However, it should be noted that there were significant limitations and possible errors in this study, and many experts disagree with these findings.

The latest research, an observational study of seventy-five thousand female nurses, published in 2014 in *Osteoporosis International*, showed that women who took 1,000 mg or more of calcium a day had a 29 percent *lower* risk of heart attack over twenty-four years.

Obtaining your calcium through diet avoids the added risk of heart disease, so that is preferred over supplementation. If you eat a diet rich in low-fat dairy products, you may not need any calcium supplementation. The studies overall show that if you take less than 1,200 mg total from both diet and supplementation, your risk of heart attack may not be elevated; so if you decide to take it, stay below that amount.

***

Strontium may be the most important alternative supplement. Strontium is an earth-based element similar to calcium. Also like calcium, it is a significant component of bone; in fact, 99.9 percent of the strontium in the body is in your bones. The STRATOS study published in 2004 in the *New England Journal of Medicine* demonstrated that strontium prevents bone loss, increases bone formation, and also strengthens the bone.

The authors stated that strontium "leads to early and sustained reductions in the risk of vertebral fractures and…may be as effective as current drug therapy without the side effects." A more recent study (2008) was the first to prove strontium reduces the risk of spine (39 percent) and hip (36 percent) fractures, and numerous studies in Europe have shown that it delays bone breakdown, promotes bone growth, and reduces hip and vertebral fractures in older women. It may be even more effective for the very elderly. The ranelate form (340 mg [active strontium] twice daily) is the one used in most studies but is not available in the United States. However, other salt forms (such as citrate) may be as beneficial. It may take three years for its full effect. Unfortunately, most doctors are not aware of strontium because it is sold OTC and not marketed by drug companies. Side effects may include diarrhea and possible blood clots or seizures, although these are rare.

Warning: The European Medicine Agency warned that strontium increases the risk for DVT (blood clots) and cardiac events, so it should not be used in patients at risk for DVT (those who are immobilized; or those with history of heart attacks, stroke, or uncontrolled high blood pressure). It also may have serious skin reactions. Be aware, however, that this is the ranelate salt, which is not used in the United States. There have not been many studies on the citrate form.

Avoid Large Amounts of Vitamin A

One supplement that should *not* be taken if you have osteoporosis in large amounts is vitamin A. This vitamin has been shown to increase the risk of fractures by weakening the bones. You should avoid taking more than 3,000 mg of vitamin A, including from multivitamins. This occurs only with preformed vitamin A: Beta-carotene, which breaks down into vitamin A, is considered the safest form and can be taken without increasing risk.

Natural progesterone (50–100 mg twice daily in oral form, 20–40 g daily if in cream) is another alternative supplement that can increase bone density in both men and women, because numerous studies reveal that it stimulates osteoblasts, the cells that make new bone. This is not the same as the *synthetic* progesterone that drug companies manufacture; the latter drugs are chemicalized, which prevent them from having the same benefit. Natural progesterone can be taken orally via capsule, by troches (which dissolve in your gums), or by topical cream. It can be found in health food stores or compounded by trained pharmacists.

Other supplements have also been shown to benefit osteoporosis. *Ipriflavone* is a synthetic isoflavone (plant estrogen, 600 mg daily) that can significantly reduce or prevent postmenopausal bone loss, especially when combined with 1,000 mg of calcium. A study performed in 1999 and published in the journal *Menopause* showed that ipriflavone both reduces bone loss and increases bone density.

In addition, a combination of *fish oil* and *evening primrose oil* when taken with calcium has been shown to decrease bone turnover and increase bone density, as reported in 2004 by the US Agency for Healthcare Research and Quality.

Your Empowered Patient Action Plan for Treating Osteoporosis

Important Note*: It is not necessary to treat osteopenia. If you have this diagnosis and do want to strengthen your bones, use Steps 1 through 4.*

Step #1: Exercise, using resistance type exercises, should be done whether you have osteoporosis or want to prevent it.

Step #2: Obtain calcium, vitamin D and magnesium through your diet. Supplements may not be necessary.

Step #3: Take strontium to increase your bone density. This is preferred over conventional drugs because it makes new bone and strengthens bone, which conventional drugs don't do. It is also much cheaper with fewer side effects. It is best to take it at least two hours away from taking calcium as the two are structurally similar and compete for absorption.

Step #4: Take ipriflavone and fish oil if your bone density has not returned to normal.

However, you can take it with Step #2.

Step #5: Take natural progesterone if you still have poor bone density. Note that men can also take this hormone.

Marilyn is a sixty-three-year-old woman who had severe osteoporosis. She had been prescribed bisphosphonates and took calcium, magnesium, and vitamin D, all which improved her bone density, but did not bring it back to normal. She also had acid reflux disease, and the bisphosphonates made her symptoms much worse, although her doctor insisted she take it anyway. One day, Marilyn slipped on ice and fell, fracturing two vertebrae in her spine. Her doctor then prescribed calcitonin, but unfortunately, another fall caused a hip fracture. Her bone density was still abnormal.

When I examined her, she admitted that she loved carbonated colas and caffeine, and I asked her to eliminate or at least decrease the amounts she drank. Because she was also having menopausal symptoms, I placed her on natural progesterone cream along with strontium and krill (fish) oil. Six months later, her bone density was much improved. She discontinued the bisphosphonates on her own due to the side effects. Another bone-density test a year later revealed only osteopenia. She has not had any further fractures.

Step #6: **Try Evista** (women only) if you are menopausal and continue to lose bone mass.

Step #7: **Take a bisphosphonate** if you still continue to have osteoporosis. Take the form that you are most likely to stay adherent with. After taking for five years, ask your doctor about discontinuing the drugs for another three to five years.

Step #8: **Try topical nitroglycerin** if you still have moderate osteoporosis.

Step #9: **Take prescription calcitonin** if you still have osteoporosis that has not responded to the above steps or you have had serious side effects with those medications.

Step #10: **Try Denosumab or zoledronic acid** if you still have poor bone density and have had fractures.

Step #11: **Take prescription parathyroid hormone injection** (PTH) if you still have osteoporosis and have had fractures.

Expected Outcome

With these steps, you should be able to reverse osteoporosis, return to normal bone mass, and prevent fractures. Just remember that although BMD may improve, that doesn't necessarily mean your fracture risk will go down.

Chronic Pain (Including Fibromyalgia)

What You Need to Know

Surveys show that 9 percent of the population suffers from moderate to severe non-cancer-related pain and that 56 percent of these patients have suffered for at least five years. (Seventy-five percent of cancer patients suffer from chronic pain). The problem is worse among elderly and chronically ill patients, with estimates of 48 to 80 percent suffering from pain.

Chronic pain can be caused by many problems, such as arthritis or injuries (see those sections), but in addition, there are generalized pain conditions such as fibromyalgia. Numerous other factors can cause pain, including various diseases (such as cancer, lupus, etc.), poor posture, and psychological problems. Chronic pain is actually a condition in itself and has specific treatments, which is why this section is included.

Pain Symptoms May Not Correlate with Physical Findings

Too often, doctors doubt that you have chronic pain of any severity because physical findings of pain from pressure (palpation) may be absent, even if you "feel" pain. Historically, when this "disconnect" has occurred, doctors think the pain is psychological.

In fact, psychological factors explain very little of the variance between symptoms and structural problems. There is no chronic pain state in which the degree of tissue damage or inflammation in the periphery relates well with the pain you feel.

The reason for this is that although pain may originate from receptors in the periphery, nerves in the central nervous system and brain nearly always play a role in individual differences in pain sensitivity. Some of these actions are genetically determined, so you may not have a say in the pain you may feel.

This does not mean, however, that psychological treatments will not help…it's just that they may not be causing your pain.

Pain is considered chronic if it has been present for more than three to six months. Chronic pain is very different than acute pain, both in how the body reacts to it and how it is treated. When pain becomes chronic, there are many changes that occur in the brain and body tissues that can perpetuate the pain. These include a heightened sensitivity to pain in both the spinal nerves and brain and an increase in particular chemicals (NMDA, Substance P) that increase the pain messages going to the brain. In addition, receptors in your soft tissues that usually detect painless stimuli (such as wetness, heat, cold, light touch) may be converted into pain receptors, which is why such stimuli often cause your pain to worsen.

Obese People Suffer More from Pain

According to a survey conducted by the journal *Obesity*, obese people are much more likely to experience pain than thinner people. The mechanism appears to be increased inflammation in the body as well as depression, both of which can cause increased pain.

Not only do obese people feel pain more, but obesity also contributes to conditions that cause pain, such as arthritis and back problems. To complicate matters, pain can then limit physical activity, which makes these problems worse, so it's a vicious cycle. The answer? Lose weight, of course.

———

There are also many psychological factors that play a role in pain, such as stress, mood, emotion, and motivation; and in reverse, chronic pain can also cause psychological problems. Because of these factors, treatment for chronic pain involves much more than just giving pain medications. In fact, pain medication can perpetuate and even worsen chronic pain.

———

Chronic Pain Impacts Overall Brain Function

A new study revealed that people with chronic pain have alterations in certain areas of the brain unrelated to pain, which probably accounts for symptoms that often accompany pain, including depression, anxiety, sleep disturbances, and decision-making abilities.

———

Treatments for Chronic Pain

The Preventive Approaches

Diet: There are many foods that can affect pain both positively and negatively. Foods that contain tryptophan can increase a brain neurotransmitter, serotonin, which can block pain. Foods high in tryptophan include turkey, chicken, cheddar cheese, halibut, eggs, peanuts, and nuts. Foods containing omega-3 fatty acids, such as cold-water fish (e.g., mackerel, tuna, salmon, herring, cod, trout, and halibut), have natural anti-inflammatory properties. Foods high in calcium and magnesium, such as dairy products, salmon, and whole grains, can relax muscles.

Avoid saturated fats because they contain prostaglandins, which increase the inflammatory response. One may also have food sensitivities or intolerances that, over time, can increase inflammation in the body, causing pain. You can visit with your dietitian about consideration of an elimination diet to find the foods that affect you adversely.

Regular **exercise** is very important in reducing chronic pain. Exercise stimulates large neurons (brain cells) to help reduce the perception of pain and stimulate the production of natural painkillers from the brain. Inactivity causes increased stiffness and loss of muscle tone, which can increase and perpetuate the pain. Aerobic, resistance, and stretching exercises are all important, and you should perform all three types at least three times a week. You may feel that you cannot perform exercises because of the pain, but you will find out that exercise will eventually decrease your pain. Even with disabilities, there are exercises that you can do.

The Conventional Approaches

Chronic pain can cause a variety of psychological problems, especially anxiety, frustration, anger, and depression. **Psychotherapy** with a therapist who works with chronic pain patients can help you learn to cope better with your chronic pain, so you can participate in more activities and generally feel better. It also helps improve your relations with family, friends, and work. This does not mean that you are "crazy" or that your pain is caused by psychological factors; simply that you need help in dealing with the changes that are inevitable with chronic pain. Often, your pain will also decrease as a result of dealing with your emotions.

Medications are usually a mainstay of conventional treatment for chronic pain. It is, of course, better if you can get by with taking less potent medications that have fewer long-term side effects. OTC *naproxen* and *ibuprofen* are the safest long-term and should be tried first when other methods fail to relieve your pain, but they may not be effective if your pain is severe or has been present a long time. *Caution*: These drugs can cause stomach inflammation when taken long-term, and you may need to take proton pump inhibitors (acid reflux drugs) along with them. Avoid high doses of acetaminophen long-term as it can cause liver problems.

Stronger NSAIDs such as naproxen [Naprosyn], meloxicam [Mobic], piroxicam [Feldene], oxaprozin [Daypro], nabumatone [Relafen], ketoprofen [Orudis], diclofenac [Cataflam], and diclofenac/misoprostol [Arthrotec]) are commonly used when milder OTC drugs aren't helpful. These NSAIDs are more powerful but also have higher risk of side effects, primarily stomach irritation and bleeding. NSAIDs called Cox-2 inhibitors (such as celecoxib [Celebrex]) have a lower risk of stomach problems, although they are more expensive and may slightly increase your risk for heart attack if you have heart disease.

Caution: In July, 2015, the FDA started requiring NSAIDs to carry a warning of increased risk of heart attacks, stroke and heart failure. This is especially evident when taken long term, at higher doses, or by people with pre-existing heart disease. The risks can increase as early as the first weeks of NSAID use. However, ibuprofen and naproxen do not appear to increase the risk, so are the safest and preferred NSAIDs.

All NSAIDs have equivalent effectiveness, although people tend to respond better to some brands than to others. If one doesn't work for you, try another (ask your doctor for samples). It can take three weeks or longer for these drugs to decrease your pain. *Helpful tip*: Be sure to take PPIs (e.g., Nexium, Prevacid, Prilosec) if you have stomach irritation.

Low-dose antidepressants, such as amitriptyline (Elavil) 25–50 mg daily or trazadone (Desyrel) 50–150 mg daily, can decrease chronic pain for some people through effects on the pain center (hypothalamus) and neurotransmitters in the brain. It may take four to six weeks for your pain to decrease if they work.

Several medications have potencies midway between NSAIDs and narcotics. *Tramadol* (Ultram) is a nonnarcotic pain reliever that often is effective when NSAIDs are not and has less addiction potential. Both *pentazocine* (Talwin) and *butorphanol* (Stadol) are quite effective and can be given intramuscularly or intravenously. The latter two are in a category called kappa opiates, which have been shown to be far more effective in relieving pain in women than in men.

If these medications fail to relieve your pain, stronger pain relievers (*narcotics/opioids*) are usually prescribed. However, these drugs do have significant side effects, can be addictive, and can actually increase your pain in the long term. You should use them only if the other methods are not effective and your pain prevents you from engaging in your usual activities.

In regard to opioids, most doctors start with codeine-containing drugs, which range in potency from Tylenol with codeine (Tylenol #3) to hydrocodone (Lortab, Vicodin, Norco) to oxycodone (Percocet, OxyContin). You may be able to decrease your dosage of these narcotics by taking acetaminophen (Tylenol) or ibuprofen with them or between doses. Codeine-containing drugs may cause stomach irritation in many patients. Highly potent narcotics (morphine, Demerol, Fentanyl, dilaudid, methadone, etc.) should be reserved for the worst cases. A lesser-known drug, levorphanol, has less development of tolerance than other opioids, is low in cost, and has no serious side effects, but it may not be as effective for severe pain. *Warning*: All these drugs can cause constipation when used long-term and are highly addictive. The hydrocodone drugs may contain acetaminophen (often in high doses), and you should avoid such combination drugs them if you have liver disease.

Narcotic medications can be applied in numerous forms, including oral, sublingual (under the tongue), buccal (next to the gums), by patch, intranasal, by spray, and of course by intramuscular or intravenous injection. There are several devices, including patient-controlled pumps (PCA), which can allow continuous control of pain for people who require frequent potent narcotics, such as cancer patients.

Important Note
Men and Women Experience Pain Differently

It is well recognized that men and women experience pain, especially *chronic* pain, differently. Women appear to recover more quickly from pain, seek help more quickly for their pain, and are less likely to allow pain to control their lives. These factors may be due in part to hormonal effects, especially estrogen.

In addition, the ability of narcotic (opioid) medications to relieve pain also differs between men and women. Narcotics that are referred to as *kappa-opiates* are more effective in women, apparently due to having more kappa receptors in an area of the brain that perceives pain. Such medications include *nalbuphine* (Nubain) and *butorphanol* (Stadol). Though these medications are not prescribed for most chronic pain, they are currently used for relief of labor pain and in general work best for short-term pain.

Nonnarcotic medications: For fibromyalgia or myofascial-type syndromes, gabapentin (Neurontin), pregabalin (Lyrica), pramipexole (Mirapex), and duloxetine (Cymbalta) have been found to be beneficial in some people. Cymbalta was also recently approved for use in chronic musculoskeletal pain, including low back and osteoarthritis pain. Gabapentin and pregabalin are often prescribed for chronic nerve pain. **Warning**: A recent study from *Neurology* found that significant neurotoxicity and negative cognitive (thinking) effects occurred with use of pregabalin, especially using over 600 mg a day.

A recent study in *JAMA* showed that *tricyclic antidepressants* (such as amitriptyline, nortryptiline) reduce pain, fatigue, and sleep disturbances in fibromyalgia better than other classes of antidepressants. One study showed that the combination of gabapentin with nortryptiline (an antidepressant) is better than one drug alone.

A new drug indicated for fibromyalgia is *milnacipran* (Savella), also an antidepressant. However, the absolute differences between placebo and treated groups, ranged only between 7% and 9% (i.e., more than 90% of patients received no benefit from the drug beyond what they would have gotten from a placebo). It can have serious side effects, including hypertension, increased heart rate, and increased suicidal ideation.

In a 2011 meta-analysis ***comparing antidepressants*** used in fibromyalgia, the significant effects of amitryptiline (AMX) and Duloxetine (DLX) were small and those of milnacipran (MLN) not substantial. In adjusted indirect comparisons, AMX was superior to DLX and MLN in reduction of pain, sleep disturbances, fatigue and limitations of quality of life (QOL). DLX was superior to MLN in reducing pain, sleep disturbances and limitations of QOL. MLN was superior to DLX in reducing fatigue.

For problems with muscle spasm, *baclofen* may be beneficial. ***Important note***: Muscle relaxants (e.g., Flexeril, Soma) are ineffective long-term and are usually not effective in chronic pain syndromes.

Many Pain Patients Do Not Take Their Prescriptions

In a study of 240,000 long-term chronic pain patients, it was found that 30 percent of patients were not taking the medications they were prescribed. Another 30 percent were using prescription drugs that were not prescribed by the patient's doctor. Not taking medications as prescribed will result in worsening of pain and less response to medications as well.

People with chronic pain, especially fibromyalgia, have difficulty sleeping or do not sleep restfully, so a conventional medication to help sleep is often beneficial. This can be an actual sleep medication, such as Ambien, Restoril, or Sonata, or a mild antidepressant such as amitriptyline (Elavil) or trazadone (Desyrel) (see section on *Insomnia*).

For medication management of chronic pain, I highly recommend that you be evaluated and treated by a **physiatrist** or a **pain management specialist**, especially if controlling your pain requires more potent pain medications.

Pain Medication Too Often Underprescribed

Many doctors are hesitant to provide adequate pain relief for fear of retaliation from the authorities and also due to not being well trained in appropriate prescribing of pain medications. Many doctors are fearful of causing addiction, but for many patients, that is simply a consequence of the treatment. Surveys show that 50 percent of patients change doctors in their quest for pain relief because the doctors were unwilling to treat pain aggressively, failed to take the pain issue seriously, or had a lack of knowledge about pain management.

Physical Therapy may be of help using movement therapy, individualized exercises, and electrical stimulation. Physical therapy modalities such as traction or ultrasound are usually not beneficial.

Multidisciplinary pain programs are beneficial in treating all aspects of chronic pain and may decrease the need for pain drugs. Although such programs are not designed to reduce pain specifically, they do improve functional and back-to-work ability and teach you how to cope better with your pain. They usually include evaluation and treatment by pain-management specialists, physical and occupational therapists, and psychologists or psychiatrists.

Unfortunately, many people with chronic pain become addicted to medications they take for pain relief. Pain medications, especially narcotics, can actually cause an increase of your pain perception through their effect on the brain, making you feel *more* pain, not less. Reducing the amount of medication you take can often reduce your pain, but this can produce psychological difficulties and physical withdrawal. If you are dependent on or addicted to pain medication, a **drug addiction program** may be necessary to help you reduce your dependence.

The Alternative Approaches

I always recommend **acupuncture** first for chronic pain because it can address both the area of pain and the part of the brain that perceives pain (the hypothalamus). There are styles of acupuncture that can provide immediate relief by stimulating production of endorphins (your own internal pain relievers), but this provides only temporary relief. I prefer to address the chronic underlying condition because it then provides longer-term relief or at least reduction in the pain and, thus, the amount of drugs you require. Always seek evaluation and treatment from a practitioner certified in acupuncture. You should notice initial improvement within two to six acupuncture treatments but might need additional sessions for maximum benefit. Since acupuncture often can address the underlying cause of the pain, it can provide long-term relief when successful.

There are several **Chinese herbal formulas** that can be used together with acupuncture to help reduce symptoms. *Yan Hu So Wan* ("stop pain tablets") can help acute pain. Common formulas include *Huo Luo Dan* in combination with either *Gui Pi Tang* or *Huo Luo Xiao Lin Dan*. Consult a practitioner qualified in Chinese herbal medicine to determine if these Chinese herbal formulas are the best for your particular syndromes, especially for chronic pain. You should feel better within three to six weeks but may need to take these remedies longer, depending on your condition.

Low level energy laser ("cold" laser or LLEL) is excellent at reducing chronic pain in the spine or joints (degenerative disc disease or osteoarthritis). It is also excellent at reducing pain from trigger points or chronic nerve injuries. It can also be used to stimulate acupuncture points if needle acupuncture is not available.

Tai chi *and* **qigong** are also beneficial for chronic pain. A study in the *NEJM* showed improvement in physical function and quality of life in patients with fibromyalgia using these Chinese exercises.

Often, chronic pain is a result of imbalance of peripheral nerve and muscle feedback connections with the brain. Certain **bodywork** methods address these imbalances. The *Feldenkrais method, Alexander technique,* and *Rolfing* are the most common forms of bodywork that might relieve chronic pain that doesn't respond to other treatments. *Bowen work* (uses gentle movement/ technique) can also be effective.

Bodywork involves realigning, rebalancing, and retraining the structures of the body, which have become dysfunctional due to pain, injury, disuse, or misuse. The Feldenkrais method focuses on retraining how you move your body in order to interrupt unhealthy patterns of movement that have become habits. The Alexander technique concentrates on correcting faulty posture in daily activities (sitting, standing, and moving). Rolfing involves manipulating and stretching the body's fascial tissues (deep connective tissues that hold your body together), thus allowing correct realigning of the body. These bodywork methods require a therapist certified in these techniques (see Chapter 4 for additional discussion of these methods).

Mind-body methods are also very effective in reducing chronic pain. *Meditation* is excellent for reducing stress and providing relaxation, which increases endorphin production. *Hypnosis* can reduce pain by addressing the emotional and psychological aspects that can either cause pain or make it worse. If hypnosis works, it can do so quickly, often in two to three sessions. *Guided or interactive imagery* can influence the amygdala, the area of the brain that receives pain messages, teaching the brain not to perceive the pain. This method may take several weeks to months to be effective (see chapter 4 for more information).

Yoga promotes relaxation and stretching, both of which are important in healing and preventing pain. A pilot study from the University of Oregon showed that eight weeks of yoga significantly decreases symptoms of fibromyalgia. Because there are many different types and different levels of yoga, with some better for chronic pain than others, I recommend working with a qualified yoga instructor. It may take several months (sometimes less) to notice improvement from yoga. Yoga done incorrectly may increase your pain.

Nutritional supplements: In people with fibromyalgia, serotonin levels may be deficient, so supplements that raise serotonin levels may help relieve symptoms. A combination of 5-HTP (100 mg daily), in combination with St. John's wort (300 mg three times a day containing 0.3 percent hypericin content), magnesium (150–250 mg three times daily), and malic acid (1,200 mg daily) may be helpful. You should notice improvement within one to two months. ***Caution***: Be careful with St. John's wort if you are taking other medications as this herb interacts with many other drugs.

Vitamin D Deficiency May Be Related to Chronic Pain

Several studies have shown that many patients with unexplained musculoskeletal pain have vitamin D deficiency, although taking additional vitamin D did not seem to reduce their pain. Another study revealed that people with vitamin D deficiency must take higher doses of narcotics and for longer periods. For these people, supplementation is worth a try.

For fibromyalgia, **guaifenesin** (such as Humibid), an expectorant also used in many OTC cough remedies (such as Robitussin), has been purported to be beneficial in reducing symptoms of fibromyalgia. If you decide to try it, you must take high doses, and it usually takes several months to be effective. It can, and usually does, cause a much more severe increase in pain in the initial few weeks of treatment. A prescription is required at a dosage of 600 mg twice daily.

Topicals: It should be noted that capsaicin has often been used as a topical cream to control pain. There is now a pharmaceutical 8 percent capsaicin patch called Qutenza, which is given over a one-hour period, but can provide pain relief for up to three months. Studies show a greater than 30 percent decrease in pain reduction at each week during the three-month period. However, this patch can cause significant burning when applied. Topricin (homeopathic cream), Traumeel cream tablets, or the Chinese herbal topical Zheng Gu Shui may be able to give temporary relief.

There are many **other methods and supplements** that may be beneficial to reduce pain. A summary of these and the above methods is found in the following chart.

Alternative Pain Treatments

Vitamins	D_3, B_{12}, C, folic acid
Minerals	Magnesium, copper, calcium
Amino Acids	Taurine, phenyalanine, glycine GABA, tryptophan
Herbal/plant and animal Products	Milk thistle, Boswellia, aloe vera Krill oil, rosemary, ginger, turmeric
Temperature agents	Ice, heat, infrared, warm water

Creams/lotions	Menthol, capsaicin, salicylates, Boswellia, AloeVera
Oral anti-inflammatories	Glucosamine, chondroitin, MSM
Active exercise	Tai chi, yoga, pilates, qigong, Feldenkrais
Passive exercise/manipulation	Massage, chiropractic, osteopathic
Electric palliation	Acupuncture, magnets, acupressure, Ultrasound, copper jewelry, Mineral baths
Neuropathway retraining	Biofeedback, hypnosis, imagery, Meditation
Light therapy	Laser (cold), UV lamps

From *Pain Management*, Jan/Feb 2009

Your Empowered Patient Action Plan for Treating Chronic Pain

Step #1: Most of you with chronic pain will already have been ***prescribed medications***. If you must take medications, start with the ones that have the least potential for side effects or harm, such as NSAIDs or tricyclic antidepressants. Avoid narcotics if at all possible. You can also try alternative topicals (Topricin, Traumeel) or the Qutenza patch. If the medications are helping, continue taking them while undergoing the following steps and discontinue them when the steps are effective. If they have not helped, the following steps should help relieve your pain.

Step #2: ***Undergo acupuncture and take appropriate Chinese herbal formulas*** for long-term relief or significant reduction in pain.

Amy began having pain on the left portion of her face, which then spread to her left arm, left leg, and eventually her entire body, over the course of several months. She had been evaluated by numerous doctors, including physiatrists, neurologists, pain specialists, and a psychiatrist, none of whom could tell her why she was hurting. She was eventually diagnosed as having polyneuritis, a widespread inflammation of the nerves throughout her body. After two years the pain had worsened to the point that Amy was unable to engage in any activity. She had to quit her job, could not maintain a sexual relationship, and could not engage in any social activities. She literally became an invalid. I performed acupuncture based on her underlying Chinese diagnoses. After the first acupuncture, she was pain-free for the first time in two years and went out partying to celebrate. The pain did return within a few days, but it was not as severe. She continued acupuncture on several more occasions, and eventually her pain went away for good.

⌘

Rachel had fibromyalgia for twelve years, with pain throughout her body that never let up. She was unable to participate in most activities or even go shopping for more than a few minutes at a time. She had taken numerous conventional medications, had undergone trigger point injections and physical therapy, and had also tried various topical creams and ointments. I started her on acupuncture as well as a combination of Chinese and Western herbs. After two months, nearly all of her symptoms had gone away, and she felt better than she had in years. She has continued receiving acupuncture every few months for flare-ups.

⌘

Step #3: *Receive hypnosis, guided imagery, and/or interactive imagery* to help control or reduce your pain.

⌘

Betty is a forty-eight-year-old patient of mine who would develop pain in different areas of her body at different times (migrating pain). She had been prescribed pain medications, which did control the pain temporarily but did not resolve her problems. I felt that there was an underlying psychological basis for the pain and performed interactive imagery. After several sessions, she began having repressed memories, revealing that a close relative had abused her physically, mentally, and emotionally when she was a child. Each time a particular memory occurred, she would report pain in some area of her body, which correlated with the abuse (for example, she would have pain in her arm and remember her relative twisting her arm). The pain would continue or worsen until she dealt with the memory, at which time the pain would disappear. After several months of therapy, her pain finally stopped for good.

⌘

Step #4: *Undergo psychological counseling* to help you cope with your pain and address emotional or psychological issues related to the pain.

Step #5: *Undergo physical therapy* for a trial of electrical stimulation and movement therapy.

Step #6: *Enter a multidisciplinary pain program* to help you cope with your pain and improve your QOL.

Step #7: *Undergo the Feldenkrais method, Alexander technique, Bowen technique, or Rolfing* to rebalance your nerve, muscle, and brain connections.

Step #8: ***Practice appropriate yoga postures*** to reduce pain.

Step #9: ***Take herbal combinations*** as outlined above to control symptoms of fibromyalgia or other chronic pain syndromes not relieved by the previous steps.

Step #10: ***Try pregabalin, duloxetine, or pramipexole*** if you have fibromyalgia pain not relieved by the above steps.

Step #11: ***Take conventional sleeping medication*** for insomnia due to pain.

Step #12: ***Try high-dose guaifenesin*** if you still have fibromyalgia symptoms.

Step #13: ***Attend a drug addiction program*** if addicted to narcotic pain relievers or alcohol due to chronic pain. Reducing narcotic medications may actually decrease your pain.

Ed is a forty-five-year-old patient of mine who had chronic arthritic pain for over fifteen years. Conventional therapies had been ineffective, and during the previous three years, his pain was controlled only by large doses of hydrocodone. I treated him with acupuncture, which totally relieved his pain within ten treatments. However, he had been so used to taking the hydrocodone that he could not stop taking it because of psychological addiction, even though he knew he didn't need it anymore. I tried to wean him off the drugs and gave him withdrawal medications, but he felt that he "needed" more. I referred him to an outpatient addiction center, and with extensive counseling, he was finally able to discontinue the medications in six weeks.

Expected Outcome

Chronic pain is a difficult condition to resolve completely, but with the addition of alternative methods, it can be controlled much more easily and, in some cases, resolved long-term. Certainly, pain management may be necessary, but by using alternatives, you may not have to rely on medications. You should not have to let chronic pain control your life if you use the above methods.

Parkinson's Disease and Essential Tremor

What You Need to Know

Parkinson's disease develops gradually, often starting with a barely noticeable tremor in just one hand. But while tremor may be the best-known sign of Parkinson's disease, the disorder also commonly causes a slowing or freezing of movement. Parkinson's symptoms tend to worsen as the disease progresses.

Besides Parkinson's, there are other causes of tremor, the most notable called essential tremor, which is the most common movement disorder in the world. It is three times as common as Parkinson's. Other neurological disorders can mimic symptoms of Parkinson's, so it is important to obtain a proper diagnosis.

Delayed Orthostatic Hypotension: A Possible Warning Sign of Parkinson's

Many people as they age can become lightheaded when they first stand up or stand up too quickly, which is called orthostatic hypotension (OH). Many physicians don't realize that OH can develop several minutes after standing, referred to as Delayed Orthostatic Hypotension (DOH).

A 2015 study on DOH indicated that DOH may progress to OH and can be an early manifestation of Parkinson's disease.

Treatments for Parkinson's Disease and Essential Tremor

The Preventive Approaches
Correctable causes: Antipsychotic medications, such as chlorpromazine (Thorazine) and haloperidol (Haldol), and antinausea drugs like prochlorperazine (Compazine) or metoclopramide (Reglan), can all cause Parkinson's-type symptoms, but they can be reversed when you get off the drug as soon as they occur.

Exposure to carbon monoxide, cyanide, or certain other toxins can produce symptoms similar to Parkinson's disease, so rule out these causes before being treated.

Beware of Falls after Eating

Many people with Parkinson's may develop low blood pressure after eating. If this occurs, you should try drinking more water before meals and eating six smaller meals a day rather than three large ones.

It has been noted that drinking alcohol can decrease essential tremor, but this effect wears off as the alcohol diminishes in the bloodstream.

Exercise is important for general health, but especially for maintaining function in Parkinson's disease.

The Conventional Approaches
For Parkinson's

Medications can help manage problems of Parkinson's with walking, movement, and tremor. Your initial response to Parkinson's drugs can be dramatic, but over time, the benefits of drugs frequently diminish or become less consistent, although symptoms can usually still be fairly well controlled.

Levodopa is the most effective Parkinson's drug and is combined with *carbidopa* to create the combination drug *Sinemet*. As the disease progresses, the benefit from levodopa may decrease, with a tendency to work intermittently, requiring medication adjustments. *Eventually, all patients will need to take Sinemet.* **Important notes**: These drugs should not be taken with meals. Take at least one hour before or two hours after meals. There also may be periods of time were blood levels are too low for effectiveness, so timing of dose is important. There are several side effects, such as nausea, hallucinations/delusions, orthostatic hypotension (dizzy upon standing), and dyskinesias (unusual movements of the muscles). These all can and should be addressed.

Dopamine agonists (pramipexole [Mirapex], ropinirole [Requip], bromocriptine [Parlodel], pergolide [Permax], apomorphine [Apokyn], and rotigotine patch [Neupro]) are not nearly as effective as the above drugs in treating the symptoms of Parkinson's disease. However, they last longer and are often used to smooth the sometimes intermittent effect of levodopa. These drugs have many side effects, including confusion, delusions and hallucinations, involuntary movements called dyskinesia, and even compulsive behavior changes (compulsive gambling, hypersexuality, shopping sprees).. These side effects resolve with dose reduction—but sometimes at the expense of reduced symptom control.

Other medications, including *MAO-B inhibitors* (selegiline [Eldepryl], rasagiline [Azilect]) and *Catechol O-methyltransferase (COMT)* inhibitors such as entacapone [Comtan] or tolpacone [Tasmar], prolong the effect of carbidopa-levodopa therapy and are now combined with these other drugs in a medication called Stalevo.

Anticholinergics have been used for many years to help control the tremor associated with Parkinson's disease, but they have only modest benefits and numerous side effects such as confusion, hallucinations, severe constipation, and urine retention, particularly in people over the age of seventy.

Antivirals such as amantadine (Symmetrel) can provide short-term relief of mild, early stage Parkinson's disease and can be added to carbidopa-levodopa therapy for people in the later stages of Parkinson's disease, especially if they have problems with involuntary movements (dyskinesia) induced by carbidopa-levodopa.

Medications for nonmotor (movement) symptoms of Parkinson's: these include sildenafil (Viagra) for erectile dysfunction, polyethylene glycol for constipation, modafinil (Provigil] for excessive daytime sleepiness, and methylphenidate (Ritalin) for fatigue. A newly approved drug, droxidopa (Nothera) can treat symptoms of orthostatic hypotension (dizziness upon standing), but there are questions regarding how effective it is, and blood pressure may increase when lying down.

Can Nicotine Help Parkinson's?

In an interesting study in 1966, an epidemiologist at the NIH noted that death due to Parkinson's disease occurred at least three times as often in nonsmokers as in smokers, indicating that smoking somehow might be beneficial for Parkinson's. This was confirmed by another study in 1971. Later it was determined that it was the nicotine alone that was beneficial by increasing levels of dopamine in the brain, which helps control movement.

A 2007 paper from the Parkinson's Institute in Silicon Valley showed that in monkeys administered nicotine, there were 50 percent fewer tremors and tics, and dyskinesia was reduced 35 percent even in those already on L-dopa. Currently, studies are being conducted on humans at Vermont College of Medicine.

Does this mean you should start smoking if you have Parkinson's? At this time, the evidence is not available to recommend it. If it is proven beneficial, you don't have to smoke; you can simply use nicotine patches. And you won't have to worry about addiction because studies reveal that nicotine does not cause addiction when used to treat disease (it's the other chemicals in tobacco that do so).

Caution: Nicotine may interfere with blood pressure medications.

Physical therapy has not been found to improve function for activities of daily living, according to a 2016 study in *JAMA Neurol*. However, it may be beneficial for specific problems such as a shortened stride or reduced arm swing.

There are also some **surgeries** available for Parkinson's. *Deep-brain stimulation* (DBS) is the most common; it involves implanting an electrode deep within the parts of your brain that control movement. Deep-brain stimulation is most often used for people who have advanced Parkinson's disease and have unstable medication (levodopa) responses, but it isn't beneficial for people who don't respond to carbidopa-levodopa. Tremor is especially responsive to this therapy. Deep-brain stimulation doesn't help dementia and may actually make that worse. Two recent studies reveal that deep-brain stimulation may be superior to medications in many people with Parkinson's, but side effects are much more frequent. Risks of this surgery include brain hemorrhage, stroke-like problems, and infection.

Studies on using **stem cells** to treat Parkinson's disease are underway and may be beneficial in the future.

For essential tremors,

The most common **medication** is *propranolol* (Inderal), but other medications that may help include *mysoline* [Primadone], *topiramate* [Topamax], and *alprazolam* [Xanax], the latter two of which are uncommonly used due to side effects and addiction potential, respectively. Many patients obtain better results using a combination of propranolol and mysoline.

Botox has also been used, primarily for limb tremor, but it can cause weakness in the limb.

Two **surgeries** can be successful for essential tremors. *Thalotomy* has a 60–90 percent efficacy but has many side effects. The best, as with Parkinson's, is *deep-brain stimulation*, which has a 65–90 percent efficacy and long-term results.

The Alternative Approaches

There are several **nutritional supplements** that may be of benefit for Parkinson's, including the following:

- *Essential fatty acids* may be helpful due to their anti-inflammatory properties. A mix of omega-6 and omega-3 may be the best, but don't mix these from separate sources. Krill oil contains the exact ratio of omega-3 to omega-6 that the body requires and may be the most potent.
- *Antioxidants* vitamin C (1,000 mg three times a day), vitamin E (400–800 IU per day), and the trace mineral selenium (200 mcg) may slow progression of Parkinson's. Other antioxidants commonly used are alpha-lipoic acid, grape-seed extract, and pycnogenol, but it is not known whether they help Parkinson's.
- *Coenzyme Q10* has been found to be low in people with Parkinson's and may be of some benefit. It appears to be most beneficial using higher doses earlier in the disease (1,200 mg daily, if tolerated)
- *Glutathione* (200 mg daily) is found to be deficient in patients with Parkinson's, so it may be of benefit to supplement.
- *Vitamin B$_6$* (100 mg per day) helps nerve function and may help with symptom control, but it should be given with *zinc* (30 mg per day). However, zinc should not be continued longer than six months due to adversely affecting copper levels.

Important note: Early animal studies indicated that *creatine* may delay the progression of Parkinson's. However, a 2015 study in *JAMA* showed that creatine has no effect on Parkinson's.

Acupuncture cannot resolve Parkinson's, but it is very effective at reducing many of the symptoms, including tremor, rigidity, slow movement, imbalance, fatigue, depression, and incontinence. It is also very beneficial for reducing or resolving essential tremors. You should observe benefits within six to eight treatments but may need maintenance therapy long-term.

A **Chinese herbal formula** called *Du Zhong Pian* may be effective as well.

Massage therapy can reduce muscle tension and promote relaxation, so it is beneficial to reduce muscle rigidity in Parkinson's.

Qigong/tai chi helps improve flexibility and balance and can be done at any age and in any condition. It helps to improve postural stability when performed for sixty minutes twice weekly for twenty-four weeks. It is important to be instructed by a trained professional.

Yoga also increases flexibility and balance, but depends on your physical stamina.

Homeopathic remedies may be of benefit to reduce various symptoms. These include:

- *Argentum nitricum* may be helpful for cerebellar ataxia (loss of muscle coordination), painless paralysis, staggering gait, twitches, and tremor.
- *Causticum* may be beneficial for Parkinson's with restless legs at night, contractures, or paralysis.
- *Mercurius vivus* for Parkinson's that is worse at night, especially with panic attacks. However, mercurius in general can be a good remedy for hand tremors.
- *Zincum metallicum* is useful for great restlessness, twitches and jerks, and depression.

Your Balanced Healing Action Plan for Treating Parkinson's

Step #1: Take the appropriate medications to reduce symptoms and slow progression.

Step #2: Undergo acupuncture to reduce symptoms. You may be able to decrease or discontinue some of the medications in step #1 if acupuncture is successful.

Step #3: Exercise and use qigong/tai chi and/or yoga to improve flexibility and balance.

Step #4: Take various nutritional supplements to help reduce symptoms. Again, this may be able to help you decrease the medications in step #1.

Step #5: Undergo homeopathy to reduce symptoms if the above steps have not helped.

Step #6: Undergo surgery if you have advanced Parkinson's and are resistant to the above medications.

Your Empowered Patient Action Plan for Treating Essential Tremor

Step #1: Undergo acupuncture to reduce tremors.

Step #2: Take propranolol with or without mysoline (Primadone) if Step #1 is not beneficial.

Step #3: Undergo deep-brain stimulation for severe symptoms unresponsive to the other steps.

Expected Outcome

Parkinson's disease and essential tremor cannot be cured, and medications are not always beneficial, or they may have side effects. You can improve your quality of life, however, by using additional alternative methods.

Plantar Fasciitis/Heel Spurs

What You Need to Know

Foot problems are some of the most common problems that we encounter as we age. In fact, more than 75 percent of all people eventually develop foot problems.

There are many causes of foot problems, including "wear and tear" from years of walking and running; structural deterioration of the arch or bones of the foot; and alignment problems with the hips, pelvis, or knees that can cause compensatory damage to the feet.

For several foot conditions, such as calluses, bunions, corns, and hammertoes, surgery is the usual treatment, and you should seek the care of a podiatrist. For arthritis of the ankle or foot or for tarsal tunnel, see the sections on *Osteoarthritis* or *Compressive Neuropathies*.

In this section, I will discuss two conditions that do not necessarily require surgery and are some of the most common foot conditions as we age. Plantar fasciitis and heel spurs are actually caused by the same underlying causes and are a continuum. That is, most people develop plantar fasciitis (inflammation of the connective tissue in the arch to heel), which, if left untreated, progresses to heel spurs, which are composed of calcium deposited in an area of inflammation in the heel.

Most people do not realize that spurs are usually not the cause of the pain. The pain is caused by the inflammation, and for this reason, you must treat the inflammation, not the spur. However, if they continue to grow, spurs can put pressure on other tissues, eventually causing pain and additional problems and thus requiring removal of the spur. If treated early, however, surgery is not necessary.

Once inflammation occurs, the body may not be able to resolve it on its own. This is especially true in the foot because there is not a large amount of blood circulation in those tissues. Once it starts, it continues to progress unless treated. Even so, these conditions can last for years even with common treatments.

Treatments for Heel Spurs and Plantar Fasciitis

The Preventive Approaches

Correctable causes: The inflammation that causes spurs is usually due to injuries, which can occur at one time or gradually, due to repetitive trauma. The best way to prevent them is to *treat injuries early* and thoroughly. Unfortunately, many people just let injuries take their course and don't treat them. When this occurs, the initial symptoms may resolve, but chronic inflammation can be the result, and the symptoms may return years later.

Poor posture is often a cause of heel spurs and plantar fasciitis, due to abnormal pressure being exerted on the area. Often, there is a problem in the pelvis (such as misalignment) that goes uncorrected, placing more pressure on only part of the foot or on one foot more than the other. Thus, if you have pelvis, hip, knee, or back pain that causes limping or abnormal pressure on one lower extremity, foot conditions can be a result if those problems remain uncorrected.

The Conventional Approaches

Most doctors (and podiatrists) will start with **medications** if your symptoms are mild. *Acetaminophen* (Tylenol) is usually the first tried, but *NSAIDs* (such as naproxen [Naprosyn], meloxicam [Mobic], piroxicam [Feldene], oxaprozin [Daypro], nabumatone [Relafen], ketoprofen [Orudis], diclofenac [Cataflam], diclofenac/misoprostol [Arthrotec] or celocoxib [Celebrex]) are more potent. These drugs will not cure the condition unless it heals on its own over time (often one to two years).

Caution: In July, 2015, the FDA started requiring NSAIDs to carry a warning of increased risk of heart attacks, stroke and heart failure. This is especially evident when taken long term, at higher doses, or by people with pre-existing heart disease. The risks can increase as early as the first weeks of NSAID use. However, ibuprofen and naproxen do not appear to increase the risk, so are the safest and preferred NSAIDs.

Many podiatrists will prescribe an **orthotic** (a lift or insert for your shoes) as heel spurs and plantar fasciitis may be caused by weakness in portions of your feet, especially the arches. Studies show that orthotics may produce small, short-term benefits in function and small reductions in pain but do not have long-term beneficial effects for these conditions compared with sham devices. *Helpful tips*: There are both prefabricated (drugstore) and customized orthotics (molded to your feet); the latter are much more expensive (usually around $500) but may have similar effectiveness, so you might try the prefabricated ones first. A 2015 study showed that the customized orthotics may decrease pain on walking better than prefabricated ones but doesn't improve function and quality of life. Also, avoid wearing high heels and poorly supported shoes.

⸺⸺

Stretches for Plantar Fasciitis

If your heel spur or plantar fasciitis is mild, along with anti-inflammatory medications, you may be treated with *stretching and ice*. There are two main stretching exercises.

For one type of stretch, you hold on to something (such as a chair, table, or wall) and keep your entire foot on the ground. Keeping your knee locked straight, lean forward slowly. You will feel the stretch of your Achilles tendon (in back of your lower leg/ankle). Hold this for five to ten seconds, and then stand again. Repeat this five times, and then apply ice to the back of your lower leg and heel for twenty minutes. Do this every day. You should feel better within a few weeks if it is successful.

For another type of stretch, sit and cross your foot over the knee of the other leg. Grasp your toes and pull them toward your shin until you feel the stretch across the arch of your foot. Then, using the thumb of your opposite hand, massage the arch. Hold for ten seconds and repeat ten times.

⸺⸺

Physical Therapy may be beneficial for treatment in several ways. Exercises alone may help (usually passive stretching), but combining *exercise* with *manual mobilization* appears to work better. Manual therapy consists of deep soft tissue mobilization to the plantar fascia as well as joint mobilization and manipulation to the foot, ankle, knee and hip. In addition, there are certain *taping techniques* that can improve symptoms and accelerate healing as well.

Cortisone injection into the heel or arch is a common treatment for heel spurs. This may be beneficial in only a minority of people; it usually provides no pain relief in the majority of patients. Studies show that it can relieve pain at four weeks but loses its effect by eight weeks.

In a small study, **Botox** (botulinum toxin) appeared to reduce pain in the foot and increase the range of motion of the ankle and knee. However, larger confirmatory studies have not been done.

Orthotripsy (shock-wave treatment) is another common treatment for heel spurs and plantar fasciitis. In this method, sound waves are transmitted through your heel, involving a series of about 1,500 shocks. However, most studies show disappointing results from this procedure, with only about 15 to 34 percent of patients improving and placebo treatments often being just as effective. In fact, one study showed that the stretch/massage detailed above was much more effective. Shock-wave treatment also costs between $2,000 and $3,000 and is usually not covered by insurance.

Cryosurgery is another conventional treatment in which a small probe freezes (and kills) the nerve fibers. It costs from $500 to $600. The nerves regenerate in about six months. Although it can reduce pain, most people still retain some residual pain. The major problem is that there have been no good placebo studies proving that it is beneficial.

Surgery should be the last resort and done only for severe, unrelenting problems that are not controlled by any other method. In actuality, as the pain from heel spurs usually comes from the inflammation, surgery may not relieve the pain unless the inflammation is also eliminated. This is why such surgery may have a high failure rate. For plantar fasciitis, a portion of the fascia is cut, but it has a long recovery period and can sometimes result in flat feet. If you undergo surgery on your foot, it may take several months of recovery before you can walk normally again.

The Alternative Approaches

Most alternative approaches are designed to eliminate the inflammation, not just treat the symptoms. As a result, you may obtain long lasting resolution.

The **low level energy laser** (*LLEL* or "cold" laser) is a device that can directly break up inflammatory cells and heal surrounding tissue. It is very successful in treating spurs and fasciitis in the majority of patients and can do so quite quickly in many cases (2-6 treatments). (See chapter 4 for further discussion of cold laser).

Acupuncture is also quite successful at reducing the inflammation causing spurs in all areas and can be used with the laser for accelerated results. You should feel less pain within six acupuncture treatments, but additional sessions may be necessary for maximum benefit.

As mentioned above, underlying structural problem (bones, ligaments, tendons, joints, and/or muscles not working correctly) may cause abnormal pressure on the spine, hips, knees, or feet and cause inflammation/spurs of the feet. These alignment abnormalities can cause you to walk incorrectly, resulting in heel spurs and plantar fasciitis. **Osteopathic evaluation and mobilization** (OMT) is the best therapy to uncover and correct these underlying problems although chiropractic may also be beneficial. In addition, direct mobilization of the plantar fascia may also be helpful.

Your Empowered Patient Action Plan for Treating Plantar Fasciitis and Heel Spurs

Step #1: Wear shoe orthotics for heel spurs if evaluation shows structural abnormalities of the feet (such as flat feet or fallen arches). Remember that less-expensive store orthotics may be just as beneficial as special-order orthotics.

Step #2: ***Use stretching and apply ice*** for mild plantar fasciitis and heel spurs. This may be able to resolve the condition without further treatments.

Step #3: ***Undergo LLEL therapy*** for long-term relief of either heel spurs or plantar fasciitis. This is the most cost-effective and successful treatment.

Step #4: ***Undergo osteopathic or chiropractic evaluation*** if you have problems with the spine, hips, or knees, whether or not the above steps have been effective. If misalignment is found, then undergo corrective manipulation to prevent reoccurrence.

Stephanie came to me with a heel spur on her left foot. She had previously had a heel spur on the right foot removed by surgery, but she still had some residual pain and numbness in that foot. She didn't want another surgery for the new bone spur on her left foot. She first received osteopathic evaluation, which indicated a problem with the pelvis that caused her to favor the left foot. She underwent four sessions of OMT to correct the underlying problem. At the same time, I gave her laser therapy for the current pain and inflammation, which resolved after six sessions. Stephanie has not had any further problems with her feet.

Step #5: ***Undergo physical therapy techniques*** to both treat the condition and prevent its recurrence.

Step #6: ***Undergo acupuncture*** for long-term relief of heel spurs and plantar fasciitis if the laser has not helped within six to eight treatments. This step can be used with the laser for faster results.

Step #7: ***Take a prescription NSAID*** for temporary relief if the above steps have not helped.

Step #8: ***Receive a cortisone injection*** for temporary relief if you still have foot pain despite the above steps.

Step #9: ***Undergo a Botox injection*** for reduction of symptoms if the above steps have still not helped.

Step #10: ***Undergo orthotripsy*** to avoid surgery, although it only helps in 15 percent of patients.

Step #11: ***Undergo cryosurgery,*** if the above steps have still not worked, to avoid major surgery.

Step #12: ***Undergo surgery*** as a last resort, which can be done by a podiatrist or an orthopedic surgeon specializing in foot disorders.

Step #13: ***Use cold laser therapy*** after surgery to accelerate healing.

Expected Outcome

With the application of alternative methods, plantar fasciitis and heel spurs can be resolved within a few weeks or months rather than a few years—and without surgery in most cases.

Prostate (Benign Prostatic Hypertrophy or BPH; Prostatitis or Chronic Pelvic Pain Syndrome)

What You Need to Know about BPH

Prostate enlargement is quite common with advancing age and typically starts appearing after the age of forty-five. The cause of prostate enlargement is usually hormonal; as you age, your testosterone levels decrease, but other hormone levels increase, resulting in an increase of a more powerful derivative of testosterone. This derivative causes prostate cells to grow and enlarge, thus constricting the urethra (the tube that leads from your bladder through your penis).

Symptoms of BPH can wax and wane. BPH may cause blockage of the urinary tract, which can lead to infection, bladder failure, and kidney problems.

Dr. A's Suggestions:
Prostate Cancer versus BPH

Because BPH symptoms can be the same as prostate cancer, it is important that you have a prostate examination (digital rectal exam) on a yearly basis and PSA (prostate-specific antigen) blood level (see chapter 2 for specific guidelines). You need to understand that PSA levels can be elevated in both BPH and prostate cancer, and the larger your prostate becomes, the higher the PSA levels can be. A good way to make a distinction is to obtain a *Free PSA* level and compare it to a *Total PSA* level. When total PSA is in the range of 4.0-10.0 ng/mL, a free:total PSA ratio < or =0.10 indicates 49 percent to 65 percent risk of prostate cancer depending on age; a free:total PSA ratio >0.25 indicates a 9 percent to 16 percent risk of prostate cancer, depending on age. If the ratio is questionable or your total PSA is greater than >10, you should undergo a prostate biopsy to rule out cancer.

Never diagnose and treat yourself! If your exam and testing are negative for cancer, you can then follow the steps listed in this section.

Treatments for BPH

The Preventive Approaches

Correctible causes: OTC antihistamines containing diphenhydramine (Benadryl), chlorpheneramine, hydroxyzine, or cyproheptidine can cause prostate enlargement as well as urinary slowing in some men because they cause retention of urine. Stop taking them; and if these medications are causing your prostate enlargement, your symptoms should improve within a few days to a few weeks. If you have COPD or emphysema, inhaled anticholinergics can also cause urinary retention.

Cut down on fluids, especially alcoholic beverages, in the evening to reduce nocturia (frequent urinating at night). Caffeinated drinks (coffee, tea, colas) have a mild diuretic effect, so they can increase the need to urinate.

Cold weather leads to urine retention and increases the urgency to urinate in some people, so try to stay warm.

Having **regular sex** is one of the best (and most enjoyable) ways of preventing prostate problems. Several studies have shown that men who have more sex may have less incidence of BPH as well as less prostate cancer.

Staying **physically active** has been shown in a 2014 study to decrease nocturia, especially severe nocturia (waking two or more times per night to urinate).

The Conventional Approaches

Medications: If your symptoms continue, your doctor may prescribe an *alpha-blocker* (doxazosin [Cardura], tamsulosin (Flomax), terazosin [Hytrin], or silodosin [Rapaflo]). These drugs have possible side effects of dizziness, weakness, rhinitis (runny nose), postural hypotension (dizziness when standing up), and reduced sexual function and desire. *Warning*: Alpha-blockers can also cause serious side effects when taken with erectile dysfunction (ED) drugs.

If these drugs do not work, your doctor may prescribe a *5a-reductase inhibitor* (finasteride [Proscar]), dutasteride [Avodart]) as the next step for mild to moderate prostate enlargement. Dutasteride will become a generic in 2015. These medications also may reduce sexual function and desire and cause low blood pressure and dizziness. *Warning*: Proscar may cause decreased libido that persists post-treatment.

Important Note: Alpha-blockers and 5a-reductase inhibitors are primarily used for relieving obstructive symptoms, such as incomplete emptying and weak stream.

Another older class of drugs used for BPH is *anticholinergics*, such as oxybutynin (Ditropan) or tolterodine (Detrol). These drugs are used primarily for patients with "storage" problems, that is, symptoms of frequency, urgency, or nocturia. However, they can have side effects of dry eyes, dry mouth, heartburn, fatigue, and urinary retention, which is why the above medications are often preferred.

Important notes: A combination of all these types of drugs appears to work no better than each alone. It should be noted as well that these drugs only decrease nocturia (needing to urinate at night) in a minority of patients. A 2013 study in the *Journal of Urology* showed that the combination of alpha-blockers and anticholinergics is only slightly better than each alone (and many experts think there is no advantage at all). In fact, overall effectiveness is lacking: The American Urologic Association rates alpha-blockers as giving a 12–16 percent improvement and 5a-reductase drugs as a 4–6 percent improvement. The new alpha-blocker, Rapaflo, may be somewhat better, but is more expensive. ***Warning***: The FDA announced in June 2011 that these drugs are associated with increased risk for more aggressive prostate cancer at time of diagnosis.

In October 2011, the FDA announced that *tadalafil* (Cialis, 5 mg daily) has been approved to treat BPH and provides significant improvements. Studies comparing it to the above drugs do show comparable benefits.

Some physicians have used **Botox injections** into the prostate, but a 2014 study in the *Journal of Urology* showed that this is no better than placebo.

If drugs don't work, **surgery** is the last resort, but there are numerous types of surgery, as follows:

- *Transurethral prostatectomy* (TURP) is the standard and does not increase the risk of ED or incontinence. Bleeding and infection are the possible complications for an open procedure. However, it can also be done by laparoscopy, which is helpful for selected patients with large-volume, obstructive BPH.
- *Robotic simple prostatectomy* is relatively new. Studies show this alternative to have less surgical time and minimal side effects. The limitation is the experience and training of the surgeon.
- *Laser vaporization* removes prostate tissue using low-energy plasma radiation. There are several types of laser that can be used:
  - Coagulative laser: neodymium: yttrium–aluminum–garnet (Nd:YAG), diode laser;
  - Cutting laser: holmium:YAG (Ho:YAG) and thulium:YAG (Tm:YAG);
  - Vaporizing laser: Nd:YAG, Ho:YAG, diode, KTP (potassium–titanyl–phosphate) and lithium triborate (LBO).
  - Green laser vaporization

A review of the vaporization procedure in 2011 in *Therapeutic Advances in Urology* concluded that bipolar vaporization of the prostate is safe and effective, providing low complication rates at a significantly reduced cost per procedure. However, other studies showed it to not to be lasting and effective enough compared with the gold standard TURP. Laser treatment is primarily suitable for patients with cardiac pacemakers, bleeding disorders, or those under anticoagulant therapy, for which TURP may be contraindicated.

- *Holmium laser enucleation* (HoLep) was developed as a more efficient and cost effective method of surgery for BPH than laser vaporization and resection techniques; it mimics open prostatectomy and is as long lasting. Multiple studies report that it is a safe and effective procedure for treating symptomatic BPH, independent of prostate size, and with low risk of side effects and a short hospital stay. The limitation of this technique is the experience and training of the surgeon.
- There are several *minimally invasive procedures* that can be done, including balloon dilatation, stents, transurethral needle ablation (TUNA), transurethral microwave thermotherapy (TUMT), and high-intensity ultrasound. These procedures have not been fully researched in comparison to each other or TURP. It is important to evaluate these procedures and obtain second opinions before undergoing them.
- *Open prostatectomy* is the surgery of last resort, involving the removal of the prostate externally. Minimally invasive procedures have led to higher rates of urinary incontinence and ED than open prostatectomy. All these surgeries can have potential side effects involving sexual dysfunction, although they are uncommon in the hands of a skilled surgeon.

The Alternative Approaches

Acupuncture may help many men with prostate enlargement and can reduce symptoms of slow stream and nocturia. It usually takes 4-6 treatments to see benefit but the results can be long lasting.

Nutritional supplements may be very helpful for reducing symptoms or enlargement of the prostate. These include:

- *Saw palmetto* (160 mg twice a day, standardized to contain 85–95 percent fatty acids and sterols) is similar in action to finasteride, and is the most commonly used herb for BPH. It has been shown in some studies to be effective for mild to moderate BPH, but other studies have shown no benefit. If it hasn't worked within four to eight weeks, it probably won't work.
- *Pumpkin seed* (5 g twice daily) and *pygeum* (100–200 mg of standardized lipophilic extract twice daily, containing 0.5 percent docosanol and 14 percent triterpenes) are contained in many herbal prostate formulas, although they may be effective at reducing prostate enlargement by themselves.
- *Cernilton* (60–120 mg, two to three times daily), an extract of flower pollen, has been used in Europe for thirty-five years and reduces symptoms in 70 percent of patients. You should notice improvement within three to four weeks.

- *African wild potato* (containing 60–130 mg of beta-sitosterol divided into two to three doses daily) is another herb that has shown effectiveness in studies. Beta-sitosterol is also found in pumpkin seeds and saw palmetto.
- *Cranberry powder* (500 mg three times a day) may significantly reduce BPH and lower PSA levels according to a recent study.
- *Other nutritional supplements* have been shown to decrease prostatic enlargement, increase urine flow, and decrease most symptoms of BPH. They include:
  - *Zinc* (45–60 mg per day)
  - *Flaxseed* (1 Tbsp daily, freshly ground)
  - *Amino acids*, a daily combination of 200 mg of each: glycine, glutamic acid, and alanine

These nutrients can be taken together if one does not completely eliminate your symptoms. You should notice improvement within four to six weeks with these supplements.

A **Chinese herbal formula**, called *Ba Zheng San*, can often help relieve the symptoms of BPH. *Rhabdosia Prostate Formula* is effective for many prostate symptoms.

Your Empowered Patient Action Plan for Treating BPH

Step #1: Undergo acupuncture for long term resolution. This may be the most cost-effective treatment for resolving your BPH, although it doesn't work in everyone.

Herb was a sixty-seven-year-old man who tried to be active but was limited by his BPH. He had to urinate numerous times during both the day and night and was not getting restful sleep. His doctor prescribed several types of medications, but none worked very well. I performed acupuncture for eight sessions, which resolved his symptoms completely. Afterward, I suggested he take ground flaxseed to maintain prostate function and improve his circulation.

Step #2: Take various nutritional supplements to reduce symptoms if acupuncture is not beneficial. Start with cernilton, cranberry powder, African wild potato, or a combination of saw palmetto with pygeum/pumpkin seed. These have less side effects than conventional medications.

Step #3: Take tadalafil (Cialis) if you still have symptoms and especially if you have ED as well (it may help both at the same time).

*Step #4: **Take zinc, flaxseed oil, and/or amino acids*** to help reduce symptoms if you are still having BPH symptoms.

*Step #5: **Take Ba Zheng San*** to reduce symptoms if the above steps have not helped.

*Step #6: **Take an alpha-blocker or a 5a-reductase drug*** to reduce symptoms if the above steps still have not worked.

*Step #7: **Undergo surgery as a last resort:*** TURP is still the most common surgery, although there are types to choose from. Be sure to obtain a second (or even third) opinion to find the best procedure for your combination of symptoms and physical findings.

Expected Outcome

BPH is a very common condition and one for which conventional drugs may not be very successful at relieving symptoms and can have significant side effects. Although surgery can resolve symptoms, it has possible side effects; and with alternative methods, relief may be obtained in most men without the need for surgery and side effects.

Prostatitis (Chronic pelvic pain syndrome)

What You Need to Know

Prostatitis has been described as an inflammation of the prostate (thus the term "itis"), but only two types can actually cause inflammation: acute or chronic bacterial infection. However, these types are the most uncommon causes of actual prostatitis: Most prostatitis is nonbacterial, and in fact, recent studies have shown that it really does not involve inflammation. For this reason, no one really knows what causes it, and most conventional treatments are ineffective as a result. Many physicians refer to chronic prostatitis as chronic pelvic pain syndrome.

Treatments for Prostatitis

The Preventive Approaches

Both urination and ejaculation flush the urethra and thus may provide a defense against prostatic infection and irritation. The prostate also secretes an antibacterial substance known as prostatic antibacterial factor into the seminal fluid (semen), which helps to fight infection. For this reason, **drinking increased fluids** and having **sex** regularly may help prevent prostatitis.

Sex Is Beneficial for Treating Prostatitis

In one preliminary study, unmarried men with nonbacterial prostatitis who had avoided sexual activity for personal or religious reasons and who had not responded to medication were encouraged to masturbate at least twice a week for six months. Seventy-eight percent experienced moderate to complete relief of symptoms.

To avoid infection of the prostate, you should practice good hygiene and keep your penis clean. You should also seek early treatment of any possible urinary tract infection.

Smoking tobacco reduces the zinc content of prostatic fluid and may therefore reduce natural immunity to prostate infection. No research has investigated the effect of smoking cessation on the prevention of prostatitis, but it is still a good idea to stop.

The Conventional Approaches

Medications are the primary conventional treatments for prostatitis, although they have only modest effects at best. For *bacterial prostatitis* (diagnosed by urine culture), antibiotics are used to cure the infection. If you have acute bacterial prostatitis, you may need to be hospitalized for a few days to receive antibiotics intravenously, and you may need oral medication for a few weeks. How long you take antibiotics depends on how well you respond to the drug.

Chronic bacterial prostatitis is more resistant to antibiotics and takes longer to treat. You may need to continue taking medication for as long as six to twelve weeks. In some cases the infection may never be eliminated, and you could have a relapse as soon as the drug is withdrawn. If this happens, you may need to take a low-dose antibiotic indefinitely.

For *nonbacterial prostatitis/chronic pelvic pain* syndrome, some doctors may prescribe an antibiotic to see if symptoms improve. For unknown reasons, some men with this condition seem to benefit from a continuous low dose of an antibiotic, but usually it does not respond.

Other medications are used for control of various symptoms:

- *Alpha-blockers.* If you're having difficulty urinating, your doctor may prescribe an alpha-blocker, an oral medication that helps relax the bladder neck and the muscle fibers where your prostate joins your bladder (includes doxazosin

[Cardura], tamsulosin (Flomax), terazosin [Hytrin], or silodosin [Rapaflo]). These medications may help you urinate more easily and empty your bladder more completely. ***Important note***: Recent studies show that alpha-blockers do not help prostatitis symptoms any better than placebo.

- *Pain relievers.* Sometimes OTC pain relievers, such as aspirin or ibuprofen (Motrin, Advil, others), are used to make you more comfortable. Keep in mind, however, that taking too much of any of these medications may cause side effects.
- *Muscle relaxants.* A combination of a muscle relaxant medication and other medications used to treat prostatitis may be helpful because spasms of the pelvic muscles can accompany prostatitis.

Special exercises and relaxation techniques can improve symptoms of prostatitis in some men. Common techniques include:

- *Exercise.* Stretching and relaxing the lower pelvic muscles, along with heat to make the muscles more limber, may help relieve your symptoms. Contact a physical therapist with training in these exercises.
- *Sitz baths.* This type of bath simply involves soaking the lower half of your body in a tub of warm water. Warm baths can relieve pain and relax the lower abdominal muscles.
- *Prostate massage.* Prostate massage may help relieve congestion by unplugging the small ducts blocked by inflammation. The massage is performed using a gloved finger, similar to what is done during a digital rectal exam. However, this procedure is not performed much anymore.

Surgical removal of the infected part of the prostate is an option in a few severe cases of bacterial prostatitis when other treatments don't work. However, the chances of responding to a major surgical procedure for any type of prostatitis are quite low. For this reason, most doctors are very hesitant to perform surgery for these conditions and generally discourage surgery even as a last resort.

The Alternative Approaches

Acupuncture is the best alternative treatment for prostatitis and may be able to resolve the symptoms completely and for long term. It usually takes six to eight treatments for initial benefits although more treatments may be necessary for maximum benefit.

A **Chinese herbal formula** such as *Ba Xheng San* may also be helpful in reducing symptoms. *Tian Wang Bu Xin Dan* tonifies and calms the body but should not be used if you have Spleen Qi Deficiency (consult a TCM practitioner)

Biofeedback is a mind-body technique that teaches you how to control certain body responses, including relaxing your bladder muscles. During a biofeedback session, a trained therapist applies electrodes and other sensors to various parts of your body. The electrodes are attached to a monitor that displays your heart rate, blood pressure, and degree of muscle tension. You'll see changes on the monitor and learn to control these changes on your own.

There are several **nutritional supplements** that have been used for prostatitis. Taking *quercetin* (500 mg twice daily) orally seems to reduce pain and improve quality of life but does not seem to affect voiding dysfunction in patients with chronic, nonbacterial prostatitis. *Saw palmetto* and *zinc* have been used but don't appear to be beneficial.

Your Empowered Patient Action Plan for Treating Prostatitis

Step #1: Take antibiotics only if urine cultures show a bacterial cause.

Step #2: Undergo acupuncture to obtain long lasting relief. This is probably the most effective (and cost-effective) treatment.

Step #3: Take Ba Xheng San to control symptoms. You can take this Chinese herbal along with acupuncture as well.

Step #4: Take quercetin if you continue to have symptoms despite the above steps.

Dwayne is a sixty-two-year-old patient of mine who had suffered from chronic prostatitis for six years. He had intermittent severe pelvic pain and frequent urination, which woke him up at night several times. The pain increased when he had sex and had caused problems with his marriage. He had taken years of antibiotics, tried alpha-blockers and other drugs, and tried saw palmetto, all to no benefit. I placed him on quercetin and performed acupuncture. In eight treatments, his symptoms had vanished.

Step #5: Undergo biofeedback to control symptoms if you still have problems.

Step #6: Undergo physical therapy involving pelvic-floor exercises to reduce symptoms if none of the above has helped.

Step #7: Take sitz baths to relieve pain.

Step #8: Try alpha-blockers if you have difficulty urinating.

Step #9: Take muscle relaxers if you have bladder spasms.

Expected Outcome

Prostatitis can be a chronic and unrelenting condition that does not often respond well to conventional methods. With some alternative approaches, however, it may be controlled or even resolved.

Restless Legs Syndrome (RLS)

What You Need to Know

RLS is a syndrome in which your legs feel very uncomfortable while they are at rest, and moving them often resolves the symptoms. Because it happens frequently at night, it can definitely interfere with sleep, but it can also occur during the day.

RLS is often thought of as causing involuntary twitching or kicking of the legs, but that condition is called periodic limb movements of sleep (PLMS). However, 80 percent of people with RLS also experience PLMS, and the treatments are the same.

Important Information
RLS Can Be Associated with Stroke and Heart Disease

A study published in *Neurology* revealed that RLS is associated with a significantly increased risk for strokes and heart disease. This association was strongest for those who had at least sixteen episodes a month and for those who had more severe symptoms. The reasons for this association may include poor quality of sleep as well as recurrent increases in blood pressure and heart rate when these leg movements occur. Some people have as many as two to three hundred periodic leg movements every night.

Many Doctors Ignore RLS Symptoms

A recent study in the *Archives of Internal Medicine* revealed that 81 percent of patients with RLS symptoms at least twice a week reported discussing their symptoms with their primary care physicians, but only 6.2 percent had received a diagnosis of RLS. Because RLS may be associated with strokes and heart disease, it is important for your doctor to address this condition.

———— ⸘ ————

Treatments for Restless Legs Syndrome

The Preventive Approaches

Correctible causes: There are several other conditions that may cause or exacerbate RLS, so controlling these conditions may help relieve RLS. These conditions include peripheral neuropathy (from alcoholism), iron deficiency, and kidney failure.

Relaxation may lessen the symptoms as stress tends to worsen RLS symptoms.

Pregnancy can also temporarily worsen RLS symptoms, but they usually disappear after delivery.

Some **medications** may worsen the symptoms of RLS, most notably antidepressants and some antinausea drugs. Avoiding these drugs may help reduce symptoms.

There are several **lifestyle changes** that can help prevent worsening of RLS symptoms. These include:

- *Exercise* may relieve symptoms, but don't overdo it or work out late in the evening.
- *Taking baths and massages* to relax your muscles.
- *Applying warm or cold packs* (or alternating) can lessen the sensations in your legs.
- *Avoiding caffeine* can sometimes reduce symptoms. This includes coffee, tea, soft drinks, and chocolate.
- *Cut back on alcohol and tobacco*, which can aggravate RLS symptoms.

The Conventional Approaches

Medications: There are several pain relievers that can help reduce the uncomfortable feeling. Sometimes, OTC drugs such as ibuprofen (Advil, Motrin, etc.) may help when the symptoms begin.

Other prescription medications can be useful if the minor analgesics are not, especially for symptoms of PLMS. The primary drugs are ones actually used for Parkinson's disease. These include *pramipexole* (Mirapex), *ropinirole* (Requip), and a combination of carbidopa and levodopa (*Sinemet*). A generic of ropinirole has now been approved for use in RLS and is less expensive. **Caution**: Pramipexole and ropinirole can have side effects of impulse control disorders (compulsive gambling, hypersexuality, shopping sprees) and may worsen symptoms in the long term.

Some *drugs used for seizures* may also help, including *gabapentin* (Neurontin) and *pregabalin* (Lyrica). A recently approved drug (in 2011) is *gabapentin enacarbil* (Horizant), which is a precursor of gabapentin but carries the same side effects such as drowsiness, dizziness, and increased risk for suicidal thoughts. A 2014 study in the *NEJM* showed that pregabalin and pramipexole are equally effective, but the latter is more likely to augment RLS.

Sometimes, doctors prescribe *benzodiazepines* (Valium, Xanax) to help you sleep better at night. However, these drugs do not reduce the leg sensations and may cause daytime drowsiness. If symptoms are severe, *narcotic medications* may be prescribed. However, they are highly addictive and can have significant side effects.

If one of the above medications doesn't work, a combination might. However, sometimes a medication that has worked for you may become ineffective after a prolonged period of time, or you may find your symptoms starting earlier than normal. Another medication will have to be substituted if that occurs. *Caution*: Some of these drugs may initially help but may worsen the condition over time.

Relaxis is the first device to help improve quality of sleep in patients with RLS and was approved in 2014. It uses a low-profile pad, which you place your legs on and which provides counter stimulation that gradually ramps down and shuts off. It has been shown to be as effective as medications and superior to placebo. *Caution*: Relaxis may worsen symptoms of RLS, but this is reversible upon discontinuing use of the device.

The Alternative Approaches

Acupuncture is the best alternative treatment for RLS and may reduce or resolve symptoms long-term. You should obtain initial benefits within six to eight treatments, although more treatments may be necessary for maximum benefit.

Chinese herbal formulas may also be helpful. *Feng Shi Pian* ("rheumatism tablets") or *Xuan Bi Tang Wan* may be recommended by a TCM practitioner.

Several **nutritional supplements** may be of value in RLS:

- If you are iron-deficient, taking *iron* supplements may improve your condition and has been shown equivalent to taking pramipexole. If you are not iron-deficient, it won't help.
- *Magnesium* (300 mg each evening for four to six weeks) improves sleep efficiency in patients with RLS.

- *Vitamin E* (400 IU daily) has been shown in one small study to eliminate symptoms in 80 percent of the subjects but takes at least three months to do so. It can also help control nocturnal leg cramps.
- *Folic acid* in high doses (5,000–30,000 mcg daily) may be beneficial in people who have a genetic form of RLS. Due to the high doses, these amounts should be taken under the supervision of a healthcare provider.

Your Empowered Patient Action Plan for Treating RLS and PMLS

Step #1: Undergo acupuncture for long-term relief. This is the best and most cost-effective treatment.

Step #2: Use various lifestyle changes as mentioned above to reduce symptoms while undergoing acupuncture and to prevent reoccurrence.

Step #3: Try the Relaxis device since it has minimal side effects compared to medications.

Step #4: Take magnesium and vitamin E to reduce or eliminate symptoms and improve sleep if the above steps have not helped.

Step #5: Try appropriate prescription medications to control symptoms if the above steps have not been effective. Start with Parkinson's-type medications and then try antiseizure medications.

Step #6: Take narcotic medications for severe pain under the direction of a pain management specialist if you still have symptoms.

Step #7: Take folic acid if RLS runs in your family.

Expected Outcome

It is important to effectively control restless legs syndrome to reduce risk for other conditions. With the above steps, most people can adequately control or even resolve their symptoms.

Rheumatoid Arthritis (RA)

What You Need to Know

Unlike *osteo*arthritis, rheumatoid arthritis is caused by dysfunction of the immune system, which makes cells (antibodies) that can destroy your joints and other tissues. This disease can be variable and unpredictable, causing flare-ups and remissions, or it can be progressive.

Rheumatoid arthritis can cause significant structural damage to your joints (gnarled and misshapen joints) and can have systemic effects leading to damage of other organ systems, including heart, lungs, eyes, nerves, and muscles.

Those with rheumatoid arthritis have substantially reduced life expectancy because of heart disease and also have increased in-hospital deaths following acute respiratory failure.

Interestingly, women who live in New England have a 37–43 percent elevated risk of RA compared to those living in the West. The reasons are unknown.

Procalcitonin: Ruling Out Infection

Patients with autoimmune diseases such as rheumatoid arthritis will often have fevers caused by the disease. However, infections also are common in such patients, due both to the disease and some of the treatments.

The question is whether fever indicates a potentially serious infection or is a manifestation of the disease. Procalcitonin is made by certain organs in the body and has been shown to help differentiate between an autoimmune flare and an infection (if elevated, it indicates probable infection).

Treatments for Rheumatoid Arthritis

The Preventive Approaches

Food allergies have been implicated as a possible cause of RA, and an **elimination diet** is helpful for determining if any foods are contributing to your condition. The most common foods causing inflammation are wheat, corn, milk, and foods from the nightshade family, such as potatoes, eggplant, tomatoes, peppers, and tobacco. Beef protein, especially, may be implicated.

Diet: Foods that help reduce RA symptoms include beans, fruits and vegetables, flavonoid-containing berries (cherries, blueberries, blackberries), and cold-water fish (mackerel, herring, halibut, trout, cod, sardines, and salmon). The use of olive oil (3 Tbsp per day) is also excellent at reducing inflammation and symptoms of rheumatoid arthritis. When cooking, the use of ginger and turmeric also aids in decreasing joint inflammation.

A recent study has found that **vitamin D** deficiency is very common in almost 85 percent of patients. Whether supplementation will help your symptoms is unknown, but you should have your blood levels measured and correct them if you are insufficient.

A recent study showed that personal use of **insecticides** may also increase the risk for rheumatoid disease, so avoid exposure to them.

The Conventional Approaches

Medications: The first purpose of treatment in RA is to control your symptoms and inflammation of the joints. Treatment with powerful medications is geared to four different categories of disease activity: low/moderate, moderate (with poor prognostic factors [PPF]), high without PPF, and high with PPF (see chart below for PPF).

—☙—

Poor Prognostic Factors in Rheumatoid Arthritis

Morning stiffness lasting longer than 1 hour

Arthritis involving more than 3 joints

More than 8 swollen, tender joints

Rheumatoid nodules

Anti-CCP antibodies (blood)

Presence of vasculitis (blood vessel inflammation)

Internal organ involvement (eye, lung)

Symmetric arthritis

Arthritis affecting the hands

High Rheumatoid factor (blood test)

High levels of CRP or ESR (blood)

Bone/cartilage erosions on x-ray

—☙—

Salicylates (aspirin compounds) are the primary drugs initially to control pain and stiffness in *mild* rheumatoid arthritis. ***Important note***: If you take aspirin, you should avoid taking ibuprofen, which blocks the blood-thinning effects of aspirin. If you must take ibuprofen, take the aspirin first and wait at least two hours to take the ibuprofen so that the aspirin has time to exert its beneficial effects. Take as few ibuprofen as you can as three doses will negate 90 percent of aspirin's effects, even if taken after the aspirin dose. You should also take vitamin C (600 mg daily) as a supplement as aspirin can deplete vitamin C levels in the body.

If aspirin is not helpful, *NSAIDs* (such as naproxen [Naprosyn], meloxicam [Mobic], piroxicam [Feldene], oxaprozin [Daypro], nabumatone [Relafen], ketoprofen [Orudis], diclofenac [Cataflam], or diclofenac/misoprostol [Arthrotec]) are given to relieve inflammation and pain. OTC NSAIDS (ibuprofen, naproxen) are usually not as effective as the prescription NSAIDs. These medications may take at least three weeks to be effective. They may cause stomach irritation and bleeding, and if this occurs, you can try the Cox-2 inhibitor, celecoxib (Celebrex), which has less risk of these side effects.

Warnings: Studies show a small increased risk of heart attack in patients who use Cox-2 inhibitors. In July, 2015, the FDA started requiring all NSAIDs to carry a warning of increased risk of heart attacks, stroke and heart failure. This is especially evident when taken long term, at higher doses, or by people with pre-existing heart disease. The risks can increase as early as the first weeks of NSAID use. However, ibuprofen and naproxen do not appear to increase the risk, so are the safest and preferred NSAIDs.

Caution: Many patients are given opioids to control pain. However, a Cochrane review showed that they are of weak benefit, and the harms outweigh the risks.

The most potent weapons in the medical arsenal for moderate to severe or progressive rheumatoid arthritis are medications called *DMARDs*—disease-modifying antirheumatic drugs. Doctors usually prescribe these in combinations, depending on your category of severity. Methotrexate, minocycline, hydroxychloroquine sulfate, sulfasalazine, and auranofin (oral gold) are all beneficial and have similar effects to each other. *Methotrexate* is usually the first line drug prescribed.

A recent study showed that another DMARD, *leflunomide* (Arava), is more effective than methotrexate. However, a recent review by the FDA shows that it can cause severe liver injury, including liver failure. (This risk is higher for those using other liver-toxic drugs or who have liver disease). Methotrexate, however, can cause serious infections, although not commonly.

These powerful, toxic drugs *should be used under the supervision of a rheumatologist* and may need to be started as the first step (within the first year) if you have moderate to severe disease at the onset. Each drug may have potentially significant side effects. *Warning*: The risk of cancer is almost 50 percent higher in people treated with DMARDs.

A newer drug is *tofacitinib* (Xeljanz). This is the first new DMARD for RA in more than ten years and will be the first RA treatment in a new class of medicines known as janus kinase (JAK) inhibitors. Benefits include being an oral medication, with negatives being the cost ($30,000 annually). A 2014 study showed that it improved clinical response much better than methotrexate and modestly slowing joint deterioration, but has more toxicities, including shingles and cancers (lymphomas primarily). It may be covered by insurance only after failure of other drugs.

There are also *stronger DMARDs* that are used as a last resort. Because of their possible side effects, you should use these drugs only if the previous medications are ineffective. These include penicillamine, azathiaprine, cyclophosphamide, and cyclosporine.

Another beneficial class of drugs is referred to as *biologics or tumor-necrosis factor antagonists* (etanercept [Enbrel], infiximab [Remicade]). These drugs are given intravenously and can prevent erosion of your joints when your rheumatoid arthritis is severe (high activity with PPF). You must use these along with methotrexate (or one of the other DMARDs) to avoid the formation of cells (antibodies) that can destroy these drugs. These are powerful drugs with potentially serious side effects (life-threatening infections, including tuberculosis), so discuss them with your doctor.

Rheumatoid arthritis may continue to progress, causing destruction of your joints. If you have significant erosions of your bones, you can undergo **joint replacement** by a qualified orthopedic surgeon.

The Alternative Approaches

Acupuncture can address the entire body as well as improve immune system dysfunction. It is very good for decreasing symptoms of RA but not necessarily controlling joint destruction. You should notice improvement within six to ten acupuncture treatments, but you will most likely need additional sessions for maximum benefit.

Chinese herbal formulas can be beneficial in treating the underlying immune dysfunction and some of the symptoms of rheumatoid arthritis and can be used along with acupuncture. *Shu Jing Huo Xue Tang* or *Du Huo Luo Dan* may be helpful. You should notice improvement within three weeks, but you may need to take them longer for full relief. A Chinese herb called *Tripterygium wilfordii* (also known as thunder god vine or lei gong teng) has been shown to be more effective than sulfasalazine, according to a study in the *Annals of Internal Medicine*.

Qigong/tai chi is excellent at reducing joint pain and also has a beneficial effect on the immune system. It may take three months for maximum effects, but you should see initial results in two to four weeks. There are qigong exercises that can be performed sitting or lying down.

If you have specific joints that are affected, **low level energy laser** ("cold" laser or *LLELs)* can be very beneficial as well. These lasers reduce swelling and stiffness and give long-lasting pain relief in many patients. They are called "cold" lasers, because they do not produce heat like the hot lasers used in surgical procedures and have few to no side effects. You should notice improvement within six to nine treatments (two to three weeks). (See chapter 4 for more information on cold lasers).

Several **nutritional supplements** may help reduce symptoms of rheumatoid arthritis.

- *Omega-3 fatty-acid supplements* flaxseed (freshly ground) or fish oil have anti-inflammatory properties. Both of these oils have been shown to potentiate the effect of NSAIDs as well as decrease the need for NSAIDs. A 2015 study showed that the addition of fish oils to DMARDs lowered the risk of treatment failure. It may take about one to two months to observe an effect with flaxseed or fish oil.

- *Important notes*: There are problems with fish oil that you need to be aware of. You must take *at least* 1,500 mg daily to obtain benefits. Many studies were done using 3,000–4,000 mg, especially with RA. Many fish oils also deteriorate very rapidly (three months); so by the time you buy them, they may already be partially deteriorated. Krill oil may be more potent and stable, contains two natural antioxidants, and has few to no side effects. However, krill oil products differ in their concentrations of omega-3s and combinations with other ingredients, so check the label.
- *Sea cucumber* (500 mg) is another potent anti-inflammatory that has been shown in Australian studies to be very effective in reducing symptoms in most people with RA. You should take four per day for the first two weeks and then take two per day. You should notice improvement within one to two months.
- You can also take *mucopolysaccharides* (such as beta 1,3/1,6 glucan, 1 daily), special carbohydrates that can trap antibodies and thus may help prevent destruction of the joints.
- *Borage oil* (1,500 mg daily), an omega-6 fatty acid that has anti-inflammatory properties, is another supplement that can be beneficial. Mucopolysaccharides and borage oil may take six to eight weeks to be beneficial.

If you suspect food allergies, **NAET** combines acupuncture, kinesiology, chiropractic, herbs, and nutrition to desensitize you to foods you are allergic to. It may take several months to notice improvement, depending on how many allergens are sensitizing you (see Chapter 4 for more discussion on this method).

Your Empowered Patient Action Plan for Treating Rheumatoid Arthritis

- *For moderate to severe rheumatoid arthritis, go to steps 10–13; then return to step 3 when your symptoms stabilize. Depending on the benefits of the first steps, you may then be able to decrease or discontinue the stronger medications.*

Step #1: Take aspirin for temporary relief of *mild* symptoms.

Step #2: Take prescription NSAIDs for temporary relief of *mild to moderate* symptoms.

Step #3: Take omega-3s to potentiate NSAIDs and decrease inflammation for mild disease.

Step #4: Participate in qigong/tai chi to reduce symptoms, improve immune system function, and help prevent progression of the disease along with other steps.

Step #5: Undergo acupuncture for longer-term relief and control of flare-ups.

Step #6: *Receive LLEL treatment* for long-term relief on specific joints. This treatment can be very effective.

———❀———

Roxanne had severe rheumatoid arthritis for more than forty-five years. Over the years, she had been prescribed steroids and numerous DMARDs, which would only give her moderate relief from her pain and stiffness and to which she would become resistant after a year or two. She had significant destruction of her finger joints and was unable to even pick up a piece of paper. I placed her on Krill oil and provided cold laser treatment. After just seven treatments, she was able to not only pick up a piece of paper but also open jars. Her deformities could not be corrected, but her pain and stiffness were reduced significantly.

———❀———

Step #7: *Take sea cucumber, mucopolysaccharides, and/or borage oil* to significantly reduce symptoms if the above methods have not resolved all your symptoms.

———❀———

For a long time, Betty was able to control her mild rheumatoid arthritis with aspirin. Her symptoms began worsening, and she was prescribed several NSAIDs, but they did not control the symptoms. I placed her on sea cucumber and krill oil and then gave her cold laser and acupuncture treatments. Within one month, all her symptoms had resolved. I continued her on the Krill oil and I advised her that she might have flare-ups, which should respond to additional laser treatment and sea cucumber.

———❀———

Step #8: *Take Chinese herbal remedies Shu Jing Huo Xue Tang or Du Huo Luo Dan* to reduce symptoms if you still have pain and stiffness.

Step #9: *Use the NAET* if food allergies are a suspected cause or precipitating factor.

Step #10: *Take low-dose prednisolone* if you continue to have symptoms or your disease is moderately severe.

Step #11: *Take prescription DMARD medications* to control moderate to severe symptoms and retard the disease if it has progressed. Take omega 3's with them.

Step #12: *Receive etanercept or infiximab by injection* if the above step is not effective or, for some people, in place of the above step.

Step #13: *Take stronger DMARDs* if the disease continues to progress.

Step #14: *Undergo surgery* to replace destroyed joints if indicated.

Expected Outcome

Rheumatoid arthritis is a very difficult disease to conquer, and it cannot be cured. However, it can be controlled sufficiently to decrease symptoms significantly and improve quality of life in most patients.

Sciatica (Acute)

What You Need to Know

Sciatica is one of the most common nerve conditions and can occur at any age. It involves irritation, damage, or inflammation of the sciatic nerve, a large nerve that comprises several nerves from the lower lumbar and sacral levels of the spinal canal. These nerves combine together in the pelvic region, enter the leg, and then branch out into separate nerves once again.

Often, sciatica occurs in people who have degenerative disc disease (arthritis of the spine), and doctors may conclude that it is your disc deterioration that is causing your symptoms, sometimes recommending invasive treatments (including surgery). However, this nerve can be adversely affected by other causes (such as piriformis syndrome or pelvic structural dysfunction), so it may not be the disc disease causing your symptoms. It is important to follow the steps below and not rush into an invasive procedure that may not help—or even make you worse.

Often, sciatica may occur but then resolve on its own after a few days or weeks. However, it can become chronic and last for years. I will discuss treatments for both. This section will discuss *acute* (recent) onset sciatica.

Important Information:
Most Doctors Ignore National Guidelines for MRI Scans

MRI scans are performed and repeated much too often for sciatica. Studies show that there is a minimal chance of any significant change within a year of doing an MRI scan, but many doctors repeat them before then because they own their own MRI scan centers or are worried that they will miss something.

The national guidelines for spine pain recommend against ordering imaging or other diagnostic tests unless severe or progressive neurological defects (e.g., paralysis, loss of bladder/rectal control) are present or a condition such as cancer is suspected. Furthermore, MRI should be done only if surgery or epidural injections are considered. Based on the steps below, most MRIs are not needed and do not improve outcome.

⸺∞⸺

Treatments for Acute Sciatica

The Preventive Approaches
Sitting, lifting, and performing activities properly are very important factors in both preventing and treating sciatica. For example, many people walk hunched over or sit stooped over a computer. You might lift without using your legs. *Back schools* or *physical therapists* who teach proper posture and techniques can benefit most people with sciatica. These schools also teach you dozens of ways to avoid worsening and flare-ups of back pain and further injuries.

Exercise is a mainstay of prevention for sciatica. Proper stretching and resistance exercises are the most important, along with exercises specifically designed for the spine.

The Conventional Approaches

⸺∞⸺

Dr. A's Suggestions:
Avoid Treatments That Don't Work

For *acute* sciatica, many treatments are given that have been proven not helpful by numerous studies and thus are not recommended. These include traction, prescription antidepressants, lumbar supports, and TENS units (small devices that conduct electricity to the superficial soft tissues).

⸺∞⸺

Medications: If your symptoms are mild, NSAIDs are usually started to help control your symptoms while the body has time to heal the nerve itself. OTC NSAIDs (ibuprofen, naproxen) are recommended first, but if not helpful, your doctor may prescribe stronger NSAIDs (such as naproxen [Naprosyn], meloxicam [Mobic], piroxicam [Feldene], oxaprozin [Daypro], nabumatone [Relafen], ketoprofen [Orudis], diclofenac

[Cataflam], or diclofenac/misoprostol [Arthrotec]). These NSAIDs all have equivalent effectiveness, but one particular form may be more effective than another for you; so you may need to try several to find the one that works best for you (ask your doctor for samples).

These NSAIDs are more powerful than the OTC variety but also have higher risk of side effects, primarily stomach irritation and bleeding. If stomach irritation occurs, an NSAID known as a Cox-2 inhibitor (Celebrex) has a lower risk of stomach problems, although it is more expensive and may not be covered by many insurance plans. *Caution*: Studies show a small increased risk of heart attack in patients who use Cox-2 inhibitors, so caution is advised if you have heart disease. In July, 2015, the FDA started requiring all NSAIDs to carry a warning of increased risk of heart attacks, stroke and heart failure. This is especially evident when taken long term, at higher doses, or by people with pre-existing heart disease. The risks can increase as early as the first weeks of NSAID use. However, ibuprofen and naproxen do not appear to increase the risk, so are the safest and preferred NSAIDs.

These medications are used to control your pain while the body heals itself and may not help if the condition is more severe. However, if your pain continues after several weeks, your doctor can prescribe stronger pain medication temporarily until your symptoms improve. *Tramadol* (Ultram) is a common choice of doctors, and if that isn't effective, propoxyphene is another option. *Warning*: Propoxyphene is not indicated for elderly people.

If your pain is more severe, *narcotic medications* may be prescribed, starting with codeine-containing compounds (hydrocodone, oxycodone) up to morphine or dilaudid. *Warning*: These medications are highly addictive and should be used only temporarily.

Muscle relaxers (such as Flexeril, Soma, Zanaflex, or Robaxin) can be used in conjunction with these medications for extra relief, but they may make you drowsy. As with the above medications, the use of muscle relaxers is to allow time for your body to heal itself, but you can become dependent on some of these medications, so you don't want to take them long-term. *Helpful tip*: Most studies show that muscle relaxers lose their effectiveness after a few days to a week.

Oral steroids are commonly given for acute sciatica, but a 2015 study showed that although there was some improvement in function, its clinical importance was marginal and it did not relieve pain nor decreased the likelihood of surgery. It did appear to improve disability scores but also had twice as many side effects as placebo. Overall, one out of seven people may benefit, but not to a great degree.

Other medications are commonly used to reduce the nerve pain running down your leg. The most common are *gabapentin* (Neurontin) and *pregabalin* (Lyrica), and they can help some patients but may cause drowsiness. They are not beneficial in the majority of people. *Warning*: The FDA has also warned that such drugs may cause suicidal behavior.

Physical therapy modalities are often provided in *acute* sciatica to help your nerve heal faster. However, many physical therapists also use exercises for treatment, which may make acute sciatica worse. Treatment modalities that are given include therapeutic massage and electrical current (both direct current and alternating current can be applied to the painful areas; I prefer alternating, which can project deeper into the tissues without burning the skin). These modalities increase blood flow and oxygen delivery to the damaged tissues, helping them heal faster. Other modalities include hot packs (dilate blood vessels and increase blood flow to the damaged area) and cold packs (for swelling and spasm). Ultrasound (high-frequency sound that projects heat into the deep tissues) can be used for some patients, but it can be irritating if there is inflammation present.

An **epidural steroid injection** is commonly given in the first six to eight weeks after onset if a herniated or bulging disc is suspected of causing the sciatica. The intended purpose of an epidural injection is to reduce the inflammation and allow the nerve to heal. If the first injection is not beneficial, you can repeat it once or twice, but no studies have shown benefit if the first is not effective.

Important note: Several studies, including a 2012 meta-analysis of 23 studies, have shown that epidural steroid injections are no better than placebo injections for sciatica or have little effectiveness (only in the short term, if at all). In addition, some doctors recommend injection of etanaercept, a tumor-necrosis factor used in rheumatoid arthritis, but this is even less effective than steroids. *Warning*: In rare cases, epidurals can cause blindness, stroke, paralysis, or death.

Surgery may be necessary if your nerves are being pinched by a ruptured disc and the previous steps are ineffective, and/or if you have neurological symptoms (loss of knee reflex, paralysis of the leg, or loss of bladder or bowel control). Surgery may also be necessary if you have intolerable pain going down your leg. If MRI does not show a significant disc problem correlated with neurological signs (such as leg weakness, sensory loss, or reflex loss), have further testing (myelogram) before you consider surgery.

Spinal Fusion: Overused and Abused

Spinal fusions have witnessed an explosive increase; estimates have placed the increase at 200 percent. The reason for this increase is due to new surgical techniques but above all, money.

Several studies have been done on spinal fusions, most with poor results, especially in acute sciatica. It should be noted that these studies have also not compared fusion to nonsurgical treatments including alternative methods. In a landmark study published in February 2011 in the *Annals of Rheumatic Disease*, it was proven that the invasive and high cost fusion procedure did not afford better outcomes as compared with a significantly lower-cost conservative treatment approach (education, support, and physical training sessions over three weeks).

The conclusion is that spinal fusion is tremendously overused and abused and is unnecessary in the majority of cases of acute sciatica, as well as being extremely expensive. If surgery is necessary, simple discectomy/ laminectomy may be just as beneficial and much cheaper. Unfortunately, fusion is considered standard practice and continues to be paid for by Medicare and insurance, unnecessarily increasing the costs of medical care.

The Alternative Approaches

Acupuncture is the best treatment to reduce or resolve sciatica. You should notice improvement within six acupuncture treatments, but you might need additional sessions for maximum benefit. Because acupuncture addresses the underlying cause, I can provide long-term resolution.

Along with acupuncture, a **Chinese herbal formula** called *Yan Hu Suo Wan* ("stop pain tablets") may help with acute pain.

Low level energy lasers *("cold" lasers or LLELs)* are also very effective and can be used with acupuncture. The laser appears to help heal the tissue (including nerves and spinal discs), reduce the inflammatory response, and give long-lasting relief for many nerve problems. These lasers are called "cold" lasers, because they do not produce heat like the hot lasers used in surgical procedures. You should notice improvement within three to nine treatments (two weeks). (See chapter 4 for more in-depth discussion of cold laser).

Several **topical solutions** can give temporary relief when applied over the painful area. These include Zheng Gu Shui (a topical Chinese liniment), EMU oil (usually combined with MSM and aloe vera), long crystal menthol, Biofreeze, capsaicin, glucosamine/MSM, and other herbal combinations. These topicals are not curative but may provide pain relief for two to eight hours and have minimal side effects (skin allergy or sensitivity are the most common). Some of these may work better than others on different people, so you may have to try several to find the best one. In my clinic, I applied samples to my patients so they would know whether a product works before purchasing it. Encourage your doctor or practitioner to do the same.

Infrasound, or low-frequency sound therapy, can also be helpful. Infrasound works by increasing the local circulation of blood, lymph, and the activity of the nervous system to accelerate the healing process. It not only can reduce pain but also decreases spasms and swelling. Numerous chiropractors, naturopaths, acupuncturists, and a few doctors use infrasound.

Because the sciatic nerve passes through the pelvis, misalignment problems involving your piriformis muscle, spine, pelvis, sacrum, and/or sacroiliac joint can be pinching, stretching, or irritating the nerve. If this is the case, **manual therapy** is necessary to correct the condition. For acute sciatica, chiropractic or osteopathic manipulation can help. With any type of manipulation, your pain should start decreasing in three to six treatments, although additional treatments may be necessary to achieve maximum benefit. If your pain is still present after ten to twelve treatments, further evaluation or a different method may be necessary.

A **homeopathic remedy**, Hypericum (30c three times daily for one week) may be helpful for nerve pain. If this is going to help, it should be evident within the first week of taking it.

Your Empowered Patient Action Plan for Treating Acute Sciatica

- **Warning**: *If you have worsening severe back pain with radiation down the leg, paralysis, or inability to urinate or have a bowel movement, you should obtain emergency medical attention and diagnostic testing such as MRI or myelogram (start with step 7).*

Step #1: *Apply Zheng Gu Shui, EMU oil, long crystal menthol, Biofreeze, capsaicin, or other topical solutions* for temporary pain relief *while using the following steps.*

Step #2: *Take medications* for temporary relief of mild pain while your nerve heals if step 1 doesn't help. Start with the least potent medications, but increase as needed.

Step #3: *Undergo alignment evaluation and receive manual manipulation* if findings show structural misalignment.

Step #4: *Undergo acupuncture* to resolve sciatica long-term if there are no alignment problems. This is the best and most cost-effective treatment for nerve pain.

Step #5: *Undergo LLEL* to resolve sciatica if you still have pain. This is the best and most cost-effective treatment for spinal disc derangement. It can be used with acupuncture for faster results.

Wayne had acute sciatic pain from lifting a heavy object. He had tried various NSAIDs and mild pain relievers, which helped control the pain. However, when he tried to stop taking the medications, his pain would return. His doctor sent him for physical therapy, but he was given exercises and traction only, which made his symptoms worse. I started him on cold laser and also performed acupuncture. His pain steadily decreased and was totally gone in three weeks.

—∞∞∞—

Step #6: ***Try Hypericum*** for at least three weeks if you still have pain.

Step #7: ***Undergo MRI scan*** to determine structural damage if the pain has continued.

Step #8: ***Try an epidural injection*** if the above step is positive and symptoms are persistent but not considered an emergency. If the first injection doesn't help, it is unlikely that further injections will help.

Step #9: ***Undergo surgery*** (discectomy/laminotomy) if you have a ruptured disc and continue to have severe pain and disability despite the above steps or neurological symptoms have developed. Avoid fusion surgery.

Step #10: ***Use cold laser treatment after surgery*** to accelerate healing and decrease scarring.

Expected Outcome

With acute sciatica, patience is advised. Although it may take several weeks or months, most sciatica can be resolved with various alternative methods, without the need for rushing into surgery.

Sciatica (Chronic)

What You Need to Know

Sciatica is one of the most common nerve conditions and can occur at any age. It involves inflammation of the sciatic nerve, a large nerve that is comprised of several nerves from the lower lumbar and sacral levels of the spinal canal. These nerves combine together in the pelvic region, enter the leg, and branch out into separate nerves once again.

Often, sciatica occurs in people who have degenerative disc disease (arthritis of the spine), and doctors may conclude that it is your disc deterioration that is causing your symptoms, sometimes recommending invasive treatments. However, this nerve can be irritated by other causes (such as piriformis syndrome or structural pelvic abnormalities), so it may not be the disc disease causing your symptoms. It is important to follow the steps below and not rush into an invasive procedure that may not help or may make you worse.

Although most sciatica can resolve on its own within a few weeks or months, it can become chronic, especially if underlying conditions exist as causes. This section deals with *chronic* sciatica.

Important Information:
Beware MRI Results for Chronic Sciatica

Treatments for chronic sciatica are often based on testing, such as MRI scan. Studies show that 75 percent of people with no back pain will have abnormalities on MRI, meaning that *just because you have an abnormality does not mean that is what is causing your sciatica.*

Unfortunately, many invasive procedures and surgeries are done based on the MRI, resulting in high failure rates and continuation or worsening of chronic pain. In fact, many surgeries are repeated due to failure, yet those have even a higher failure rate.

Treatments for Chronic Sciatica

The Preventive Approaches
Sitting, lifting, and performing activities properly are very important factors in both preventing and treating sciatica. For example, many people walk hunched over or sit stooped over a computer. You might lift without using your legs. *Back schools* or *physical therapists* who teach proper posture and techniques can benefit most people with sciatica, especially the chronic type. These schools also teach you dozens of ways to avoid worsening and flare-ups of back pain and further injuries.

Exercise is a mainstay of prevention for chronic sciatica. Proper stretching and resistance exercises are the most important, along with exercises specifically designed for the spine.

Ergonomic Products and appliances: There are many products that can help reduce chronic sciatica. This is in the realm of ergonomics, which is the design of such things as safe furniture and easy-to-use interfaces to machines and equipment. Proper ergonomic design is necessary to prevent repetitive strain injuries and other musculoskeletal disorders, which can develop over time and can lead to long-term disability. Such equipment includes special beds, mattresses, and pillows; back supports; and ergonomic chairs, desks, and recliners. You need to realize, however, that many companies make such products and you should always comparison shop to obtain the best product for you. These products can make your life much easier and less painful. *Helpful tip*: When purchasing such products, make sure you can return them if they don't help.

The Conventional Approaches

Dr. A's Suggestions:
Many Medical Procedures Ineffective for Chronic Sciatica

In the 2008 guidelines established by the American Pain Society, it was stated that local injections, Botox injections, facet joint injections, sacroiliac joint injections, and radiofrequency ablation "are not supported by convincing consistent evidence." Unfortunately, they continue to be done nevertheless.

Analgesic Medications: Usually, by the time your sciatica has become chronic, you have already tried less potent analgesics such as NSAIDs or pain relievers such as Tramadol (Ultram). You may have also tried muscle relaxants, but they have not been found to be beneficial in chronic sciatica.

Narcotic medication may be given to control the pain with continued symptoms. These stronger narcotics should be used only a short time due to their addiction potential but are often given long term by pain management specialists for severe chronic sciatica. The most common include Tylenol with codeine, hydrocodone, and oxycodone, but for more severe pain, morphine, dilaudid, fentanyl, or methadone may be prescribed. You should always obtain these medications from a *pain management specialist*.

Other medications are commonly used to reduce the nerve pain running down your leg (radiculopathy). The most common are *gabapentin* (Neurontin) and *pregabalin* (Lyrica), and they can help some patients but may cause drowsiness. However, no large randomized studies have been conducted to prove their efficacy. One study showed that gabapentin was no better than epidural steroid injections, which other studies have shown to be poorly effective as well (see below). *Warning*: The FDA has also warned that such drugs may cause suicidal behavior.

For some people, *low-dose antidepressants* such as amitriptyline (Elavil, 25 to 50 mg daily) or trazadone (Desyrel, 50 to 150 mg daily) can decrease chronic sciatic pain through effects on the pain center (hypothalamus) and neurotransmitters in the brain. It may take several weeks to a month before you notice improvement.

Physical therapy/modalities are often provided but are really not much help in chronic sciatica. However, specific *exercises* may help chronic sciatica. You should perform them under the auspices of a knowledgeable physical therapist.

Epidural steroid injections are commonly given for chronic sciatica but are *rarely helpful*, and no studies have supported their use. If the first injection is not beneficial (relief lasting several months), most of these doctors will advise undergoing two more, but again, no studies have shown benefit if the first is not effective. ***Warning***: In rare cases, epidurals can cause blindness, stroke, paralysis, or death.

Important Information:
Study Shows Epidural Steroid Injection to Be No Better than Placebo

Despite epidural steroid injections being routinely done for chronic sciatica, a study performed in Canada was the first one to compare these injections to one using only salt water (placebo). The results showed that the placebo injection was just as effective as the steroid injection. This study was totally ignored by doctors because epidural steroid injections are tremendous money-makers, costing up to $2,500 for a fifteen-minute procedure. The study was criticized for not including a series of three injections, yet no high quality study has been done to show that three injections are superior to one.

A meta-analysis of 23 studies published in 2012 showed that epidurals injections were ineffective for radiculopathy, at the most providing some short-term relief, but no long-term benefit. Epidural steroid injection is largely a wasteful and unnecessary procedure for most people with chronic sciatica.

Surgery is often done as a last resort, but like epidural injections, it has a very high failure rate for *chronic* sciatica. An increasingly common surgery for chronic sciatica is spinal fusion, in which your spinal bones (vertebrae) are fused together using bone from your hip (done by neurosurgeons) or with instrumentation (rods, screws, and/or cages, done by orthopedic surgeons). Sometimes, a 360-degree fusion is done, fusing the vertebrae from front *and* back.

Important Information:
Spinal Fusion: Overused and Abused

Spinal fusions have witnessed an explosive increase of 200 percent (from recent estimates). The reason for this increase is due to lingering symptoms, new surgical techniques, and, above all, money.

Several studies have been done on spinal fusions, most with poor results. For specific abnormalities such as spondylolisthesis and spinal stenosis, surgery may improve pain, function, and disability at two years for selected patients, but not in a majority of cases. For degenerative disc disease without radicular symptoms, less than half of patients experience optimal outcomes (optimum defined as reducing pain and increasing function by 50 percent). The rate of repeat surgery after the initial surgery is around 25 percent over four years.

It should be noted that these studies have not compared fusion to non-surgical treatments. In a landmark study published in February 2011 in the *Annals of Rheumatic Disease*, it was proven that the invasive and high-cost fusion procedure did not afford better outcomes as compared with a significantly lower-cost conservative treatment approach (education, support, and physical training sessions over three weeks). It should further be noted that fusion has never been compared to alternative methods as well.

The conclusion is that spinal fusion is tremendously overused and abused and is unnecessary in the majority of cases, as well as being extremely expensive. Unfortunately, it is considered standard practice and continues to be paid for by Medicare and insurance, unnecessarily increasing the costs of medical care.

A fusion done at one level, which is common in sciatica, exerts more pressure on the spinal disks above and below the fusion, typically causing them to deteriorate within two to five years. This is why many people have persistent or recurrent spine pain after such surgeries and end up undergoing many more surgeries. Additional fusion surgeries usually have very poor outcomes. Fusions for chronic sciatica should be done *only* for unrelenting pain with evidence of structural deterioration of the discs and/or additional or worsening neurological signs.

Less complex and less expensive surgeries can be done, although they also don't have very good outcomes for chronic sciatica. *Discectomy with laminectomy* (taking out the disc and cutting bone away to free the nerve, also referred to as "decompression") is the most common, although studies show that nonsurgical, alternative interventions (see below) are just as effective.

Important Information:
Be Careful What You Hear from Spine Surgeons:
The Last-Resort Fallacy and More

Spine surgeons commonly give you several reasons for undergoing spine surgery that are often misleading. The most common is that surgery is a "last resort" as "conservative treatment hasn't helped."

First, does a "last resort" mean it's effective? If it was *that* effective, it wouldn't be a last resort! Second, the treatments usually done before surgery don't include alternative treatments, which could help avoid most back surgeries.

Another common warning is that if you don't have the surgery, you could become paralyzed. This complication is extremely rare, and I have never seen it happen in thirty-nine years of practice.

The bottom line is that surgery, especially fusion, is very lucrative for the surgeon, costing you (or your insurer) $80,000-100,000 on average. The *bottom line* is don't rush into surgery, especially if they try to scare you.

The Alternative Approaches

Acupuncture is the best treatment to reduce or resolve sciatica. You should notice improvement within six acupuncture treatments but might need additional sessions for maximum benefit. Because acupuncture addresses the underlying cause, it can provide long-term relief.

A ***Chinese herbal formula***, *Jin Gui Shen Qi Wan*, may be useful in many chronic conditions that require "kidney energy."

Low level energy lasers ("cold" lasers or *LLELs)* are also very effective and can be used with acupuncture. The laser appears to help heal the tissue (including nerves and spinal discs), reduce the inflammatory response, and give long-lasting relief for many nerve problems. You should notice improvement within six to nine treatments (two to three weeks). The laser also provides long-term healing as it addresses the underlying cause rather than just treating symptoms.

Infrasound can also be helpful. Infrasound works by increasing the local circulation of blood, lymph, and the activity of the nervous system to accelerate the healing process. It can not only reduce pain but also decrease spasms and swelling. Numerous chiropractors, naturopaths, acupuncturists, and a few doctors use infrasound.

Because the sciatic nerve passes through the pelvis, misalignment problems involving your piriformis muscle, spine, pelvis, sacrum, or sacroiliac joint can be pinching, stretching, or irritating the nerve. If this is the case, **manual therapy** is necessary to correct the condition. For chronic sciatica, osteopathic manipulation may be preferred, although some chiropractic methods may help as well. With any type of manipulation, your pain should start decreasing in three to six treatments, although additional treatments may be necessary to achieve maximum benefit. If your pain is still present after ten to twelve treatments, further evaluation or a different method may be necessary.

Manual therapy includes **Bodywork**—but in different forms. There are several techniques, the most common being Rolfing, the Feldenkrais method, the Bowen technique, and the Alexander technique. Bodywork involves realigning, rebalancing, and retraining the structures of the body, which have become dysfunctional due to pain, injury, disuse, or misuse. The Feldenkrais method focuses on retraining how you move your body in order to interrupt unhealthy patterns of movement that have become habits. The Alexander technique concentrates on correcting faulty posture in daily activities (sitting, standing, and moving). Rolfing involves manipulating and stretching the body's fascial tissues (deep connective tissues that hold the body together), thus allowing correct realigning of the body. These bodywork methods require a therapist certified in these techniques.

Yoga may be successful in reducing chronic sciatica symptoms as well. Yoga promotes relaxation and stretching, both of which are important in healing and preventing sciatic pain. Because there are many different types of yoga, I recommend working with a qualified yoga instructor. The wrong type or doing it poorly can result in more pain, not less.

For residual pain or flare-ups of pain, several **topical solutions** can give temporary relief when applied over the painful area. These include Zheng Gu Shui (a topical Chinese liniment), EMU oil (usually combined with MSM and aloe vera), long crystal menthol, Biofreeze, capsaicin, glucosamine/MSM, Topricin cream, and other herbal combinations. These topicals are not curative but may provide pain relief for two to eight hours and have minimal side effects (skin allergy or sensitivity, most commonly). Some of these may work better than others on different people, so you may have to try several to find the best one. In my clinic, I applied samples to my patients so they can know whether a product works before purchasing it. Encourage your doctor or practitioner to do the same.

Your Empowered Patient Action Plan for Treating Chronic Sciatica

Step #1: Apply Zheng Gu Shui, EMU oil, long crystal menthol, Biofreeze, capsaicin, or other topical solutions for temporary pain relief in chronic sciatica while following the next steps.

Step #2: Undergo alignment evaluation and undergo mobilization if findings are positive.

Step #3: Undergo acupuncture to resolve sciatica long term if there are no alignment problems. This is the best and most cost-effective treatment for chronic sciatica.

Step #4: Undergo LLEL to resolve sciatica if you still have pain—and especially if you have low back pain along with the leg pain. It can be used with acupuncture for faster results.

Teresa injured her back several years ago, causing sciatica. After trying several conservative measures (medications and physical therapy), an MRI scan showed a bulging disc that was touching a nerve, and she underwent surgery. She had relief for about a year, but the pain returned. She was told that she had developed scar tissue and underwent another surgery to remove the scarring and fuse the bone. This surgery only helped for about a month, after which time she was told that another surgery may be necessary.

Her doctor placed her on low-dose antidepressants and narcotic pain relievers. She had tried biomagnets and several topical salves, but they only gave her relief for an hour or two. I recommended mobilization because I felt that her sacroiliac joint was dysfunctional. Sure enough, the exam showed not only sacroiliac joint dysfunction but also facet joint dysfunction in her entire lumbar area. After five treatments, her pain was much improved but still present. I then performed a combination of acupuncture and cold laser, which ended her remaining pain in seven treatments.

Step #5: Receive physical therapy exercises if you are still having pain.

Step #6: Undergo the Feldenkrais method, Alexander technique, or Rolfing to help relieve chronic sciatic pain if the above steps have not been beneficial.

Step #7: Practice appropriate yoga postures to help relieve chronic sciatic pain.

Step #8: Take low-dose prescription antidepressants to control chronic pain if the above steps have not helped.

Step #9: Take appropriate narcotic medications to control your pain, under the guidance of a doctor who specializes in pain management, if your symptoms continue.

Step #10: Undergo surgery only if you have a ruptured disc and continue to have severe pain and disability after following the above steps.

Step #11: Use cold laser treatment after surgery to accelerate healing and decrease scarring.

Expected Outcome

Chronic sciatica can be a persistent problem for years, but it doesn't need to be. With the advent of various alternative methods, it is potentially resolvable in the majority of patients. Laser and acupuncture can help prevent the need for surgery in the majority of cases.

Sexual Dysfunction in Men

What You Need to Know

As noted in chapter 2, sexual function is important, no matter what our age. In fact, surveys have shown that sexual activity often persists into the eighth decade, although sex with a partner declines to about 38 percent at that age.

In men, impotence and inability to maintain an erection (erectile dysfunction or ED) are the major problems. Physical factors are the primary cause (especially atherosclerosis) 90 percent of the time. Smoking, diabetes, obesity, metabolic syndrome, and increasing age are all contributing factors in decreasing testosterone levels.

Frequent Ejaculation Associated with Lower Prostate Cancer Risk

Sex is important not only emotionally and mentally but also physically. Several studies have shown that frequent ejaculation (with a partner or self) decreases the risk of prostate cancer.

ED May Indicate Other Medical Problems

Most men with ED don't realize that it is a sign of elevated risk for heart disease. In addition, a 2015 study revealed that men with erectile dysfunction had more than double the odds of having undiagnosed diabetes. So, if you have ED, have your heart checked and be screened for diabetes. The good news is that, with some lifestyle changes and integrative treatments, both problems can be helped.

Treatments for Sexual Dysfunction in Men

The Preventive Approaches
Correctible causes: Atherosclerosis of the penile artery is present in over half the men over the age of fifty who have erectile dysfunction. A study from the *Archives of Internal Medicine* in 2011 showed that reducing heart disease risk factors with either lifestyle changes or lowering cholesterol increased sexual functioning.

In addition, **alcohol and tobacco** use can both inhibit sexual function and should be avoided. In obese men, **losing weight** improves sexual function in about a third of men with ED.

There are also a large number of **medications** that can cause ED. These include anti-hypertensives, diuretics, anti-depressants, anti-seizure and anti-anxiety drugs, antihistamines, Parkinson's drugs, some ulcer drugs (H_2 –receptor antagonists), muscle relaxants, prostate cancer drugs, some chemotherapy agents, and even some NSAIDs. Discontinuing, lowering the dosage or changing these drugs may reverse E.D.

A **diet** rich in whole foods, antioxidants and adequate protein can help improve erectile function. The best protein sources are fish, chicken, turkey, and lean cuts of meat. Special foods recommended for enhanced virility include liver, oysters, seeds and legumes, due to their zinc content. A 2011 study showed that pistachio nuts (100 grams daily) increased erectile performance by 150 percent. In addition, antioxidant-rich foods that contain vitamins C and E produce sperm with less DNA damage. Watermelon contains phytochemicals that can enhance performance.

Sexual enhancement is noted in men who regularly **exercise** and is correlated with the degree of individual improvement in fitness. Light exercise has no effect, so moderate intensity or greater is required. I especially recommend aerobic exercise, which improves oxygen flow to the genitalia and may also stimulate production of sex hormones. Studies show that physically active men have better-formed and faster-swimming sperm as well as hormone values that are more favorable for sperm production.

Regular Intercourse Can Help Prevent ED

A recent study revealed that having intercourse regularly protects against the development of erectile dysfunction in men ages fifty-five to seventy-five. Use it or lose it?

The Conventional Approaches

Medications: The greatest advancement for ED has been medications that increase blood flow to the penis and traps it there temporarily, called phosphodiesterase-5 *(PDE-5) inhibitors*. The three main drugs are sildenafil [Viagra], vardenafil [Levitra], tadalafil [Cialis] and avanafil (Stendra). They work in most men, but some men do not respond (about 20 percent). *Warning*: These drugs can cause heart attacks and death in men who have heart disease and/or are taking nitrates, and they can interfere with drugs for prostate problems; so take it only under a physician's direction and have your heart function checked before taking them.

These medications have various differences as to how fast they work and how long they last, as well as possible side effects (other than heart issues) and interference with food, as follows:

	Avanafil	Sildenafil	Vardenafil	Tadalafil
Onset of action	15-30 minutes	30-60 minutes	30-60 minutes	60-120 minutes
Duration of action	Up to 6 hours	Up to 12 hours	Up to 10 hours	Up to 36 hours
Effect of food intake	Not affected	High-fat meals decrease efficacy	High-fat meals decrease efficacy	Not affected
Unique side effects		Vision abnormalities (PDE6)	Vision abnormalities (PDE6)	Back pain, myalgias

The only other medication used in ED is *testosterone*. If your testosterone level is low, testosterone supplementation may be of some benefit, primarily in libido or erectile function. Testosterone may be provided in many different forms, including pills, injection, skin gel, and a recently approved nasal gel. It can also be compounded by a pharmacist. ***Warning***: Overtreatment may be dangerous: A recent study published in the *NEJM* showed that use of a testosterone gel might increase risk for heart disease as well as respiratory and dermatologic disorders. Side effects include worsening prostate cancer, increasing red blood cells, sleep apnea, gynecomastia (enlarged breasts), fluid retention, and skin/hair changes.

Statins Helpful in ED

A study published in 2014 in the *Journal of Sexual Medicine* reviewed eleven clinical trials and found that men who took statin drugs (for cholesterol) had 24 percent better erectile function. This makes sense because statin drugs are indicated for heart disease, which can be a cause of ED. Although statins are not recommended as a treatment for ED, they provide 30–50 percent of the effect of ED medications.

There are several **invasive methods** used if medications are not effective.

- *Vacuum pump*: You insert your penis into a plastic tube and use a hand-held vacuum pump to draw blood into the penis. A constriction device placed around the base of the penis prevents blood from leaking out. You then remove the plastic tube for intercourse. You must remove the constriction device within thirty minutes.
- *MUSE intraurethral suppository*: You insert an ultrathin applicator into the tip of your penis and gently push a plunger that releases a small, rice-size pellet of prostaglandin E1 (Alprostadil). This medication dilates the blood vessels, causing an erection within ten to fifteen minutes. The primary and most bothersome side effect is penile aching.

- *Injection therapy*: You inject Alprostadil directly into your penis. Erection again occurs within ten to fifteen minutes and lasts forty-five to sixty minutes. A rare side effect is priapism (an erection lasting more than four hours), which can damage your penis and requires prompt medical attention.
- *Surgical implants*: There are several mechanical devices that can be implanted into the penis. The most popular is an inflatable implant that is activated by squeezing a pump in the scrotum. These implants are not visible and are much like breast implants. This method requires a surgical procedure, which is covered by Medicare.

The Alternative Approaches

Chinese herbal formulas have been used for centuries and have the advantage of not needing to plan sexual activity and have little to no side effects. A common formula is *You Gui Wan*. However, you have to take it continuously for best results. *Li Wu Jia Pian* restores Jing (spirit). *Cong Rong Bu Shen Wan* and *Tai Pan Tang Yi Pian* are other possibilities. *Caution*: Formulas in these categories may contain animal parts and natural hormones.

There are several **nutritional supplements** that can be effective in erectile dysfunction, including:

- *Yohimbe* is the Chinese herbal equivalent of PDE-5 inhibitors. Look for a product that contains a standardized 15 mg content of yohimbine (the active ingredient), and take it two to three times per day. (There is a prescription form of 5.4 mg tablets.) The advantage of yohimbe is that you don't have to plan your sexual encounters, but you do have to take it daily. It increases blood flow to the penis, thus improving erections, and may be good for erectile dysfunction caused by antidepressants. *Cautions*: Yohimbine can negate the effects of hypertensive medications and can enhance tricyclic antidepressants such as amitriptyline and nortriptyline. Yohimbe can also lower blood glucose, so use it with caution if you have diabetes. Yohimbine can also induce anxiety, panic attacks, and hallucinations in some individuals, as well as elevated blood pressure, high heart rate, dizziness, headache, and skin flushing. *Warning*: *Do not use* yohimbe if you have heart disease or angina (much like the PDE-5 inhibitors), have kidney or liver disease, or are a woman.
- *Korean red ginseng* increases nitric oxide and also works like PDE-5 inhibitors.
- *Gingko biloba* is usually used for memory but also increases blood flow to the penis. Although it takes about eight weeks to be effective, half of the patients regain normal potency.
- *Muira puama* (1 to 1.5 grams of 4:1 extract) is a Brazilian herb that has been used in Europe for some time. It is effective in helping increase sexual desire as well as attaining and maintaining an erection. The action of the muira puama herb is not fully understood, but it seems to assist with both the psychological as well as the physical aspects of sexual function.

- *L-arginine* (5 g per day) increases blood flow to the penis by increasing nitric oxide like the PD5 Inhibitors, but it is much weaker.
- *DHEA* (50 mg daily) has also been shown to improve all aspects of sexual function but may take three to six months to become effective. ***Important note***: You should avoid wild yam and soy products labeled as "natural DHEA" because they do not break down into DHEA in the body. ***Warning***: Do not use if you have asthma.
- *Maca*, a root from Peru, can be used to help with sexual desire and helping with integrity of an erection, and it can also increase fertility.

Several other herbs may be advertised to improve erectile function but have no scientific support. These include saw palmetto, deer horn, horny goat weed, wild oat, stinging nettle, damiana, sarsaparilla, kola nut, L-citrulline, maca, and puncture weed.

Caution **If Using Enzyte**

Enzyte is a supplement advertised for sexual enhancement. It contains several herbs, including horny goat weed, Korean red ginseng, Tribulus terrestris, L-arginine, and many others. Recent research shows that taking Enzyte can cause an abnormality in the electrical conduction of the heart (prolonged QT interval as seen on an EKG), which is a risk factor for sudden cardiac death. It should be avoided if you take other drugs that can lengthen QT interval, the most common of which are amiodarone (Cordarone), sotalol (Betapace), and thioridazine (Mellaril), although there are others (check with your doctor).

Acupuncture has also been used for centuries to correct certain underlying problems causing erectile dysfunction. Acupuncture can give you longer-lasting results and decrease or eliminate the need to take drugs or supplements. You should notice improvement within six to eight acupuncture treatments but might need additional sessions for maximum benefit.

Avoid Some "Natural" Erectile Dysfunction Supplements

The FDA has warned against unapproved supplements for erectile dysfunction, stating that most contain ingredients similar to the conventional drugs (such as PDE-5 inhibitors). The problem is that men taking these supplements may not be aware that the same side effects and risks occur in these supplements as with conventional drugs. Some of these products include Blue Steel, Hero, any of the Shangai supplements, Strong Testis, and Xiadafil.

Your Empowered Patient Action Plan for Treating Sexual Dysfunction in Men

Step #1: **Take a PDE-5 inhibitor** if you do not have any contraindications. These drugs are the most scientifically proven, although they are expensive. You may be able to obtain generic versions from Canadian pharmacies.

Step #2: **Take muria puama** in place of step 1 if you prefer an herbal remedy and if you need an increase in sexual desire as well as erections. *Maca* may also be helpful.

Step #3: **Try panax ginseng and/or gingko biloba** if the other steps have not worked.

Step #4: **Take testosterone supplements** if you have low testosterone.

Step #5: **Take Chinese herbs** (prescribed by a TCM practitioner) to further enhance sexual function.

Jay was able to get an erection but could not keep it long enough to complete intercourse. He had been prescribed Viagra, but it hadn't helped. He had also tried testosterone, which was not effective. I prescribed a Chinese herbal formula to increase his kidney yang; and within one week, his wife related that their sex life had improved dramatically.

Step #6: **Undergo acupuncture** if you still have erectile problems.

Step #7: **Try L-arginine and/or DHEA** if you still have problems with sexual dysfunction. These herbs may take longer to have a beneficial effect than the steps above.

Step #8: **Try an herbal product** containing a combination of Ginseng, saw palmetto, wild oat, stinging nettle, damiana, yohimbe, sarsaparilla, kola nut, and/or puncture weed to improve sexual function if the above steps are still not effective.

Step #9: **Take yohimbe** if you still have problems but undergo appropriate medical supervision due to adverse side effects, some of which can be harmful.

Step #10: **Try other conventional methods or devices** as a last resort.

Expected Outcome

Sexual dysfunction is common in men especially as they age but can be appropriately managed in most men using the above steps.

Sexual Dysfunction in Women

What You Need to Know

In women, sexual dysfunction is much more complicated than in men; it can involve decreased libido (sexual desire and sexual arousal), lack of lubrication, as well as decreased ability to have orgasms. Another problem that is rarely discussed is vulvodynia, chronic vulvar pain without identifiable cause; it is estimated that 28 percent of reproductive-aged women have been affected by vulvodynia, and this condition often increases as women age; yet about 40 percent of these women do not seek treatment.

There are several sex hormones and neurotransmitters involved in sexual functioning, which suggests that different treatments may or may not work depending on the mechanism (see sidebar below).

Sex Hormones and Neurotransmitters Involved in Sexual Function

Substance	Sex Function Affected	Type of Effect
Estrogen	Arousal, desire	Positive
Progesterone	Receptivity	Positive
Testosterone	Desire, initiation of sex activity	Positive
Dopamine	Desire, arousal	Positive
Nitric oxide	Vasocongestion of clitoris	Positive
Norepinephrine	Arousal	Positive
Oxytocin	Receptivity, orgasm	Positive
Prolactin	Arousal	Negative
Serotonin	Arousal, desire	Positive and negative*
Vasoactive intestinal Peptide	Vasocongestion of clitoris	Positive

* May facilitate uterine contractions during orgasm but may also inhibit orgasm by different mechanism

---

Certainly, menopause is one of the primary causes of sexual dysfunction in women, but other causes exist as well. Hysterectomy alone has not been shown to be associated with sexual dysfunction.

Treatments for Sexual Dysfunction in Women

The Preventive Approaches

Correctible causes: There are a number of *medications* that can decrease libido. Blood-pressure medications that may *negatively* affect sexual function include diuretics (such as HCTZ, Diuril, Lasix), alpha-agonists (such as prazosin [Cardura]), and beta-blockers (such as atenolol [Tenormin], metoprolol [Lopressor]). Calcium antagonists (such as nifedipine [Procardia], amlodipine [Norvasc], verapamil [Calan], diltiazem [Cardizem]), and ACE inhibitors (such as captopril [Capoten], lisinopril [Prinivil]) have only *minor negative* effects. Angiotensin II antagonists (such as losartan [Cozaar]) appear to *improve* sexual function.

The SSRI antidepressants (see section on *Depression*) also can decrease libido, which may complicate your treatment of menopause-related depression. SSRIs will cause this effect in 30–60 percent of women. Other classes of antidepressants, including bupropion (Wellbutrin, Zyban), nefazodone (Serzone), and mirtazapine (Remeron) have minimal effects on sexual function.

If you have decreased libido and are on any of the above medications, consult with your doctor to see if changing medications will help. Also, taking Gingko biloba (120–240 mg daily) may reverse these side effects.

Reversing Sexual Dysfunction Caused by Antidepressants

Sexual dysfunction is a major side effect of antidepressants, occurring in both men and women. Taking gingko biloba (180–240 mg daily) or sildenafil (Viagra), tadalafil (Cialis), or vardenafil (Levitra) may reverse this effect in women and is worth a try. If not, there are other drugs that may be helpful.

A 2012 study showed that regularly scheduled exercise improves sexual functioning in women taking antidepressants. Of note, simply scheduling regular sexual activity improved orgasm, whereas scheduling exercise, especially just before sexual activity, increased desire. However, improvement of sexual function with exercise at least six hours before sex was not statistically significant, but within thirty minutes it was.

Kegel Exercises May Help Sexual Function and Orgasm

For women, Kegel exercises have been found to be of benefit for enhancing or stimulating orgasm by strengthening the pelvic floor muscles.

To perform the classic Kegel exercise, first find the muscle. Stop the flow while you are urinating to feel this muscle; however, do not exercise the muscle during urination. You can also place your finger inside your vagina and squeeze down; the muscle will tighten. Once you learn which muscle it is, you can voluntarily contract and relax this muscle whenever you want. The more you exercise it, the stronger it will become.

You can perform these exercises lying down (easiest initially), seated, or standing. Contract the muscles for 3 seconds and relax for three seconds; repeat ten to twelve times. Gradually work up to ten-second contractions. Don't use other muscles (abdominal, buttock, thigh) during this time and don't hold your breath.

There are other Kegel exercises that you can do, which are easy to find when searching the Internet.

Difficulty Achieving Orgasm? Try Additional Clitoral Stimulation

Achieving orgasm may be difficult in some women and one reason may be mechanical. Although most people think that orgasms are a result of stimulation of the vagina alone, the vagina actually contains few nerve endings. The clitoris forms a continuum with the vagina and usually must be stimulated along with the vagina to achieve orgasm. During sexual intercourse, the vagina and clitoris both swell; the vagina extends upward and the clitoris changes position due to swelling as well. So basically, the vagina and clitoris work in concert to produce an orgasm. However, if the clitoris is not stimulated enough during intercourse, a woman may not be able to achieve orgasm.

If this occurs, there are some simple actions you and/or your partner can take during intercourse, which involves additionally stimulating the clitoris directly. Such stimulation can be enhanced naturally in certain positions (especially woman on top) if the man's pubic bone can rub against the clitoris. Otherwise, the clitoris can be stimulated using fingers or a vibrator simultaneously with intercourse.

The Conventional Approaches
There are several **medications** that have been tried for sexual dysfunction in women, but most do not work well.

Viagra has been shown in a few small studies to improve orgasm and sexual enjoyment, but not arousal, and is better at increasing lubrication. It may help some women who have decreased desire due to antidepressant therapy. However, most women don't benefit from these types of drugs.

Testosterone has been commonly used and may provide some benefit in some women. However, there are side effects associated with testosterone, primarily facial hair growth and, possibly, breast cancer (although rare). Testosterone can be prescribed both conventionally and alternatively (through a cream made by compounding pharmacists).

A new drug called *flibanserin* (Addyi) was recently approved by the FDA. The drug was originally tried as an antidepressant but women reported higher levels of sexual satisfaction, so it was re-studied. Research shows that women reported 0.5-1 more sexually satisfying events per month and scored higher on questionnaires measuring desire and scored lower on stress scales. ***Warnings***: There are some safety issues especially low blood pressure and fainting (the FDA had rejected the drug twice but approved it after intense marketing directed by the drug company). It can interfere with some commonly-used medications and side effects are increased when used with alcohol. It is only indicated for women who are pre-menopausal.

Psychotherapeutic methods: For orgasmic disorders, directed masturbation, cognitive behavioral therapy, and sensate focus may all help. *Cognitive therapy* focuses on decreasing anxiety and promotes changes in sexual attitudes and thoughts. *Sensate focus* guides a woman and her partner through a series of exercises, moving from nonsexual to sexual touching. *Directed masturbation* works for those women who cannot achieve vaginal orgasm: By stimulating the clitoris during intercourse, orgasm can be achieved more easily.

Estrogen replacement alone can be given if sexual dysfunction is caused by menopause-induced vaginal atrophy. There is also a new drug, *ospemifine* (Osphena), that is used to treat women who have painful intercourse from vaginal atrophy. *Warning*: Ospemifine can cause thickening of the endometrium, so you should consult with a doctor if bleeding occurs. Ospemifine, however, has a lower risk of strokes and blood clots than estrogen therapy. It can also potentially be used in breast cancer survivors.

For vaginal dryness, **lubricants** such as KY moisten the vagina and allow for non-painful intercourse. They do not interfere with achievement of orgasm.

Beware of Vaginal Rejuvenation Procedures

There are several vaginal cosmetic surgeries such as that are purported to enhance sexual gratification and genital appearance altered by childbirth and aging. These include "designer" vaginoplasty (tightens the vaginal muscles), clitoral unhooding, labiaplasty (reduce the size of the labia…the outer "lips" of the vagina) and G-spot amplification (injecting a filler into the supposed G-spot, although researchers are not sure if or where it exists). You should be aware that there are potential complications, including infection, altered sensation, adhesions, and scarring. The American College of Obstetricians and Gynecologists caution that there have been no reliable studies on the safety or effectiveness of these procedures.

The Alternative Approaches

There are several alternative methods that may work much better than conventional approaches.

Nutritional supplements: *DHEA* (25–50 mg daily), a precursor of sex hormones, has been shown in some studies to improve sexual performance as well as help libido. Although natural testosterone has been used as well, DHEA seems to work much better. ***Important note***: You should avoid wild yam and soy products labeled as "natural DHEA" because they do not break down into DHEA in the body

Herbs that may be beneficial include damiana, Siberian ginseng, wild yam, licorice, sarsaparilla, saw palmetto, wild oat, kola nut, ginger, and puncture weed. These are usually combined together in one product. Maca, a Peruvian herb, is purported to restore hormonal imbalance and related sexual desire and fertility, although there are no studies supporting this indication.

Probiotics (Ultimate Flora for Vaginal Support, which includes *L. rhamnosus, L. acidophilus*, etc.) may be very helpful with vaginal dryness.

Vitamin E (vaginal) suppositories for one week can also help with lubrication and healing the tissue.

Auricular (ear) acupuncture can help a number of women increase desire and arousal by stimulating a point actually called the "sexual desire point." It may take several sessions of acupuncture, although ear seeds can be placed in this point and remain for one to two weeks. For vulvodynia, both body and ear acupuncture may be helpful.

Gui Pi Wan is a safe **Chinese herbal formula** for an underlying syndrome that affects many women's sexual desires. *Yang Rong Wan* is another possibility. Consult with a TCM practitioner for best results.

USE IT OR LOSE IT: MAINTAIN
LUBRICATION THE NATURAL WAY

You may think that you need hormones such as DHEA or testosterone to increase your vaginal lubrication and maintain sexual function, but studies have shown that, for many women, having sex several times a week will stimulate the vagina, produce natural lubrication, and maintain sexual desire, without the need for supplemental hormones.

Important note: For additional treatments for sexual problems caused by menopausal problems, such as vaginal dryness, see section on *Menopause*.

Your Empowered Patient Action Plan for Treating Sexual Dysfunction in Women

Step #1: **Discontinue any medications** that may be causing sexual dysfunction.

Step #2: **Undergo auricular (ear) acupuncture** to increase libido if the DHEA hasn't helped.

Step #3: **Practice Kegel exercises or additional clitoral stimulation** to achieve or enhance orgasm.

Step #4: **Take DHEA** to restore libido.

Step #5: **Use the EROS machine** to initiate and enhance orgasm.

Step #6: **Undergo directed masturbation, cognitive behavioral therapy, or sensate focus** to increase sexual arousal and enhance orgasm if the above steps are not beneficial.

Step #7: **Use vitamin E, probiotics or estrogen** cream for vaginal dryness.

Step #8: **Try Viagra** if you still have sexual problems.

Step #9: **Consider testosterone** if all else has failed. Use natural testosterone cream rather than synthetic.

Step #10: **Try flibanserin** to increase sexual desire if no other steps have worked.

Expected Outcome

Sexual dysfunction is common in both menopausal and premenopausal women. With the above steps, however, sexual dysfunction can be reversed in most women, and you can achieve a satisfactory sex life.

Shingles (Herpes Zoster, Acute)

What You Need to Know

Shingles is actually a direct descendent of the chicken pox virus, which lies dormant in nerves until something triggers it to become active again. It then breaks out in sores along a nerve. It is usually seen along the trunk, but can occur in the face, eye, or anywhere there are nerves. Occasionally, the sores aren't evident; you may have a rash or just pain along the nerve branch.

The incidence of shingles is estimated at 10–20 percent of people but increases as one ages. In a significant amount of elderly people, it is refractory to treatment and has a poor outcome.

The lesions of shingles can last up to a month, but pain can last for several months and be quite debilitating as well as causing fatigue and sleep disorders. Even after the infection is gone, you may still have pain from damage of the nerves, called postherpetic neuralgia. This complication occurs in up to 70 percent of patients (for treatment of this and other neuralgias, see the section on *Neuralgia*).

The main goal is to treat this infection as soon as possible, which will minimize the complications and improve your quality of life (QOL).

Treatments for Shingles

The Preventive Approaches

The best method for preventing shingles is to take the **vaccine**, Zostavax. However, the vaccine is not effective in preventing the acute infection in all people; it is 70 percent effective in people 50 to 59, 64 percent in those 60 to 69 and only 38 percent effective in those 70 and older. It helps prevent postherpetic neuralgia in 66 percent of patients. Nevertheless, it is recommended for everyone over the age of sixty and is also recommended if you have already had shingles because it can decrease the recurrence rate or minimize symptoms if it does reoccur. *Helpful Tip*: A recent study shows that the vaccine is not cost-effective for people under age 50. *Warning*: Zostavax contains live virus and should never be used in immunocompromised patients.

A new vaccine (called HZ/su) is twice as effective as Zovirax, protecting 97.2 percent of people at all ages (including at age 50). It has the same side effect profile as Zovirax, primarily pain at the injection site. Its advantages include not being live (so it can be used in immunocompromised patients) and it does not lose its effectiveness with age. It is currently undergoing the FDA approval process.

The Conventional Approaches

Several medications have been used to treat shingles although they may not be very effective. *Antivirals* are the primary medications, but they must be started within seventy-two hours of the initial outbreak (rash) to be effective. Even so, the use of antivirals reduces the duration of the outbreak by only one or two days. The primary antivirals used are *famciclovir*, *valacyclovir*, and *acyclovir*. However, use of antivirals for a week along with gabapentin (an antiseizure medication used for nerve pain) may reduce the occurrence of postherpetic neuralgia by 77 percent, according to a recent study.

In combination with antivirals, *corticosteroids* have also been used to treat shingles but have not shown any reduction in the incidence of post herpetic neuralgia. However, it appears to improve QOL (activity, sleep).

Analgesics such as aspirin or NSAIDs seem to have little to no value in controlling pain, so *narcotics* are usually necessary. However, even narcotics may not be of much benefit.

The Alternative Approaches

There are several alternative approaches that are much more helpful for resolving shingles than conventional treatments.

Low level energy laser ("cold" laser or *LLEL)* may be the best treatment for both the acute stage of shingles and postherpetic neuralgia. It usually takes one to four treatments for the acute stage and six to ten treatments for the chronic form. These lasers have minimal to no side effects.

Acupuncture can reduce both the duration and severity of shingles, usually within two to six sessions, which can be done every day. It is also one of the best treatments for postherpetic neuralgia.

Along with acupuncture, there are several **Chinese herbal formulas** that have potent antiviral benefits and may also reduce the duration of the condition. The primary formula should contain astragalus and isatis and is usually combined with a different formula that reduces "heat" in the system, called *Long Dan Xie Gan Tang*. If "cold" signs are found by your acupuncturist, then several *medicinal mushrooms* with immune benefits are indicated (Ganoderma, Tremella, Poria, Polyporus). Another commonly used formula is Chuan Xin Lian Pian. For best results, these herbs should be taken as soon as possible after the breakout of lesions.

There are several **topical pain relievers** that also may help relieve pain temporarily. A topical suspension of two five-grain aspirin tablets crushed and dissolved in 15 ml of chloroform can give relief for several hours. Topicals containing cayenne or peppermint oil can also help relieve the pain.

There are several **homeopathic remedies** that have been used with moderate success, depending on the various symptoms. These include:

- *Arsenicum album*: If a person feels chilly, anxious, restless, and exhausted during fever—and the burning pain of the eruptions is relieved by heat—this remedy may be indicated. Discomfort is often worse around midnight.
- *Apis mellifica*: Swelling around eyes, tender eruptions with burning, stinging pain, and itching. Symptoms are aggravated by warmth and relieved by cold applications or exposure to cool air.
- *Clematis*: Red, burning, blister-like eruptions, made worse from washing or contact with cold water.
- *Iris versicolor*: For herpes zoster infection that is accompanied by stomach problems with burning sensations and nausea. Eruptions may appear, especially on the right side of the abdomen.
- *Mezereum*: Intense burning is followed by bright red eruptions that itch intolerably. The local pain of the eruptions is worse from heat and relieved by cold applications.
- *Ranunculus bulbosus*: Intense itching of shingles on the ribcage (either on the back or chest), which are also very sore and worse from motion and from contact with clothing or any kind of touch. The blisters may look bluish.
- *Hypericum*: Postherpetic neuralgia with sharp shooting pains.

Finally, there have been small studies indicating that **hypnosis** may help reduce or resolve shingles, often in only one or two sessions.

Your Empowered Patient Action Plan for Treating Shingles

Step #1: Obtain a shingles vaccine if you are over the age of sixty. The vaccine is also still useful even if you have already had an attack of shingles.

Step #2: Try topical solutions to relieve pain temporarily while the following steps are being applied.

Step #3: Use LLEL, which can heal the lesions quickly as well as help prevent and/or treat postherpetic neuralgia.

Step #4: Undergo acupuncture and take Chinese herbs to reduce or resolve the condition more quickly. It is also helpful for postherpetic neuralgia. It can be used along with the laser.

Step #5: Take antivirals within seventy-two hours of initial rash, along with gabapentin, to reduce the risk of postherpetic neuralgia. These can be taken with the following steps.

Step #6: Undergo hypnosis to more quickly resolve shingles if the above steps have not helped or along with the acupuncture and/or laser.

Step #7: Take homeopathic remedies if the above steps have not been effective.
Step #8: Take narcotic medications for pain relief if you still have pain.

Note: For pain after shingles (postherpetic neuralgia), see section under *Neuralgia*.

Expected Outcome

With the advent of the shingles vaccine, this disease can be prevented in half of those who take it. If you do get the infection, there are methods that can reduce the duration and severity, but the quicker the use of these methods, the better the results. Alternative methods are especially fast at resolving the infection and other symptoms.

Sinusitis (Acute and Chronic)

What You Need to Know

Sinusitis is an inflammation of the sinus cavities, which are air-filled areas in the facial bones. Sinusitis can be acute, usually caused by viral infection, or chronic, caused by continued inflammation, scarring, allergies, or obstruction of the sinus openings (called ostia). With chronic sinusitis, you can develop outgrowths of tissue, called polyps, which may cause obstruction.

Most people think that sinusitis is a bacterial infection that requires antibiotics, but in fact, antibiotics rarely resolve sinusitis unless it has been present over a week, at which time bacteria can enter the sinuses and continue the symptoms or make them worse. With chronic sinusitis, *antibiotics are not indicated and won't help.* **Helpful Tip**: It should be realized that there is no reliable sign or symptom (such as facial pain or colored discharge) that can distinguish if sinusitis patients would benefit from antibiotics.

Although it has been reported that 90 percent of *chronic* sinusitis patients have fungi in their sinuses, it is not known whether the fungi is a result of or a cause of sinusitis.

Often, allergies play a significant role in chronic sinusitis.

As acute and chronic sinusitis can require different approaches, they will be discussed separately.

Treatments for Acute Sinusitis

The Preventive Approaches

If you can prevent infections from entering the sinuses, you can prevent many sinusitis problems or reoccurrences. Here are some ways to do so:

- Improve household ventilation by opening windows whenever possible.
- Use a humidifier in the home or office when you or a family member has a cold.
- Sleep with the head of the bed elevated. This promotes sinus drainage.
- Use decongestants with caution.
- Avoid air pollutants (such as tobacco smoke) that irritate the nose.
- Eat a balanced diet and exercise.
- Minimize exposure to persons with known infections.
- *Treat cold symptoms immediately*. Drink plenty of fluids and keep your nasal passages clear when you contract a cold.

The Conventional Approaches

OTC **decongestants** (such as Triaminic, Dimetapp, or Sudafed) can reduce swelling and help unclog the sinuses but should be used sparingly since they can make sinusitis worse.

Many doctors prescribe **antibiotics** but should do so only if your symptoms continue after seven days and you have purulent nasal drainage, facial pain, or tooth pain/tenderness. Narrow-spectrum antibiotics such as amoxicillin, doxycycline, or trimethoprim-sulfamethoxazole are the most appropriate. If you are allergic to penicillin, erythromycin or a cephalosporin (Keflex, Ceclor) is the next choice. *You do not usually need more powerful, broad-spectrum antibiotics such as cipro or a Z-pak..*

Important Information:
Antibiotics, Nasal Steroids, and X-Rays
Usually Don't Help Acute Sinusitis

A recent study published in *JAMA* confirmed what many previous studies have concluded: Antibiotics and nasal steroids do not improve symptoms of acute sinusitis. Unnecessary use of antibiotics can increase resistance, so they should not be used initially.

In another study, antibiotics did not affect the course of sinusitis and abnormal x-rays did not provide any information about its prognosis (end result).

Surgery may be performed for some people who have persistent or recurrent sinusitis. If the cause of sinusitis is blockage of drainage, the obstruction may need to be removed so the sinus can drain. Most surgeries are done when medical treatment has failed.

Surgery should definitely be done for complete obstruction by polyps; spread of infection into the brain, eye, or frontal sinus; fungal sinusitis; or tumor. Surgery is usually done as an outpatient, with most patients going home the same day. The surgery itself usually takes one to two hours, and a similar amount of time is spent in the recovery room. Surgery is typically done using a rigid metal endoscope, which allows the surgeon to view the inside of the nose while performing surgery at the same time.

The Alternative Approaches

Acupuncture can be invaluable for decreasing inflammation as well as accelerating healing with sinusitis. It is also very effective if allergies are an underlying problem. It may take only a few acupuncture treatments to benefit you.

Low level energy laser ("cold" laser or *LLEL)* can also be very useful to reduce or resolve symptoms, and can potentiate the benefits from acupuncture. This type of laser reduces sinus inflammation and is applied directly over the sinuses. It has no known side effects when treating sinusitis.

Nutritional supplements: A combination of wet heat with *vitamin C* (500 mg every two hours), *bioflavonoids* (100 mg per day), and *bromelain* (250–500 mg between meals) may effectively resolve acute sinusitis. Vitamin C and bioflavonoids work through their antioxidant effects and bromelain is an expectorant. This combination is very effective in reducing symptoms and healing the inflammation.

Echinacea (2–4 ml of tincture [1:5] or fluid extract [1:1] three times daily) may be helpful in reducing symptoms and the duration of the condition, if viral infection is involved. *Warning*: Do not use echinacea if you have any immune or systemic diseases (such as tuberculosis, lupus, multiple sclerosis, scleroderma, or AIDS). You should not take echinacea more than eight weeks as it can suppress the immune system if taken long-term.

Chinese herbal formulas can be very effective in reducing or resolving acute sinusitis. Formulas are determined based on the color of your sputum (phlegm) and other findings. *Qing Bi Tang* and *Long Dan Xie Gan Tang* are commonly used with fever, and *Xiao Qing Long Tang* is used if there is no fever. *Bi Yan Pian* can be used for bacterial infection and *Cang Er Zi San* for congestion, but these formulas should not be taken long-term. You should notice improvement within a few days to a week, but you may need to take them longer for full relief.

Homeopathy uses several different remedies to control and resolve acute sinusitis:

- *Mercurius vivus* (30c) is used twice daily for facial pain, yellow-green discharge, and alternating chills and sweats.
- *Nux vomica* (30c) is used twice daily for clear, thin discharge, sneezing, headache, and nasal stuffiness at night and sneezing and runny nose in the morning.

- *Kali bichromicum* (30c) is used one to two times daily for thick, stringy mucous and pain in the cheeks or nose. ***Important note***: You may have a cough, which is worse in the morning.
- *Pulsatilla* (30c) is used twice a day for light yellow or green discharge accompanied by lack of thirst and low spirits.
- *Allium cepa* is used in allergic and infectious nasal discharge.
- *Arsenicum:* watery for acrid nasal discharge, although the nose is completely obstructed.

Consult a qualified homeopathist for guidance on which remedies will be most beneficial and for proper dosages. You should notice improvement within one to three days.

Finally, many people have begun to use **neti pots**, or nasal irrigation (available OTC), which has been shown useful to clear the sinuses and soothe cold and allergy symptoms and decrease sinus infections. ***Caution***: Preliminary research, however, now shows that *continuous* irrigation may actually increase the risk for sinus infections. This may be caused by contaminated neti pots and rinse bottles, so you should wash them with soap regularly and never share them. You should limit nasal irrigation to once or twice daily. ***Caution***: Do not use tap water!

Your Empowered Patient Action Plan for Treating Acute Sinusitis

- *Important Note: If symptoms are severe, persist for at least seven days and includes purulent nasal drainage, facial pain, or tooth pain/tenderness, go to step 8 first.*

*Step #1: **Undergo acupuncture** for faster resolution of your symptoms. This can be done while undergoing the following steps, but may be all you need.*

*Step #2: **Apply wet heat and take vitamin C, bioflavonoids, and bromelain** to help resolve the condition.*

*Step #3: **Use a neti pot** short-term for immediate relief. Keep your pot clean and don't use tap water!*

*Step #4: **Undergo LLEL** treatment, with or without acupuncture if your symptoms persist.*

*Step #5: **Take the Chinese herbal remedies Qing Bi Tang, Long Dan Xie Gan Tang, or Xiao Qing Long Tang** to resolve the condition if you still have symptoms.*

*Step #6: **Take an appropriate homeopathic remedy** if the above steps have not helped.*

*Step #7: **Take an OTC decongestant** to control continued symptoms.*

Step #8: Take prescription antibiotics if symptoms have persisted and worsened or you have additional symptoms indicative of bacterial infection. Undergo cultures from nasal swabs to detect bacteria before treatment is started with antibiotics.

Step #9: Try echinacea if the above steps have still not resolved your symptoms.

Treatments for Chronic Sinusitis

The Preventive Approaches

One way to prevent chronic sinusitis is to treat acute sinusitis quickly and effectively. In addition, the same preventive measures used for acute sinusitis should be used for chronic sinusitis, including:

- Improve household ventilation by opening windows whenever possible.
- Use a humidifier in the home or office when you or a family member has a cold.
- Sleep with the head of the bed elevated. This promotes sinus drainage.
- Use decongestants with caution.
- Avoid air pollutants (such as tobacco smoke) that irritate the nose.
- Eat a balanced diet and exercise.
- Minimize exposure to persons with known infections.
- Treat cold symptoms immediately. Drink plenty of fluids and keep your nasal passages clear when you contract a cold.

The Conventional Approaches

Inhaled nasal steroids can be helpful in reducing chronic inflammation for persistent sinusitis, with or without polyps. It may take one to three weeks for inhaled steroids to be effective. Steroids are more effective if used with saline irrigation. ***Important note***: Although some physicians use oral steroids, a study published in the *Annals of Internal Medicine* showed that the side effects and potential harm outweigh any benefit, so they shouldn't be used unless no other medications have helped or for intermittent or rescue therapy for those with nasal polyps.

Leukotriene antagonists (Montelukast) are recommended in guidelines for maintenance (long-term) therapy in patients with polyps.

Short-term antibiotics and long-term macrolide antibiotics are recommended in guidelines for those without polyps, although they frequently are not effective.

Surgeries: For chronic, persistent sinusitis that does not respond to other measures, endoscopy to clean the sinuses may be indicated. Other surgeries are done to remove polyps and open up "windows" for drainage. Surgery should be the last resort and does not always resolve your sinusitis. In fact, in 20 percent of cases, continued medications and repeat surgeries are necessary.

The Alternative Approaches

Acupuncture is the most effective method for resolving chronic sinusitis, whether due to allergies or other causes. You should notice improvement within three to four acupuncture treatments, but you might need additional sessions for maximum benefits. Because acupuncture addresses the underlying cause, you can obtain long-term relief.

Chinese herbal formulas are excellent at reducing the symptoms, as well as the underlying causes of chronic sinusitis, and can be used along with acupuncture. *Qing Bu Tang*, *Xiao Qing Long Tang*, and *Wen Dan Tang* are all beneficial. There are several other formulas that address allergic causes, such as *Yu Ping Feng San*. Consult a practitioner qualified in Chinese herbal medicine to determine which Chinese herbal formulas are the best for your particular syndromes. You should notice improvement within one to three weeks, but you may need to take them longer for complete relief.

Low level energy laser ("cold" laser or *LLEL)* can also be very useful to reduce or resolve symptoms and can potentiate the benefits from acupuncture. This type of laser reduces sinus inflammation and is applied directly over the sinuses. It has no known side effects when treating sinusitis.

If allergies are a suspected cause (either food and/or airborne), the **NAET method** may help. It combines acupuncture, kinesiology, chiropractic, herbs, and nutrition to desensitize you to substances you are allergic to. It may take several months for its effectiveness to be observed, depending on how many allergens are sensitizing you.

If the bones in your face and cheek are not aligned correctly, they can cause obstruction of the sinuses. If this is a possibility (especially with previous face or head trauma), **osteopathic** evaluation and treatment are indicated. If structural problems are evident, then they must be corrected before other treatments, or your symptoms may continue to reoccur. A specific type of osteopathic treatment is necessary, called *cranial-sacral* manipulation. ***Important note***: Make sure you find a practitioner who is qualified and certified in cranial sacral manipulation.

Butterbur is the alternative herb that has the mechanism of a leukotriene inhibitor (which is recommended in conventional guidelines)

Your Empowered Patient Action Plan for Treating Chronic Sinusitis

- *Important Note*: *Although your drainage may be colored, antibiotics are usually not indicated in chronic sinusitis and should be avoided.*

Step #1: *Undergo acupuncture* to resolve chronic sinusitis. This is the most effective and cost-effective treatment for long term resolution.

Step #2: *Take the Chinese herbal remedies Qing Bu Tang, Xiao Qing Long Tang, Wen Dan Tang, or Yu Ping Feng San* to more quickly resolve the condition, along with acupuncture.

Step #3: *Undergo LLEL* with or without acupuncture. It can also provide long-term relief.

Step #4: *Try butterbur or Montelukast* if you still have symptoms.

Step #5: *Undergo the NAET* if allergies are suspected as the cause.

Step #6: *Undergo cranial-sacral evaluation and manipulation for structural problems* if you have had facial or head trauma and your symptoms haven't responded to the above steps.

Becky came to my clinic for treatment of constant migraine headaches. She had been treated by several neurologists for years, but nothing relieved her symptoms. Because migraine headaches are rarely present on a continuous basis, I evaluated her further and found that her problem was chronic sinusitis, caused by allergies. The sinus inflammation was causing her headaches.

Because one of the standard Chinese herbal formulas contains cinnamon, which she was allergic to, a specific formula was designed for her. She also underwent twelve acupuncture sessions. These two methods significantly decreased her symptoms and her flare-ups, but she still had some residual problems. I suggested that she undergo osteopathic evaluation, and she underwent cranial-sacral manipulation. She did receive additional benefit from this technique, and her residual symptoms are now easily controlled by the Chinese herbal formula alone.

Step #7: *Take inhaled steroids* if the above steps have still not helped.

Step #8: *Consider sinus surgery* if drainage is obstructed and none of the above steps has resolved the condition.

Expected Outcome

Chronic sinusitis is more difficult to treat successfully than acute sinusitis, but using the above steps, you should be able to resolve the condition long-term.

Sprains, Strains, Muscle Tears

What You Need to Know

The most common result of injury is sprain or strain of "soft" connective tissues (ligaments, tendons, muscles), in which these tissues tear. Because soft tissues do not have a large blood supply, they often take long periods of time to heal. Any soft tissue can tear, but there are different degrees of tears, from first-degree to third-degree, with the latter being a complete tear.

A tear of *ligaments* is referred to as a *strain* or *sprain* injury. If in the knees, it may involve the medial and lateral collateral ligaments (on each side of the knee) and/or the anterior cruciate ligament (ACL), which runs through the knee from front to back. The knee also contains cartilage that can tear, called menisci, which serves as padding for the knee. Ligaments can be torn in the hands/wrists and feet/ankles as well. Often, shoulder injuries result in what's called "impingement syndrome," most likely representing small ligament tears that cause swelling and compression.

The most common *tendon* tears in older people occur in the shoulder rotator cuff (a group of five tendons) but can also occur frequently in the heel (Achilles). *Muscle* tears can also occur, most commonly in the biceps (arm) and hamstrings (leg).

Beware of Blood Clots Following Injury

A recent study published in the *Archives of Internal Medicine* revealed that leg injuries, including muscle or ligament ruptures and sprains, are associated with significantly increased risk of blood clots in the legs. The association is the strongest in the month following the injury.

Injuries to soft tissues can occur from numerous sources, and even minor objects can cause injuries, the most common being beds and bedding, household containers, sofas, and footwear. Of course, as we age, many of us still think we can do activities we've always been able to do, but overdoing can have consequences as well.

Knee Buckling: What Does It Mean?

Twelve percent of people report at least one episode of a knee buckling or "giving way." This occurs more often during activities such as walking, stair climbing, and twisting or turning. Pain in the knee, being overweight, poor physical function, and weakness of the thigh muscles can predispose people to this feeling.

Knee pain is often associated with knee buckling, but most people who have buckling do not have arthritis evident on x-rays. About 12 percent of people will have tears of their ACL, but most people have no particular abnormalities.

One possible cause that was not considered and is not understood by doctors but can cause buckling is called the "tib-fib" syndrome, in which the two calf bones can become misaligned. This is an osteopathic diagnosis and is treated using osteopathic manipulation.

Treatments for Sprains/Strains/Tears

The Preventive Approaches

Warming up followed by *stretching properly* before sports activities or exercise is a primary method of preventing soft-tissue tears. Many people only stretch before exercise but this may actually cause more strains and sprains. Of course *avoiding falls* is another important method of preventing tears.

Falls Common as We Age

One of the most common problems as we age is falling, due to weakness, balance problems, blood pressure problems (including orthostatic hypotension), and other causes, including wearing multifocal glasses. About one in six adults over the age of sixty-five falls every three months, and one-third of those who fall sustain injuries. Therefore, in general, preventing falls is the best way to prevent injuries. The CDC describes fourteen effective fall-prevention strategies in a new publication, *Preventing Falls: What Works* (http://www.cdc.gov/ncipc/PreventingFalls/).

In addition, taking vitamin D (800 mg daily) has been shown to prevent falls as well. A recent study showed that elderly people who fell and had access to an alarm system did not use the alarm in 80 percent of cases. Using the alarm is a must because prolonged time on the floor after falling is associated with greater injury and hospitalization.

One uncommon cause of falls is decreased blood pressure after eating, which occurs with many elderly patients. If that should occur, increased water intake before eating or eating six smaller meals a day rather than three large ones can help prevent this.

———

Several studies have revealed that the use of a certain class of antibiotics, called flouroquinolones, can increase the risk for tendon rupture. These antibiotics all end in the wording floxacin (such as ciprofloxacin). Patients at higher risk include those over the age of sixty, those taking steroids, and those undergoing organ transplants.

The Conventional Approaches

For mild to moderate problems, conventional methods start with the **RICE protocol**:

- *Rest* the joint: avoid using it, especially for strenuous activities such as lifting (shoulder) or walking/climbing (knee, hip).
- Apply *ice* to the affected area: you can use commercial ice packs sold in drugstores or wrap a towel around some ice. Do not apply it for more than twenty minutes every hour.
- *Compress* the joint: wrap the joint with an elastic bandage such as an ACE wrap, but don't tighten it to the degree that your circulation is cut off.
- *Elevate* the affected limb: keep the joint elevated, perhaps by placing your knee on some pillows.

———

Ice versus Heat

Should you use heat or ice if you've sustained an injury? In general, it is recommended to use ice for an acute injury with swelling. Heat should be applied after the swelling has subsided and if you are sore or achy; it can worsen inflammation if applied too soon. Whatever method is used, do so for only twenty minutes every two to three hours while awake. If overused, it can worsen your symptoms and slow the healing process.

———

Medications: OTC *NSAIDs*, such as ibuprofen or naproxen (Aleve), are helpful for short-term pain relief and to reduce inflammation while the tissues heal naturally, if you have a mild to moderate tear. You should obtain relief within a few days from these drugs. If these are not effective, *other NSAIDs* (such as naproxen [Naprosyn], meloxicam [Mobic], piroxicam [Feldene], oxaprozin [Daypro], nabumatone [Relafen], ketoprofen [Orudis], diclofenac [Cataflam], and diclofenac/misoprostol [Arthrotec]) are more powerful and may work if the OTC drugs don't. Any NSAID should be used short-term to relieve pain and swelling. These drugs may cause stomach irritation and bleeding, and if this occurs, you can try the Cox-2 inhibitor Celebrex, which has a lower risk of these side effects. *Warning*: Studies show a small increased risk of heart attack in patients who use Cox-2 inhibitors, so caution is advised, especially if you have heart disease.

Caution: In July, 2015, the FDA started requiring NSAIDs to carry a warning of increased risk of heart attacks, stroke and heart failure. This is especially evident when taken long term, at higher doses, or by people with pre-existing heart disease. The risks can increase as early as the first weeks of NSAID use. However, ibuprofen and naproxen do not appear to increase the risk, so are the safest and preferred NSAIDs.

Physical therapy modality treatments are often done for these conditions but have a variable success rate. These treatments include electrical stimulation (passing direct or alternating low-voltage current through the painful joint), ultrasound, and iontophoresis (application of a topical steroid solution through the skin into the affected joint). Exercises may cause a worsening of the tear.

Corticosteroid injections may also be administered for some of these injuries, especially impingement syndrome. However, a 2014 study in the *Annals of Internal Medicine* showed that steroid injection and physical therapy are equally effective, but steroid injection users were more likely to need additional therapies.

Surgery is often done for certain tears when the above treatments don't work. Surgeries are commonly done for rotator cuff tears and Achilles tendon tears. Ligament tears such as the ACL and meniscal tears in the knee usually have good results from surgery, but collateral ligaments do not. *Important note*: A 2014 study in *CMAJ* showed that arthroscopic knee surgery for meniscal tears may not be effective if you have no or minimal arthritis.

Asymptomatic Tears Common in Knees and Shoulders: You May Not Need Surgery!

Patients often obtain MRI scans to evaluate injuries to various joints, especially shoulders and knees. However, tears may be present but are not causing any symptoms—and thus may not need treatment. A study on shoulders revealed that 34 percent of people overall have asymptomatic tears of the rotator cuff—54 percent of people older than sixty. Because tears are common but may not cause any symptoms, just because a tear is identified does not mean you necessarily need to undergo surgery. Other treatments may be beneficial and can be tried first.

Another interesting study revealed that meniscal tears of the knee are sometimes noted in knees that have no symptoms. Only certain types of tears (full thickness, radial, and displaced) are greater in symptomatic knees, with horizontal or oblique tears similar in symptomatic and asymptomatic knees.

What this means is that, depending on what type of tear you have, just because the MRI shows a tear does not mean that it is causing your symptoms. This may be why knee and shoulder surgeries sometimes do not resolve the symptoms. In fact, a 2015 study revealed that surgery for non-traumatic rotator cuff tears was no better than physical therapy alone.

Muscle tears are often not helped by surgery. Surgeries done for impingement of the shoulder and *partial* tendon tears may not be necessary if you use alternative methods.

The Alternative Approaches

For partial tears of most soft tissues, alternative methods often accelerate healing faster than conventional methods.

Low level energy laser (*LLEL* or "cold laser") is the best alternative method. It appears to help heal the tissue directly, reduce the inflammatory response, and increase blood flow to the injured tissue. It often accelerates healing two to three times as fast as conventional methods, and side effects are minimal. You should feel better within two to nine treatments (two weeks).

Acupuncture can also be used for partial tears, appearing to increase blood flow, reduce swelling and inflammation, and accelerate healing. You should feel better within two to eight acupuncture treatments. It can be used with the laser for faster results.

Infrasound appears to work better than ultrasound. Infrasound works by increasing the local circulation of blood and lymph, thereby accelerating the healing process. It decreases swelling as well. Infrasound is used by numerous chiropractors, naturopathic doctors, and acupuncturists—and a few doctors.

For temporary relief, there are several **topicals** that can provide reduction of pain and inflammation for several hours. These include the Chinese herbal formula Zhen Gu Shui, Biofreeze, capsaicin, and many others. Traumeel cream and the oral tablets can be used to alleviate bruising, swelling, and pain.

Other **Chinese herbal formulas**, containing numerous herbs including *San Ji*, can be taken orally or applied locally to enhance the healing response. *Jin Gu Die Shang Wan* can be taken internally and *White Flower Topical Liniment* can be applied topically for muscle-level pain.

In addition, there are several **nutritional supplements** that are beneficial in healing sprains and minor tears, which can be used with the above treatments. The most common are *arnica* and *comfrey*, both of which can be used in compresses and applied directly to the area of injury. *Caution*: Comfrey should not be used over an open wound.

Your Empowered Patient Action Plan for Treating Soft-Tissue Tears

- *Important Note: If you have a complete tear, go first to step 8*

Step #1: Use the RICE method if you have mild symptoms.

Step #2: Use herbal topicals and/or Traumeel oral tablets for temporary control of pain and inflammation while awaiting the following steps to resolve the condition.

Step #3: Receive LLEL therapy for accelerated healing. The laser should heal and strengthen the tissues quickly unless they are completely torn.

Step #4: Undergo acupuncture for accelerated healing. Use with step 3 if both are available.

Step #5: Use compresses containing arnica and/or comfrey to enhance the healing process.

Step #6: Take an NSAID if pain and swelling continue despite the above measures.

Step #7: Try physical therapy modalities if you still have symptoms and you don't have a complete tear.

Step #8: Consider surgery if nothing else has worked or of you have a complete tear.

Expected Outcome

Tears of soft tissues can generally heal sufficiently with conventional and/or alternative methods. Certain tears, especially complete tears, may require surgery.

Stroke (Cerebrovascular Accident [CVA], Cerebrovascular Insufficiency [CVI], Transient Ischemic Attack [TIA])

What You Need to Know

Cerebrovascular insufficiency (CVI) means that there is not enough blood flow and delivery of oxygen to the brain. It is caused most frequently by atherosclerosis (hardening/clogging of the arteries), either in the arteries of the brain, or the carotid artery in the neck. Stroke (cerebrovascular accident, CVA) occurs when the blood supply is cut off completely and the brain cells start dying.

Stroke Affecting More People Every Year

The good news is that death from stroke has declined over the past two decades. The bad news is that the absolute number of people afflicted by stroke is high and continues to increase. This, of course, causes more complications and long-term disability.

"Ministrokes," called TIAs (transient ischemic attacks), may cause symptoms similar to stroke, but these symptoms disappear in one to twenty-four hours. TIAs can be a precursor or warning sign of impending stroke. In fact, 4–20 percent of patients with TIAs end up having strokes.

Strokes More Common in the American Southeast

Several studies have noted that the risk of having a stroke (and dying from it) has been higher in the American Southeast than any other region. This includes eleven states: Arkansas, Louisiana, Mississippi, Alabama, Georgia, the Carolinas, Tennessee, Virginia, Kentucky, and Indiana, now referred to as the "stroke belt." Despite a thirty-year search for an explanation, no reason has been found.

In addition, African Americans have double the risk of stroke of other groups; and if they live in the stroke belt, it is even higher.

Eighty percent of the time, a stroke is due to a clot obstructing the artery, called *ischemic* stroke. The other major causes of stroke are when the arteries bleed, usually due to high blood pressure (called *hemorrhagic*) or when a blood vessel bursts (*aneurysm*)).

Testing for Stroke

The two main types of stroke, ischemic strokes and bleeding strokes, must be treated differently. Therefore, diagnostic testing (MRI, MRA or CT scan of the brain) can be crucial in determining which type of stroke has occurred.

However, studies show that when trying to identify stroke in patients with symptoms of syncope (fainting) or altered mental status, CT scans are unnecessary in most cases and will not yield good information. They are also costly and emit high radiation doses.

Half of all strokes occur after the age of seventy. Women generally suffer more strokes than men, but they recover just as well or better; and men are twice as likely as women to die from a stroke. Stroke is the third leading cause of death and is the leading cause of disability in this country.

Unfortunately, many Americans are unaware of the warning signs of stroke. A recent survey revealed that only 44 percent of people could recognize the five main warning signs of stroke, as follows:

- Sudden numbness or weakness of the face, arm, or leg
- Sudden confusion or trouble speaking
- Sudden difficulty walking, dizziness, or loss of balance
- Sudden trouble seeing
- Severe headache

It is very important to know these warning signs because the faster you get treatment for stroke, the better the outcome (see sidebar below).

Fast Diagnosis and Treatment... Can Fifteen Minutes Make a Difference?

In general, most authorities recommend treatment as quickly as possible for stroke to reduce brain damage, especially preventing further damage in areas around the initially damaged region. For ischemic strokes, it is recommended to receive clot-busting drugs within three hours to prevent long-term complications, although some patients can obtain the same benefit up to 4.5 hours; after that, they are not very effective. However, a recent study revealed that stroke can cause brain damage within three minutes, so there always may be some residual damage.

The *bottom line* is that the faster you get treated, the less the damage. A 2013 study in *JAMA* showed that with each fifteen-minute decrease in time to treatment, patients were significantly less likely to die in the hospital or experience brain bleeding.

Important Information:
Hospitals Differ in Stroke Treatment and Outcome

It is important to know that where you are hospitalized for stroke can make a significant difference in survival. An analysis of a registry of more than ninety thousand stroke patients revealed that 26 percent of Medicare beneficiaries die, and 36 percent must be readmitted within one year of stroke. There was marked variation among hospitals in rates of death and readmission. This was thought to be due to differences in care processes and systems of care in the hospital, during transition of care, and during postdischarge management (follow-up). Be sure to follow the recommendations on hospitalization found in chapter 3.

Treatments for Stroke

The Preventive Approaches
Correctible causes: *Smoking* and *high blood pressure* are two of the major causes of CVI and stroke. If you smoke, it is essential that you quit (see chapter 2). Have your blood pressure checked every six to twelve months. If you have high blood pressure, one of the best antihypertensive medications to take for preventing strokes is a thiazide diuretic (such as Diuril, hydrodiuril, or HCTZ). If these do not control your blood pressure, see the *Hypertension* section for more specific recommendations.

Other conditions that can cause stroke include uncontrolled diabetes and high cholesterol. (See the sections about these conditions for more information on treatment.)

Certain medical conditions can predispose patients to releasing clots into the brain. The most common conditions are atrial fibrillation (AF) and carotid artery stenosis. Controlling these conditions will reduce the risk of stroke (see *Heart Disease: Arrhythmias* and *Arterial Stenosis* sections for treatments of these conditions).

Risk Factors for Stroke

Nine factors *that you can modify* account for 90 percent of all strokes:

High blood pressure

Smoking

Low waist-to-hip ratio

Unhealthy diet

Lack of regular exercise

Diabetes

Moderate or high alcohol intake

Stress

Depression

If you are a postmenopausal woman on standard doses of estrogen, the risk of stroke increases between the third and fourth year you are taking them, especially if you smoke. If your doctor recommends hormone replacement, I recommend taking very low-dose estrogen (primarily transdermal), raloxiphene, or natural estrogens, as there is lower risk of stroke from these forms of estrogen. (See the section on *Menopause* for further information and treatment guidelines.)

Diet plays a significant role in both causing and preventing stroke as with any blood vessel disease caused by atherosclerosis. In fact, obesity accounts for the largest rise in stroke occurrence. Eating more fruits and vegetables is the best way of preventing stroke. A balanced diet, with not more than 30 percent of calories from fat and less than 10 percent of those fat calories from saturated fat (use polyunsaturated and monounsaturated fat preferably), can decrease blood-cholesterol levels. If you have very high blood-cholesterol levels, you should restrict your fat intake to 20 percent of calories, and even 10 percent for the best results. Also, avoid cholesterol-containing products. Use plant-based butter spreads, such as Take Control and Benecol, which can reduce cholesterol by an additional 10 percent.

In addition, soy products are excellent at reducing cholesterol levels, as is black tea. Avocado is very potent at reducing cholesterol levels. Increasing the fiber in your diet can also decrease cholesterol levels. (See section on *Cholesterol* for further information and guidelines).

Eat at least two meals of fish per week (cold-water fish such as mackerel, salmon, halibut, tuna, herring, or cod) to reduce or prevent cholesterol buildup in the brain arteries. Lastly, adding ground flaxseed to your salads, oatmeal, and other baked items helps reduce inflammation and provides additional fiber to reduce cholesterol levels.

High Vitamin C Levels Decrease Stroke Risk

An analysis from the European Prospective Investigation into Cancer (EPIC) showed that people with high blood levels of vitamin C had a 42 percent reduced risk for stroke compared to those in the lowest quartile. What this indicates is that people eating more fruits and vegetables have lower stroke risk. Taking supplements with vitamin C has *not* been shown to decrease risk, so you need to get it from food.

Drinking one glass of **wine** daily with meals appears to be preventive of stroke. Wine, especially red, has powerful antioxidant properties and has been shown in numerous studies to decrease the risk of stroke. However, other alcoholic beverages have nearly the same preventive capabilities, if consumed moderately. Drinking adequate amounts of **water** daily is also very important.

Physical activity can also significantly decrease the risk of stroke. Walking a brisk pace for thirty minutes a day is all that is required, although more strenuous aerobic exercise is even better—but get checked by a doctor before beginning strenuous exercise.

Stroke Risk in Women Plummets with Healthy Lifestyle

A study published in the August 2008 issue of *Circulation* revealed that women who pursue healthy habits had a 79 percent reduced risk of any type of stroke and an 81 percent decreased risk of ischemic stroke. The habits are:

- Not smoking
- Maintaining a healthy weight
- Exercising regularly
- Drinking moderate amounts of alcohol

Taking *aspirin* (81 mg daily) is quite effective for preventing ischemic stroke if you are at high risk, have TIAs, or have other vascular (blood vessel) problems (25 percent risk reduction).

The Conventional Approaches

For ischemic strokes

There are several **medications** that are beneficial both during and following ischemic strokes. *Anticoagulants* (blood thinners) can break up the blood clot (a process referred to as thrombolysis) if given promptly. Studies show that these agents (urokinase, streptokinases, or recombinant tissue plasminogen activators [rt-Pas]) taken shortly after ischemic stroke reduce overall death and disability in the long term and increases the chance of a good outcome by 30–40 percent. These drugs do have a 2–6 percent increased risk of brain hemorrhage (with greater than 50 percent mortality), but the benefits definitely outweigh this risk. It is not known which people are most likely to benefit, and this therapy must be given within four and a half hours of stroke onset (the sooner, the better). *Warning*: These agents should not be used in bleeding strokes.

Helpful Tip: Following an ischemic stroke, you may need treatment with *cholesterol-lowering drugs and antihypertensive* (see sidebar below for caveat), which have been shown to reduce death after stroke and prevent reoccurrences. Unfortunately, studies show that a majority of patients never receive these medications.

Important Information
Hypertension Can Be Overtreated in Ischemic Stroke

Although very high blood pressure in patients with ischemic stroke should be lowered, a study published in *Neurology* stated that up to 65 percent of patients with ischemic stroke are likely to be *inappropriately* treated for hypertension during the first four days of hospitalization. This is important because, unless blood pressure is very high, lowering the pressure can aggravate stroke symptoms and worsen both short-term and long-term outcomes.

Another study in the *NEJM* showed that angiotensin receptor blockers (ARBs -- given for hypertension) failed to lower stroke recurrence after an ischemic stroke.

One *aspirin* a day (81 mg) is the primary medication doctors use to prevent *ischemic* stroke recurrence. *Important notes*: Ibuprofen blocks the blood-thinning effects of aspirin, so try not to take it if you are taking aspirin. If you must take ibuprofen, take the aspirin first and wait at least an hour to take the ibuprofen, and take the lowest ibuprofen dose you can (three doses will negate 90 percent of aspirin's effects). Aspirin use can also deplete body stores of vitamin C, so make sure you get at least 600 mg of vitamin C per day through your diet or by taking a supplement. If aspirin bothers your stomach, your doctor may prescribe the drug ticlopidine instead, or use OTC PPIs (generically end in "prazole, such as omeprazole: most popular name brands include Prilosec, Prevacid, Nexium, Dexilant, Protonix and Aciphex) to protect the stomach.

Aspirin Resistance: Real or Not?

Some patients, however, are thought to have aspirin resistance, in which aspirin does not have the antiplatelet effect to prevent clots. People who are nonresponsive to aspirin have a fourfold increased risk of adverse coronary events. However, a recent study revealed that 90 percent of patients who are unresponsive to aspirin have simply not taken their aspirin on a regular basis. You can find out if you are truly aspirin resistant by undergoing arachidonic acid testing.

A very new drug, *cilostazol (Pletal)*, has been shown in a Japanese study to be more effective than aspirin in preventing second strokes and has less risk of bleeding. ***Caution***: Drug side effects occur more often with cilostazol than aspirin (except bleeding), and it costs more.

The prescription drugs *dipyridamole* (Persantine) or *clopidrogel* (Plavix) are effective alternatives for those who cannot take either aspirin or ticlopidine. It is usually given if aspirin is not helping or you can't take it. ***Helpful tip***: A study from the *NEJM* showed that dipyridamole with either aspirin or clopidrogel are equally effective at preventing stroke recurrence and may be a little better than aspirin alone.

Stenting for Atherosclerosis Now May Be Useful

Atherosclerosis of the large arteries in the brain is the major cause of ischemic stroke. A procedure that has been tried to prevent stroke is placing stents in these arteries, much like stenting coronary arteries in heart disease and for heart attack.

However, two major trials in 2013 showed that stenting cerebral arteries caused more harm than benefit and was significantly worse than medical treatment.

However, five studies published in 2015 showed that a stent could be placed in the obstructed artery, expand within the clot, and then be withdrawn, pulling the clot with it. Outcomes were significantly improved. Patients who received benefit had clots within specific arteries, had the procedure done within 6 hours from stroke onset, and had already received tissue plasminogen activators (see above).

Caution: Understand that these procedures are done in a limited number of stroke centers at this time.

For hemorrhagic strokes

You must reduce or eliminate the factors causing the bleeding, the primary one being elevated blood pressure; it must be reduced as quickly as possible. However, it cannot be reduced too low because more ischemia may result. A systolic (higher number) pressure of 150 has been shown to be adequate in recent studies.

Avoid Statins in Hemorrhagic Stroke

Statins are often used to prevent ischemic strokes due to high cholesterol, but a study in *Neurology* found that patients with a history of a recent stroke or TIA are more likely to suffer a subsequent hemorrhagic stroke. (See *Cholesterol* section for alternatives to statins.)

Treatment After Strokes:

After a stroke occurs, **intensive rehabilitation** in a specialty stroke rehabilitation center is essential. The activities and exercises that you undergo in rehabilitation re-teach healthy parts of your brain to take over damaged functions.

A recent study from *Lancet Neurology* reports that the SSRI **fluoxetine** (Prozac) might reduce motor disability after stroke.

Patients with strokes often are bedridden for long periods and may not be able to walk, thus increasing the risk for deep vein thrombosis (DVT) or leg clots. *Helpful tip*: A recent study showed that compression stockings are not beneficial in stroke patients for preventing DVT, and you should use **low-molecular-weight heparin** (LMWH) or pneumatic compression devices instead.

If you have atrial fibrillation, **warfarin** (Coumadin) is the most common drug to re-duce the risk of stroke, but newer drugs such as dabigatran have also been approved for this indication and do not require monitoring like warfarin does, so they are now preferred (see section on Arteries: Peripheral Artery Disease and Stenosis for further discussion).

Many Stroke Survivors Don't Take Their Medications

A report in the *Archives of Neurology* found that one-fourth of stroke survivors say they stopped taking at least one of their medications within three months of their stroke. The authors reported that the numbers are probably higher since these numbers came from hospitals participating in a national stroke program.

For treatment of aneurysms causing strokes
Although a ruptured aneurysm causing a stroke has a high risk of mortality before treatment is attempted, **surgery** is usually necessary in those who survive, depending on the size of the aneurysm. There are two types of surgery: *Surgical clipping* (a clip is placed across the neck of the aneurysm) and *endovascular coiling* (Platinum coils are inserted into the aneurysm causing a clot that then forms around the coils, obliterat-ing the aneurysmal sac). In many cases, anatomic considerations, such as size, location, other morphological features determine which treatment is most appropriate for the patient. In centers with available expertise and in patients with blood vessel-accessible lesions, short term outcomes appear to be improved with endovascular coiling as com-pared to surgical clipping. *Helpful Tip:* Treatment at specialized neurosurgical centers performing high volumes of cerebral aneurysm procedures is associated with better outcome compared with treatment at lower volume centers. (For more information on aneurysms, see section on *Arteries: Aneurysms and Dissection*).

The Alternative Approaches
Acupuncture is supported by the NIH and the World Health Organization for aid-ing in recovery of function, sensation, and extremity strength following stroke, as well as cognitive functions such as speech and vision. The sooner you begin acupuncture after the stroke, the more effective it is, although good results can be obtained even years after the stroke. You should see improvement within six to eight acupuncture treatments but will probably need additional sessions for maximum benefit. Often, it

may take up to thirty treatments to obtain good benefits. It should be noted that both auricular (ear) and body acupuncture are beneficial.

Nutritional supplements: If you are having symptoms of CVI or TIAs, *gingko biloba* (160–240 mg per day, containing 24 percent gingko flavonglycosides) may help reverse many of the symptoms including impaired mental performance. It improves blood flow, oxygen flow, and glucose utilization and protects brain cells. Gingko can also thin your blood, so be aware that you may bleed or bruise more easily if you take aspirin and gingko together.

If you have a transient ischemic attack (TIA), *aortic glycosaminoglycans* improve blood flow in both the brain and the extremities and seem to reduce ischemic events. It should be used for at least six months after a TIA. Dosage is 100 mg per day.

Fish oil is both a blood thinner and anti-inflammatory and may help prevent strokes as well as decrease recurrences. ***Important notes***: There are problems with fish oil that you need to be aware of. Although regular fish oil can decrease cholesterol levels and protect the heart, you must take *at least* 1,500 mg daily to obtain benefits. Many studies were done using 3,000–4,000 mg. Many fish oils also deteriorate very rapidly (three months); so by the time you buy them, they may already be partially deteriorated. Krill oil may be more potent and stable, contains two natural antioxidants, and has few to no side effects. However, krill oil products vary in their concentrations of omega-3s and combinations with other ingredients, so check the label.

Dr. A's Suggestions:
Vitamin E Not Helpful to Prevent Stroke

A study by the National Cancer Institute and another study published in *BMJ* showed that vitamin E supplements have no effect on overall stroke, significantly increase the risk for hemorrhagic stroke by 22 percent, and show a mild decrease (10 percent) in the risk of ischemic strokes. Indiscriminate use of vitamin E supplements is not advised by experts.

Your Empowered Patient Action Plan for TIA, CVI, and *Prevention* of Strokes

*Step #1: **Take an aspirin a day or alternative medications*** to thin your blood. Consult with your doctor.

*Step #2: **Lifestyle changes*** are extremely important, including dietary changes. Appropriate water intake is crucial, and mild exercise like walking is beneficial.

*Step #3: **Treat other medical conditions*** that can lead to stroke, especially hypertension and high cholesterol.

*Step #4: **Take fish oil*** to decrease inflammation, help brain function, and help prevent strokes or their recurrence.

*Step #5: **Take gingko biloba*** if you have CVI or TIAs to improve blood flow in the brain and improve cognitive functions.

*Step #6: **Take aortic glycosaminoglycans*** if you have a TIA to increase blood flow in the brain.

*Step #7: **Take transdermal estrogen replacement or raloxiphene (postmenopausal women)*** if you must take hormone replacement therapy.

Your Empowered Patient Action Plan for *Treating* Acute Stroke

- *Important Note: If you have any of the symptoms listed in the introduction, go immediately to an emergency room, preferably at a hospital that has a stroke unit.*

For ischemic stroke

*Step #1: **Take thrombolytic drugs*** to break up clots within four and a half hours of stroke but sooner if possible.

*Step #2: **Consider an endovascular procedure*** if it is available and you fit the specific criteria.

*Step #3: **Take aspirin*** or other indicated blood thinners to prevent recurrence.

For bleeding (hemorrhagic) stroke

*Step #1: **Reduce blood pressure*** if elevated.

*Step #2: **Consider surgery*** to repair aneurysm if present.

*Step #3: **Avoid taking statin drugs*** so as to reduce the risk of recurrence of hemorrhagic stroke.

For all post-stroke patients

*Step #1: **Enter a specialized stroke rehabilitation program*** to regain function as soon as you have recovered.

Step #2: Undergo acupuncture to accelerate return of function and begin as soon as possible for maximum benefit.

Suzanne's bleeding stroke four years previously left her with severe weakness and pain in her right arm and leg. She had a "claw" hand (meaning it was in a fist and the fingers could not be extended voluntarily). She walked with a limp and needed a cane for assistance. She also had memory and concentration difficulties. After three acupuncture treatments (using both body and ear points), her concentration and memory were restored almost completely. With twelve sessions, she could voluntarily open her hand and no longer needed a cane to walk. Her strength began returning, and her pain resolved. She continued receiving acupuncture on a monthly schedule, and her improvement continued.

Step #3: Take fish oil, gingko biloba and/or glycosaminoglycans to improve blood flow and function in the brain as well as prevent recurrence.

Step #4: Take statins if indicated to prevent recurrence of ischemic stroke.

Step #5: Take antihypertensive medications if indicated to prevent recurrence of hemorrhagic stroke.

Step #6: Take aspirin or alternative medications to thin your blood after an ischemic stroke.

Expected Outcome

Strokes can be devastating and cause long-term brain damage and poor quality of life. The most important aspect is to prevent strokes in the first place, but if you have a stroke, time to treatment is of the essence. After stroke, preventing recurrence and using complementary methods to rehabilitate are the main goals to reduce long-term complications.

Thyroid (Hypothyroidism, Subclinical Hypothyroidism)

What You Need to Know

The diagnosis of thyroid hormone imbalances is based on measuring blood levels of thyroid hormones, but some results can be misleading due to interference from other medical conditions or medications (for example, the primary thyroid hormone, T_4, can be falsely elevated if you take birth-control pills or synthetic hormones). The TSH level (thyroid stimulating hormone, a pituitary hormone that stimulates production of thyroid hormones) is considered a more reliable test: above-normal levels usually indicate hypothyroidism (low thyroid function).

Thyroid Tests May Be Misleading

Although TSH, T_4, and T_3 are the tests used by most doctors, there are problems. TSH and T_4, which are measured in the blood, are actually poor indicators of thyroid levels *in the tissues*, which is more important for health.

T4 is measured while bound to protein, which prevents it from exerting effects in the tissues. Free T4 does get into the tissues, and this test (and free T3) is more indicative of thyroid function.

Another less frequently used test is the reverse T_3 (rT_3) and the ratio of T_3 to rT_3, which may be the best indicators of tissue levels of thyroid, according to a recent study in the *Journal of Clinical Endocrinology and Metabolism*. This study showed that increased T_4 and rT_3 levels and decreased T_3 levels are associated with hypothyroidism at the tissue level with diminished physical functioning. Thus, it is important to obtain an rT_3 level and a T_3/rT_3 ratio.

Subclinical hypothyroidism is a condition that is being diagnosed more often and may increase as we age. In this condition, the TSH is borderline high, but the actual thyroid hormone (T_4) level is normal. People may not have any symptoms of low thyroid, but others may complain of low energy, memory problems, or weight gain. A recent study from the *JAMA* revealed that subclinical hypothyroidism can increase the risk of heart events up to 89 percent and heart deaths by 58 percent. Another study in *Archives of Internal Medicine* reveals that it can increase the risk for osteoporosis and fractures. It is estimated that nearly 20 percent of people may have subclinical hypothyroidism, most of them women.

The question is whether people with this diagnosis should be treated, and this is controversial. Benefits of treatment include preventing progression of hypothyroidism, improvement in symptoms, decreased cholesterol, helping the heart work better, and decreasing the increased risk detailed above. Negatives are that many people do not benefit at all, and overtreatment can cause additional problems. In fact, a 2012 study showed that many of these patients (especially the elderly) revert back to normal without treatment. Another study showed that there is no correlation between this condition and mood disorders or cognitive deficiencies in people older than sixty-five. A consensus of endocrinologists recommends treatment if TSH is over 10 mIU/L. However, some people with symptoms of low thyroid have a TSH lower than that level, and treatment may still benefit them.

The major cause of hypothyroidism, both clinical and subclinical, is Hashimoto's thyroiditis. This is an autoimmune condition in which your body makes antibodies that eventually destroy your thyroid cells. There are blood tests to help you determine this condition, but TSH may remain normal during the early stages.

Important note: Many people think that you can take your basal body temperature (your temperature when taken first thing in the morning), which reflects your metabolic rate. If low (usually and consistently below 98 degrees), it is thought that the thyroid is not working well. However, the metabolic rate is not solely dependent on thyroid hormones, so other factors may be causing the lowered body temperature as well as other symptoms.

Thyroid Nodules: Cause for Concern?

It is quite common to have cysts and nodules in your thyroid gland, and you might worry that you have thyroid cancer. What should you look for?

Most commonly, a thyroid uptake scan using radioactive iodine can help determine the possibility of cancer. Cysts are rarely cancerous but if a nodule is not stimulated by the iodine ("cold nodule"), it needs to be biopsied, especially if you're a man.

Another good test is ultrasound, which is easy to do and inexpensive. A 2013 study in *JAMA Internal Medicine* showed that three characteristics of ultrasound, taken together, predict the likelihood of cancer and the need for biopsy. They are as follows:

- Microcalcification in a nodule
- Nodules greater than 2 cm in diameter
- Entirely solid nodules

Biopsies are indicated if two out of the three characteristics are found. In addition, biopsy should also be done for the following:

- Nodules greater than 5 mm in patients who have had neck radiation exposure or positive family histories of cancer
- Solid nodules greater than 10 mm
- Cystic-solid nodules greater than 20 mm

You should understand that your basic thyroid tests may be normal even if you have thyroid cancer.

—∞—

Treatments for Hypothyroidism

The Preventive Approaches

Diet: Certain foods may need to be avoided in hypothyroidism; cabbage, peaches, soybeans, spinach, peanuts, and radishes can all interfere with the production of thyroid hormones.

On the other hand, there is some evidence that suggests that supplementing your diet with coconut oil can help thyroid function and may possibly boost your metabolism, which can help with the weight problems that so many hypothyroid patients encounter. The oil can be used in cooking or taken by the spoonful as a supplement.

Exercise stimulates the production of thyroid hormones and increases tissue sensitivity to the hormones. It is especially important to exercise if you are trying to lose weight and are hypothyroid, because dieting can cause a slowing of your metabolic rate, thus making your symptoms worse; exercise may prevent this from occurring by stimulating your metabolic rate.

The Conventional Approaches

Synthetic thyroid hormones (such as levothyroxine) are the most commonly prescribed medications for hypothyroid. Most contain only one form of thyroid, T_4, which is converted in the body to the other (active) form of thyroid, T_3, but some thyroid medications contain both. Some studies have shown that they may increase the risk of prostate cancer, but overall, they are relatively safe, have been used for decades, and are effective.

However, a recent study showed that T_4-only preparations (Synthroid, Levoxyl) may be inadequate for restoring normal thyroid hormone *in the tissues* (you may still have symptoms of low thyroid), and TSH cannot be relied upon to detect this (see sidebar above regarding rT_3). Therefore, prescription medications that contain both T_4 and T_3 may work better. However, you can also take your T_4 medication along with a T_3 drug (Cytomel).

—∞—

Elderly People May Need Less Thyroxine (T4)

A 2011 study published in *BMJ* revealed that elderly patients receiving levothyroxine have an increased risk of fractures, with the risk becoming higher as the dosage gets higher. It was pointed out by editorialists that the risk is still small, but elderly people may need relatively low thyroxine doses.

⸻ ◦◦◦ ⸻

Even though you replace your thyroid hormones with synthetic thyroid, your symptoms may still not seem to improve, or your tests may still indicate low thyroid. This could be due to interference with other drugs or food, protein binding, or poor absorption (see sidebar below). Many people also don't seem to absorb thyroid well or may be so sensitive that they become symptomatic if they miss a dose. It is advisable to consult with an endocrinologist if these problems occur.

⸻ ◦◦◦ ⸻

Dr. A's Suggestions:
Warning: **Coffee, Food, and Medication**
Can Interfere with Absorption of Thyroid Medications

A recent study revealed that drinking coffee delays the time to peak concentrations and decreases levels by 27–36 percent by binding thyroid in the gut. You should therefore take thyroid medication an hour before drinking coffee.

Another study showed that taking thyroid medications with meals also lowers the amount that is absorbed. It is recommended that you take your thyroid medications an hour before breakfast after fasting all night, or at least take it several hours apart from meals. You can also take your thyroid medication at bedtime.

Finally, a 2014 study showed that taking PPIs (for acid reflux) can decrease absorption of thyroid taken in tablet form. Thyroid in solution is not affected but is also not available in the United States. There is a softgel capsule that is unaffected by PPIs, but is more expensive than generic.

If you are taking higher-than-expected doses of thyroid hormone, check with your endocrinologist and make sure your absorption is not being blocked by these other factors.

⸻ ◦◦◦ ⸻

The Alternative Approaches
Desiccated ("natural") thyroid (Armour thyroid, Westhroid) is derived from animals rather than from synthetic sources and contains both forms (T_4 and T_3) of thyroid hormone. Studies have shown them to have the same benefits of just taking T_4, and as the above discussion reveals, they are sometimes more effective than just taking conventional T_4-only products. These are available only by prescription and are regulated by the FDA. *Caution*: Understand that the T_3 in natural hormones may only last for four to six hours. It may be prudent to use a split dose. *Warning*: As desiccated thyroid is foreign to our bodies, you should avoid its use if you have an active autoimmune disease. (*Caution*: Hashimoto's and Grave's diseases are autoimmune causes of hypothyroidism. You should not take desiccated thyroid while these conditions are ongoing. You can check a thyroid peroxidase antibody level to make sure.) *Important note*: Many endocrinologists do not like or use desiccated thyroid, although no studies have shown them to be inferior. If you take synthetic thyroid and still have symptoms, you may want to try taking natural thyroid instead.

Dr. A's Suggestions:
Diagnosing and Treating Iodine Deficiency

An important aspect of thyroid function is iodine. The main function of iodine in the body is for thyroid hormone production, and too little iodine may cause symptoms of hypothyroidism. Tincture of iodine (costs about eighty-seven cents) can be used to both diagnose and treat iodine deficiency: Place it on a patch of skin (thigh is best) about one inch square. If the iodine disappears before twenty-four hours, you may not be obtaining enough iodine. If it lasts much longer than twenty-four hours, you may be taking too much iodine, either in food or supplements. If deficient, you can apply iodine to the skin until it lasts more than 24 hours.

However, it is always a good idea to corroborate iodine deficiency by undergoing a blood test to determine iodine level.

Warning: Be careful of *iodine supplements* because they may contain too much iodine. The upper limit of normal is 1,100 mcg daily, and many supplements contain much more than that. The RDA for iodine is only 15 mcg a day. Obtaining iodine from the diet is much better (iodized salt, seafood, and dairy foods). Taking iodine in high doses or for prolonged periods of time can lower serum thyroid hormone and cause elevated TSH. In addition, it can cause or exacerbate thyroid hyperplasia, Grave's disease, or goiter.

There are several **nutritional supplements** that may be of benefit. *Kelp* and *bladder wrack* are from seaweed and contain large amounts of iodine. *Coleus foreskohloii* (1–2 ml three times per day) stimulates thyroid hormone production.

L-tyrosine (500 mg no more than twice daily) is actually a component of your T_4 and T_3 thyroid hormones. Any deficiency in this amino acid can interfere with the healthy function of your thyroid. ***Caution***: Supplementation may increase high blood pressure.

Health food stores sell *thyroid extracts* that are milder forms of desiccated thyroid. They can ease symptoms of mild hypothyroidism, but their purity and potency are not consistent from product to product and from bottle to bottle, even when you use the same brand. ***Caution***: Taking such extracts may cause more harm than good if you don't have your thyroid function monitored by a physician.

Your Empowered Patient Action Plan for Treating Hypothyroidism

Important note: *If your TSH is greater than 10 mIU/L, start at step 5.*

Step #1: Use tincture of iodine and/or a blood test to determine and treat deficiency of iodine.

Step #2: Measure your free T_4, free T_3, or reverse-T_3 level to determine if you are subclinically hypothyroid.

Step #3: Try coleus foreskohloii to increase thyroid hormone production if you have mild subclinical hypothyroidism.

Step #4: Consider taking L-tyrosine if you still have symptoms of mild subclinical hypothyroidism, but monitor your blood pressure.

Step #5: Take desiccated (natural) thyroid containing both T_3 and T_4, to resolve symptoms of low thyroid if your TSH is still elevated.

Step #6: Take synthetic thyroid hormone supplement(s) to lower TSH and resolve symptoms if you don't tolerate the natural thyroid in step 4 or in place of it.

Expected Outcome

Hypothyroid symptoms may be caused by other conditions so you should always check the thyroid hormone levels discussed above. If abnormal, your symptoms should fully resolve by using the above steps.

Tinnitus

What You Need to Know

Tinnitus is a noise heard inside your ear caused by damage to the cochlea, a small organ in the internal ear. The most common cause of tinnitus is chronic and loud noise exposure, but it can also be associated with other diseases (such as Meniere's disease) and often occurs with hearing loss but is not caused by it.

Other causes may include heavy metal toxicity, postchemotherapy damage (i.e., from cisplatin or other platinum containing drugs), wax blockage, infection, allergies, and tumor of the auditory nerve.

Treatments for Tinnitus

The Preventive Approaches

As with hearing loss, the best preventive is to **avoid loud noises**, even after tinnitus begins.

Correctible causes: In addition, there are over two hundred medications (including nonprescription) that can cause tinnitus, especially aspirin, some antibiotics, and quinine. If you are taking any medications, check the *PDR* to see if that medication can cause tinnitus.

Too much salt intake, caffeine, alcohol, and smoking can make tinnitus worse and should be reduced or eliminated.

The Conventional Approaches

Conventional medicine primarily uses **devices**, such as tinnitus maskers, that are designed to block out the tinnitus by making different sounds, but they can sometimes be more irritating than the tinnitus.

Another method, called **auditory habituation**, uses a device that generates "white noise," teaching the brain to ignore the tinnitus. Consult an ear specialist (otologist) for further information and guidance.

Tinnitus Retraining Therapy (TRT) is offered at specialized centers and is used in over 20 countries. TRT is a method aimed primarily at habituating tinnitus-evoked reactions of the brain and body, and secondarily, at habituation of tinnitus perception (i.e., you become more accustomed to the tinnitus). As a result, successful TRT patients may not be bothered by their tinnitus, even though they are aware of it. Additionally, the amount of time the successful TRT patient perceives tinnitus is decreased. The two main components of TRT are educational counseling (which is intensive, individualized and interactive) and sound therapy.

Medications may help some people. These include dexamethasone (a steroid), alprazolam (Xanax) and misoprostol (Cytotec). ***Caution***: Be aware that these medications may all have side effects and may not be very effective in most patients.

The Alternative Approaches

Acupuncture may resolve or reduce tinnitus long-term. However, the longer the tinnitus has been present, the more difficult it is for acupuncture to be effective. You should notice improvement within six acupuncture treatments, but you might need additional sessions for maximum benefit. Acupuncture is especially beneficial for Meniere's disease (see *Hearing Loss* section).

Along with acupuncture, **Chinese herbal formulas** called *Er Ming Zuo Ci Wan* ("tinnitus kidney yin pills") or *Er Long Zuo Ci Wan* may be helpful.

Homeopathy has had success in reducing several types of tinnitus, and the remedies differ depending on the type of sound being heard:

- *Chininum sulphuricum* is used for violent ringing (ringing as of bells) and tingling in ears. It is used in Meniere's syndrome.
- *Salicylium acidum* is used for roaring and ringing sounds or noises in ears like swarms of bees or buzzing.
- *Kali iodatum* is used for ringing sounds, tearing in the ear, which is sensitive in evening, or darting in ear.
- *Barboneum sulphuratum* is used for roaring sounds accompanied by the feeling that your ears are blocked and tingling sensations.

You should consult a qualified homeopathist for guidance on which remedies will be most beneficial and for proper dosages. You should notice improvement within one to two months.

Some **nutritional supplements** may also be of value. *Feverfew* (50–125 mg standardized to contain 0.6–0.7 percent pathenolide) and *gingko biloba* (160–240 mg daily) may be effective in some patients, the latter especially if a circulation problem is causing your tinnitus. It may take several weeks to two months to observe results.

Some people have structural problems involving the bones of the face and surrounding the ear. If so, you can undergo an osteopathic technique called **cranial-sacral manipulation**, in which the bones of the face and skull are realigned. You should notice improvement within two to three treatments. Be sure to find a qualified/ certified practitioner in cranial-sacral manipulation.

Your Empowered Patient Action Plan for Treating Tinnitus

*Step #1: **Undergo acupuncture*** to obtain long-lasting relief if the tinnitus has been present less than a year or two.

*Step #2: **Take an appropriate homeopathic remedy*** if acupuncture has not worked.

*Step #3: **Take feverfew or gingko biloba*** if the above steps haven't helped, especially if you have circulation problems.

*Step #4: **Undergo osteopathic evaluation and receive cranial-sacral manipulation*** if a structural problem is diagnosed.

*Step #5: **Undergo Tinnitus Retraining Therapy*** if you still have symptoms.

*Step #6: **Use a sound-masking device*** if nothing else helps and you are exceedingly bothered by the tinnitus.

Leroy had constant tinnitus, which he described as "crickets" in his ears all the time. The tinnitus had worsened over fifteen years and was worse in the right ear than the left. I started him on acupuncture, as well as some of the herbal remedies (step #3), and the tinnitus in his left ear improved, but not the right ear. I wondered if there might be a structural problem with the right ear, and he underwent osteopathic evaluation. At that time, he remembered having had an accident twenty years before in which he struck the side of his head and sustained a concussion. He underwent treatment using cranial-sacral techniques, and after only two sessions, the tinnitus in his right ear was completely gone.

Expected Outcome

Tinnitus is a very difficult condition to resolve or reverse, especially if it has been present a long time. However, there are some alternative methods that may be able to reduce the severity and frequency.

Urinary Tract (Bladder) Infections (Acute, Chronic, Recurrent)

What You Need to Know

A urinary tract infection (often called UTI) is an infection that begins in your urinary system, which is composed of the kidneys, ureters, bladder, and urethra. Any part of your urinary system can become infected, but most infections involve the bladder (called cystitis) or the urethra (connects the bladder to the outside of the body).

Diagnosing and Treating Urinary Tract Infections Yourself

According to a 2014 meta-analysis, as well as numerous guidelines, you may not need to see a doctor to diagnose a urinary tract infection. According to the study, urinary tract infections can be diagnosed if exhibiting at least two out of three cardinal symptoms: dysuria (burning on urination), urgency (feeling an urgent need to go), and/or frequency (frequent urination), along with no vaginal discharge in women.

Second, telephone-based protocols for treatment have outcomes similar to office-based diagnosis and treatment. Patients with histories of uncomplicated infections can be taught to diagnose and initiate therapy themselves.

If you fit into these categories, talk with your doctor to make diagnosis and treatment more efficient and less costly.

Urinary tract infections occur primarily in women—rarely in men. If persistent, they can lead to permanent damage in the urinary tract, which can lead to kidney damage and failure. They also can be a sign of sexually transmitted disease that can affect other pelvic organs (e.g., uterus, ovaries, fallopian tubes) and cause sterility.

If a man has a urinary tract infection, it *always* needs to be evaluated by a urologist for underlying structural problems. Women who have *recurrent* bladder infections (more than two or three in a year) also should be evaluated by a urologist.

Dr. A's Suggestions:
Don't Treat Urine Bacteria If You Don' Have Symptoms

Sometimes, a routine urine sample will show *traces* of bacteria. A study in 2012 in *Clinical Infectious Disease* showed that this should *not* be treated with antibiotics—and, in fact, antibiotics can lead to dramatically higher recurrence rates. This includes older people, diabetics, those with spinal cord injuries, and healthy young women. Treatment is not indicated unless symptoms are present, or during pregnancy, or before urinary instrument procedures.

Treatments for Urinary Tract Infections

The Preventive Approaches

Correctible causes: Some women develop infections after sexual intercourse, especially when not well lubricated. Proper lubrication and urinating after intercourse can help prevent these problems.

Medications: OTC antihistamines that contain Benadryl, chlorpheneramine, hydroxyzine, or cyproheptidine can underlie recurrent urinary tract infections in some women because they cause retention of urine. Discuss discontinuing them with your doctor.

Drinking large quantities of **fluids** (water, juices, or tea are preferred) can help prevent urinary tract infections. Avoid fluids that irritate the bladder, including alcohol, coffee, black tea, peppers, chocolate milk, carbonated beverages, and citrus juices.

For recurrent infections, drink sixteen ounces per day of unsweetened 100 percent **cranberry juice** to help prevent bacteria from adhering to the bladder's walls. Try to avoid sweetened juice as sugar can decrease resistance to the bacteria. *Important note*: If you have diabetes, remember to include juice when counting your carbohydrates.

The Conventional Approaches

Antibiotics are the usual treatment for *acute* urinary tract infections and there is a large variety of antibiotics that can be effective. Guidelines recommend one of the common antibiotics, such as sulfamethoxazole, or trimethoprim-sulfamethoxazole (Bactrim or Septra) or nitrofurantoin, which usually resolves the infection. If these are not effective, or you are allergic to sulfa, other antibiotics, including amoxicillin, fluoroquinolones (Cipro, Levaquin), and others, are often used. In general, seven days are an adequate duration of treatment.

Flouroquinolone Treatment Often Inappropriate

Recent studies reveal that flouroquinolone antibiotics (those ending with the term "floxacin") have become the most commonly prescribed antibiotics for uncomplicated urinary tract infections. Use of these antibiotics can increase bacterial resistance, and they should be used only if testing shows the bacteria being resistant to nitrofurantoin or sulfa drugs (occurring in 12–22 percent nationwide). They are also much more expensive than these older antibiotics.

Warning: The FDA states that fluoroquinolones may cause possible permanent peripheral neuropathy, which may occur rapidly. Stop taking this drug immediately if you start getting pain, numbness, tingling, or loss of strength in your hands or feet. Flouroquinolones may also increase the risk for rupture of tendons when taken orally. These side effects are seen primarily in people over the age of sixty, those taking corticosteroids, or recipients of organ transplants.

If a bladder infection recurs or does not respond to initial antibiotics, your urine needs to be tested for the type of bacteria and its resistance to various antibiotics. Then your physician will know and prescribe the antibiotic that will kill the specific bacteria causing the infection.

If you still have *recurrent or chronic* urinary infections, long-term antibiotics are often prescribed. There are several antibiotics that are used for this purpose, the major ones being sulfa drug combinations (trimethoprim-sulfamethoxazole) or nitrofurantoin.

Important notes: Taking antibiotics can predispose many women to vaginal yeast infections. There are many OTC products that can resolve yeast infections within one to seven days, and taking probiotics may prevent these as well (see below).

Important Information:
Chronic Urinary Tract Infections in Men:
Longer Treatment Unnecessary

Urinary tract infections in men are not as common as in women. Both men and women with *chronic* infections often get long-term antibiotics. A 2012 study in the *Archives of Internal Medicine* showed that long-term antibiotic use for male urinary tract infections was not associated with a reduction in early or late recurrence and is unnecessary. In fact, using them increases the risk of developing *C. difficile* infections (see section on *Dangerous Infections*).

The Alternative Approaches

There are several **Chinese herbal formulas** that are very effective in reducing symptoms and helping to alleviate urinary tract infections. *Ba Zheng San* is a common formula, and *Bi Xie Sheng Shi Wan* may be indicated for cloudy urine and a feeling of cold lower-abdominal pain relieved by warmth. Burning and yellow urine symptoms require a different formula.

Acupuncture is exceptional for significantly reducing or eliminating *recurrent* bladder infections. It takes four to twelve treatments, on average, to obtain this effect.

There are several **Western herbs** that can help reduce or prevent recurrent cystitis:

- *Uva ursi* (bearberry or upland cranberry), an herb that has antiseptic effects, has shown benefits in preventing recurrent bladder infections. Take it three times a day as a tea (2–4 g; prepare tea with cold water to minimize the tannin content), tincture (1:5, 4–6 ml), or fluid extract (1:1 in 25 percent alcohol, standardized to 20 percent arbutin, 0.5–4 ml). *Caution*: This herb should not be used for more than one week at a time and should not be used more than 5 times per year due to hydroquinone constituent.
- *Dandelion* (no typical dosage determined) also has antiseptic effects. Several products combine dandelion with uva ursi.
- *Juniper* (1–2 tsp of herb placed in 150 mL boiling water, seep for at least ten minutes) can be prepared as an herbal tea taken two to three times daily.

Alkalinizing the urinary tract can sometimes prevent bladder infections. Potassium or sodium citrate solutions are recommended, 125–250 mg orally three to four times per day. You can obtain these solutions at your local pharmacy. *Warning*: However, *do not self-treat* with these solutions if you have high blood pressure or heart failure, as they can make these conditions worse by causing fluid overload.

A study published in the *Archives of Internal Medicine* showed that **probiotics** *Lactobacillus rhamnosus* and *L. reuteri* were as effective as the antibiotic trimethoprim/sulfamethoxazole in *preventing* recurrent infections. A study in the *Journal of Infectious Disease* showed that using vaginal suppositories containing *L. crispatus* decreased recurrent urinary tract infections by half, comparable to taking antibiotics. *L. rhamnosus* and *L. reuteri* are also helpful for the urinary tract. Probiotics also have the advantage of not causing antibiotic resistance. Probiotics can be very helpful to prevent recurrent yeast infections as well, especially when caused by other treatments—especially antibiotics. (See chapter 2, under *Probiotics*, for a more detailed discussion.).

Your Empowered Patient Action Plan for Treating *Occasional* Urinary Tract Infections

- *If bladder infection symptoms are moderate to severe, or have been present for several days, go to step 3.*

Step #1: Increase your fluid intake: After the first signs of bladder infection (within twenty-four hours), drinking lots of water (twelve ounces daily) and/

or ***unsweetened cranberry juice*** (sixteen ounces daily) may alleviate the symptoms.

Step #2: Take the Chinese herbal remedy Ba Zheng San when you start getting symptoms to prevent progression.

Step #3: Take prescription antibiotics if symptoms continue or worsen.

Step #4: Take probiotics if yeast infections occur as a result of antibiotic use.

Your Empowered Patient Action Plan for Preventing or Treating *Recurrent* Urinary Tract Infections

Step #1: Drink cranberry juice regularly to prevent recurrent urinary tract infections.

Step #2: Undergo acupuncture to resolve recurrent urinary tract infections long-term.

Step #3: Take probiotics. Intravaginal suppositories have shown benefit, but oral probiotics may also help. Lactobacilli have been proven to be beneficial.

Step #4: Take the Western herbal remedy uva ursi (bearberry) to reduce the frequency of recurrent urinary tract infections if the above steps have not helped.

Step #5: Make your urine more alkaline to reduce recurrent cystitis, but do so under a doctor's direction, if you still have recurrent infections.

Step #6: Take long-term prescription antibiotics to control recurrent urinary tract infections if the above steps have not been beneficial. Take probiotics any time you take antibiotics.

Expected Outcome

An occasional urinary tract infection is not dangerous and usually can be resolved very quickly. Recurrent urinary tract infections may cause harm to urinary organs and need to be controlled. With alternative methods, recurrent urinary tract infections can be alleviated long-term, which is better than taking antibiotics.

Varicose Veins, Venous Insufficiency, and Venous Ulcers

What You Need to Know

Varicose veins are swollen veins that protrude just beneath the skin (superficial veins). They are generally caused by stress on the walls of the veins, which then thicken and dilate, secondarily damaging the valves that regulate flow and causing reflux (blood backing up into the vein).

Venous insufficiency occurs in deeper veins and has similar causal mechanisms; stress on the walls cause progression of venous hypertension (VH), leading again to thickened walls and damaged valves which then leads to disturbances and reflux of blood flow. Treatments are similar for both conditions.

Severe venous insufficiency can result in *venous ulcers*, which are difficult to treat because of lack of blood supply. This complication can occur in 10–15 percent of men and 20–35 percent of women.

Treatments for Vein Problems

The Preventive Approaches

Diet: As obesity is one of the primary predisposing factors for varicose veins, a balanced diet for weight management is important (see *Weight Loss* section for further treatment guidelines). In addition, because excessive pressure from straining can worsen or cause incompetent veins, a high-fiber diet is beneficial in making bowel movements easier. Foods high in antioxidants, especially berries, garlic, onions, ginger, and cayenne, are very helpful in maintaining the structure of the veins.

Exercise is very important to prevent and treat venous dysfunction. Aerobic exercises such as walking, biking, and jogging are especially beneficial since they help contract the leg muscles, which then squeeze the veins and push the blood up your legs. Resistance exercises can help as well, as long as you don't overstrain.

The Conventional Approaches

A common conventional recommendation for ***venous insufficiency*** is to wear **elastic support stockings,** which can help blood circulation in the legs and prevent pooling of blood in the veins. These stockings should fit snugly, but if they are too tight, they can cause more discomfort and restrict the veins even more. Such stockings can also help the healing of venous ulcers.

For severe ***varicose veins*** that are very painful and swollen, the primary treatment is **surgery**. There are several procedures that may help and are comparable to each other. The most common uses a *high-energy ("hot") laser* that ablates (destroys) the vein. However, veins can grow back, and there is a 16 percent recurrence rate. Reflux occurs more commonly after laser treatment.

The next most common surgery is *vein stripping* (also called surgical ligation), followed by the injection of sclerosing agents into the veins (foam sclerotherapy). The latter procedure can result in continued pain, tenderness, staining of the skin, and inflammation. A newer procedure uses vein stripping but applies a tourniquet to the thigh. It has been found to have no early failures compared to a failure rate of 8–15 percent with standard vein stripping. Overall, recurrence is 23 percent with stripping.

Comparison of surgeries: A 2014 study in the *NEJM* showed that laser ablation appeared to have a better balance of benefits and complications than surgical ligation or foam sclerotherapy.

In February 2015, the FDA approved an **adhesive** that permanently "seals" superficial varicose veins (VenaSeal). It is indicated for patients whose varicose veins cause blood clots, mild to moderate pain, and skin ulcers. It has been shown to be as effective and safe as radio-frequency ablation.

__For venous ulcers__, several studies have shown benefit from taking low-dose *aspirin* (*Lancet* 1994), *pentoxifylline* (*Cochrane* database 2012), and *topical beta-blockers* (*Journal of the American Academy of Dermatology* 2013).

Simvastatin (a cholesterol lowering drug) with compression heals ulcers greater than twofold better than placebo, according to a study in 2014 in the *British Journal of Dermatology*.

Therapeutic ultrasound has been recommended to help heal hard-to-heal venous ulcers, but a 2011 study in *BMJ* showed that it added no benefit to standard care.

The Alternative Approaches

- *Caution: If you have swelling of your extremity, make sure a Doppler test is done to rule out a blood clot before self-treating.*

There are a number of **nutritional supplements** that are very effective in enhancing the structure, function, and tone of veins and can be effective in six to eight weeks. They can be used alone or together. They include the following:

- *Horse chestnut* (extracts or pills containing 50 mg escin, twice daily).
- *Butcher's broom* (100 mg containing 9–11 percent ruscogenin, three times a day). This supplement is often combined with hesperidin and vitamin C.
- *Gotu kola* (30–60 mg of triterpenic acids daily).
- *Aortic GAGs* (100 mg daily).
- *Hydroxyethylrutosides (HER)* (1,000–3,000 mg daily).
- *Bilberry with flavonoids* (80–160 mg, containing 25 percent anthocyanosides, three times daily).
- *Bromelain* (500–750 mg, containing 1,200–1,800 mcu, 2–3 times a day between meals).
- *Grapeseed or pine bark extract* (150–300 mg, containing at least 95 percent procyanidolic oligomers, daily).
- *Pycnogenol* (50 mg three times daily or 45–90 mg once daily).

For venous ulcers, a recent study demonstrated that *pycnogenol* tablets, and powder applied topically, can accelerate healing of venous ulcers due to its effect of increasing blood circulation. Optimum healing time is six weeks. (Pycnogenol is basically the same as pine bark extract.)

Acupuncture can provide long-lasting relief from by increasing blood flow, improving venous function, and decreasing swelling and pain. You should notice initial improvement within six to eight treatments. **A *Chinese herbal formula*** called *Tao Ren Wan* may also be beneficial.

The **low level energy laser** ("cold" laser or *LLEL)* may be even better for healing venous ulcers. This is a "cold" laser, which accelerates the healing process directly by stimulating new cell growth but also increases blood flow. Ulcers can heal in as little as three weeks. This laser has minimal side effects.

Homeopathic remedies have also been used effectively for vein problems. *Pulsatilla* is one that is often prescribed for long-term relief. For short-term symptoms, you can try OTC remedies, including the application of *Hamamelis cream* (6x to 15c) to bruised or bluish areas that are sore and *belladonna* (12x or 12c) four times daily for red, hot, swollen, and tender veins. You should consult a qualified homeopathist for guidance on which remedies will be most beneficial and for proper dosages. You should notice improvement in one to two months.

Your Empowered Patient Action Plan for Treating Varicose Veins, Venous Insufficiency, and Venous Ulcers

Step #1: Take various herbal extracts to reduce swelling, pain, and varicosities. Butcher's broom and horse chestnut are the best and most researched, with aortic GAGs, gotu kola, and HER next best, but others can be helpful if these two do not help. You can take these herbs in various combinations.

Step #2: Wear support stockings that are fit correctly to improve circulation in venous insufficiency if Step #1 has not helped you.

Step #3: Undergo acupuncture to reduce symptoms and improve circulation if you still have vein problems.

Step #4: Take an appropriate homeopathic remedy for short- or long-term relief of symptoms if the above steps have not been of benefit.

Step #5: Use the cold laser to rapidly heal venous ulcers.

Step #6: Take pycnogenol tablets and apply topical powder to heal venous ulcers more rapidly (use along with conventional treatments for open wound healing). They can be used with the laser for faster results.

Step #7: Use VenaSeal for varicose veins with ulcers, blood clots and/or pain.

Step #8: Undergo surgery to remove varicose veins as a last resort.

Step #9: Use aspirin, pentoxifylline or topical beta-blockers for venous ulcers if the above Steps have not been beneficial.

Expected Outcome

Varicose veins are unsightly, and venous insufficiency can be painful and cause swelling or ulcers. With the use of either herbs or surgery, you can improve your venous system significantly and remove unsightly varicosities. Using the laser and pycnogenol can rapidly heal difficult-to-treat venous ulcers. However, surgery is beneficial if it is needed.

Deep-Venous Thrombosis (DVT) and Pulmonary Emboli (PE) (Blood Clots); Superficial Venous Thrombosis (SVT)

What You Need to Know

Deep-venous thrombosis (DVT) is a condition in which a blood clot forms in a vein that is deep inside the body. *Superficial venous thrombosis* (SVT) occurs in the veins just under the skin. They can occur in the arms and legs; intravenous (IV) infusions are the usual cause in the arms and varicose veins predispose to SVT in the legs. SVT rarely causes emboli but may develop into DVT (see sidebar below).

SVT May Increase Incidence of DVT and Blood Clots

Most authorities state that SVT rarely causes any complications or blood clots but a 2015 study showed this not to be accurate; the study showed that 9.4% of patients with SVT had extension to the deep veins. The association was stronger in men than women and there was increased risk of pulmonary embolism. The rates of adverse reactions were highest in the first three months after SVT and declined gradually thereafter. It was also noted that SVT increased the risk of arterial blood clots as well, in turn increasing risk for heart attacks and ischemic strokes. The *bottom line* is that you should not ignore SVT: get it treated!

DVT mainly affects the veins in the lower leg and thigh, but it can affect the upper limbs and even large internal veins as well, depending on its cause. A clot (thrombus) forms in the veins of the area and can interfere with blood flow. The biggest danger is that a portion of the clot may break off and travel through the bloodstream (embolize). The traveling blood clot (embolus) can lodge in the lungs (called pulmonary embolus or PE), severely damaging that organ as well as potentially causing death. The treatments for PE are basically the same as for DVT. DVT is most common in adults over age sixty, but it can occur in any age group.

Pulmonary Embolism: Overdiagnosed and Overtreated?

The introduction of computed tomographic pulmonary angiography (CTPA) has increased the diagnosis of pulmonary embolism (PE) significantly (by 81 percent). However, much like all advanced technology, undergoing such tests may not translate to better outcomes.

A study published in the *Archives of Internal Medicine* in May 2011 showed that despite the increased diagnosis of PE, death from PE has changed little. This means that many of the patients treated for PE may not need treatment at all. In fact, complications associated with treatment rose by 71 percent after introduction of CTPA.

The authors conclude that CTPA has created overdiagnosis and overtreatment. Although some of these patients may benefit from therapy, it is not currently known who will and who won't. It's a quandary that will need much more research to understand.

Risks for DVT include prolonged sitting (such as on long plane or car trips) or bed rest. It also may be caused by recent surgery (especially hip, knee, or female reproductive organ surgery), fractures, childbirth within the last six months, and the use of medications such as estrogen and birth-control pills. Even minor injuries can cause DVT. Excess body weight is a risk factor for recurrent DVT. Twelve percent of patients with COPD have DVT (see section on COPD).

Cancer and DVT/SVT

People who are apparently healthy but develop DVT for no specific reason (such as injury or poor circulation) may have an occult (hidden) cancer. Limited screening tests are indicated if this occurs, such as basic blood testing, chest x-ray and tests such as mammogram, pap test and prostate screening depending on age and gender. Some doctors order CT scans of the body, but a 2015 study showed that they did not improve detection of cancer. About 25 percent of cancers will be discovered by either of these actions. If testing is normal, it is recommended to have a one year follow-up but if any other symptoms occur within that time, you should obtain further evaluation.

On the other side of the coin, you should also be aware that having cancer can predispose you to developing DVT, and you should consider prophylaxis if you are at high risk (see below and in section on *Cancer*).

There is a form of SVT that is a warning sign for cancer. Called *Trousseau's Syndrome* (migratory thrombophlebitis), episodes of SVT occur recurrently or appear in different locations over time, especially in unusual areas such as the chest wall and arms. The clot is just under the skin and usually tender. The syndrome has been associated with gastric and lung cancers but particularly pancreatic cancer and can appear months or even years before the cancer is detected.

Some people may have chronic pain and swelling in the leg after the DVT is treated successfully, known as *post phlebitic syndrome* (treatment is the same as with venous in-sufficiency, so refer to that Section).

DVT Increases Risk for Other Conditions

It is well recognized that pulmonary emboli are the primary complication of DVT, but recent studies have shown that venous blood clots may also pose a strong risk of heart attack or stroke within one year.

Treatments for DVT and SVT

The Preventive Approaches
Obesity is a primary cause of DVT as well as SVT, and so **weight loss** is very important. In addition, **exercise** can increase the venous circulation and is highly recommended. Smoking also predisposes to both SVT and DVT and should be discontinued.

Especially after major surgery, **early walking** is essential to prevent DVT, and for low-risk surgical patients, ambulation is better than drug prophylaxis. ***Important note***: You are at higher risk to develop DVT after hip (and perhaps knee) surgery and should be given medical (drug) prophylaxis after the surgery. If you already have vein problems, compression stockings may help prevent DVT as well.

Important note: Patients with *strokes* are often bedridden for long periods and may not be able to walk. A recent study showed that compression stockings *are not* beneficial in stroke patients for preventing DVT, and you should use blood thinners (see below) or pneumatic compression devices instead.

If you take a long airplane flight or car trip, you should get up, move, and stretch frequently. Also, keep hydrated as dehydration may predispose to leg clots. Eating dark chocolate (1/2 ounce) has been shown to reduce the incidence of DVT on long trips as it has actions as a weak blood thinner.

Since SVT is most often caused by varicose veins, see the previous section to treat that condition. If a catheter or IV is placed in your arm and it becomes red, swollen or painful, tell your doctor immediately.

The Conventional Approaches

If you have a condition that predisposes you to DVT, such as certain types of cancer, COPD, or obesity; have undergone certain surgeries; or have had an embolism previously, you may need to take medication long-term to prevent DVT (called *prophylaxis*). This is especially true if you have these conditions in addition to prolonged bed rest or sitting or have major trauma. If you have three risk factors from the list in Table 1, prophylaxis should be considered by your doctor.

Table 1
<u>Risk Factors for Blood Clots</u>

Age over 60	Leg swelling, ulcers, varicose veins
Estrogen therapy (HRT)	BMI greater than 29 (see *Weight Loss* section)
Smoker	Family history of blood clots
Surgery within 30 days	Documented history of blood clots
Nephrotic syndrome	Inflammatory bowel disease
Acute respiratory failure	Congestive heart failure or heart attack
Severe COPD (emphysema)	Hip, pelvis, or leg fracture
Malignancy and/or chemotherapy	Major trauma or spinal cord injury
Sepsis (blood borne infection)	Stroke with paralysis
Anticipated bed confinement or immobilization greater than 24 hours	

Medications are the most common prophylaxis. An oral medication called *warfarin* (Coumadin) is the standard and has been used for decades. However, warfarin requires frequent dose adjustments and can be affected by numerous foods (mainly veggies) and drugs (especially antibiotics) and thus must be monitored frequently (see sidebar below).

Factors That Alter the Effects of Warfarin

When thinning the blood with warfarin, you need to be monitored week-ly because results can vary from several factors. Certain antibiotics (le-vofloxacin [Levaquin], trimethoprim-sulfamethaxazole [Bactrim/Septra], and others), NSAIDs (including naproxen [Naprosyn], meloxicam [Mobic], piroxicam [Feldene], oxaprozin [Daypro], nabumatone [Relafen], ketopro-fen [Orudis], diclofenac [Cataflam], celecoxib [Celebrex] or diclofenac/misoprostol [Arthrotec]), Tylenol (acetaminophen), steroids, pain relievers, stomach remedies (including Tagamet, Alka Seltzer, Pepto Bismol), mul-tivitamins, green tea, gingko, quercetin, and other herbs; and alcohol can often increase blood thinning (some can also decrease it, such as green leafy vegetables).

Most patients need to undergo a blood test to determine the required level of blood thinning (the test is called an INR and the therapeutic level needs to be between 2.0 and 3.0). Recently, new instrumentation is avail-able for use at home, using fingerstick determinations (as is done with diabetics).

Warning: Some doctors may prescribe antiplatelet agents (aspirin and clopidogrel [Plavix]) along with warfarin. This significantly raises the risk for serious and some-times fatal bleeding and most of the time should not be used together, except in spe-cific cases.

Another option to warfarin is *Low Molecular Weight Heparin (LMWH)*, which is injected under the skin. Although you can take LMWH every day, you don't need repetitive blood tests to make sure your blood is thinned enough; however, it may be expensive and may not be covered by insurance.

Statins May Help Prevent DVT in Cancer Patients

Multiple studies have documented that people taking statins (used for lowering cholesterol) have a decreased incidence of DVT. In cancer patients, Coumadin is often not used prophylactically because of risk of bleeding, but because statins do not cause bleeding and have minimal side effects, they may still provide some protection for cancer patients. However, they have not yet been approved for this indication.

Warning: Because of the blood-thinning effects of statins, if you are on warfarin and take a statin, you can also have a higher risk of gastrointestinal bleeding. Pravastatin has not been associated with increased risk and is the preferred statin in these situations.

If you develop DVT or pulmonary emboli

Heparin, given intravenously, is an older blood thinner that is still effectively used if you develop a blood clot, but it has a higher risk of bleeding than newer blood thinners. At present *LMWH* is often considered better, but again, it is expensive. An alternative is to take LMWH for three to four days to immediately thin your blood while taking warfarin at the same time, which takes about four days to thin your blood. You can then stop the LMWH and continue the warfarin long-term. Warfarin or LMWH should be taken for at least six to twelve months, depending on the cause of the DVT/PE and whether that cause has been resolved.

Warfarin Discontinuation Is Too High

Patients who have blood clots should be started on warfarin (or LMWH) immediately and continue it usually for at least twelve months. This does not occur in the real world, however. A February 2014 study presented at the AHA scientific sessions revealed that less than half of patients with clots started therapy within ten days, and 75 percent discontinued it before one year. This was more common in patients with fracture, pregnancy, or hormone therapy, as well as atrial fibrillation (heart arrhythmia).

There is no reason to delay starting therapy; a delay is most likely a doctor issue. Most patients discontinue warfarin when their original condition is past and because it is difficult to maintain at the indicated blood level. They may discontinue LMWH due to the cost and the inconvenience and side effects of the injections (most commonly bruising). However, this may be dangerous as blood clots can be lethal (it is the most common preventable cause of death in hospitalized patients.) Fortunately, there are alternatives (see below), so talk with your doctor if you are on warfarin and want to quit taking it.

There are three relatively **new blood-thinning drugs** that have significantly changed the treatment for DVT/PE: *dabigatran* (Pradaxa), *rivaroxaban* (Xarelto), and *apixaban* (Eliquis). Pradaxa has a different mechanism of action than the others, but they all have essentially equal or better outcomes than warfarin or LMWH but with less risk of bleeding. An advantage is that they are fixed doses, so they do not require blood monitoring or dose adjustments. One downside is that they are expensive, but they are often covered by insurance or Medicare. Another downside was that there was no known antidote for their blood-thinning effects, but a new drug called *idarucizumab* (Praxbind) has been approved as an antidote for dabigatran. However, the wholesale price is $3500. *Caution*: The FDA will be performing a new assessment of dabigatran, due to persistent concerns on its safety, but not on the other two medications.

If you have recurrent DVT and emboli to your lungs that can't be controlled by medications, or if the medications cause too many bleeding complications, a **vena cava filter** can be placed in a large vein going to the heart (the vena cava) to catch these clots. *Cautions*: A recent study in the *Archives of Internal Medicine* found that some of these filters are prone to break, causing emboli themselves, and too many of these devices are being left in patients after the threat of embolism has passed (many of the filters are retrievable). In addition, a 2015 French study showed that there may be no benefit in adding a filter in patients with severe pulmonary emboli who are already on blood thinners.

Do You Need to Be Hospitalized If You Have a Blood Clot?

Most doctors hospitalize patients who have DVT or PE. However, this is now changing. According to a study in *Lancet* in July 2011, stable, low-risk patients (which comprise the majority of patients) do not need to be hospitalized.

For SVT

Warm compresses and *NSAIDs* (such as naproxen [Naprosyn], meloxicam [Mobic], piroxicam [Feldene], oxaprozin [Daypro], nabumatone [Relafen], ketoprofen [Orudis], diclofenac [Cataflam], diclofenac/misoprostol [Arthrotec] or celecoxib [Celebrex]) are usually effective for superficial thrombosis, with or without elastic support. *Caution*: In July, 2015, the FDA started requiring NSAIDs to carry a warning of increased risk of heart attacks, stroke and heart failure. This is especially evident when taken long term, at higher doses, or by people with pre-existing heart disease. The risks can increase as early as the first weeks of NSAID use. However, ibuprofen and naproxen do not appear to increase the risk, so are the safest and preferred NSAIDs.

If SVT persists, taking out the clot (*thrombectomy*) under local anesthetic may be necessary. *Anticoagulants* can be used but are rarely necessary.

The Alternative Approaches

Nutritional supplements: Some studies have shown that taking *pycnogenol* or *grape-seed extract* can help prevent DVT if you are at greater risk. These herbs contain the same ingredients, but grape-seed extract is much less expensive.

Caution: You should avoid the supplement Quercetin if you are taking warfarin (Coumadin) as it decreases its blood thinning effect.

Your Empowered Patient Action Plan for Preventing and Treating DVT

*Step #1: **Keep hydrated and exercise*** or ambulate to *prevent* DVT if you are at higher risk to develop this condition.

*Step #2: **Take LMWH*** to *prevent* DVT if you are at high risk or after certain surgeries.

*Step #3: **Take pycnogenol or grape-seed extract*** to help prevent DVT if you are at high risk.

*Step #4: **Eat 1.2 ounce of dark chocolate*** if you take a long trip by car or plane to help prevent clots.

*Step #5: **Take anticoagulants*** (LMWH, or one of the oral medications) to *treat* DVT/PE. These are the best and most proven treatments. Discuss which medication will be best for your situation with your doctor and make sure it is covered by your insurance.

*Step #6: **Wear compression stockings*** if you have recurrent problems with DVT.

*Step #7: **Undergo surgical placement of a vena cava filter*** if you have recurrent pulmonary emboli that are not prevented by the above steps and cannot take blood thinners.

Expected Outcome

Many DVTs resolve without a problem when treated properly, but they can recur, especially with some chronic underlying conditions. A pulmonary embolus can be life-threatening; recognition and rapid treatment of DVT or PE helps prevent this. Since SVT can lead ro DVT, it should be treated promptly and should resolve within one to two weeks.

Vertigo and Meniere's Disease

What You Need to Know

Vertigo is a type of dizziness in which you or your surroundings seem to spin. Many people think of dizziness as imbalance or lightheadedness (see sidebar below) but vertigo is due to problems in the inner ear and should be distinguished from these other symptoms.

Lightheadedness, Imbalance Is Not Vertigo

Many older people have symptoms of lightheadedness, but this is different than the "spinning" sensation of vertigo. Lightheadedness in seniors is most often caused by orthostatic hypotension, in which blood pools in the legs; and when you stand quickly after sitting or lying for a period of time, the blood doesn't return fast enough to the brain. The symptom usually goes away from a few seconds to a minute when the blood reaches the brain. This is very common, and if it happens, you should always stand up slowly. There are other causes of lightheadedness, such as anemia, dehydration, and diabetes; and Parkinson's can lead to orthostatic hypotension.

Other people have symptoms of imbalance, either falling to the side falling forward or backward. If caused by an abnormality in the brain (stroke, brain tumor, and so on), it is referred to as *ataxia*. However, other conditions, such as neuropathy of the feet, can cause you to stumble and/or lose your balance due to loss of feeling in your feet.

You should always be checked by a doctor to rule out underlying causes of these symptoms.

The most common cause of vertigo is BPPV (benign paroxysmal positional vertigo), in which certain positions such as lying down or turning your head quickly will elicit a spinning sensation. It is caused by debris collecting in the semicircular canals of the middle ear.

Testing Overused in Vertigo

Often, numerous tests are performed to find out the cause of vertigo, but most are entirely unnecessary. Most vertigo can be diagnosed by history and physical examination. One test, magnetic resonance angiography (MRA), is done for isolated vertigo of unknown origin, but the majority of such tests will not find abnormalities and are not needed.

—⚭—

Meniere's disease is a specific disorder of the inner ear in which there is too much endolymph, the fluid that fills the inner ear. Besides dizziness, Meniere's disease can cause hearing loss, tinnitus (ringing in the ears), feeling of fullness in the ears, poor job performance, accidents, and psychological disorders. Whereas BPPV is a self-limited disease (it can last a few days to a few months), Meniere's may last for years.

Treatments for Vertigo and Meniere's Disease

The Preventive Approaches

Stress and anxiety can precipitate attacks of Meniere's disease, and it can also be a result of the disease. *Relaxation* methods can help prevent attacks and recurrences by decreasing your stress and anxiety level.

Also for Meniere's, *restricting salt* intake may lessen the frequency and number of attacks in some people and decrease the feeling of fullness in the ears.

The Conventional Approaches

There are several **physical maneuvers** that may be helpful in relieving BPPV effectively and quickly. They are done with the assistance of health professionals (usually chiropractors or physical therapists) and work by moving debris from the semicircular canals into other areas of the ear. The *Semont* and *modified Epley* maneuvers (also referred to as otolith or cannalith repositioning) are the most common; and a single ten- to fifteen-minute session usually is all that is needed, although for some people, several sessions may be necessary. However, these maneuvers are for debris in the posterior (back part) of the canals, not the front (anterior) or horizontal areas, so some people may not obtain relief.

<u>The Semont Maneuver:</u>

- You are seated, and the health professional turns your head forty-five degrees horizontally toward the unaffected ear.

- The health professional tilts you 105 degrees so that you are lying on the side of the affected ear with your head hanging and your nose pointed upward. You remain in this position for three minutes. The debris should move to the apex of the canal.
- The health professional then moves you quickly through the seated position, holding your head in place, until you are lying on the side of the affected ear with your nose pointed to the ground. You remain in this position for three minutes. The debris should move toward the exit of the canal.
- The health professional then slowly moves you back to the seated position. The debris should fall into the utricle of the canal, where it will not cause vertigo.

The Modified Epley Maneuver:

- You are seated, and the health professional turns your head forty-five degrees horizontally toward the affected ear. You should hold the health professional's arms for support.
- The health professional tilts you backward to a horizontal position with your head kept in place at a forty-five-degree turn, hanging. An attack of vertigo is likely as the debris moves toward the apex of the canal. You are held in this position until the vertigo stops, usually within a minute.
- The health professional turns your head ninety degrees toward the unaffected ear. The health professional then rolls you onto the side of the unaffected ear so that you are now looking at the floor. The debris should move in the canal again, possibly provoking another attack of vertigo. You should remain in this position until the vertigo stops, usually within a minute.
- The health professional helps you back to a seated position. Then the health professional tilts your head down thirty degrees, which allows the debris to fall into the utricle of the canal, where it will not cause vertigo.

Sometimes these maneuvers are performed while you wear a *vibrating headband*. The vibration can help move the debris into an area of the inner ear where it will not affect balance.

Other than these maneuvers, the most common conventional treatment involves **medications**. *Meclizine* (Antivert) is the first drug of choice for vertigo, and some doctors use *Valium*. *Diuretics* such as HCTZ can decrease swelling in the inner ear, which may be helpful in Meniere's disease. You should feel relief within a few hours to a few days.

If these medications don't work, *promethazine* and *dimenhydrinate* can sometimes help reduce symptoms of vertigo. Other drugs that have been used include betahistine and trimetazidine, but benefits are questionable. All these drugs may give temporary relief but do not cure the condition.

To try to eliminate the dizziness for Meniere's, an **antibiotic** called gentamicin can be injected into the eardrum. Hearing loss can occur but is usually temporary.

There are also several **surgeries** performed for vertigo, and they may have good results. Dizziness is completely resolved in 47 percent of patients undergoing endolymphatic mastoid shunt, 71 percent undergoing neurectomy (cutting the nerve), and 95 percent of those who undergo labyrinthectomy (removal of part of the inner ear). The latter procedure causes total hearing loss, however.

The Alternative Approaches

Acupuncture is very effective in reducing the symptoms and resolving both BPPV and Meniere's long-term, since it addresses the underlying cause(s). You should notice improvement within six acupuncture treatments, but often only two or three treatments are necessary. BPPV responds more quickly than Meniere's to acupuncture.

Chinese herbal formulas are also effective at controlling symptoms of dizziness as well as the fullness in the ear and are most effective when you take them along with receiving acupuncture. Some formulas include *Wen Dan Tang, Chai Hu Long Mu Li Wan*, and *Wu Ling San*.

Several **homeopathic** remedies (12c or 30c, one to three times per day) can reduce or control persistent symptoms. These include:

- *Bryonia* for headache, dizziness, buzzing, humming, or a roaring in the ears.
- *Conium* for sensitivity to light and increased symptoms when lying down or turning over.
- *Cocculus* for dizziness and nausea.

You should notice improvement in one to two months.

Your Empowered Patient Action Plan for Treating Vertigo and Meniere's Disease

Step #1: Undergo physical maneuvers for relief of BPPV. This is the fastest and easiest method for possibly resolving BPPV.

Step #2: Undergo acupuncture for long-term relief. This method is the best for resolving BPPV if the above steps don't help, and it can potentially resolve Meniere's even if it has been present for years.

Step #3: Take meclizine and/or diuretics for initial short-term relief: However, if you don't obtain relief quickly, they won't work.

Step #4: Take the Chinese herbal remedies Wen Dan Tang or Wu Ling San, which are especially helpful for relieving fullness in the ear and help you hear better if you have Meniere's. You can take these with step #3.

Jeff had Meniere's disease for fifteen years, with a feeling of "fullness" in his ears as well as dizziness and ringing in his ears. He had taken meclizine and diuretics, but these drugs did not help. I started him on Wen Dan Tang, which quickly resolved the ear "fullness" within three days. I then provided acupuncture, and after five sessions, the remainder of his symptoms resolved.

Step #5: Take an appropriate homeopathic remedy: If the above steps don't work, it's worth a try. If they don't work within a week or two, discontinue them.

Step #6: Take the prescription medications promethazine or dimenhydrinate for temporary relief if the above steps have not relieved your symptoms.

Step #7: Undergo surgery as a last resort.

Expected Outcome

Vertigo is potentially curable very quickly in most cases by using alternative methods or physical maneuvers. Meniere's disease is more difficult to resolve, but most cases can be resolved or significantly improved by using alternative methods.

Weight Loss

What You Need to Know

Obesity is a significant problem in our country, and the United States is rated as the "fattest" among thirty-three advanced countries. Two-thirds of Americans are overweight, and one-third are obese (roughly thirty pounds overweight).

Obesity is defined as a body-fat percentage greater than 30 percent for women and 25 percent for men (measured by various instruments), or weighing 20 percent more than your ideal body weight (based on insurance charts). At present, most doctors and researchers use the BMI, a calculation using your height and weight (see Table 1 for calculation). A BMI of 25 to 29 is considered overweight, and a BMI greater than 30 indicates obesity. Studies show that the death rate is lowest in people with baseline BMIs of 22.5 to 25.

Table 1
BMI Calculation

Step #1: Multiply your weight (in pounds) by 703

Step #2: Multiply your height (in inches) by your height (in inches) (inches squared)

Step #3: Divide your answer in step 1 by your answer in step #2

More recently, researchers have described two body types using waist-to-hip ratio (WHR), which appears to be a better predictor of future chronic medical problems than BMI. If your *shape* is like an apple (more abdominal or 'belly' fat…called central obesity), you have an increased risk of heart disease, stroke, diabetes, hypertension, weakened bones and muscles, and some cancers. If your shape is like a pear (fattest in buttocks, hips, and thighs), you have fewer risks; it may actually be protective.

Central Obesity and Normal Weight: Still a Risk

You might think that if you have a normal weight, you do not have an elevated risk for various diseases. A 2015 study showed this to not be accurate; researchers found that people who have normal BMI but have central obesity (tummy fat) are at higher risk for cardiovascular death.

In the study, WHR but not BMI was associated with a higher overall mortality risk. Among men, the risk was 87% higher and in women, the risk was 48% higher. That is why shape is important to consider as well as height and weight.

Are You an Apple or a Pear?
Calculating Waist-to-Hip Ratio (WHR)

Step #1: Measure waist at navel

Step #2: Measure hips at the greatest circumference around the buttocks

Step #3: Divide waist measurement by hip measurement.

A result greater than 0.9 for men and 0.8 for women: above average risk

A result above 1.0 for men and 0.9 for women: high risk

Although WHR is a better predictor of future medical conditions associated with being overweight than BMI, both measurements have downsides. The BMI does not consider body composition and shape. So no matter if your body fat is 10 percent or 40 percent, the BMI would be the same if the height and weight was the same. The WHR describes shape, but not body composition. To combine all these elements, another way to measure fat is called ABSI (A Body Shape Index), which uses height, weight, and waist circumference. It has proven to more accurately predict health consequences in obese patients; people with an ABSI in the top 20% had death rates 61% higher than those with an ABSI in the bottom 20%. In general, you should have a body fat percentage below 25 percent. At this time, however, not many doctors or researchers are using the ASBI.

Poor Diet and Lack of Exercise
May Not Be the Only Causes of Weight Gain

There's no question that poor diet and lack of exercise are the main contributors to weight gain, but increased exercise and a better diet alone may not cure weight problems. Several other factors may play a part in how we gain weight and how we can lose it. Some of these factors include:

- *Inadequate sleep*: Sleep deprivation influences two hormones that affect appetite, leptin and ghrelin, causing increased appetite and increased BMI.
- *Stress*: Psychological factors such as anxiety, stress, and depression are noted in many people to cause increased weight gain and may also do so by influencing the appetite hormones.
- *Hot and cold*: An environment that is either too hot or too cold makes the body expend calories to balance temperature. High temperatures seem to kill appetite, so turn up the air conditioner.
- *Medications*: A variety of medications can cause weight gain, including antidepressants, hormone medications (including birth-control pills), diabetic drugs, and hypertensive drugs.
- *Environmental toxins*: various toxins in water, soil, air (pollution), and food can accumulate in the body and interfere with hormones that can lead to fat accumulation.
- *Genetics*: A field called epigenetics has shown that under stress, chemicals called methyl groups can attach to our DNA and change the way our genes express. Not only can this contribute to poor eating habits and weight gain, it can also be passed down through many generations (see chapter 2 for more discussion on epigenetics).

Certain Bodily Processes and Other Factors Implicated in Weight Gain

New studies have discovered some interesting findings about weight gain and loss. The first showed that eating fructose, a sugar that "saturates" the American diet, can actually trigger changes in the brain that may *lead to* over-eating. Unlike simple glucose, the brain doesn't register the feeling of being full after fructose consumption. Fructose is often added to processed foods and beverages, especially in the form of high-fructose corn syrup.

Second, three 2013 studies published in *Nature* and *Science* revealed that the *bacteria* found in our guts influence obesity. These studies show that the composition of bacteria in our gut can affect whether we are obese as well as whether we develop obesity-related metabolism traits. They also indicate that *what we eat* can affect our gut bacteria and thus cause a vicious cycle. The studies don't prove that altering the composition of our guts (with probiotics, for example) will improve health but many researchers are already delving into the possibilities.

Finally, an intriguing study from Spain demonstrated that the *timing of your eating* may affect weight gain or loss. The study, published in the *International Journal of Obesity*, showed that eating earlier in the day can lead to more weight loss, even with the exact same calorie intake and diet composition. This is an area called *chronobiology*, which is showing that not only do we have a "clock" that regulates our normal activities (circadian rhythm) but there are also "clock genes" in the gut and the liver that can affect how much fat is absorbed and metabolized and how carbohydrates are metabolized. This may help to explain why shift workers tend to gain weight. For this reason, eating earlier in the day and avoiding late-night meals may help you lose weight.

So, in general, there are many factors involved in weight control, including physiological, environmental, psychological, and societal (influence of your particular culture).

———

Obesity and being overweight places you at much greater risk for developing a variety of diseases, including cancer (especially uterus, gall bladder, kidney, cervix, thyroid, colon, ovary, breast, liver, and leukemia), heart disease, hypertension, gallstones, stroke, colonic adenomas (precursor to colon cancer), joint arthritis, sleep apnea, blood clots, diabetes, and also premature death.

A recent study revealed that people who are overweight during midlife have a 20–40 percent increase in the risk of death, even if they are healthy and have never smoked. In these people, for every unit of BMI greater than 25, odds for disease-free survival at age seventy is decreased by 12 percent.

Although obesity and being overweight may result in various diseases and increased mortality, it is not the extra weight alone that is harmful to your body. It is what you eat or don't eat and what activity you do or don't do that may help determine if your body's tissues are harmed. Those are the factors that cause you to gain weight in the first place, but they also cause damage to your body at the same time. *Just losing weight, without changing those lifestyle factors, may not protect your body from damage.* In fact, studies show that even if you don't achieve an "ideal" weight, but you have a healthy lifestyle, you do not have as high a risk for chronic diseases and mortality.

Obesity, Metabolic Syndrome, and Heart Disease

Most obese persons may also develop high blood pressure, high cholesterol, and high blood glucose and/or triglycerides, what is referred to as *metabolic syndrome*. Metabolic syndrome has definitely been linked to increased heart disease, which is one reason why obesity increases mortality rates.

However, don't think that being obese yet having a *normal* metabolic profile is protective. An analysis of observational studies with at least ten years of follow-up showed that such patients had a 24 percent increased risk for heart disease and death.

Thus, an important issue to be considered in obese people is not just weight itself but also the *changes in body composition* from obesity. The good news is that treating these accompanying medical conditions can help decrease your risk of dying.

The Overweight Paradox: Less Risk for Heart Disease and Death?

In a well-publicized study from *JAMA* in 2013, researchers pooled data from three million people and surprisingly found that overweight people (BMIs between 25 and 35) had a 6 percent lower overall death rate than normal weight people. This was most notable in people over sixty-five. Another December 2013 study in the *Annals of Internal Medicine* showed that metabolically healthy *overweight* people did not have adverse heart disease outcomes, but obese people did. That certainly seems to contradict the studies in the previous sidebar. What gives?

The good news is that fewer Americans are dying of obesity-related illnesses because doctors are more aggressive at treating these factors, and medical care is better at treating heart attacks and strokes and keeping people alive.

The bad news is that numerous disorders can still be caused by even mild obesity, including heart attacks, strokes, kidney disease, diabetes, and arthritis of the knees and hips, which impair your quality of life, increase disability, and increase health care costs. *So, you may live longer but be more miserable.* It also *does not mean* that overweight people are at lower risk for developing high blood pressure and diabetes:

To complicate matters, it may also be that using BMI to determine death rates is not as accurate as other measurements, which may explain some of these discrepancies. Besides the downsides discussed above, BMI does not account for demographic, racial, and other differences in how fat is stored or for the association with cardiorespiratory fitness.

Finally, another study published in the *NEJM* in early 2014 showed that mortality is not lower among diabetics who are overweight. The authors opined that previous studies of this paradox were limited by short follow-ups and few deaths.

So, the *bottom line* still is that there is no such thing as "benign" obesity. In the long run, being overweight is not beneficial for your health.

Overall, as you try to lose weight, remember these important acknowledgments:

- *Obesity is a disease*
- *Environment influences obesity*
- *Weight loss is a process*
- *Help is available*

Treatments for Weight Loss

Weight-Loss Myths

Most of the most firmly held beliefs about weight loss are actually either untrue or unproven. In a January 2013 article in *JAMA*, it was noted that these myths were untrue:

- Small changes in food intake and/or exercise will produce long term weight changes. This doesn't take into account that as weight is lost, it takes increasingly more exercise and reduced intake to continue the loss.
- Realistic weight goals will keep people motivated. Studies actually show that people with very ambitious goals lose more weight.
- A bout of sexual activity burns 100–300 kcal per person. In actuality, based on the average time of sex and orgasm, only about 14 kcal are expended.

The authors also recorded some presumptions that have neither been proven nor disproven, including:

- Eating breakfast prevents obesity. Actually, two studies showed no effect versus skipping breakfast.
- Adding fruits and veggies to the diet results in weight loss. This still adds calories that can add weight *if no other changes are made.* However, fruits and vegetables are healthier than many other foods.
- Yo-yo dieting increases mortality. The studies showing this have had too much bias.

Rapid Weight Loss Better than Gradual Weight Loss?

It has long been thought that gradual weight loss works significantly better than rapid weight loss, but a recent study showed that people who lose weight quickly are more likely to lose weight than those in gradual weight-loss programs. In this study, 85 percent of the rapid-weight-loss patients lost 15 percent of their baseline weight versus 48 percent on the gradual-loss diet.

Two reasons can explain this. First, patients see better results quicker and therefore have more motivation to continue. Many patients on gradual weight loss become disheartened and stop their diets.

Second, losing weight causes changes in several hormones. One major change is called ketogenesis—substances called ketones are produced with rapid weight loss, and this leads to the release of cholecystokinin (CCK), which *reduces hunger.* A rapid-weight-loss diet causes ketogenesis by day three or four. Gradual weight-loss patients do not undergo ketogenesis until about the fifth week, so their weight loss starts to level off too early, and they get hungrier.

However, there are several *caveats*. First, this study used a diet that was low carb and low fat and was nine hundred calories a day, which is a difficult diet to follow. Second, patients with rapid weight loss are more likely to gain more weight back—and do so more quickly. Several studies show that if you lose 20 percent of your weight on a very-low-calorie diet over six months compared with 10 percent of your weight on a gradual-loss plan, over the long term, you end up at the same place. The authors of the first study did state that to keep the weight off after rapid weight loss may require taking drugs that help maintain weight.

The Preventive Approaches

Obviously, the best preventive approach (and treatment) involves **lifestyle changes—** basically diet and exercise.

All **diets** that reduce calories, regardless of their composition, may result in some weight loss. What matters more is that you maintain the weight loss and establish eating habits that are healthy for you in the long run. There are two important considerations that you must incorporate into your life if you want to lose weight, maintain that loss, and be healthy for the rest of your life.

- *Make a long-term commitment to change your lifestyle.* Short-term dieting (yo-yo dieting) not only doesn't work for long, but you may regain lost weight quickly and usually put on even more. The only proven way to lose weight and keep it off is to make permanent lifestyle changes.
- *Lose any weight you can.* The worse problem with being overweight is that you usually continue to gain weight. It becomes a vicious cycle. So reverse that cycle—even losing ten pounds can make a difference in the outcomes of being overweight.

An Important Step: Admit You're Overweight

Being overweight has negative health implications, but if you don't perceive yourself as overweight, you may not be motivated to change it. A 2008 study in the *British Medical Journal* showed that 25 percent of people who are overweight or obese do not describe themselves as such.

It is also important to realize that it's not just *what* you eat but also *how* you eat that can help you lose weight. Here are some additional recommendations:

- Plan your meals every morning. This includes times when you are traveling or having a luncheon at work.
- Eat more frequent meals. People who have been most successful losing weight and keeping it off average five mini-meals per day. This is because the more meals you eat, the less total fat is absorbed into your body.
- When you eat a meal, do not engage in another activity. Studies show that watching TV or reading while eating definitely increases weight gain because your digestion slows down, allowing more fat to be absorbed into your body.
- Be aware that eating with friends make you eat more—35 percent more.
- Eat *slowly*. The faster you eat, the more calories you consume. It takes twenty minutes of eating to tell your brain that you are satiated (have had enough food), so eating too fast thwarts you from feeling full.
- Stop eating *before* you are full. Studies show that eating until you're full is associated with weight gain. Remember again that it takes time for the stomach to cue the brain that you are "full."
- Avoid drinks that have high fructose corn syrup. Experts state that such drinks are a major cause of increased obesity rates in this country.

Liquid Calories Worse than Solid

If you get calories from liquids, you will tend to consume more than if you get the same calories from food. This is because liquid calories do not make you feel as full as solid foods. It also doesn't matter if the liquids are high in fat, sugar, or protein. Beverages supply 20 percent of the calories in US diets.

- Use smaller dishes so portions look larger.
- Write down everything you eat (food diary). This feedback helps you determine areas that you might be able to cut to aid in achieving your goals quickly.
- MyFitnessPal.com is a good online tool to help monitor calories/meals.

The Health Halo Effect from Fast Food

Just because you eat at a "healthy" restaurant does not mean you'll eat fewer calories. People who go to healthier restaurants often end up eating more calories than at more traditional fast food places. This is called the health halo effect—underestimating the amount of calories in healthy foods and then indulging elsewhere by ordering calorie-rich side dishes, larger drinks, and dessert.

The *balance* of foods that you eat, both in quality and quantity, may also affect whether or not you will lose weight. Some general suggestions:

- Substitute as many fruits and vegetables as possible for meat and starches. Adding these foods may still increase weight without other changes, but substituting them for high-calorie foods will help you lose weight as well as decrease risk of chronic diseases.
- Of total calories, less than 30 percent should come from fat, 20 percent from protein, and 50 percent from carbohydrates for the best balance.
- When eating fat, aim for polyunsaturated or monounsaturated, which do not elevate your cholesterol levels. Saturated fats are not all bad, but they should not exceed 10 percent of your total calories to prevent increasing your blood-cholesterol level. Some saturated fat is OK, especially in place of other harmful products such as fructose and corn syrup. Regular fruit does not contain much fructose, but sodas, fruit drinks, and some canned fruits may.
- When using oils, use olive oil, preferably, with canola oil second. These oils are monounsaturated, so they don't elevate cholesterol levels like other oils do.

Eating *Low*-Fat May Not Be the Best

Advice can be quite confusing when it comes to what types of fat to eat. Some facts to contemplate include the following:

Do you think that eating low-fat products will help you lose weight? Not always! In fact, it may have the opposite effect. Many low-fat products contain as many calories as their regular-fat counterparts. People tend to eat larger amounts of low-fat products, thinking they won't do any harm, yet again adding to their weight problems. In addition, beneficial fats (primarily fatty acids, such as omega-3) are eliminated in low-fat products. Low-fat products also usually contain increased sodium or sugar. Be sure to read the labels on low-fat products to check the calories, added ingredients, and serving size.

Data recovered from an old study (Sydney Diet Heart Study) revealed that substituting dietary omega-6 linoleic acid for saturated fats (advised by the AHA) *increases* risk of heart disease.

Obesity rates paradoxically have increased in the face of a concurrent reduction in saturated-fat consumption. Because taking fat out of food causes it to taste worse, the food industry replaced saturated fat with added sugar, especially fructose, which is a worse culprit. (Excerpted from an editorial in the *BMJ*.)

Gender May Make a Difference When Eating Fats

Research shows that there are some differences in how different genders process fats and carbohydrates. Some of the findings:

- A diet low in saturated fat and cholesterol may be more effective in men (but still benefits both sexes).
- A low-fat diet may reduce HDL ("good") cholesterol more in women.
- Women are better at converting omega-3 fats found in plant foods into the heart-healthy omega-3s found in fish.

- The US government in 2015 advised that there should not be any limitations placed on dietary cholesterol, as it actually plays an insignificant role in determining blood levels of cholesterol.
- Avoid trans fats, which are contained in processed (packaged) and fried foods. Trans fats are much worse for your health than saturated fats. In fact, the Institute of Medicine reported that *no* level of trans-fatty acid is safe to consume.
- Consume 25–35 grams of fiber daily. You can obtain this amount by eating lots of fruit, vegetables, ground flaxseed, and whole grains.

Why Europeans Are Thinner than Americans:
It's in the Food

In general, Europeans are much thinner overall than Americans. Many people think this is because Europeans walk and exercise more, which is a factor, but it is more than that.

European nations have much greater restrictions on what can be in their food. For example, foods cannot contain dyes and especially corn syrup, the latter being one of the major causes of obesity in this nation. Even snacks such as gummy bears in Europe don't contain the unhealthy ingredients that they contain in America.

Efforts such as those in New York City to restrict sugary drinks have been much opposed and ruled unconstitutional. As a nation, if we want to control obesity, we will have to control what we put into food and drink. In the meantime, you need to watch what you imbibe.

- When eating grains, choose whole rather than refined grains. The refining process removes most of the beneficial nutrients and vitamins in the grains. If you eat refined grains, make sure they are enriched.
- When eating protein, restrict animal fats, which cause increased cholesterol. If you eat animal protein, consume more seafood, chicken, and turkey than red meat. If you eat red meat, use lean cuts only. Eat more plant protein (legumes, beans) than animal protein.
- When eating carbohydrates, eat complex carbohydrates (beans, whole-grain foods, nuts), which are absorbed better into your system, are more nutritious, contain more fiber, and do not put more weight on you like simple carbs (soft drinks, sweetened prepared foods) and refined carbs.
- Snacking is fine; just eat healthy snacks such as fruit (especially berries), vegetables, nuts, or low-fat popcorn. High-protein snacks stave off hunger and reduce food intake at the next meal.
- Take a multivitamin while dieting to make sure you are receiving all the essential nutrients (see chapter 2 under "Multivitamins" for recommendations).

Drinking lots of **water** can also help you lose weight. Try for at least half of your body weight in ounces (e.g., if you weigh 140 pounds, you would aim to consume seventy ounces per day at least). However, drinking water before meals may work even better. A 2015 study in the journal *Obesity* showed that those drinking 500 ml of water thirty minutes before eating had a two pound greater weight loss at twelve weeks.

Other than your diet, **exercise** is the most important aspect for losing weight, but even if you don't lose weight, exercise may protect you from developing chronic diseases. *If you are" fat but fit", you may live longer than if you are normal weight but not fit, but only if your BMI is less than 35.* You will lose more weight and be much healthier if you combine exercise with diet. And without exercise, 95 percent of all people on weight-loss diets regain the pounds they lose.

More Exercise Needed to *Maintain* Weight Loss

An *Archives of Internal Medicine* study revealed that of women who lost 10 percent of their weight over six months, by two years, only 25 percent had maintained that weight loss. Those who did had increased their leisure time physical activity to approximately 275 minutes per week, more than the 150 minutes currently recommended. There was no difference between vigorous and moderate intensities of activity.

Aerobic exercise is important, but resistance exercise (weight lifting) is crucial if you want to lose body fat. Sustained exercise may be difficult for many people to accomplish or become motivated, but a recent Italian study revealed that exercising three times a day for four minutes each time is the equivalent to thirty minutes on a treadmill. The key is that you need to get your heart rate up to 90 percent of maximum during those 4 minutes. **Important Note**: A 2015 study showed that *too much* exercise can be harmful to you (see chapter 2 for more discussion). **Caution**: Be sure to have your heart checked first before you start exercising if you haven't exercised in a while.

Middle-Aged Women Ward Off Weight Gain through Exercise

A recent study in *JAMA* showed that one hour of moderate exercise daily is needed to prevent weight gain in middle-aged women. However, this association was observed only among women with a BMI less than 25. Among women who were already heavy, there was no relation. This means that if your BMI is greater than 25, controlling caloric intake is important along with exercise.

Another study in *Obesity* showed that people who lift more weights (strength training) averaged smaller gains in waist size than those just doing aerobic exercise. So both types are important to keep that weight off as you age.

If you do use a treadmill, use interval training programs, which vary the speed and height. This type of training is better for all-around endurance as well as weight loss.

Standing Can Fight Obesity

Standing versus sitting is also important for fighting obesity. A 2015 study found that standing at least 25 percent of their day lowers the risk for obesity 32 percent for men and 35 percent for women. Standing for half the day reduced the risk to 47 percent for men and 59 percent for women. So if you have a sedentary job, use a raised desk to work if possible.

This is important because the effects of so-called "sitting disease" (see Chapter 2 for more discussion) may not be reversed by exercise alone.

Lifestyle intervention and counseling has been shown to have the most far-reaching effects if implemented. The gold standard of therapy is on-site, high-intensity (e.g., at least fourteen sessions over six months) provided in individual or group sessions by a trained interventionist. You might be able to lose weight alone, but most people need outside support and help.

Genetic Testing to Determine Diet and Exercise: Not Ready for Prime Time

There are several companies that promote testing your genes to determine personalized exercise regimens and diets that ostensibly work more specifically for you. Companies who perform the tests (which can range in cost from $100 to $400), state that their tests look at how your environment interacts with your genes, thus allowing doctors to personalize your diet and exercise.

At this time, these tests have not been validated as providing beneficial outcomes. Although it is known that we all have different variations on our genes that can predispose us to weight gain, no studies have proven that you can achieve better or faster weight loss by testing your genes. Until such studies have been done, you may be wasting your time and money.

The Conventional Approaches

Can Obese People Attain Normal Body Weight?

In a 2015 study from the United Kingdom, obese patients were followed for 9 years to determine how many could attain normal weight and how many could decrease weight by 5%. They analyzed data for 76,704 obese men and 99,791 women.

The results showed that in simple obesity (BMI 30-35), 1 in 210 men and 1 in 124 women attained normal weight. One in 8 men and 1 in 7 women with morbid obesity achieved a 5% reduction in weight.

These are obviously depressing statistics. The conclusion was that current obesity treatment frameworks, grounded in weight management programs accessed through primary care, were unsuccessful in reducing weight in most obese patients.

On the other hand, there were 1283 men and 2245 women who did attain normal weight and the percentages were much higher for those reducing their weight, so it *can* be accomplished. However, the study unfortunately did not investigate any differences in those who were successful and those who weren't.

The study also excluded patient undergoing bariatric surgery (see below), which may be superior to the usual medical weight loss programs.

Nevertheless, any weight that can be reduced is healthy. And if you are not yet obese, the chances are greater that you can attain a normal weight.

The best advice I can give you about diet is to consult with a registered dietician. Most people do better if they have help and guidance; a knowledgeable practitioner can be the difference between failure and success. The *next best advice is that "one size does not fit all"*: the best diet and exercises are the ones with which you can comply and maintain and which work for *you*. In fact, a 2015 study from Israel demonstrated that the way people metabolize food can vary dramatically from person to person, so no one diet can work for everybody. Again, that's why you should obtain a personalized diet plan. That being said, the following provides some general information on dieting and diets.

Certainly, you can follow the above general diet suggestions, but for many people, a **specific diet or program** is necessary for support and guidance. There are several that have been extensively studied and have potential to be beneficial for both weight loss and improving health as well as preventing diseases such as diabetes. These include:

- *The Mediterranean diet*
- *The DASH diet*

- *Low-carbohydrate diet* (Atkins, the Zone, The South Beach)
- *The New American Plate diet*
- *Low-fat diet* (Ornish, Pritikin, and others)

Commercial Weight-Loss Programs Effective...If Used

Eating prepared foods is an easy way to lose weight. Most studies do confirm that they help lose weight and maintain weight loss, but these studies provide the food free. In the "real world," these structured commercial diet programs are expensive, so most people do not adhere to the program long-term and thus may not benefit.

Currently, insurance companies will often cover the cost of bariatric surgery, estimated at $19,000 to $29,000 per patient, but do not cover the cost of commercial weight loss programs, which are estimated at $1,600 for twelve weeks of the food and the program. Based on this, insurers providing such food free to participants could be a cost-effective method for losing weight.

There are several commercial weight loss programs available, including Weight Watchers, Jenny Craig, the Biggest Loser diet, Slimfast, HMR, Nutrisystem and others. Although healthy, they utilize prepackaged foods, some of which can be expensive. My Fit Foods is a commercial program that makes fresh food locally (although it is not available in many states).

A 2015 study compared various commercial weight loss programs and concluded that some weight loss programs may be slightly better than others, but overall "weight loss is modest and likely below patients' expectations". Weight Watchers and Jenny Craig were the best with nutrisystem showing promise. Others seemed not to maintain weight loss as well after 6 months. Overall, highly structured programs with in-person support seem to be the best

Be Sure to Get Enough Protein and Calcium

Recent studies have shown that many diets can cause bone loss, primarily due to not containing enough protein or calcium. Thus, you should check your diet to make sure it contains enough calcium (lean meats and low-fat dairy provide enough calcium). Otherwise, you will need to supplement.

Comparison of established diets

The *Mediterranean diet*, with its emphasis on plant-based foods, fish and olive oil, appears to have the most beneficial outcomes of the established diets. Studies have shown that this diet not only decreases the risk of heart disease but also may help prevent cancer (especially breast). A meta-analysis in 2011 showed that the Mediterranean diet has the best effects for lowering heart-disease risk factors and inflammatory markers. Another study in 2014 demonstrated that this diet increases telomere length, which is associated with longer life expectancy and lower risk for chronic diseases (telomeres are at the ends of chromosomes and protect them from degeneration).

The *low-fat diet* is proven beneficial but is strict and more difficult to follow. A recent study published in the *JAMA* showed that the *low-carb diet* has greater weight loss at two and six months than the Zone, Ornish, or LEARN diets and increases HDL, the "good" cholesterol. On the other hand, another study showed that the low-carb Atkins diet increases LDL (the bad cholesterol), increases a marker for heart disease, and may in fact increase the risk for cardiovascular disease. A study published in 2015 from Spain on over 7000 people showed that a high protein diet (low-carb) may lose weight initially, but was linked to a 90 percent risk of regaining more than 10 percent of body weight in the long run and a 59% higher risk of death from any cause (**Note**: the study found an association between these factors but not a cause-and-effect link).

The low-carb diet also decreases widening of arteries (thus decreasing arterial flow), compared to no change on the low-fat diet. On the other hand, the low-carb diet has beneficial effects on diabetes and on energy expenditure, which is a factor in regaining weight; the low-fat diet had the worst effect on energy, predicting more weight regain.

You should note that there are *differences even among low-carb diets*. Those that emphasize animal sources of fat and protein are associated with higher all-cause cancer and heart-related mortality, whereas diets that emphasize vegetable sources are associated with lower all-cause and heart-related mortality.

A study from the *Annals of Internal Medicine* concluded that both low-carb and low-fat diets are safe and effective, with weight loss of about 11 percent of initial weight at the end of one year and roughly 7 percent at the end of two. However, in the study, both groups received more than thirty-five group behavioral treatments. Without those, you should realize that most studies reveal that weight loss from these diets is minimal (average 6.4 pounds for low fat, 9.7 for Mediterranean, and 10.3 pounds from low carb); and most people regain one-third to one-half the weight after the first five months.

A study in November 2014 showed that the Atkins, South Beach, Zone, and Weight Watchers diets produce only modest long-term benefits, with few differences across the four. Data out to two years indicated that some of the weight was regained. (Weight Watchers seemed to be the best, but weight-loss difference was minimal).

Diet versus Diet: *Adherence* the Most Important Factor

There are lots of different types of the low-fat and low-carb diets, each differing in macronutrient composition. There have also been hundreds of studies comparing these diets (see above), some of which are good and some that compare "apples to oranges" to promote their own type. So how do you know which one is the best?

What you should know is that the differences in weight loss and metabolic risk factors are small (a difference of only two pounds) as well as inconsistent. The only consistent finding among these trials is that adherence to the diet is the most important factor in losing weight and becoming more healthy.* A 2014 meta-analysis in *JAMA* showed that significant weight loss can be observed with any low-fat or low-carbohydrate diet.

The *bottom line* is that the best diet for you is the one to which you can adhere for a long period of time. By following a good, healthy diet, along with exercise and lifestyle changes (behavioral modification), you will lose weight and keep it off. Trying every fad diet that becomes popular (see below) may be a road to failure.

*From S. Pagoto, PhD, and B. Appelhans, *JAMA*, August 2013

Other Diets: There are many diets that are promoted as unique, often supported by celebrities or by doctors calling themselves experts. In general, many of these "fad" diets may have potential harm and long-term ineffectiveness. Many have not been well researched and thus lack scientific credibility. Just because a book or celebrity promotes a new type of diet or it's a unique approach does not mean it will be effective or healthy.

However, there are two diets that don't have as much research support as the above but hold promise for helping you lose weight:

The Fast Metabolism Diet: Most people would love a diet that loses weight rapidly, doesn't cause cravings or hunger and can be used to maintain weight loss. You also want a diet that, as mentioned above, you can adhere to as well as one that can be flexible. To do so requires a diet based on long-term changes in eating patterns as well as a different approach than the standard diets, all of which have proven to lack long term success. *The Fast Metabolism Diet* by Haylie Pomroy may achieve these goals. Just a few of the ways this diet program differs from others is as follows:

- It is based on manipulating your metabolism (increasing it) to lose fat rather than limiting your calories (and counting calories).
- It promotes eating more food, not less, by modifying meal placement and timing.
- It promotes getting pleasure from the food you eat rather than eating bland diets that are unmotivating and thus likely to fail.
- It teaches you how to burn fat rather than store it.
- It demonstrates how starving your body or chronic dieting actually slows your metabolism, preventing continued weight loss.

This program has been designed to help lose ten to twenty pounds in the first month, and then continue to lose weight at a steady rate, and finally to maintain the weight loss. But you have to be committed to following her recommendations. In addition, since not every person responds the same, you may have to make specific (but minor) modifications in the food you eat.

The Fast Metabolism Diet has not been as well researched or compared to the standard diets mentioned above. However, I have observed its benefits in several people. You can purchase her book (same name) or go to her website: www.hayliepomroy. com.

The Paleo Diet is modeled after our ancestors, primarily hunter-gatherers. Evidence shows that hunter-gatherers did not suffer from the chronic disease of affluent societies, including atherosclerosis, angina or heart attacks, hypertension and perhaps diabetes. Although critics state that our ancestors did not live long enough to develop these diseases, that contention has been disproved: if they survived infancy, many lived to at least 70 and in good health (according to evolutionary biologists).

The Paleo diet includes lean meats, fruits and vegetables, healthy fats from nuts, seeds, avocados, grass-fed meats, olive oil and fish oil. It avoids legumes, dairy and processed foods. Although there is a belief that prehistoric people did not eat grains, it has recently been discovered by paleontologists that they did collect wild oats and used stone tools to make a type of flour. Critics have stated that the historical basis stated by the proponents of the Paleo diet are not completely accurate but there have been some studies showing that the Paleo diet may decrease lipids and can help lose weight. Just reviewing the foods that are consumed may indicate that it may be a healthy diet.

However, you also need to realize that our ancestors had to engage in strenuous exercise simply hunting for food. At the same time, paleontologists relate that they balanced the exercise with needed rest. So if you undergo a Paleo diet, as with any other diet, you should also exercise as well as spend time "chilling out".

A newly coined diet is the *"Pegan"* diet, which takes the best of the Paleo and Vegan diets and may be superior to each one while supplying foods that are not included in the other.

There are also several **medications** that are commonly prescribed for weight loss, but they have not been proven very effective for most people. They can be used as an adjunct to diet and exercise but *should not be used as a replacement for lifestyle changes*. Medications include:

- *Phentermine* is a stimulant (amphetamine) that acts as an appetite suppressant and has been used for decades. Although it can be used as a single agent, it is most often used in combination with other weight-loss drugs. Being a stimulant, it can increase heart rate and blood pressure and should be used with caution.

- *Topiramate* (Topamax), an anti-seizure medication, has been shown to cause decreased appetite. Almost 75 percent of patients have shown weight loss (5–16.5 percent from baseline). **Caution**: There may be significant side effects, especially at the higher dosages.

- The FDA has just approved a combination of the above two drugs... *phentermine with controlled-release Topiramate* (formerly Qnexa, now called *Qsymia*), thinking that lower doses of both will be synergistic with fewer side effects. A study in *Lancet* in April 2011 showed that the combination does increase weight loss (10.2 kg high dose, 8.1 kg low dose), but there were significant side effects of dry mouth, constipation, paresthesia, loss of taste, dizziness, and irritability. However, it was shown to decrease hypertension and triglycerides and is beneficial for those with prediabetes. Notwithstanding these benefits, it may lose effectiveness after one year.

- *Orlistat* (Xenical) is a frequently used primary weight-loss drug. Unlike other weight-loss drugs, it works on the digestive tract, not the central nervous system, preventing about one-fourth of the fat you eat from being absorbed. It can now be purchased OTC (Alli). However, it does have several GI side effects that occur if you eat too much fat; if you adhere to eating less than 30 percent fat, you are less likely to have the side effects and will lose more weight. Orlistat reduces weight only an average of 2.9 kg (7 pounds), which is meager. In addition, recent reports indicate possible adverse reactions including pancreatitis, kidney stones, and kidney failure.

- *Bupropion* (Wellbutrin, Zyban) is an antidepressant used to help quit smoking that has also been shown to help you lose weight. It can help you lose up to 10 percent of your body weight, when given with exercise and proper diet, by reducing the flow of certain hormones in the brain that affect behavior. However, if you use this medication, lose weight, and then regain the weight, taking it again may not be as effective the second time.

- *Contrave* was approved by the FDA in September 2014. It is a combination of naltrexone and bupropion and is indicated in patients who have one weight-related condition, such as hypertension, diabetes, or hyperlipidemia. It may decrease body weight by 5 percent in 25 percent of patients compared to placebo. If you haven't lost at least 5 percent of your weight in twelve weeks, you should discontinue it. However, in an interim analysis of data called the *LIGHT* trial, neither benefit nor harm could be determined.

- *Lorcaserin* (Belviq) is a new drug recently approved, which has been shown by the manufacturer to help lose up to 4 percent of your weight (a mean weight loss of twelve pounds). The FDA commented that the weight loss was negligible and was concerned about possible heart valve problems. However, it does not increase blood pressure and can also be effective in diabetics. It may lose effectiveness after one year and has a long list of possible side effects.

- *Liraglutide* (Saxenda) has been approved for weight loss by the FDA as of December 2014. It is a diabetic drug (Victoza) that was found to help 64 percent patients lose 5 percent of their weight, and 33 percent lost at least 10 percent. It should be discontinued after sixteen weeks if 4 percent weight loss has not been achieved. **Caution**: This drug has significant gastrointestinal side effects (40 percent nausea, 16 percent vomiting). **Warning**: This drug carries a serious warning about the increased risk of medullary thyroid cancer and warnings about gall bladder disease, pancreatitis, hypoglycemia, and kidney impairment. Other side effects include increased heart rate. This drug is expensive ($1100 monthly) and must be injected subcutaneously daily.

- Some weight doctors also prescribe *thyroid*, designed to increase metabolism. In general, thyroid is not very effective unless you are hypothyroid. There are many people who have subclinical hypothyroidism, in which thyroid blood tests are borderline or normal, yet you have symptoms of low thyroid. Several studies have shown a correlation between thyroid levels and obesity but have not proven that giving thyroid can lessen obesity. You can take a trial of thyroid if you have subclinical hypothyroidism (see *Thyroid* section), but if you don't see benefits within two months, it won't help you.

Intra-abdominal vagal nerve blockade was developed because of this nerve's influence on satiety (feeling full). In this procedure, electrodes are placed on the nerve and are programmed to deliver blockade for at least twelve hours daily. Although some studies have reported minor benefits, there are serious adverse side effects, and thus it is not recommended.

However, the FDA approved an **implantable device** in 2015 that uses the same mechanism to lose weight. Called the *Maestro System*, it blocks the vagal nerve and thus reduces hunger and increases the feeling that you are full. Studies show that patients with the device lost 8.5 percent more body weight, and about half the group lost at least 20 percent of their excess weight. There are some contraindications to its use, and it has an adverse-event rate of 8.6 percent, but it can be turned off.

Bariatric surgery has become a viable option for very obese people. In fact, bariatric surgery has been shown to actually resolve diabetes in many obese patients as well as improve cardiac function. It has also been found to improve sexual functioning. *Important note*: Bariatric surgery is only indicated for severely obese patients who have exhausted all other options. It is most indicated if you have a poor metabolic profile, poor cardiac function and structure, and related disorders such as diabetes, high lipids, liver disease, hypertension, and/or sleep apnea. There are thirty million people who meet the criteria.

There are four main types of bariatric surgery, all of which can be done through a laparoscope, which is less invasive than open surgery. The first type promotes weight loss by decreasing food intake (restriction): *Gastric banding* (lap band) and *vertical-banded gastroplasty (VBG)* are surgeries that limit the amount of food the stomach can hold by closing off or removing parts of the stomach. VBG is the most commonly used, from which 30 percent of patients achieve normal weight, and 80 percent achieve some degree of weight loss. However, the weight loss may not be as great as with other surgeries. The FDA has lowered the indications for lap band to patients with BMIs of 30, but only if you have associated severe conditions such as heart disease or diabetes. It is indicated for BMIs greater than 40 even without other conditions. As with any surgery, infection and even death are risks. The devices can shift after surgery, losing their effectiveness, and no one knows how long they will last in the body (they're made of silicone).

The second type of surgery causes food to be poorly digested and absorbed (malabsorption): *Gastric bypass (Roux-en-Y)* is the primary surgery that provides malabsorption. Most patients undergoing bypass lose two-thirds of their weight within two years. Bypass surgery has been shown to not only resolve diabetes in many patients (62 percent) and cut heart disease in half but also reduce long-term total mortality. *Caution*: Obese patients *without* diabetes who undergo gastric bypass have a high prevalence of developing hypoglycemia (low blood sugar) starting about a year after the surgery. This effect does not occur if you have diabetes. *Caution*: Gastric bypass can also cause vitamin and mineral deficiencies within the first year due to the changes in absorptive areas in the GI tract.

With either of these first two types of surgery, most patients lose weight rapidly and do so until eighteen to twenty-four months after the procedure. Most patients then start to regain some of the lost weight, but few regain it all. *Warnings*: Ten to 20 percent of patients require follow-up operations to correct complications, one-third develop gallstones, and 30 percent develop nutritional deficiencies (must take vitamin and mineral supplementation). To prevent these issues, it is important to continue to work with a registered dietitian.

Comparison of these two surgery types: Of these two types of surgery, there are tradeoffs. Studies in the *NEJM* and *JAMA Surg* showed that bypass confers greater long-term weight loss and twice as much weight loss as does banding. However, bypass has higher short-term complication rates and longer-term hospitalizations from the surgery. *Important tip*: A recent study showed that patients discharged within a day after bypass surgery had at least a twofold increased risk for thirty-day mortality than those discharged two days after surgery.

Beyond thirty days, though, complication rates (obstruction or reoperation) become higher with banding. Both surgeries have an operative mortality between 0.1 percent and 2 percent and can have complications of blood clots in the lungs, leaks from surgery, bleeding strictures, ulcers, hernias, and behavioral maladaptation.

Important Information

Gastric Bypass Appears to Be More Effective than Lap-Band

A study from Belgium (April 2011) showed that the long-term outcomes of lap-banding are relatively poor. Findings included only 43 percent maintaining weight loss, 60 percent requiring reoperation, and obesity-related diseases such as diabetes, hypertension, and sleep apnea persisting.

In Europe, there has been a marked shift in treatment away from lap-banding toward gastric bypass, but the opposite trend has occurred in the United States, despite some experts contending that lap-banding can result in "a mediocre quality of life and significant number of complications, as well as a tendency to regain weight after some years."

Bypass and banding are by far the most common types of bariatric surgery, but there are two more types. The third is called *sleeve gastrectomy* (SG), removal of part of the stomach (called the greater curvature). The rates of complications, weight loss, and favorable health effects of SG fall between those of banding and bypass (see chart below). A 2015 study showed that SG patients experience weight loss and short-term decrease of diabetes and hypertension, but these benefits may decline with time (diabetes resolved in 93 percent at year 1 and dropped to 80 percent at year 5; hypertension resolved in 78 percent at year 1 and fell to 55 percent at year 5). *Caution*: A February 2014 report in *JAMA Surgery* showed that patients with SG could continue having acid reflux in 84 percent or worsen or cause symptoms of reflux in 9 percent. With gastric bypass, reflux was actually resolved in 63 percent. You should avoid SG if you have severe reflux.

Comparing Three Types of Bariatric Surgery

	Bypass	Sleeve Gastrectomy	Banding
Complication rate	10%	6.3%	2.4%
Percent of excess weight loss at one year	69%	60%	34%
Diabetes Remission			
At year 1	80%	93%	60%
At year 5 or 6	*	80%	*

*Long-term studies have shown overall remission rates of 72% after 2 years and 30.4% after 15 years. I have not been able to find specific breakdowns for each type of surgery.

Combining a restrictive component with a malabsorptive is the fourth type of surgery, called *duodenal switch (DS)*, which uses a partial gastrectomy (partial stomach removal) with a rearrangement of the small intestines. A recent study published in the *Annals of Internal Medicine* in 2011 showed that DS had greater weight loss and greater reductions in cholesterol but almost double the adverse side effects (primarily malnutrition). There have not yet been studies done comparing DS directly against the other types. However, DS was shown to be the best at diabetes remission at least in the short-term (95 percent).

Weight-Loss Surgery Can Lead to Bone Loss

Weight loss following surgery induces a drop in bone density and increases the risks for falls. So be aware of these problems and take precautions. (See section on *Osteoporosis* to normalize bone density.)

Care after Bariatric Surgery Important

Roughly 20–25 percent of lost weight from surgery will be regained over the following ten years. To avoid this, the following recommendations should be followed with the help of your registered dietitian:

- You should undergo dietary counseling, behavior modification, drug therapy and undergo physical activity at least 150 minutes weekly.
- You should eat 60–120 grams of protein daily and supplement with vitamins and minerals.
- For bone health, if you undergo bypass, you should check blood levels of vitamin D, calcium, phosphorus, parathyroid hormone, and alkaline phosphatase every six months and check bone density every year.
- To assess nutritional deficiencies, you should check ferritin, vitamin B_{12}, folate, vitamin D, and calcium levels every six months for the first two years and then yearly after that.

Another procedure approved by the FDA in July, 2015 is called the *ReShape Balloon*. This device is inserted endoscopically into the stomach through the mouth and then filled with saline. It is temporarily implanted and works by triggering a feeling of fullness. It should be removed after 6 months and is meant to jump-start weight loss. This technique has been used in several countries since 2011 and most patients lose about 14.3 pounds on average and keep off an average of 9.9 pounds at the end of the 6 months. *Caution*: This technique cannot be used if you have had previous bariatric or stomach surgery or have certain inflammatory or infectious stomach conditions. Side effects include nausea, vomiting, abdominal pain, gastric ulcers and feelings of indigestion.

The Alternative Approaches

Acupuncture can be effective for weight loss as an adjunct to diet and exercise and can be done along with conventional methods. Two forms of acupuncture are usually done; ear acupuncture, using press tacks, is the easiest. These are small needles that are embedded in an adhesive bandage and then are pressed in specific points in the ear. These needles remain in the ear for as long as possible (on average, one week) and are replaced when they fall out. There is a point called the "appetite control point," which helps reduce cravings. For better results, you can tap on the needle several times a day to stimulate the point. There are several protocols for body acupuncture, all designed to regulate the stomach and intestines, increase metabolism, and decrease water retention. Acupuncture can be done up to several times a week and then less often as you lose weight.

There are also several **Chinese herbal formulas** that can help curb appetite and improve digestion. *Fang Feng Tong Sheng San* is a common formula that can be used with various sweet-tasting diet teas. *Bo Jenmi Chinese tea* is popular and is carried in some Asian grocery and health-food stores. However, other formulas depend on why you "hold on to" weight.

⁓⊗⊗⊗⁓

Do Ear Staples Work?

Although many people have given testimonials for ear staples, there has been no scientific proof that they work—and for most people, they don't. Ear staples are placed in two acupuncture points in the ear to suppress appetite, but in fact, those two points are actually not appetite suppression points according to Chinese medicine. In addition, they are deeply placed in cartilage for long periods of time and have a high incidence of infection and scarring. True ear acupuncture, using press tacks or seeds, is much more effective, with relatively no side effects.

⁓⊗⊗⊗⁓

There are several **nutritional supplements** that may also help with various aspects of weight loss, but most studies are very small or poorly done. They include:

- *7-keto DHEA* (50 mg daily) has been shown in studies to decrease abdominal (midline) fat in postmenopausal women and significantly increase insulin sensitivity (which decreases fat) in the elderly. ***Important note***: You should avoid wild yam and soy products labeled as "natural DHEA" because they do not break down into DHEA in the body
- *5-HTP* (50–100 mg 30 minutes before meals) may reduce appetite, promotes weight loss, and reduces carbohydrate cravings. This supplement can cause nausea initially, but this side effect will usually resolve within six weeks. ***Caution***: Do not exceed 500 mg daily.
- *Green tea* (tea or extract) has fat-burning (thermogenic), insulin-regulating, and cholesterol-lowering effects; and studies have shown it to decrease weight, BMI, body fat mass, subcutaneous fat, and waist circumference. However, weight loss is usually minimal.
- *CLA* (Conjugated linoleic acid, 3.5 grams daily) improves body composition, that is, it converts fat into lean body mass but may not actually decrease body

weight. It appears to reduce hunger and improve satiety. CLA is especially beneficial if you exercise a lot.

- *Hoodia* has been shown in small studies to decrease appetite through effects on the midbrain and to increase energy. In most people, this is a very mild effect.
- *Garcinia cambogia* (500 mg with 60 percent hydroxycitric acid three times daily) may suppress appetite in some patients.
- *Irvingia gabonensis* (150 mg twice daily) is a relatively new product derived from a tree in Africa. It works as a bulk-forming laxative and can reduce weight by about six pounds in ten weeks.
- Taking a tincture of *gymnema sylvestre* may decrease sugar cravings.
- *Bach flower remedies* may help decrease cravings due to emotional eating issues.
- *Chlorogenic acid* (green coffee beans) had been demonstrated to reduce BMI, increase lean body mass, and reduce blood sugar and weight loss of about 1.5–2.5 kg over one to two months. However, the research showing this was retracted in October 2014 because the study was fraudulent and flawed.

You can take supplements separately or in combinations. As every person is different, you may benefit from one or several of these supplements, so you should try to understand what each does and whether that mechanism will be helpful to you. Give each of them a month or two to work—and if they don't, discontinue it.

—∞∞∞—

HCG: Effective or Misleading?

HCG (human chorionic gonadotropin) is actually a hormone secreted in pregnancy. The HCG weight-loss protocol consists of a very low-calorie diet (500 calories) accompanied by treatments of HCG, either oral or injected.

HCG is thought to cause the hypothalamus (an area of the brain that regulates certain metabolic processes) to mobilize fat out of the fat storage locations in your body so that it's available for use. The weight lost may come directly from adipose fat tissue rather than lean muscle, so the weight lost comes directly from unhealthy fat and does not strip the body of much needed muscle, vitamins, or minerals essential to maintain good health. At the same time, it releases excessive amounts of fat-stored nutrients into the blood stream to be absorbed by the body.

The average HCG dieter ostensibly experiences rapid weight loss from 0.5 pound a day to 3+ pounds a day, although that can also be due to the very low calories in the diet. It is common to have mild hunger during the first few days; however, this usually passes and, by the second week, appears to resolve. This is partly due to the hypothalamus adjusting metabolic rate, but also due to the amount of calories circulating in your system from the fat being released.

Many dieters modify the amount of calories (usually to 750–1,000), which will decrease the rate of weight loss. Factors that help accelerate weight loss include increasing vegetable intake and mixing salad with each meal. Fiber intake is extremely important, as is water intake. Taking HCG orally (usually sublingual drops) appears to be as effective—and less costly—than injections.

There have been no major side effects reported from this diet, so it appears safe, although it can cause ovarian hyperstimulation. Realize that there are no definitive studies that support its benefits, and the FDA does not approve its use. Remember also that you can lose a significant amount of weight just by undergoing the 500 calorie diet. I have experience with many dieters who have had success with this diet, but others who have not. You can find the products, protocols, and even recipe books on the Internet, but prices vary, and you need to be wary.

Watch For Tainted Weight-Loss Products

An FDA analysis showed that many advertised weight-loss products contain active pharmaceuticals or chemicals that can be harmful to the body, including phenytoin (used for seizures), sibutramine (an anti-obesity drug that can cause high blood pressure, seizures, fast heartbeat, palpitations, heart attacks, and stroke, and has now been taken off the market), riminabant (an anti-obesity drug not approved in the United States), phenolphthalein (a possible cancer-causing agent), fenproporex (an amphetamine derivative that can cause arrhythmias), fluoxetine (antidepressant), and furosemide (powerful diuretic). Become empowered and make sure you know the ingredients.

Beware of Promises Too Good to Be True

It is amazing how many products there are that are marketed as "miracle" weight-loss supplements or programs. Most of these have never backed up their claims and are simply money makers for the company. In fact, the Federal Trade Commission (FTC) reports that weight-loss products are the number-one type of consumer fraud in this country. To complicate matters, most people believe that these products are tested by the FDA for safety and effectiveness and must include side effect warnings…all untrue.

Many popular dietary aids and treatments can have harmful side effects. There are numerous products (pills, powders, and liquids) that may help you lose weight, but not in ways that are healthy. Many of these products (such as bitter orange) contain herbal counterparts of the conventional drug combination ephedrine and caffeine. Although they can potentially "burn fat" (called thermogenesis), they do not provide long-term weight loss and can harm the body.

Other products, such as the "cortisol blockers," are based on incorrect assumptions and are scientifically unproven, providing no real benefit. There are also some products that supposedly control appetite through enhancing your sense of smell or taste. Again, this is scientifically unproven.

Because of the above, most of these products have no basis for weight loss and promote very deceptive advertising. In fact, the FTC has investigated and fined several products in the past year, including Sensa crystals, L'Occitane skin creams, LeanSpa acai berry and "colon cleanse" supplements, and HCG Diet Direct (you can read more about these at www.tinyurll.com/FTC-diet-ads).

These products are not recommended because their promotion centers around the false premise that you can lose weight without needing to exercise, reduce calories, or eat healthy foods. *This is exceedingly dangerous* because, as mentioned above, eating unhealthy foods and not exercising causes long-term harm to your body tissues. Losing weight (if it does occur at all) with these products gives you a false sense of security. In addition, they are all expensive, rebound weight gain is common once you stop them, and they may contain other ingredients that are harmful.

Many manufacturers will state the product is "clinically proven" or highlight studies done by the product's inventor (often a doctor) or report results from an "independent" study. Unless studies have been published in a research or scientific journal, they are unreliable as they have not been peer-reviewed or subjected to critiques by the medical community. Before buying these products, request a copy of the study from the manufacturer.

Hypnosis can also be beneficial for weight loss if you have certain triggers that precipitate your desire to eat, such as loneliness, stress, or other emotions. It can also help you cut down on snacks, reinforce slower eating, and decrease or eliminate behaviors that lead to weight gain, such as eating when you're full.

Your Empowered Patient Action Plan for Achieving Weight Loss

Step #1: Make lifestyle changes (diet and exercise) that provide long-lasting weight loss and improve your health.

Step #2: ***Take part in a specific, personalized diet program*** directed by a registered dietician for best results, but at the least, reduce your caloric intake, balance your food groups, and increase fruits and vegetables.

Step #3: ***Follow the suggestions in the Prevention section*** discussed above if you don't consult with a registered dietician.

Step #4: ***Choose a specific diet program*** if Step #3 is not helpful. The best diet is the one you can stick with. Remember that not all diets work on everyone the same way.

Step #5: ***Undergo acupuncture (body and ear)*** to increase metabolism, improve energy, and decrease appetite in conjunction with exercise and diet.

Step #6: ***Undergo hypnosis*** to alter negative behaviors and triggers that instigate poor eating habits.

Step #7: ***Take various nutritional supplements*** as adjuncts to help you lose weight if the above steps have not helped or you need added help. Use the ones that have scientific support (see above).

Step #8: ***Take Chinese herbs*** as adjuncts to help you lose weight if the supplements have not helped.

Step #9: ***Try bupropion*** to help decrease your appetite and lose weight if the above steps have not been sufficient to help you lose weight.

Step #10: ***Try the ReShape Balloon Device*** to jumpstart more weight loss if you are obese and the previous Steps have not been effective.

Step #11: ***Try OTC orlistat (Alli)*** if the above steps have not worked.

Step #12: ***Try other prescription medication*** to suppress your appetite and increase your metabolism if you still can't lose weight. Do so under the guidance of a bariatric physician.

Step #13: ***Consider surgery*** for gross obesity if the above steps have not helped and you have other serious medical conditions. Make sure you obtain a second opinion before deciding on the type of surgery.

Sandy is a thirty-four-year-old woman who had gained over sixty pounds during her two pregnancies, but was never able to lose the weight easily. She had tried most of the fad diets, including the Zone, Atkins, and Sugar Busters, and tried several "fat burner" formulas. She did lose weight with almost all of these, but either had various side effects, was unable to continue following them, or gained most or even more weight back when she stopped taking them. She did try orlistat but had increased gas and bloating.

I placed her on the Mediterranean diet, placed acupuncture press tacks, and gave her a hypnosis tape. I encouraged her to start exercising, which she did three times a week for thirty to forty-five minutes. I also gave her the Chinese herbal formula Fang Feng Tong Sheng San.

The hypnosis and acupuncture press tacks decreased her appetite and also stopped her from snacking. The Chinese herbs helped improve her digestion and also decreased her appetite. She lost ten pounds in the first two weeks and then an average of two to three pounds per week after that (about ten to twelve pounds per month). Within six months, she was back to her prepregnancy weight and felt great.

Two years later, she was still exercising. Every so often (mainly when stressed), she would start eating more and would gain five to eight pounds. At those times, she would listen to the hypnosis tape and take the Chinese herbal formula, and she would lose those extra pounds within two to three weeks.

Expected Outcome

Weight loss is one of the most difficult goals to accomplish and requires a significant amount of motivation, but it is extremely important because being overweight significantly increases your risks for many chronic diseases. There are many conventional and alternative methods that can serve as adjuncts to make weight loss easier. Many times, simple changes can make a huge impact.

Wounds

What You Need to Know

Injuries can occur from numerous sources, and even minor objects can cause wound injuries, the most common being beds and bedding, household containers, sofas, and footwear. Of course, as we age, many of us still think we can do activities we've always been able to do, but overdoing can have consequences as well.

Falls Common as We Age

One of the most common problems as we age is falling, due to weakness, balance problems, blood pressure problems and other causes, including wearing multifocal glasses. About one in six adults over the age of sixty-five falls every three months, and one-third of them sustain injuries. Therefore, in general, preventing falls is the best way to prevent injuries. The CDC describes fourteen effective fall-prevention strategies in a new publication, *Preventing Falls: What Works* (*http://www.cdc.gov/ncipc/PreventingFalls/*).

A recent study showed that elderly people who fell and had access to an alarm system did not use the alarm in 80 percent of cases...using it is a must because prolonged time on the floor after falling is associated with greater injury and hospitalization.

One unusual cause of falls is decreased blood pressure after eating, which occurs in many elderly patients. If that should occur, increased water intake before eating or eating six smaller meals a day rather than three large ones can help prevent this.

Because our tissues (especially skin and blood vessels) become weaker and more fragile as we age, it is more common to develop open sores and wounds that may be very slow to heal or not heal at all.

Certain patients are more predisposed to developing wounds, especially diabetics (in their feet), because of decreased blood flow. Many elderly people develop bed sores (decubitus ulcers) from prolonged bed rest, and others develop venous ulcers from poor venous circulation (see *Venous Insufficiency* section). Still others simply develop wounds from even minor injuries and cuts that can become infected.

Because chronic wounds can cause complications such as infection and spread to the bone or other areas of the body, it is important to heal them as quickly as possible.

Treatments for Wounds

The Preventive Approaches

The best way to prevent wounds is to take **appropriate care** of any scratches, cuts, scrapes, and other injuries. Diabetics especially need to be very careful with their feet because they can often have numbness and not know when a wound is developing, which may lead to their eventually developing gangrene and necessitating amputation. Wounds can become infected quite rapidly, so the earlier they are treated, the better.

You should also receive **tetanus vaccination** every ten years to prevent this particular type of bacteria from infecting wounds. If you've never had the vaccination, you need to undergo a series of three injections.

Correctible causes: There are several *medical conditions* that can predispose people to wounds and prevent normal wound healing, and these need to be addressed and controlled. Such conditions include obesity, diabetes, artery and vein problems, and heart failure. Surgery can also be a cause for wounds that do not heal.

Deficient nutrition is often overlooked as a cause of wounds and poor wound healing. It is important to increase caloric and protein intake. Minimum requirements are approximately 1.25–1.5 grams of protein per kilogram of body weight and 30–35 calories/kg, but for large wounds, you should intake more.

Taking vitamin D (800 mg daily) has been shown to prevent falls in the elderly. The majority of Americans are deficient in vitamin D, and you should undergo a blood test to check your level. Your vitamin D (25-hydroxy) blood level should be greater than 30 ug/mL, although most naturopaths recommend levels of at least 50.

The Conventional Approaches

Most minor wounds can be treated easily by just keeping them clean and placing a bandage over them. If the wound appears infected or to prevent infection, you may be prescribed *antibiotics* and/or *silver sulfadiazine or bacitracin-zinc topicals*. If the wound is minor, you can apply OTC *triple antibiotic ointment*.

If the wound is larger, more severe, or doesn't heal, then conventional care is important. First, infection must be dealt with. Wound infection may require **surgical debridement** (cleaning dead tissue so the wound can heal) and appropriate systemic antibiotic therapy. Topical antiseptics are usually avoided in these cases; they interfere with wound healing because of toxicity to healing cells.

Because collagen (a type of connective tissue) comprises a significant fraction of the dead cells in chronic wounds, the enzyme **collagenase** helps remove such tissue from the surface of wounds. Collagenase is used in addition to surgical excision.

After debridement, certain **dressings** are applied, depending on whether the wound is wet or draining. There are many different types of dressings, so your doctor should determine which type is the best for you. Many dressings allow oxygen in but keep bacteria out, which helps to accelerate healing. For deep wounds, there are dressings that can be used to pack the wound. Twice-daily dressing changes may be needed.

For infected wounds, **silver sulfadiazine** (Silvadene) is often used if the patient is not allergic to sulfa drugs. If the patient is allergic to sulfa, bacitracin-zinc ointment is a good alternative.

A new type of topical derived from genetic engineering, called **platelet-derived growth factor** (Regranex gel), has a modestly beneficial effect in promoting wound healing, especially diabetic foot ulcers. *Caution*: Using more than three tubes can increase cancer mortality (not incidence), so it should be used with caution in cancer patients.

Freeze-dried platelet-rich plasma has shown promise in a recent animal study, but hasn't been approved for humans yet.

Hyperbaric oxygen therapy (oxygen under pressure) is very effective in treating hard-to-heal wounds. Such wounds often do not heal because they have an inadequate delivery of oxygen, and this method provides the oxygen needed to stimulate and support healing the wound.

If the wound still doesn't heal, **surgery** is the last step. There are several surgical options, including skin grafting, application of bioengineered skin substitutes, and use of flap closures. Each depends on the type and location of the wound.

The Alternative Approaches

Low level energy laser *("cold" laser or LLEL)* is by far the best and fastest treatment for all types of wounds and ulcers, including those that are difficult to heal. It appears to directly stimulate the formation of new tissue and accelerate healing threefold. It has no side effects and is used directly over the wound. It can help heal wounds that have been present for months. It does not interfere with conventional wound-healing methods.

Nutritional supplements are definitely needed to help wound healing, especially when deficient.

- *Zinc* (20–40 mg elemental zinc daily) is a component of approximately two hundred enzymes in the human body, and is a very important mineral for wound healing, helping both debridement and stimulating new tissue formation. **Caution**: Avoid taking longer than three months due to its effects on copper levels.
- *Vitamin A* (10,000 IU daily) improves tissue repair, and *vitamin C* (2,000 mg daily) is required for connective tissue repair. *Vitamin E with mixed tocopherols and tocotrienols* (400 IU daily) accumulates in cell membranes, is anti-inflammatory, and may decrease scar formation. *B-complex* vitamins are cofactors or coenzymes in a number of metabolic functions involved in wound healing and should be taken as well. **Caution**: Avoid Vitamin A use in early pregnancy.
- *Bromelain* (200–400 mg daily) reduces edema, bruising, pain, and healing time following trauma.
- *Glutamine* is a very important building block for muscle mass. During times of stress, including wounds, your body's storage of glutamine can be depleted, therefore requiring supplementation. Often 10 mg three times per day is recommended to aid with healing.
- A 2015 study showed that a combination of *zinc, arginine and antioxidants* healed pressure ulcers much quicker than regular care.

Acupuncture can also be used effectively for wound healing. Both distal points that stimulate the body's healing processes and local points around the wound (which then often receive electrical stimulation) can accelerate the healing process.

In addition to acupuncture, there are **Chinese herbal formulas** that can be applied topically or taken orally to enhance the body's healing processes, depending on the type of wound. *San Qi* is the primary herb, but there are many others used in combinations with San Qi. *Nu Ke Zhen San* has the potential to speed wound healing.

Honey has been used topically for centuries to treat a wide range of medical problems like wounds, burns, skin ulcers, and scrapes. It can be effective on antibiotic-resistant strains of bacteria. The properties of honey include the release of low levels of hydrogen peroxide, some as-yet-unknown ingredients that reduce inflammation, and perhaps amino acids and vitamin C that speed the growth of healthy tissue. Honey is beneficial throughout all phases of wound healing and can be used for prolonged periods of time where other products/dressing may not be used for long periods because of concern for toxicity. There is also less discomfort during dressing changes because of honey's high sugar content, and it keeps the wound surface moist by canalizing fluids from the surrounding tissues to the wound. In addition, honey can assist with management of a foul wound odor and provide a short-acting analgesic affect to the site.

Honey is produced from many different floral sources, and its antibacterial activity varies with origin and processing. Researchers in New Zealand have found that honey made from the nectar of the tea tree (manuka honey) has special bacteria-killing properties and has worked in very desperate cases where nothing else has worked. It is sold under the name Medihoney.

Some **homeopathic remedies** can also be useful for wound healing:

- *Ledum* to help healing of with puncture wounds, bites, and stings of insects; wounds to area around nerves.
- *Traumeel* oral tablets or oral drops to help with accelerating healing; reduces inflammation and pain.

Your Empowered Patient Action Plan for Treating Wounds

- *Important Note: If the wound is deep or has not healed for over a month, consider step 11 first; then return to step 1.*
- *Most of the following steps can be combined together for faster healing.*

Step #1: Keep the wound clean and apply dressings as needed to enhance healing.

Step #2: Use honey as a topical to kill bacteria or prevent infection.

Step #3: Take appropriate antibiotics and silver sulfadiazine or bacitracin-zinc topicals if the wound is infected. If minor, apply an OTC triple antibiotic topical.

Step #4: Undergo LLEL to accelerate healing of all wounds.

Step #5: Undergo acupuncture to accelerate healing, which can be used with the laser if both are available.

Step #6: Take Chinese herbal formulas, both topically and orally, to enhance healing along with the above steps.

*Step #7: **Take vitamins A, E, and C; zinc; and bromelain*** to enhance healing if the wounds have not responded to the above steps or as an adjunct to the above methods. (***Caution***: avoid high-dose vitamin A in pregnancy.)

*Step #8: **Use appropriate homeopathic remedies*** if you still have trouble healing.

*Step #9: **Use topical platelet-derived growth factors*** if the wound is still not healing.

*Step #10: **Undergo hyperbaric oxygen therapy*** to accelerate wound healing if the wound still persists.

*Step #11: **Undergo surgical debridement with collagenase*** if the wound is large with necrotic tissue, to help promote proper healing.

*Step #12: **Use LLEL*** after surgical debridement to accelerate wound healing and decrease scarring.

Expected Outcome

There is no reason to have a nonhealing wound, even though this occurs quite commonly. With proper alternative treatments combined with conventional methods, most wounds can be healed completely and much faster than normal.

HELPFUL REFERENCES FOR
DOCTOR, SAY WHAT?
PART II
THE GUIDES:
WHAT WORKS AND WHAT DOESN'T:
STEP-BY-STEP INTEGRATIVE TREATMENTS FOR
OVER NINETY MEDICAL CONDITIONS

<u>*Important note*</u>: For all references on specific nutritional supplements, refer to www. NaturalDataBase.com.

Allergic Rhinitis

Vaidyanathan S et al. Treatment of chronic rhinosinusitis with nasal polyposis with oral steroids followed by topical steroids. **Ann Intern Med** 2011 Mar 1; 154:293.

Baroody FM et al. Oxymetzoline adds to the effectiveness of fluticasone furoate in the treatment of perennial allergic rhinitis. **J Allergy Clin Immunol** 2011 Apr; 127:927.

Carr W et al. A novel intranasal therapy of azelastine with fluticasone for the treatment of allergic rhinitis. **J Allergy Clin Immunol** 2012 May; 129:1282.

Brinkhaus B et al. Acupuncture in patients with seasonal allergic rhinitis. **Ann Intern Med** 2013 Feb 19; 158:225.

Lin SY et al. Sublingual immunotherapy for the treatment of allergic rhinoconjunctivitis and asthma. **JAMA** 2013 Mar 27; 309:1278.

Meltzer EO, et al. Oral phenylephrine HCl for nasal congestion in seasonal allergic rhinitis. **J Allergy Clin Immunol Pract** 2015 Sep/Oct;3:702.

Alzheimer's and Dementia

Singh-Manoux A et al. Timing of onset of cognitive decline: Results from Whitehall II prospective cohort study. BMJ 2012 an 5; 344:d7622.

Howard R et al. Donepezil and memantine for moderate-to-severe Alzheimer's disease. **N Engl J Med** 2012 Mar 8; 366:893.

Galasko DR et al. Antioxidants for Alzheimer disease. **Arch Neurol** 2012 Mar 19 (epub).

Vellas B et al. Long term use of standardized gingko biloba extract for the prevention of Alzheimer's disease. **Lancet Neurol** 2012 Oct; 11:851.

DeFina LF et al. The association between midlife cardiorespiratory fitness levels and later-life dementia. **Ann Intern Med** 2013 Feb 5; 158:162.

Boyle PA et al. Much of later life cognitive decline is not due to common neurodegenerative pathologies. **Ann Neurol** 2013 Sep; 74:478.

Rebok GW et al. Ten-year effects of the Advanced Cognitive Training for Independent and Vital Elderly Cognitive Training Trial on cognition and everyday functioning in older adults. **J Am Geriatr Soc** 2014 Jan; 62:16.

Dysken MW et al. Effect of vitamin E and memantine on functional decline in Alzheimer's disease. **JAMA** 2014 Jan 1; 311:33.

Alexander K et al. ABO blood type, factor VIII, and incident cognitive impairment (REGARDS study). **Neurology** 2014 Sept 10 (epub).

Tija J et al. Use of medications of questionable benefit in advanced dementia. **JAMA Intern Med** 2014 Sept 8 (epub).

Billioti de Gage, s et al. Benzodiazepine use and risk of Alzheimer's disease. **BMJ** 2014 Sep 9; 349:g5205.

Alzheimer's Disease Facts and Figures. Nearly half of Alzheimer's patients aren't told about their diagnosis. 2015, March; 11(3): 332.

Gray, S et al. Cumulative Use of Strong Anticholinergics and Incident Dementia. **JAMA Intern Med** 2015 175(3):401.

Morris MC et al. MIND diet associated with reduced incidence of Alzheimer's disease. **Alzheimer's and Dementia**. 2015 Feb 11 (epub).

Anemia

Carson JL et al. Red blood cell transfusion: A clinical practice guideline from the AABB. **Ann Intern Med** 2012 March 26 (epub).

Inrig JK et al. Effect of hemoglobin target on progression of kidney disease. A secondary analysis of the CHOIR trial. **Am J Kidney Dis** 2012 Sep; 60:390.

Villanueva C et al. Transfusion strategies for acute upper gastrointestinal bleeding. **N Engl J Med** 2012 Jan 3; 368:11.

Swedberg K et al. Treatment of anemia with darbopoetin alfa in systolic heart failure. **N Engl J Med** 2013 Mar 10 (epub).

Anxiety
Roest AM et al. Anxiety and risk of incident coronary heart disease. **J Amer Coll Cardiol**. 2010; 56, (1): 38-46.

Mackay GJ, et al. The effect of "green exercise" on state anxiety and the role of exercise duration, intensity, and greenness: A quasi-experimental study. **Psychology of Sport and Exercise**; Volume 11, Issue 3, May 2010, Pages 238–245.

Barton J et al. What is the Best Dose of Nature and Green Exercise for Improving Mental Health? A Multi-Study Analysis. **Environ Sci Technol**. 2010; 44, (10), 3947.

Huffman JC et al. Collaborative care for depression and anxiety disorders in patients with recent cardiac events: The management of sadness and anxiety in cardiology (MOSAIC trial). **JAMA Intern Med** 2014 Apr 14 (epub).

Bratman, G et al. Nature experience reduces rumination and subgenual prefrontal cortex activation, **Proceedings of the National Academy of Sciences;** DOI: 10.1073/pnas.1510459112.

Arteries: Aneurysm and Dissection
Jackson RS et al. Comparison of long term survival after open versus endovascular repair of intact abdominal aortic aneurysm among Medicare beneficiaries. **JAMA** 2012 Apr 18: 307:1621.

Lederle FA et al. Long term comparison of endovascular and open repair of abdominal aortic aneurysm. **N Engl J Med** 2012 Nov 22; 367:1988.

Reimerink JJ et al. Endovascular repair versus open repair of ruptured aortic aneurysms. **Ann Surg** 2013 Aug; 258:248.

Molyneux AJ et al. The durability of endovascular coiling versus neurosurgical clipping of ruptured cerebral aneurysms: 18 year follow-up. **Lancet** 2014 Oct 28 (epub).

Schermerhorn M, et al. Long-term outcomes of abdominal aortic aneurysm in the Medicare population. **N Engl J Med** 2015 July 2; 373:328.

Arteries: Peripheral

Ahimastos AA et al. Effect of ramipril on walking times and quality of life among patients with peripheral artery disease and intermittent claudication. **JAMA** 2013 Feb 6; 309:453.

Cooper CJ et al. Stenting and medical therapy for atherosclerotic renal-artery stenosis. **N Engl J Med** 2013 Nov 18. (epub).

LeFevre ML et al. Screening for abdominal aortic aneurysm: US Preventive Services Task Force recommendation statement. **Ann Intern Med** 2014 Jun 24 (e-pub).

Arthritis

Nuesch E et al. All cause and disease specific mortality in patients with knee or hip osteoarthritis. **BMJ** 2011 Mar 8; 342:d1165.

Sedrakyan A et al. Comparative assessment of implantable hip devices with different bearing surfaces: systematic appraisal of evidence. **BMJ** 2011 Nov 29; 343.

Nguyen U-SDT et al. Increasing prevalence of knee pain and symptomatic knee osteoarthritis: Survey and cohort data. **Ann Intern Med** 2011 Dec 6;155:725.

Costa ML et al. Total hip arthroplasty versus resurfacing arthroplasty in the treatment of patients with arthritis of the hip joint. **BMJ** 2012 April 19; 344:e1247.

Gomez-Outes A et al. Dabigatran, rivaroxaban, or apixaban versus enoxaparin for thromboprophylaxis after total hip or knee replacement: **BMJ** 2012 Jun 14; 344:e3675.

Guermazi A et al. Prevalence of abnormalities in knees detected by MRI in adults without knee osteoarthritis. **BMJ** 2012 Aug 29; 345:e5339.

McAlindon T et al. Effect of vitamin D supplementation on progression of knee pain and cartilage volume loss in patients with symptomatic osteoarthritis. **JAMA** 2013 Jan 9; 309:155.

Katz JN et al. Surgery versus physical therapy for a meniscal tear and osteoarthritis. **N Engl J Med** 2013 Mar 18 (epub).

Parkes MJ et al. Lateral wedge insoles as a conservative treatment for pain in patients with medial knee osteoarthritis: A meta-analysis. **JAMA** 2013 Aug 21; 310:722.

Messier SP et al. Effects of intensive diet and exercise on knee joint loads, inflammation, and clinical outcomes among overweight and obese adults with knee osteoarthritis (IDEA trial). **JAMA** 2013 Sep 25; 310:1263.

Uthman OA et al. Exercise for lower limb osteoarthritis. Meta-analysis. **BMJ** 2013 Sep 20; 347:f5555.

Ayers DC et al. Patient-reported outcomes after total knee replacement vary on the basis of preoperative co-existing disease in the lumbar spine and other non-operatively treated joints. **J Bone Joint Surg Am** 2013 Oct 16; 95:1833.

Ravi B et al. The relation between total joint arthroplasty and risk for serious cardiovascular events in patients with moderate-severe osteoarthritis. **BMJ** 2013 Oct 30; 347;f6187.

Juhl C et al. Impact of exercise type and dose on pain and disability in knee osteoarthritis. **Arthritis Rheumatol** 2014 Mar; 66:622.

Kwoh CK et al. Effect of oral glucosamine on joint structure in individuals with chronic knee pain. **Arthritis Rheumatol** 2014 Apr; 66:930.

Bennell KL et al. Effect of physical therapy on pain and function in patients with hip osteoarthritis. **JAMA** 2014 May 21; 311:1987.

Dunlop DD et al. Relation of physical activity time to incident disability in community dwelling adults with or at risk of knee arthritis. **BMJ** 2014 Apr 29; 348: g2472.

Nieuwenhuijse MJ et al. Appraisal of evidence base for introduction of new implants in hip and knee replacement: a systematic review of five widely used device technologies. **BMJ** 2014; 349:g5133.

Reveendhara R et al. Comparative effectiveness of pharmacologic interventions for knee osteoarthritis: a meta-analysis. **Ann Intern Med** 2015; 162:46.

Henriksen M et al. Evaluation of the benefit of corticosteroid injection before exercise therapy in patients with osteoarthritis of the knee. **JAMA Intern Med** 2015 Mar 30 (epub).

Martel-Pelletier J et al. First-line analysis of the effects of treatment on progression of structural changes in knee osteoarthritis over 24 months: Data from the Osteoarthritis Initiative Progression cohort. **Ann Rheum Dis** 2015 Mar; 74:547.

Thorland JB et al. Arthroscopic surgery for degenerative knee: a meta-analysis. 2015 June. **BMJ**; 350:h2747.

Reveendhara R et al. Comparative effectiveness of pharmacologic interventions for knee osteoarthritis: a meta-analysis. **Ann Intern Med** 2015; 162:46.

Lu N et al. Total joint arthroplasty and the risk of myocardial infarction. **Arthritis Rheumatol** 2015 Oct;67:2771.

Skou ST et al. A randomized, controlled trial of total knee replacement. **N Engl J Med** 2015 Oct 22; 373:1597.
Kim, C et al. Association of hip pain with radiographic evidence of hip osteoarthritis: diagnostic test study. **BMJ** 2015;351:h5983.

Back and Neck Pain

Wilco C. Peul, M.D., et al. Surgery versus Prolonged Conservative Treatment for Sciatica. **N Engl J Med** 2007; 356:2245; 2256.

Suri P et al. Nonsurgical treatment of lumbar disk herniation. Are outcomes different in older adults? **J Am Geriatr Soc** 2011 Mar; 59:423.

Cohen SP et al. Effect of MRI on treatment results or decision making in patients with lumbosacral radiculopathy referred for epidural steroid injections. **Arch Intern Med** 2011 Dec 12.

Bronfort G et al. Spinal manipulation, medication or home exercise with advice for acute and subacute neck pain. **Ann Intern Med** 2012 Jan 3; 156:1.

Staal et al. Spinal injection therapy for low back pain. **JAMA** 2013 Jun 19; 309:2439.

Mafi JN et al. Worsening trends in the management and treatment of back pain. **JAMA Intern Med** 2013 Sep 23; 173:1573.

Friedly JL et al. A randomized trial of epidural glucocorticoid injections for spinal stenosis. N Engl J Med 2014 Jul 3; 371:11.

C. Williams, et al. Efficacy of paracetamol for acute low-back pain: A double-blind, randomised controlled trial. **Lancet** 2014 24 July.

Friedly JL et al. A Randomized trial of epidural glucocorticoid injections for spinal stenosis. **N Engl J Med** 2014 Jul 3; 371:75.

Bronfort DC et al. Spinal manipulation and home exercise with advice for subacute and chronic back-related pain. **Ann Intern Med** 2014 Sept; 161 (6): 381.

Cohen SP et al. Epidural steroid injections, conservative treatment, or combination treatment for cervical radicular pain: a comparative effectiveness study. **Anesthesiology** 2014 Nov; 121:1045.

Nerland U et al. Minimally invasive decompression versus open laminectomy for central stenosis of the lumbar spine: pragmatic comparative effectiveness study. **BMJ** 2015; 350:h1603.

Delitto A et al. Surgery Vs nonsurgical treatment of lumbar stenosis. **Ann Intern Med** 2015 Mar; 162(7): 465.

Jarvik J et al. Association of early imaging for back pain with clinical outcomes in older adults. **JAMA** 2015 March 17; 313(11):1143.

Cohen SP et al. Epidural steroid injections compared with gabapentin for lumbosacral radicular pain. **BMJ** 2015 Apr 16; 350:h1748.

Chou r et al. Epidural corticosteroid injections for radiculopathy and spinal stenosis: a meta-analysis. **Ann Intern Med** 2015 August 25 (online).

Friedman BW et al. Naproxen and cyclobenzaprine, oxycodone/acetaminophen, or placebo for treating acute low back pain. **JAMA** 2015 Oct 20; 314:1572.

MacPherson H et al. Alexander technique lessons or acupuncture sessions for persons with chronic neck pain. **Ann Intern Med** 2015 Nov 3; 163:653.

Bursitis and Tendonitis

Yuan J, Murrell GA, Wei AQ, Wang MX. Apoptosis in rotator cuff tendinopathy. **J Orthop Res**. 2002;20:1372–1379.

Brett M. Andres, MD[a] and George A. C. Murrell, MD. Treatment of Tendinopathy: What Works, What Does Not, and What is on the Horizon. **Clin Orthop Relat Res** Jul 2008; 466(7): 1539–1554.

Coombes BK et al. Effect of corticosteroid injection, physiotherapy, or both on clinical outcomes in patients with unilateral epicondylalgia. **JAMA** 2013 Feb 6; 309:461.

Bell KJ et al. Impact of autologous blood injections in treatment of mid-portion Achilles tendinopathy. **BMJ** 2013 Apr 18; 346:f2310.

McEvoy JR et al. Ultrasound-guided corticosteroid injections for treatment of greater trochanteric pain syndrome. **AJR Am J Roentgenol** 2013 Aug; 201:W313.

Cancer

- For specific details on nutritional supplements for cancer, refer to: Lise N Alschuler, N.D., FABNO, and Karolyn Gazella, **The Definitive Guide to Cancer**. Random House, New York. 3rd Edition (2010). ISBN 978-1-58762-358-6.

Vincent DeVita and Elizabeth DeVita-Raeburn. **The Death of Cancer**. Sarah Crichton Books, New York. ISBN-13: 978-0374135607.

Siddhartha Mukherjee. **The Emperor of All Maladies: A Biography of Cancer**. Simon and Schuster, New York. ISBN-13: 978-1439170915.

Rothwell PM et al. Effect of daily aspirin on long term risk of death due to cancer. **Lancet** 2011 Jan 1; 377:31.

Jeffrey M. Peppercorn, et al. American Society of Clinical Oncology Statement: Toward individualized care for patients with advanced cancer **J of Clin Onc** February 20, 2011 vol. 29 no. 6 755-760.

Bill-Axelson A et al. Radical prostatectomy versus watchful waiting in early prostate cancer. **N Engl J Med** 2011 May 5; 364:1708.

Schutze M et al. Alcohol attributable burden of incidence of cancer in eight European countries. **BMJ** 2011 Apr 7; 342:d1584.

Wilt TJ et al. Radical prostatectomy versus observation for localized prostate cancer. **N Engl J Med** 2012 Jul 19; 367:203.

De Giorgi V et al. Influence of beta blockers on risk of melanoma recurrence and death. **Mayo Clin Proc.** 2013; 88: 1196.

Barron TI et al. Beta-blockers and breast cancer mortality: A population-based study. **J Clin Onc.** 2011; 20: 2635–2644.

Rodriguez C et al. Use of blood pressure lowering medication and risk of prostate cancer in the Cancer Prevention Study II Nutrition Cohort. **Cancer Causes Control.** 2009; 20: 671–679.

Shebl FM, Sakoda LC, Black A. et al. Aspirin but not ibuprofen use is associated with reduced risk of prostate cancer: a PLCO study. **Br J Cancer.** 2012;107:207-14.

Ruiter R et al. Lower risk of cancer in patients on metformin in comparison with those of sulfonylurea derivatives. **Diabetes Care** 2012 Jan; 35:119.

Féher J, Lengyel G. Silymarin in the prevention and treatment of liver diseases and primary liver cancer. **Curr Pharm Biotechnol.** 2012 Jan;13(1):210–7.

Fong DYT et al. Physical activity for cancer survivors: Meta-analysis. **BMJ** 2012 Jan 31; 344:e70.

Greer JA et al. Effect of early palliative care on chemotherapy use and end-of-life care in patients with metastatic non-small-cell lung cancer. **J Clin Oncol** 2012 Feb 1; 30:39.

Barry MJ et al. Adverse effects of robotic-assisted laparoscopic versus open retropubic radical prostatectomy among a nationwide random sample of Medicare-age men. **J Clin Oncol** 2012 Feb 10; 30:513.

Rothwell PM et al. Short term effects of daily aspirin on cancer incidence, mortality and non-vascular death. Analysis of the time course and benefits in 51 randomised controlled trials. **Lancet** 2012 March 21.

Sheets, N et al. Intensity-Modulated Radiation Therapy, Proton Therapy, or Conformal Radiation Therapy and Morbidity and Disease Control in Localized Prostate. **JAMA.** 2012 April; 307(15):1611.

Algra AM, Rothwell PM. Effects of regular aspirin on long-term cancer incidence and metastasis: a systematic comparison of evidence from observational studies versus randomised trials. **Lancet Oncol**. 2012 May; 13(5):518-27.

Wilt TJ et al. Radical prostatectomy versus observation for localized prostate cancer. **N Engl J Med** 2012 Jul 19; 367:203.

Gaziano JM et al. Multivitamins in the prevention of cancer in men: The Physicians Health Study II. **JAMA** 2012 Oct 17 (epub).

Nielsen SF et al. Statin use and reduced cancer-related mortality. **N Engl J Med** 2012 Nov 8; 367:1792.

Weeks JC et al. Patients' expectations about effects of chemotherapy for advanced cancers. **N Engl J Med** 2012 Oct 25; 367:1616.

Haviland JS, Owen JR, Dewar JA, et al. The UK Standardisation of Breast Radiotherapy (START) trials of radiotherapy hypofractionation for treatment of early breast cancer: 10-year follow-up results of two randomised controlled trials. **Lancet Oncol** 2013;14(11):1086-94.

Camp R et al. Qigong improves fatigue in prostate cancer survivors. **J Cancer Surv** 2013 Oct 30 (epub).

Robinson D et al. Use of 5-alpha reductase inhibitors for lower urinary tract symptoms and risk of prostate cancer in Swedish men. **BMJ** 2013 Jun 18; 346: f3406.

Hudson MM et al. Clinical ascertainment of health outcomes among adults treated for childhood cancer. **JAMA** 2013 Jun 12: 309:2371.

Li CI et al. Use of antihypertensive medications and breast cancer risk among women aged 55 to 74 years old. **JAMA Intern Med** 2013 Aug 5; (e pub).

Cook NR et al. Alternate-day, low dose aspirin and cancer risk. **Ann Intern Med** 2013 Jul 16; 159:77.

Barton DL et al. Wisconsin ginseng (Panax quinquefolius) to improve cancer-related fatigue. **J Natl Cancer Inst** 2013 Aug 21; 105:1230.

Suh E et al. General internists' preferences and knowledge about the care of adult survivors of childhood cancer. **Ann Intern Med** 2014 Jan 7; 160:11.

Memoli MJ et al. The natural history of influenza infection in the severely immuno-compromised vs. nonimmunocompromised hosts. **Clin Infect Dis** 2014 Jan 15; 58:214.

Zimmerman C et al. Early palliative care for patients with advanced cancer. **Lancet** 2014; Feb 19 (epub).

Fine Licht Dr. S et al. Hospital contacts for endocrine disorders in adult life after childhood cancer in Scandinavia. **Lancet** 2014 Feb 18 (epub).

Washington State Health Care Authority. Health care assessment of proton beam therapy, final evaluation report. March 28, 2014. http://www.icer-review.org/wp-content/uploads/2014/07/pbt_final_report_040114.pdf.

Wright AA et al. Associations between palliative chemotherapy and adult cancer patients' end of life care and place of death. **BMJ** 2014 Mar 4; 348:g1219.

Bill-Axelson A et al. Radical prostatectomy or watchful waiting in early prostate cancer. **N Engl J Med** 2014 Mar 6: 370:932.

Sooriakumaran P et al. Comparative effectiveness of radical prostatectomy and radiotherapy in prostate cancer. **BMJ** 2014 Feb 27; 348:g1502.

Cuzick J et al. Estimates of benefits and harms of prophylactic use of aspirin in the general population**; Ann Onc**, 5 August 2014.

Bhaskaran K et al. Relation between excess weight and cancer incidence. **Lancet** 2–14 Aug 14.

Allott EH et al. Serum lipid profile and risk of prostate cancer recurrence: Results from the SEARCH database. **Cancer Epidemiology, Biomarkers & Prevention,** October 2014.

Gioulbasanis I et al. Nutritional assessment in overweight and obese patients with metastatic cancer: Does it make sense? **Annals of Oncol** 2014 Oct 30 (epub).

Daenen, L et al. Increased plasma levels of chemoresistance-inducing fatty acid 16:4 (n-3) after consumption of fish and fish oil. **JAMA Oncol** 2014 April2 (Epub).

Lee RT et al. National Survey of US oncologists' knowledge, attitudes and practice patterns regarding herb and supplement use by patients with cancer. **J Clin Onc**, 2014 Nov.

Tomasetti C et al. Variation in cancer risk among tissues can be explained by the number of stem cell divisions. **Science** 2015 Jan 2; 347: 78.

Liao W-C et al. Blood glucose levels predict risk for pancreatic cancer: A meta-analysis. **BMJ** 2015 Jan 3; 349:g7371.

Lipska K et al. Potential overtreatment of diabetes mellitus in older adults with tight glycemic control. **JAMA Intern Med** 2015 Jan 15 (epub).

Klotz L et al. Long-term follow-up of a large active surveillance cohort of patients with prostate cancer. **J Clin Onc** 2015 Jan 20; 33:372.

Shanmugam, M et al. The multifaceted role of curcumin in cancer prevention and treatment. **Molecules**. 2015 Feb 5; 20(2):2728.

Pollan, M. The Trip Treatment [Psychedelics]. **Annals of Med Archives**, The New Yorker 2015 Feb 9.

Lakoski S et al. Midlife cardiorespiratory fitness, incident cancer, and survival after cancer in men. **JAMA Oncol**. 2015 March 26 (epub).

Whiting PF, et al. Cannabinoids for medical use. **JAMA** 2015.6358.

Lewis, J, et al. Pioglitazone use and risk of bladder cancer and other common cancers in persons with diabetes **JAMA**. 2015;314(3):265-277.

Eisenhardt SU eta l. Reoperation rates after breast conserving surgery for breast cancer among women in England: retrospective study of hospital episode statistics. **BMJ** 2012 July 12;345:e4505.

Ekliasson A et al. Plasma carotenoids and risk of breast cancer over 20 y of follow-up. **Am J Clin Nutr** 2015 July 15 (online).

Early Breast Cancer Trialists' Collaborative Group. Aromatase inhibitors versus tamoxifen [and bisphosphonates] in early breast cancer. **Lancet** 2015 July 23. Epub.

Prigerson HG et al. Chemotherapy use, performance status, and quality of life at the end of life. **JAMA Oncol** 2015 Jul 23; (epub).

Ali Arshad, et al. Intravenous ⊠-3 Fatty Acids Plus Gemcitabine: Potential to Improve Response and Quality of Life in Advanced Pancreatic Cancer. **Parenter Enteral Nutr** 2015 July 28, online.

Cao Y et al. Light to moderate intake of alcohol, drinking patterns, and risk of cancer. **BMJ** 2015; 351:h4238.

Narod SA et al. Breast cancer mortality after a diagnosis of ductal carcinoma in situ. **JAMA Oncol** 2015 Aug 20 (epub).

Mark A Moyad and Nicholas J Vogelzang Heart healthy equals prostate healthy and statins, aspirin, and/or metformin (S.A.M.) are the ideal recommendations for prostate cancer prevention **Asian J Androl**. 2015 Sep-Oct; 17(5): 783–791.

Gulati G et al. Prevention of cardiac dysfunction during adjuvant breast cancer therapy (PRADA). Presented at AHA 2015, Abstract 478895.

J. J. Mao, et al. Electroacupuncture versus gabapentin for hot flashes among breast cancer survivors: A Randomized Placebo-Controlled Trial. **Journal of Clinical Oncology,** 2015 Aug; DOI: 10.1200/JCO.2015.60.9412.

Carpal Tunnel and Compressive Neuropathies

Chung KC et al. Current Status of Outcomes Research in Carpal Tunnel Surgery. **Hand**. 2006 Jun; 1(1): 9–13.

Marshall SC, Tardif G, Ashworth NL. Local corticosteroid injection for carpal tunnel syndrome. **Cochrane Database of Systematic Reviews** 2007, Issue 2. CD001554. DOI: 10.1002/14651858.CD001554.pub2.

Scholten RJPM, Mink van der Molen A, Uitdehaag BMJ, Bouter LM, de Vet HCW. Surgical treatment options for carpal tunnel syndrome. **Cochrane Database of Systematic Reviews** 2007, Issue 4. Art. No.: CD003905. DOI: 10.1002/14651858. CD003905.pub3

Verdugo RJ, Salinas RA, Castillo JL, Cea JG. Surgical versus non⊠surgical treatment for carpal tunnel syndrome. **Cochrane Database of Systematic Reviews** 2008, Issue 4. Art. No.: CD001552. DOI: 10.1002/14651858.CD001552.pub2.

Day CS, et al. Carpal and cubital tunnel syndrome. Who gets surgery? **Clin Orthop Relat Res** (2010) 468:1796–1803.

Atroshi I et al. Methylprednisolone injections for the carpal tunnel syndrome. **Ann Intern Med** 2013 Sep 3; 159:309.

Cholesterol
Jackevicius CA et al. Use of fibrates in the United States and Canada. **JAMA** 2011 Mar 23/30; 305:1217.

The HPS2-THRIVE Collaborative Group. Effects of extended-release niacin with laropiprant in high-risk patients. **N Engl J Med** 2014 Jul 17: 371:203.

Keene D et al. Drugs that raise HDL cholesterol levels don't change all-cause mortality or prevent fatal cardiac-related events. **BMJ** 2014 Jul 18; 349.

Boekholdt SM et al. Association if LDL cholesterol, non-HDL cholesterol and apolipoprotein B levels with risk of cardiovascular events among patients treated with statins. **JAMA** 2012 Mar 28; 307:1302.

Wang K-L et al. Statins, risk of diabetes, and implications on outcomes in the general population. **J Am Coll Cardiol** 2012 Aug 2 (epub).

Kokkinos PF et al. Interactive effects of fitness and statin treatment on mortality risk in veterans with dyslipidemia. **Lancet** 2012 Nov 28 (epub).

Dormuth CR et al. Use of high potency statins and rates of admission for acute kidney disease. **BMJ** 2013 March 19; 346:f880.

Mansi I et al. Statins and musculoskeletal conditions, arthropathies, and injuries. **JAMA Intern Med** 2013 Jun 3; (epub).

Carter AA et al. Risk of incident diabetes among patients treated with statins. **BMJ** 2013 May 23; 346:f2610.

Mansi I et al. Statins and musculoskeletal conditions, arthropathies, and injuries. **JAMA Intern Med** 2013 Jun 5 (epub).

Patel AM et al. Statin toxicity from macrolide antibiotic coprescription. **Ann Intern Med** 2013 Jun 18; 158:869.

Leuschen J et al. Association of statin use with cataracts. **JAMA Opthalmol** 3013 Sep 19 (epub).

Stone NJ et al. 2013 ACC/AHA guideline on the treatment of blood cholesterol to reduce atherosclerotic cardiovascular risk in adults: A report of the American College of Cardiology/American Heart Association Task Force on Practice Guidelines. **J Am Coll Cardiol** 2013 Nov 12 (epub).

Shen L et al. Role of diuretics, beta-blockers, and statins in increasing the risk of diabetes in patients with impaired glucose tolerance (NAVIGATOR study). **BMJ** 2013 Dec 9; 347:f6745.

Pencina MJ et al. Application of new cholesterol guidelines to a population-based sample. **N Engl J Med** 2014 Mar 19 (epub).

Sugiyama T et al. Different time trends of caloric and fat intake between statin users and nonusers among US adults. Gluttony in the time of statins? **JAMA Intern Med** 2014 Apr 24 (epub).

The HPS2-THRIVE Collaborative Group. Effects of extended-release niacin with laropiprant in high risk patients **N Engl J Med** 2014 Jul17; 371:203.

Keene D et al. Effect on cardiovascular risk of HDL targeted drug treatments niacin, fibrates, and CTEP inhibitors. Meta-analysis. **BMJ** 2014 Jul 18; 349:g4379.

Gagne JJ et al. Comparative effectiveness of generic and brand-name statins on patient outcomes. **Ann Intern Med** Sept 2014; 161(6): 400.

Cook N and Ridker P. Further insight into the cardiovascular risk calculator. **JAMA Intern Med** 2014 Oct 6 (epub).

Rohatgi A et al. HDK cholesterol efflux capacity and incident cardiovascular events. **N Engl J Med** 2014, Nov 18 (epub).

Banach M et al. Effects of coenzyme Q10 on statin-induced myopathy: a meta-analysis. **Mayo Clin Proc** 2015 Jan; 90:24.

Taylor, BA et al. A randomized trial of coenzyme Q10 in patients with confirmed statin myopathy. **Atherosclerosis** 2015 Feb; 238:329.

DeFilippis et al. An analysis of calibration and discrimination among multiple cardio-vascular risk scores in a modern multiethnic cohort. **Ann Intern Med** 2015 Feb 17; 162:266.

Cederberg et al. Increased risk of diabetes with statin treatment is associated with impaired insulin sensitivity and insulin secretion. **Diabetologia** 2015 May; 58:1109.

Whitehead A et al. Cholesterol-lowering effects of oat ⊠-glucan: a meta-analysis. **Am J Clin Nutr** 2015 Oct 15 (epub).

Johansen ME et al. Statin use in very elderly individuals, 1999-2012. **JAMA Intern Med** 2015 Aug 15 (Online First).
Black S et al. Influence of Statins on Influenza Vaccine Response in Elderly Individuals. **J Inf Dis**. 2015 Oct 28 (Online).

Mansi I et al. Statins and new-onset diabetes mellitus and diabetic complications. **J Gen Intern Med** 2015 Nov 30; 1599.

Colds and Flu

Ray WA et al. Azithromycin and the risk of cardiovascular death. **N Engl J Med** 2012 May 17; 366:1881.

Science M et al. Zinc for the treatment of the common cold: Meta-analysis. **CMAJ** 2012 May 7; (epub).

Wise BL et al. Impact of age, sex, obesity and steroid use on quinolone-associated tendon disorders. **Am J Med** 2012 Dec; 125:1228.

Mauthuri SL et al. Impact of neuraminidase inhibitor treatment on outcomes of public health importance during the 2009–2010 influenza A (H1N1). **J Infect Dis** 2013 Feb 15; 207:553.

Bischoff WE et al. Exposure to influenza virus aerosols during routine patient care. **J Infect Dis** 2013 Apr 1: 207:1037.

Barnett ML and Linder JA. Antibiotic prescribing to adults with sore throat in the United States, 1997–2010. **JAMA Intern Med** 2013 Oct 3 (epub).

Jefferson T et al. Oseltamivir for influenza in adults and children. **BMJ** 2014 Apr 9; 348:g2545.

Heneghan CJ et al. Zanamivir for influenza in adults and children. **BMJ** 2014 Apr 9; 348:g2547.

Etminan M et al. Oral flouroquinolone use and risk of peripheral neuropathy. **Neurology** 2014 Sept 30; 83:1261.

Dobson J et al. Oseltamivir treatment for influenza in adults: A meta-analysis. **Lancet** 2015 Jan 30 (epub).

Karsch-Volk M et al. Echinacea for preventing and treating the common cold. **JAMA** 2015 Feb 10; 313 (6):618.

Cheung DH et al. Association of oseltamivir treatment with viral shedding, illness, and household transmission of influenza viruses. **J Infect Dis** 2015 Aug 1; 212:391.

Pursnani A, Massaro JM, D'Agostino RB, et al. Guideline-based statin eligibility, coronary artery calcification, and cardiovascular events. **JAMA** 2015; 314:134-141.

Pandya A, Sy S, Cho S, et al. Cost-effectiveness of 10-year risk thresholds for initiation of statin therapy for primary prevention of cardiovascular disease. **JAMA** 2015; 314:142-150.

Greenland P, Lauer MS. Cholesterol lowering in 2015: Still answering questions about how and in whom. **JAMA** 2015; 314:127-128.

Prather A, et al. Behaviorally assessed sleep and susceptibility to the common cold. **Sleep** 2015; 38(9):1353.

Black S et al. Influence of Statins on Influenza Vaccine Response in Elderly Individuals. **J Inf Dis**. 2015 Oct 28 (Online)

Constipation

Lee-Robichaud H, Thomas K, Morgan J, Nelson RL. Lactulose versus polyethylene glycol for chronic constipation. **Cochrane Database of Systematic Reviews**. 2010, Issue 7. Art. No.: CD007570. DOI: 10.1002/14651858.CD007570.pub2

Abbott R et al. Effect of perineal self-acupressure on constipation. **J Gen Int Med**. 2015 Apr; 30:434.

COPD/Bronchitis

Vogelmeier C et al. Tiotropium versus salmeterol for the prevention of exacerbations of COPD. **N Engl J Med** 2011 Mar 24; 364:1167.

Lamprecht B et al. COPD in never smokers. **Chest** 2011 Apr; 139:752.

Barnett, ML and Linder, JA. Antibiotic prescribing for adults with acute bronchitis in the United States 1996–2010, **JAMA** 2014 May 21; 311:2020.

Suzuki M et al. A randomized, placebo-controlled trial of l in patients with COPD. **Arch Int Med** 2012 May 14 (Epub).

Stefan MS et al. Association between antibiotic treatment and outcomes in patients hospitalized with acute exacerbation of COPD treated with systemic steroids. **Chest** 2013 Jan; 1432:82.

Little P et al. Amoxicillin for lower-respiratory tract infection in primary care when pneumonia is not suspected: a 12 country, randomised, placebo controlled trial. **Lancet Inf Dis** 2013 Feb; 13:123.

Schembri S et al. Cardiovascular events after clarithromycin use in lower respiratory tract infections. **BMJ** 2013 Mar 22; 346:f1235.

Vollenweider DJ et al. Antibiotics for exacerbations of COPD. **Cochrane Database Review** 2012 Dec 12; 12:CD010257.

Leuppi JD et al. Short term versus conventional glucocorticoid therapy in acute exacerbations of COPD (REDUCE trial). **JAMA** 2013 Jun 5; 309:2223.

Tse HN et al. High-dose N-acetylcysteine in stable COPD (HIACE study). **Chest** 2013 Jul: 144:106.

Llor C et al. Efficacy of anti-inflammatory or antibiotic treatment in patients with non-complicated acute bronchitis and discoloured sputum. **BMJ** 2013 Oct 4; 347:f5762.

Quint JK et al. Effect of beta blockers on mortality after myocardial infarction in adults with COPD. **BMJ** 2013 Nov 22; 347:f6650.

Kiser TH et al. Outcomes associated with corticosteroid dosage in critically ill patients with acute exacerbations of COPD. **Am J Respr Crit Care Med** 2014 May 1; 189:1052.

Celli B et al. Once daily umeclidinium/vilanterol therapy in COPD. **Chest** 2014 May; 145:981.

Barnett ML and Linder JA. Antibiotic prescribing for adults with acute bronchitis in the United States, 1996–2010. **JAMA** 2014 May 21; 311:2020.

Varraso R et al. Alternate healthy eating index 2010 and risk of COPD among US women and men. **BMJ** 2015; 350:h286.

Collins BF et al. Factotrs predictive of airflow obstruction among veterans with presumed empirical diagnosis and treatment of COPD. **Chest**. 2015 Feb; 147:369.

Regan E, et al. Clinical and radiologic disease in smokers with normal spirometry. **JAMA Intern Med** 2015 June 22; (epub).

Suissa S et al. Discontinuation of inhaled corticosteroids in COPD and the risk reduction of pneumonia. **Chest** 2015 Nov; 148:1177.

Cosmetics

American Academy of Ophthalmology. "New vision correction options for baby boomers." **ScienceDaily**. 24 October 2010.

Teri L. Hernandez, et al. Fat Redistribution Following Suction Lipectomy: Defense of Body Fat and Patterns of Restoration. **Obesity**, 2011; DOI: 10.1038/oby.2011.64

Leuschen J et al. Association of statin use with cataracts. **JAMA Opthalmol** 2013 Sep 19 (epub).

Hamann CR et al. Is there a risk using hypoallergenic cosmetic pediatric products in the United States? **J Allergy Clin Immunol**. April 2015; 135 (4): 1070–1071.

Depression

Taylor MJ, Freemantle N, Geddes JR, Bhagwagar Z. Early onset of selective serotonin reuptake inhibitor antidepressant action: systematic review and meta-analysis. **Arch Gen Psychiatry**. 2006 Nov; 63(11):1217–23.

Barber JP et al. Short-term dynamic psychotherapy versus pharmacotherapy for major depressive disorder. **J Clin Psychiatry** 2012 Jan; 73:66.

Romera I et al. Early switch strategy in patients with major depressive disorder. **J Clin Psychopharmacol** 2012 Aug; 32:479.

Wiles N et al. Cognitive behavioral therapy as an adjunct to pharmacotherapy for primary care based patients with treatment resistant depression. **Lancet** 2012 Dec 7 (epub).

Nelson JC et al. Moderators of outcome in late-life depression. A patient-level meta-analysis. **Am J Psychiatry** 2013 Jul 1; 170:651.

Driessen E et al. The efficacy of cognitive-behavioral therapy and psychodynamic therapy in the outpatient treatment of major depression, **Am J Psychiatry** 2013 Sept 1; 170:1041.

Huffman JC et al. Collaborative care for depression and anxiety disorders in patients with recent cardiac events: The management of sadness and anxiety in cardiology. (MOSAIC trial). **JAMA Intern Med** 2014 Apr 14 (epub).

Jiang H-Y et al. use of SSRIs and risk of upper gastrointestinal bleeding: A meta-analysis. **Clin Gastroenterol Hepatol** 2014 Jun 30 (epub).

Thorland K, et al. Comparative efficacy and safety of selective serotonin reuptake inhibitors and serotonin-norepinephrine reuptake inhibitors in older adults; A meta-analysis. **J Am Geriatr Soc** 2015 May; 63:1002.

Lam RW et al. Efficacy of bright light treatment, fluoxetine, and the combination in patients with nonseasonal major depressive disorder. **JAMA Psychiatry**. 2015 Nov 18 (Online First).

Shin J-Y et al. Risk of intracranial hemorrhage in antidepressant users with concurrent use of non-steroidal anti-inflammatory drugs. **BMJ** 2015; 351:h3517.

Diabetes

Lipska KJ et al. Identifying dysglycemic states in older adults. Implications of the emerging use of Hemoglobin A1c. **J Clin Endocrinol Metab** 2010 Dec; **CMAJ**; 95:5289.

Buse JB et al. Use of twice-daily exenatide in basal insulin-treated patients with type 2 diabetes. **Ann Intern Med** 2011 Jan 18; 154:131.

The ACCORD Study Group. Long-term effects of intensive glucose lowering on cardiovascular outcomes. **N Engl J Med** 2011 Mar 3; 364:818.

Loke YK et al. Comparative cardiovascular effects of thiazolidinediones: Meta-analysis. **BMJ** 2011 Mar 17; 342:d1309.

Bril V et al. Evidence-based guideline: Treatment of painful diabetic neuropathy. Report of the American Academy of Neurology, the American Association of Neuromuscular and Electrodiagnostic Medicine, and the American Academy of Physical Medicine and Rehabilitation. **Neurology** 2011 Apr 11 (epub).

Russell-Jones D et al. Efficacy and safety of exenatide once weekly versus metformin, pioglitazone and sitagliptin used as monotherapy in drug-naïve patients with type-2 diabetes (DURATION 4). **Diabetes Care** 2012 Feb; 35:252.

Karagiannis T et al. Dipeptidyl peptidase-4-inhibitors for treatment of type 2 diabetes mellitus in the clinical setting: Meta-analysis. **BMJ** 2012 Mar 12; 344:e1369.

Hemmingsen B et al. Comparison of metformin and insulin versus insulin alone for type 2 diabetes: Meta-analysis. **BMJ** 2012 Apr 19; 344:e1771.

Diamant M et al. Safety and efficacy of once weekly exenatide compared with insulin glargine titrated to target in patients with type 2 diabetes over 84 weeks. **Diabetes Care** 2012 Apr; 35:683.

Azoulay L et al. The use of pioglitazone and the risk of bladder cancer in people with type 2 diabetes. **BMJ** 2012 May 31; 344:e3645.

Gallwitz B et al. Exenatide twice daily versus glimeperide for prevention of glycemic deterioration in patients with type 2 diabetes with metformin failure (EUREXA). **Lancet** 2012 Jun 16; 379:2270.

Aschner P et al. Insulin glargine versus sitagliptin in insulin-naïve patients with type 2 diabetes mellitus uncontrolled on metformin (EASIE). **Lancet** 2012 Jun 16; 379:2262.

Wang K-L et al. Statins, risk of diabetes, and implications on outcomes in the general population. **J Am Coll Cardiol** 2012 Aug 2 (epub).

Dong H et al. Berberine in the treatment of type 2 diabetes mellitus: A systemic review and meta-analysis. **Evid Based Complement Alternat Med** 2012 Oct (Epub).

Farkouh ME et al. Strategies for multivessel revascularization in patients with diabetes. **N Engl J Med** 2012 Nov 4 (epub).

McBrien K et al. Intensive and standard blood pressure targets in patients with type 2 diabetes mellitus: meta-analysis. **Arch Intern Med** 2012 Sept 24; 172:1296.

Boyle J et al. Randomized, placebo-controlled comparison of amitriptyline, duloxetine, and pregabalin in patients with chronic diabetic peripheral neuropathic pain: Impact on pain, polysomnographic sleep, daytime functioning, and quality of life. **Diabetes Care** 2012 Dec; 35:2451.

Fernandez Juarez G et al. Effect of dual blockade of the rennin-angiotensin system on the progression of Type 2 diabetic nephropathy. **Am J Kidney Dis** 2013 Feb; 61:211.

Basu S et al. The relationship of sugar to population-level diabetes prevalence. **PLos One** 2013 Feb 27; 8:e57873.

Margolis DJ et al. Lack of effectiveness of hyperbaric oxygen therapy for the treatment of diabetic foot ulcer and the prevention of amputation. **Diabetes Care** 2013 Feb 19 (epub).

Agarwal S et al. Coronary calcium score predicts cardiovascular mortality in diabetes. Diabetes Heart Sturdy. **Diabetes Care** 2013 Apr; 36:972.

Hong J et al. Effects of metformin versus glipizide on cardiovascular outcomes in patients with type 2 diabetes and coronary artery disease. **Diabetes Care** 2013 May; 36:1304.

Scirica BM et al. Saxagliptin and cardiovascular outcomes in patients with type 2 diabetes. **N Engl J Med** 2013 Sep 2 (epub).

White WB et al. Alogliptin after acute coronary syndrome in patients with type 2 diabetes. **N Engl J Med** 2013 Sep 2 (epub).

Muraki I et al. Fruit consumption and risk of type 2 diabetes. **BMJ** 2013 Aug 29; 347:f5001.

Schellenberg ES et al. Lifestyle interventions for patients with and at risk for type 2 diabetes. A meta-analysis. **Ann Intern Med** 2013 Oct 15; 159:543.

Shen L et al. Role of diuretics, Beta blockers, and statins in increasing the risk of diabetes in patients with impaired glucose tolerance (NAVIGATOR study). **BMJ** 2013 Dec 9; 347:f6745.

Salas-Salvado J et al. Prevention of diabetes with Mediterranean diets. **Ann Intern Med** 2014 Jan 7; 160:10.

Schauer PR et al. Bariatric surgery vs. intensive medical therapy for diabetes—3 year outcomes. **N Engl J Med** 2014 Mar 31; (epub).

Roumie CL et al. Association between intensification of metformin treatment with insulin vs. sulfonylureas and cardiovascular events and all-cause mortality among patients with diabetes. **JAMA** 2014 Jun 11; 311:2288.

Sjostrom L et al. Association of bariatric surgery with long term remission of type 2 diabetes and with microvascular and macrovascular complications. **JAMA** 2014 Jun 11; 311:2297.

Larkin ME et al. Musculoskeletal complications in type 1 diabetes. **Diabetes Care** 2014 Jul; 37:1863.

Hernández-Alonso P et al. Beneficial effect of pistachio consumption on glucose metabolism, insulin resistance, inflammation, and related metabolic risk markers: A randomized clinical trial. **Diabetes Care** 2014 August 14 (epub).

Berkowitz S et al. Initial choice of oral glucose-lowering medication for diabetes mellitus: A patient-centered comparative effectiveness study. **JAMA Intern Med**. 2014 Oct 27 (epub).

Suez J et al. Artificial; sweeteners induce glucose intolerance by altering the gut microbiota. **Nature** 2014 Oct 9; 514:181.

Griebeler ML et al. Pharmacologic interventions for painful diabetic neuropathy: Meta-analysis. **Ann Intern Med** 2014 Nov 4; 161:639.

Li R, et al. Diabetes self-management education and training among privately insured persons with newly diagnosed diabetes—United States, 2011–2012. **MMWR** 2014 Nov 21; 63: 1045.

Sacks FM et al. Effects of high vs low glycemic index of dietary carbohydrate on cardiovascular disease risk factors and insulin sensitivity. **JAMA** 2014 Dec 17; 312:2531.

Ross R et al. Effects of exercise amount and intensity on abdominal obesity and glucose tolerance in obese adults. **Ann Intern Med** 2015; 162(5): 325.

Aguilar M et al. Prevalence of the metabolic syndrome in the United States, 2033-2012.**JAMA** 2015; 313(19):1973.

Metformin prescription for insured adults with prediabetes from 2010 to 2012. **Ann Intern Med** 2015 Apr 21; 162:542.

Cederberg et al. Increased risk of diabetes with statin treatment is associated with impaired insulin sensitivity and insulin secretion. **Diabetologia** 2015 May; 58:1109.

Szu-Chun Hung, et al. Metformin use and mortality in patients with advanced chronic kidney disease. **Lancet Diabetes and Endocrinology**. 2015 Jun 17; (epub).

Lewis, J, et al. Pioglitazone use and risk of bladder cancer and other common cancers in persons with diabetes **JAMA**. 2015;314(3):265-277.

Skeldon S, et al. Erectile dysfunction and undiagnosed diabetes, hypertension, and hypercholesterolemia. **Ann Fam Med** 2015 July/Aug; 13(4):331.

Golomb I, et al. Long-term metabolic effects of laparoscopic sleeve gastrectomy. **JAMA Surg** 2015 August 5; online.

Imamura F et al. Consumption of sugar sweetened beverages, artificially sweetened beverages and fruit juice and incidence of type 2 diabetes: meta-analysis. **BMJ** 2015; 351:h3576.

Erondu E et al. Diabetic ketoacidosis and related events in the canagliflozin type 2 diabetes clinical program. **Diabetes Care** 2015 July 22 (On line).

Davies MJ et al. Efficacy of liraglutide for weight loss among patients with type 2 diabetes. **JAMA** 2015 Aug 18; 314:687.

Mansi I et al. Statins and new-onset diabetes mellitus and diabetic complications. **J Gen Intern Med** 2015 Nov 30; 1599.

McCoy RG et al. HBA$_{1c}$ overtesting and overtreatment among US adults with controlled type 2 diabetes, 2001-2013: observational population based study. **BMJ** 2015 Dec; 35:H6138.

End of Life

Smith AK et al. The epidemiology of pain during the last 2 years of life. **Ann Intern Med** 2010 Nov 2; 153:563.

Greer JA et al. Effect of early palliative care on chemotherapy use and end-of-life care in patients with metastatic non-small-cell lung cancer. **J Clin Oncol** 2012 Feb 1; 30:394.

Teno JM et al. Change in end-of-life care for Medicare beneficiaries. Site of death, place of care, and health care transitions in 2000, 2005, and 1009. **JAMA** 2013 Feb 6; 309:470.

Briesacher BA et al. Antipsychotic use among nursing home residents. **JAMA** 2013 Feb 6; 309:440.

Wright AA et al. Associations between palliative chemotherapy and adult cancer patients' end of life care and place of death. **BMJ** 2014 Mar 4; 348:g1219.

Hui D et al. Quality of end-of-life care in patients with hematologic malignancies. **Cancer** 2014 May 15; 120:1572.

Seaw H et al. Impact of community based, specialist palliative care teams on hospitalizations and emergency department visits late in life and hospital deaths. **BMJ** 2014 Jun 6; 348:g3496.

Fatigue

Price JR, Mitchell E, Tidy E, Hunot V. Cognitive behaviour therapy for chronic fatigue syndrome in adults. **Cochrane Database of Systematic Reviews** 2008, Issue 3. Art. No.: CD001027. DOI: 10.1002/14651858.CD001027.pub2.

White PD et al. Comparison of adaptive pacing therapy, cognitive behavioral therapy, guided exercise therapy, and specialist medical care for chronic fatigue syndrome (PACE). **Lancet** 2011 Mar 5; 377:823.

Larun L, Brurberg KG., Odgaard⊠Jensen J, Price JR. Exercise therapy for chronic fatigue syndrome. **Cochrane Database of Systematic Reviews** 2015, Issue 2. Art. No.: CD003200. DOI: 10.1002/14651858.CD003200.pub3.

Fractures

Bischoff-Ferrari HA et al. A pooled analysis of vitamin D dose requirements for fracture prevention. **N Engl J Med** 2012 Jul 5: 367:40.

Long SS et al. Vertebroplasty and kyphoplasty in the United States: Provider distribution and guidance method. **AJR Am J Roentgenol** 2012 Dec; 199:1358.

GERD

Galmechi J-P et al. Laparoscopic antireflux surgery vs. esomeprazole treatment for chronic GERD (LOTUS trial). **JAMA** 2011 May 18; 305:1969.

Reid et al. Inappropriate prescribing of proton pump inhibitors in hospitalized patients. **J Hosp Med** 2012 May/Jun; 7:421.

Khalili H et al. Use of proton pump inhibitors and risk of hip fracture in relation to dietary and lifestyle factors. **BMJ** 2012 Jan 31;344:e372.

Reid M et al. Inappropriate prescribing of proton pump inhibitors in hospitalized patients. **J Hosp Med** 2012 May/Jun 7:421.

Shaheen NJ et al. Upper endoscopy for gastroesophageal reflux disease: Best practice advice from the Clinical Guidelines Committee of the American College of Physicians. **Ann Intern Med** 2012 Dec 4; 157:808.

Grant AM et al. Minimal access surgery compared with medical management for gastroesophageal reflux disease. Five year follow-up. **BMJ** 2013 Apr 18; 346:f1908.

Lam JR et al. Proton pump inhibitor and histamine 2 receptor antagonist use and vitamin B_{12} deficiency. **JAMA** 2013 Dec 11; 310:2435.

DuPree CE et al. Laparoscopic sleeve gastrectomy in patients with preexisting gastroesophageal reflux disease. **JAMA Surg** 2014 Feb 5; (epub).

Kapelle WFW et al. Electrical stimulation therapy of the lower esophageal sphincter for refractory GERD. **Aliment Phmacol Ther** 2015 Sep; 42:614.

Ganz RA et al. Long-term outcomes of patients receiving a magnetic sphincter augmentation device for gastroesophageal reflux. **Clin Gastroenterol Hepatol** 2015 Jun 2; [e-pub].

Lazarus B, et al. Proton pump inhibitor use and the risk of chronic kidney disease. **JAMA Intern Med**. 2016 Jan 11; Online First.

Headache

Linde K, et al. Acupuncture for migraine prophylaxis. **Cochrane Collaboration**. 2009 Jan 21. [doi:10.1002/14651858.CD001218.pub2].

Jackson JL et al. Botulinum toxin A for prophylactic treatment of migraine and tension headaches in adults: A meta-analysis. **JAMA** 2012 Apr 25; 307:17736.

Friedman BW et al. Randomised trial of IV valproate vs metoclopramide vs ketorolac for acute migraine.
Neurology 2014 Mar 18; 82:976.

Hansen JM et al. Reduced efficacy of sumatriptan in migraine without aura vs without aura. **Neurology** 2015 May 5; 84:1880.

Da Silva AN. Acupuncture for migraine prevention. **Headache.** 2015 Mar; 55(3):470-3. doi: 10.1111/head.12525. Epub 2015 Feb 16.

Heart Disease

Ronksley PE et al. Association of alcohol consumption with selected cardiovascular disease outcomes. Meta-analysis. **BMJ** 2011 Feb 22; 342:d671.

Park S et al. Randomized trial of stents versus bypass surgery for left main coronary artery disease. **N Engl J Med** 2011, Apr 4; (epub).

Borden WB et al. Patterns and intensity of medical therapy in patients undergoing PCI. **JAMA** 2011 May 11; 305:1882.

Weintraub WS et al. Comparative effectiveness of revascularization strategies. **N Engl J Med** 2012 Mar 27.

Li K et al. Associations of dietary calcium intake and calcium supplementation with myocardial infraction and stroke risk and overall cardiovascular mortality (EPIC-Heidelberg). **Heart** 2012 Jun; 98:895.

Farkouh ME et al. Strategies for multivessel revascularization in patients with diabetes. **N Engl J Med** 2012 Nov 4 (epub).

Estruch R et al. Primary prevention of cardiovascular disease with a Mediterranean diet. **N Engl J Med** 2013 Feb 25 (epub).

Mohr FW et al. Coronary artery bypass graft surgery versus percutaneous coronary intervention in patients with their vessel disease and left main coronary disease (SYNTAX trial). **Lancet** 2013 Feb 23; 381:629.

Xiao Q et al. Dietary and supplemental calcium intake and cardiovascular disease mortality: The NIH-AARP Diet and health study. **JAMA Intern Med**. 2014 Feb 4 (epub).

Michaelsson K et al. Long term calcium intake and rates of all cause and cardiovascular mortality. **BMJ** 2013 Feb 13; 346:f228.

Lamas GA et al. Effect of disodium EDTA chelation regimen on cardiovascular events in patients with previous myocardial infarction. **JAMA** 2013 Mar 27;309:1241.

Hong J et al. Effects of metformin versus glipizide on cardiovascular outcomes in patients with type 2 diabetes and coronary artery disease. **Diabetes Care** 2013 May; 36:1304.

Brilakis ES et al. Medical management after coronary stent implantation. A review. **JAMA** 2013 Jul 10; 310:189.

Eckel RH et al. 2013 AHA/ACC guidelines on lifestyle management to reduce cardiovascular risk. A report of the American College of Cardiology/American Heart Association Task Force on practice guidelines. **J Am Coll Cardiol** 2013 Nov (epub).

Stone NJ et al. 2013 ACC/AHA guideline on the treatment of blood cholesterol to reduce atherosclerotic cardiovascular risk in adults: A report of the American College of Cardiology/American heart Association Task Force on Practice Guidelines. **J Am Coll Cardiol** 2013 Nov 12 (epub).

Sorita A et al. Off-hour presentation and outcomes in patients with acute myocardial infarction: Meta-analysis. **BMJ** 2014 Jan 21; 348:f7393.

Qaseem SP et al. Treatment of anemia in patients with heart disease. A clinical practice guideline from the American College of Physicians. **Ann Intern Med** 2013 Dec 3; 159:770.

Threapleton DE et al. Dietary fibre intake and risk of cardiovascular disease. Meta-analysis. **BMJ** 2013 Dec 20; 347:f6879.

Huffman JC et al. Collaborative care for depression and anxiety disorders in patients with recent cardiac events: The management of sadness and anxiety in cardiology (MOSAIC trial). **JAMA Intern Med** 2014 Apr 14 (epub).

Mark DB et al. Quality of life after coronary artery bypass (STITCH trial). **Ann Intern Med** 2014 Sep 16; 161:362.

Mauri L et al. Twelve or 30 months of dual antiplatelet therapy after drug-eluting stents. **N Engl J Med** 2014 Nov 6 (epub).

Hira R et al. Frequency and practice-level variation in inappropriate aspirin use for the primary prevention of cardiovascular disease. **J Am Coll Cardiol** 2015; 65(2): 111.

Chomistek AK et al. Healthy lifestyle in the primordial prevention of cardiovascular disease among young women. **J Am Coll Cardiol** 2015 Jan 6; 65:43.

Luu HN et al. Prospective evaluation of the association of nut/peanut consumption with total and cause-specific mortality. **JAMA Intern Med** 2015 Mar 2; (epub).

Shaw L et al. Long-term prognosis after coronary artery calcification testing in asymptomatic patients. **Ann Intern Med** 2015; 163(1):14.

Fink H et al. Intermediate- and long-term cognitive outcomes after cardiovascular procedures in older 9adults. **Ann Intern Med**. 2015; 163(2):107.

Marijon E, et al. Warning symptoms are associated with survival from sudden cardiac arrest. **Ann Intern Med** 2015 Dec 22; Online First.

Heart Failure

Zannad F et al. Eplerenone in patients with systolic heart failure and mild symptoms. **N Engl J Med** 2010 Nov 14 (epub).

Yeh GY et al. Tai chi exercise in patients with chronic heart failure. **Arch Intern Med** 2011 Apr 25; 171:750.

Edelmann F et al. Effect of spironolactone on diastolic function and exercise capacity in patients with heart failure with preserved ejection fraction. **JAMA** 2013 Feb 27; 309:781.

Gheorghiade M et al. Effect of aliskiren on post discharge mortality and heart failure readmissions among patients hospitalized for heart failure (ASTRONAUT trial). **JAMA** 2013 Mar 20; 309:1125.

Aliti GB et al. Aggressive fluid and sodium restriction in acute decompensated heart failure. **JAMA Intern Med** 2013 Jun 24; 173:1058.

Kaluza J et al. Processed and unprocessed red meat consumption and risk of heart failure: A prospective study of men. **Circulation: Heart Failure**. 2014 June 12 (epub).

Pivetta E et al. Lung ultrasound-implemented diagnosis of acute decompensated heart failure in the ED. **Chest** 2015 July 1; 148:202.

Khan RF et al. Symptom burden among patients who were hospitalized for heart failure. **JAMA Intern Med** 2015 August (epub).

Ades P. Temporal Trends and Factors Associated With Cardiac Rehabilitation Referral Among Patients Hospitalized With Heart Failure. **J Am Coll Cardiol** 2015, August; 66(8): 927.

Pandey A/Berry JD et al. Dose Response Relationship Between Physical Activity and Risk of Heart Failure: A Meta-Analysis. **Circulation** 2015 Oct 5; *132*:1777-1779.

Imamura F et al. Consumption of sugar sweetened beverages, artificially sweetened beverages, and fruit juice and incidence of type 2 diabetes: systematic review, meta-analysis, and estimation of population attributable fraction. **BMJ** 2015;351:h3576.

Coggan AR et al. Acute Dietary Nitrate Intake Improves Muscle Contractile Function in Patients with Heart Failure: A Double-Blind, Placebo-Controlled, Randomized Trial. **Circulation: Heart Failure**. 2015 July 15 (Online).

Heart Arrhythmias

Eagle KA et al. Management of atrial fibrillation: Translating clinical trial data into clinical practice. **The Amer J Med**. 2011; 124:4.

Ionescu-Ittu R et al. Comparative effectiveness of rhythm control versus rate control drug treatment effect on mortality in patients with atrial fibrillation. **Arch Intern Med** 2012 Jul 9; 122:997.

Nielsen JC et al. Radiofrequency ablation as initial therapy in paroxysmal atrial fibrillation. **N Engl J Med** 2012 Oct 25. 367:1587.

Ulimoen SR et al. Comparison of four single-drug regimens on ventricular rate and arrhythmia-related symptoms in patients with permanent atrial fibrillation. **Am J Cardiol** 2013 Jan15:111:225.

Lamberts M et al. Oral anticoagulation and antiplatelets in atrial fibrillation patients after myocardial infarction and coronary intervention. **J Am Coll Cardiol** 2013 Sep 10; 62:981.

Ruff CT et al. Comparison of the efficacy and safety of new oral anticoagulants with warfarin in patients with atrial fibrillation: A meta-analysis. **Lancet** 2103 Dec 4 (epub).

Morillo CA et al. Radiofrequency ablation vs. anti-arrhythmic drugs as first-line treatment of paroxysmal atrial fibrillation (RAAFT-2). **JAMA** 2014 Feb 19; 311:679.

Larsson SC et al. Alcohol consumption and risk of atrial fibrillation. Meta-analysis. **J Am Coll Cardiol** 2014 Jul 22; 64:281.

Hernandez I et al. Risk of bleeding with dabigatran in atrial fibrillation. **JAMA Intern Med** 2014 Nov 3 (epub).

Washam JB et al. Digoxin use in patients with atrial fibrillation and adverse cardiovascular outcomes. A retrospective analysis of The ROCKET study. **Lancet** 2015 Mar 5 (epub).

Appelboam A et al. Postural modification to the standard Valsalva manoeuvre for emergency treatment of supraventricular tachycardia (REVERT). **Lancet** 2015 Aug 24 (epub).

Emdin, CA, et al. Atrial fibrillation as a risk factor for cardiovascular disease and death in women compared with men: a meta-analysis. **BMJ** 2016;352:h7013.

Hypertension

Myers MG et al. Conventional versus automated measurement of blood pressure in primary care patients with systolic hypertension. **BMJ** 2011 Feb 7; 342:d286.

Houston TK et al. Culturally appropriate storytelling to improve blood pressure. **Ann Intern Med** 2011 Jan n18; 154:77.

Diao D et al. Pharmacotherapy for mild hypertension. **Cochrane Database of Systematic Reviews** 2012 Nov 14 Issue 8. Online.

Makam et al. Adverse Effects of thiazide diuretics in older patients **J Am Geriatr Soc** 2014 Jun; 62:1039.

Khalesi S et al. Effects of probiotics on blood pressure. **Hypertension** July 21 2014.

Bangalore S et al. 2014 Either JNC panel recommendation for blood pressure targets revisited: Results from the INVEST study. **J Am Coll Cardiol**. 2014; 64(8):784–793.

Kovesdy CP et al. Blood pressure and mortality in US veterans with chronic kidney disease. **Ann Intern Med** 2013 Aug 20; 159:233.

James PA et al. 2014 evidence based guideline for the management of high blood pressure in adults: Report from the panel members appointed to the Eighth Joint National Committee (JNC 8). **JAMA** 2013 Dec 18 (epub).

Rapsomaniki E et al. Blood pressure and incidence of twelve cardiovascular diseases: Lifetime risks, healthy life-years lost, and age-specific associations in 1.25 million people. **Lancet** 2014 May 31; 383:1899.

Makam AN et al. Risk of thiazide-induced metabolic adverse events in older adults. **J Am Geriatr Soc** 2014 Jun; 62:1039.

Duram-Cantolla et al. CPAP as treatment for systemic hypertension in people with obstructive sleep apnea. **BMJ** 2010 Nov 24; 341:c5991.

Fralick M et al. Co-trimoxazole and sudden death in patients receiving inhibitors of renin-angiotensin system: Population-based study. **BMJ** 2014 Oct 30; 349:g6196.

Chu P et al. The effectiveness of yoga in modifying risk factors for cardiovascular disease and metabolic syndrome: A meta-analysis. **European Journal of Preventive Cardiology**. 2014 Dec 16 (epub).

Gore J et al. Dietary nitrate provides sustained blood pressure lowering in hypertensive patients. **Hypertension** 2015 Feb; 65:320.

Antoniou T et al. Trimethoprim-sulfamethaxazole and risk of sudden death among patient staking spironolactone. **CMAJ** 2015 Mar 3; 187:E138.

Johnson, S et al. Daily Blueberry Consumption Improves Blood Pressure and Arterial Stiffness in Postmenopausal Women with Pre- and Stage 1-Hypertension. **J Acad Nutri and Dietetics** 2015 March; 115(3):369.

Hermida RC et al. Sleep-time BP: prognostic marker of type 2 diabetes and therapeutic target for prevention. **Diabetologia** 2015 Sept (Online First).

Incontinence and Overactive Bladder

Bai, SW et al. Comparison of the efficacy of Burch colposuspension, pubovaginal sling, and tension-free vaginal tape for stress urinary incontinence. **International Journal of Gynecology & Obstetrics** 2005, Dec; 91, (3): 246–251.

Dmochowski R et al. Efficacy and safety of onabotulinumtoxin A for idiopathic overactive bladder. **J Urol** 2010 Dec; 184:2416.

Burgio KL et al. Behavioral versus drug treatment for overactive bladder in men: The MOTIVE trial. **J Am Geriatr Soc** 2011 Dec; 59:2209.

Shamliyan T et al. Benefits and harms of pharmacologic treatment for urinary incontinence in women: A systematic review. **Ann Int Med** 2012 Jun 19; 156(12):861.

Visco AG et al. Anticholinergic therapy versus botulinum toxin A for urgency urinary incontinence. **N Engl J Med** 2012 Nov 8; 367:1803.

Labrie J et al. Surgery versus physiotherapy for stress urinary incontinence. **N Engl J Med** 2013 Sep 19; 369:1124.

Aseem A et al. Nonsurgical management of urinary incontinence in women: A clinical practice guideline from the American College of Physicians. **Ann Intern Med** 2014; 161(6):429.

Huang A et al. A group-based yoga therapy intervention for urinary incontinence in women: A pilot randomized trial. **Female Pelvic Medicine & Reconstructive Surgery**. 2014 May/June; 20 (3):147.

Infections

Ruhnke GW et al. Marked reduction in 30-day mortality among elderly patients with community-acquired pneumonia. **Am J Med** 2011 Feb; 124:171.

Mattila E et al. Fecal transplantation, through colonoscopy, is effective therapy for recurrent *Clostridium difficile* infection. **Gastroenterology** 2012 March; 142:490.

Kullar R et al. Impact of vancomycin exposure on outcomes in patients with methicillin-resistant *Staphylococcus aureus* bacteremia. **Clin Infect Dis** 2011 Apr 15; 52:975.

Janarthanan S et al. Clostridium difficile-associated diarrhea and proton pump inhibitor therapy: a meta-analysis. **Am J Gastroenterol** 2012 Jul; 107:1001.

Johnston BS et al. probiotics for the prevention of *Clostridium difficile*-associated diarrhea. Meta-analysis. **Ann Intern Med** 2012 Nov 13; (epub).

Aburto NJ et al. Effect of increased potassium intake on cardiovascular risk factors and stroke. Meta-analysis. **BMJ** 2013 Apr 4; 346:f1378.

He FJ et al. Effect of longer term modest salt restriction on blood pressure. Meta-analysis. **BMJ** 2013 Apr 4; 346:f1325.

Brown KA et al. Meta-analysis of antibiotics and the risk of community-associated *Clostridium difficile* infection. **Antimicrob Agents Chemother** 2013 May; 57:2326.

Mancia G et al. Long term prognostic value of white coat hypertension. An insight from diagnostic use of both ambulatory and home blood pressure measurements. **Hypertension** 2013 Jul 62:16.

Li CI et al. Use of antihypertensive medications and breast cancer risk among women aged 55 to 74 years old. **JAMA Intern Med** 2013 Aug 5; (e pub).

Chambers HF. Pharmacology and treatment of complicated skin and skin-structure infections. **N Engl J Med** 2014 Jun5; 370:2238.

Postma D et al. Antibiotic treatment strategies for community-acquired pneumonia in adults. **N Engl J Med** 2015; 372:1312.

Jain S, et al. Community-acquired pneumonia requiring hospitalization among U.S. adults. **N Engl J Med** 2015 Jul 30; 373:415.

Siemieniuk RAC et al. Corticosteroid therapy for patients hospitalized with community-acquired pneumonia: a meta-analysis. **Ann Intern Med** 2015 Oct 6; 163:519.

Restrepo MI et al. Corticosteroids for severe community-acquired pneumonia: Time to change clinical practice. **Ann Intern Med** 2015 Oct 6; 163:560.

Irritable Bowel Syndrome

Pimental M et al. Rifaximin therapy for patients with irritable bowel syndrome without constipation. **N Engl J Med** 2011 Jan 6; 364:22.

IBS. Mindfulness and IBS. **Am J Gastroenterol** 2011;106; 1678–1688 (original). f/u presented at Digestive Disease Week.

Chey WD et al. Linaclotide for irritable bowel syndrome with constipation. **Am J Gastroenterol** 2012 Nov; 107:1702.

Vazquez-Roque MI et al. A controlled trial of gluten-free diet in patients with irritable bowel syndrome-diarrhea: Effects on bowel frequency and intestinal function. **Gastroenterology** 2013 May; 144:903.

Halmos EP et al. A diet low in FODMAPs reduces symptoms of irritable bowel syndrome. **Gastroenterology** 2014 Jan; 146:67.

Yoon JS et al. Effect of multispecies probiotics on irritable bowel syndrome: a randomized, double-blind, placebo-controlled trial. **J Gastroenterol Hepatol.** 2014 Jan; 29(1):52–9.

Moayyedi P et al. The effect of fiber supplementation on irritable bowel syndrome. A meta-analysis. **Am J Gastroenterol** 2014 Sep; 109:1367.

Insomnia/Sleep Apnea

Guimaraes KC et al. Effects of oropharyngeal exercises in patients with moderate obstructive sleep apnea syndrome. **Am J Respir Crit Care Med** 2009 Feb 20; 179:962.

Rondanelli M et al. The effect of melatonin, magnesium, and zinc on primary insomnia in long-term care facility residents in Italy. **J Am Geriatr** Soc 2011 Jan: 59:82.

Buysse DJ et al. Efficacy of brief behavioral treatment for chronic insomnia in older adults. **Archives Intern Med** 2011 Jan 24 (epub).

Frey DJ et al. Influence of zolpidem and sleep inertia on balance and cognition during nighttime awakening. **J Am Geriatr Soc** 2011 Jan; 59:73.

Holley AB et al. Efficacy of an adjustable oral appliance and comparison with CPAP for the treatment of obstructive sleep apnea syndrome. **Chest** 2011 Dec; 140:1511.

Buston OM et al. Adverse metabolic consequences in humans of prolonged sleep restriction combined with circadian disruption. **Sci Transl Med** 2012 Apr 11; 4:129.

Nieto FJ et al. Sleep-disordered breathing and cancer mortality. **Am J Resp Crit Care Med** 2012 May 20; 186:190.

Kripke DF et al. Hypnotics' association with mortality or cancer. **BMJ** Open 2012 Feb 27;2:e000850.

Weaver TE et al. CPAP treatment of sleepy patients with milder obstructive sleep apnea. **Am J Resp Crit Care Med** 2012 Oct 1; 186:677.

Chai-Coetzer CL et al. Primary care versus specialist sleep center management of obstructive sleep apnea and daytime sleepiness and quality of life. **JAMA** 2013 Mar 13; 309:997.

Phillips CL et al. health outcomes of CPAP versus oral appliance treatment for obstructive sleep apnea. **Am J Respir Crit Care Med** 2013 Apr 15; 187:879.

Strollo PJ et al. Upper airway stimulation for obstructive sleep apnea. **N Engl J Med** 2104 Jan 9; 370:139.

Chirnos JA et al. CPAP, weight loss, or both for obstructive sleep apnea. **N Engl J Med** 2014 Jun 12; 370:2265.

Duram-Cantolla et al. CPAP as treatment for systemic hypertension in people with obstructive sleep apnea. **BMJ** 2010 Nov 24; 341:c5991.

Qaseem A et al. Diagnosis of obstructive sleep apnea in adults: A clinical practice guideline from the American College of Physicians. **Ann Intern Med** 2014 Aug 5; 161:210.

Ieto V et al. Effects of oropharyngeal exercises on snoring. **Chest** 2015 Sep;148:683.

Kidney Disease (CKD)

Clark WF et al. Association between estimated GFR at initiation of dialysis and mortality. **CMAJ** 2011 Jan 11; 183:47.

Rosansky SJ et al. Early start of hemodialysis may be harmful. **Arch Intern Med** 2011 Mar 14; 171:396.

Inrig JK et al. Effect of hemoglobin target on progression of kidney disease. A secondary analysis of the CHOIR trial. **Am J Kidney Dis** 2012 Sep; 60:390.

Morgan K et al. Self-help treatment for insomnia treatments associated with chronic conditions in older adults. **J Am Geriatr Soc** 2012 Oct; 60:1803.

Fernandez Juarez G et al. Effect of dual blockade of the rennin-angiotensin system on the progression of Type 2 diabetic nephropathy. **Am J Kidney Dis** 2013 Feb; 61:211.

Jamal SA et al. Effect of calcium-based versus non-calcium-based phosphate binders on mortality in patients with chronic kidney disease. Meta-analysis. **Lancet** 2013 Jul 19 (epub).

Kovesdy CP et al. Blood pressure and mortality in US veterans with chronic kidney disease. **Ann Intern Med** 2013 Aug 20; 159:233.

Weich S et al. Effect of anxiolytic and hypnotic drug prescriptions on mortality hazards. **BMJ** 2014 Mar 19; 348:g1996.

Szu-Chun Hung, et al. Metformin use and mortality in patients with advanced chronic kidney disease. **Lancet Diabetes and Endocrinology**. 2015 Jun 17; (epub).

Thomas J. Hoerger et al. The Future Burden of CKD in the United States: A Simulation Model for the CDC CKD Initiative. **Am J Kid Dis** 2015 March; Volume 65, Issue 3, Pages 403–411.

Lazarus B, et al. Proton pump inhibitor use and the risk of chronic kidney disease. **JAMA Intern Med**. 2016 Jan 11; Online First.

Macular Degeneration
Wormald R, Evans JR, Smeeth LL, Henshaw KS. Photodynamic therapy for neovascular age-related macular degeneration. **Cochrane Database of Systematic Reviews** 2007, Issue 3. Art. No.: CD002030. DOI: 10.1002/14651858.CD002030.pub3.

Virgili G, Bini A. Laser photocoagulation for neovascular age⊠related macular degeneration. **Cochrane Database of Systematic Reviews** 2007, Issue 3. Art. No.: CD004763. DOI: 10.1002/14651858.CD004763.pub2.

Evans JR, Sivagnanavel V, Chong V. Radiotherapy for neovascular age⊠related macular degeneration. **Cochrane Database of Systematic Reviews** 2010, Issue 5. Art. No.: CD004004. DOI: 10.1002/14651858.CD004004.pub.

Liew G et al. The association of aspirin use with age-related macular degeneration. **JAMA Intern Med** 2013 Feb 25; 173:258.

Menopause
Freeman EW et al. Efficacy of escitalopram for hot flashes in healthy menopausal women. **JAMA** 2011 Jan 19; 305:267.

LaCroix AZ et al. Health outcomes after stopping conjugated equine estrogens among postmenopausal women with prior hysterectomy. **JAMA** 2011 Apr 6; 305:1305.

Paramsothy P et al. Bleeding patterns during the menopausal transition in the multiethnic Study of Women's Health across the Nation (SWAN). **BJOG** 2014 Apr 16 (epub).

Joffe H et al. Low dose estradiol and the serotonin-norepinephrine reuptake inhibitor venlafaxine for vasomotor symptoms. **JAMA Intern Med** 2014 May 26 (epub).

Walega DR et al. Stellate Ganglion block for menopausal vasomotor symptoms? **Menopause** 2014 Aug 15 (epub).

Harman SM et al. Arterial imaging outcomes and cardiovascular risk factors in recently menopausal women. **Ann Intern Med** 2014 Aug 19; 161:249.

Faubion S et al. Caffeine and menopausal symptoms. **Menopause** 2014 (epub).

Crandall, c et al. Associations of Menopausal Vasomotor Symptoms with Fracture Incidence. **J Clin Endocrinol & Metab**. 2014 Dec 18; 10: 2014.

Collaborative Group on Epidemiological Studies of Ovarian Cancer. Menopausal hormone use and ovarian cancer risk: A meta-analysis. **Lancet** 2015 Feb 12 (epub).

Avis N et al. Duration of menopausal vasomotor symptoms over the menopause transition. **JAMA Intern Med** 2015 Feb 16 (epub).

Neuromas

Thomson CE, Gibson JNA, Martin D. Interventions for the treatment of Morton's neuroma. *Cochrane Database of Systematic Reviews* 2004, Issue 3. Art. No.: CD003118. DOI: 10.1002/14651858.CD003118.pub2.

Thomson CE et al. Methylprednisolone injections for the treatment of Morton neuroma. **J Bone Joint Surg Am** 2013 May 1; 95:790.

Neuropathy

Bril V et al. Evidence-based guideline: Treatment of painful diabetic neuropathy. Report of the American Academy of Neurology, the American Association of Neuromuscular and Electrodiagnostic Medicine, and the American Academy of Physical Medicine and Rehabilitation. **Neurology** 2011 Apr 11 (epub).

Boyle J et al. Randomized, placebo-controlled comparison of amitriptyline, duloxetine, and pregabalin in patients with chronic diabetic peripheral neuropathic pain: Impact on pain, polysomnographic sleep, daytime functioning, and quality of life. **Diabetes Care** 2012 Dec; 35:2451.

Finnerup NB et al. Pharmacotherapy for neuropathic pain in adults: A meta-analysis. **Lancet Neurol** 2015 Feb; 14:162.

Osteoporosis

Leslie WD et al. A before-and-after study of fracture risk reporting and osteoporosis treatment initiation. **Ann Intern med** 2010 Nov 2; 153:580.

Khalili H et al. Use of proton pump inhibitors and risk of hip fracture in relation to dietary and lifestyle factors. **BMJ** 2012 Jan 31;344:e372.

Avenell A et al. Long term follow-up for mortality and cancer in a randomized place-bo-controlled trial of vitamin D$_3$ and/or calcium (RECORD Trial). **J Clin Endocrinol Metab** 2012 Feb; 97:614.

Meier RPH et al. Increasing occurrence of atypical femoral fractures associated with bisphosphonate use. **Arch Intern Med** 2012 May 21 (epub).

Li K et al. Associations of dietary calcium intake and calcium supplementation with myocardial infraction and stroke risk and overall cardiovascular mortality (EPIC-Heidelberg). **Heart** 2012 Jun; 98:895.

Anderson JJB et al. Calcium intakes and femoral and lumbar bone density of elderly US men and women. **J Clin Endocrinol Metab** 2012 Dec; 97:4531.

Xiao Q et al. Dietary and supplemental calcium intake and cardiovascular disease mortality: The NIH-AARP Diet and health study. **JAMA Intern Med**. 2014 Feb 4 (epub).

Michaelsson K et al. Long term calcium intake and rates of all cause and cardiovascular mortality. **BMJ** 2013 Feb 13; 346:f228.

Berry SD et al. Repeat bone mineral density screening and protection of hip and major osteoporotic fracture. **JAMA** 2013 Sep 25; 310:1256.

Reid IR et al. Effects of vitamin D supplements on bone mineral density. A meta-analysis. **Lancet** 2013 Oct 11 (epub).

Crandall CJ et al. Comparative effectiveness of pharmacologic treatments to prevent fractures: An updated systematic review. **Ann Intern Med** 2014 Sep 9 (epub).

Tai V et al. Calcium intake and bone mineral density: a meta-analysis. **BMJ** 2015 Sep 29; 351:h4183.

Pain, Chronic

Häuser W, et al. Comparative efficacy and acceptability of amitriptyline, duloxetine and milnacipran in fibromyalgia syndrome: a systematic review with meta-analysis. **Rheumatology** (Oxford). 2011 Mar;50(3):532-43.

Vickers AJ et al. Acupuncture for chronic pain: Meta-analysis. **Arch Intern Med** 2012 Oct 22; 172:1444.

Vickers AJ and Linde K. Acupuncture for chronic pain. **JAMA** 2014 Mar 5; 311:955.

Kappel BS, et al. Systematic review: efficacy and safety of medical marijuana in selected neurologic disorders. **Neurology** 2014; 82(12):1083.

Hill K. Medical marijuana for treatment of chronic pain and other medical and psychiatric problems. **JAMA** 2015 Jun23/30; 313(24): 2474.

Parkinson's, Essential Tremor

Quik M et al. Nicotinic receptors as CNS targets for Parkinson's disease. **Biochem Pharmacol** 2007 Oct 15; 74:1224.

Li F et al. Tai Chi and postural stability in patients with Parkinson's disease. **N Engl J Med** 2012 Feb 9; 366:511.

Tomlinson CL et al. Physiotherapy intervention in Parkinson's disease. Meta-analysis. **BMJ** 2012 Aug 6; 345:e5004.

PD MED Collaborative Group. Long-term effectiveness of dopamine agonists and monoamine oxidase B inhibitors compared with levodopa as initial treatment for Parkinson's disease. **Lancet** 2014 Jun 11 (epub).

Writing Group for the NINDS Exploratory Trials in Parkinson's Disease. Effect of creatine monohydrate on clinical progression in patients with Parkinson's disease. **JAMA** 2015 Feb 10; 313:584.

Gibbons CH et al. Clinical implications of delayed orthostatic hypotension. **Neurology** 2015 Oct 20; 85:1362.

Clarke CE, et al. Physiotherapy and occupational therapy vs no therapy in mild to moderate Parkinson Disease. **JAMA Neurol** 2016 Jan 19 (OnLine).

Plantar Fasciitis/Heel spurs
Gollwitzer H et al. Clinically relevant effectiveness of focused extracorporeal shock wave therapy in the treatment of chronic planta fasciitis. **J Bone Surg Am** 2015 May 6; 97:701.

Oliviera HAV et al. Effectiveness of total contact insoles in patients with plantar fasciitis. **J Rheumatol** 2015 May; 42:870.

Prostate
Anothaisintawee T et al. Management of chronic prostatitis/chronic pelvic pain syndrome. Meta-analysis. **JAMA** 2011 Jan 5; 305:78.

Rocco B, et al. Recent advances in the surgical treatment of benign prostatic hyperplasia. **Ther Adv Urol**. 2011 Dec; 3(6): 263–272.

Toren P et al. Effect of dutasteride on clinical progression of benign prostatic hyperplasia in asymptomatic men with enlarged prostate (REDUCE study). **BMJ** 2013 Apr 15; 346:f2109.

Robinson D et al. Use of 5-alpha reductase inhibitors for lower urinary tract symptoms and risk of prostate cancer in Swedish men. **BMJ** 2013 Jun 18; 346: f3406.

Filson CP et al. The efficacy and safety of combined therapy with alpha-blockers and anticholinergics for men with benign prostatic hyperplasia. A meta-analysis. **J Urol** 2013 Dec; 190:2153.

Roahrborn CG et al. Effects of tadalafil once daily on maximum urinary flow rate in men with lower urinary tract symptoms suggestive of benign prostatic hyperplasia. **J Urol** 2014 Apr; 191:1045.

McVary KT et al. A multicenter, randomized, double-blind, placebo controlled study of onabotulinumtoxin A 200 U to treat lower urinary tract symptoms in men with benign prostatic hyperplasia. **J Urol** 2014 Jul; 192: 150.

Wolin KY et al. Physical activity and benign prostatic hyperplasia-related outcomes and nocturia. **Med Sci Sports Exerc** 2014 Jul 9. [Epub].

Rheumatoid Arthritis

Lee EB et al. Tofacitinib versus methotrexate in rheumatoid arthritis. **N Engl J Med** 2014 Jun 19; 370:2377.

Fleischmann R et al. Placebo-controlled trial of tofacitinib monotherapy in rheumatoid arthritis. **N Engl J Med** 2012 Aug 9; 367:495

Di Guiseppe D et al. Long term alcohol intake and risk of rheumatoid arthritis in women. **BMJ** 2012 Jul 10; 345:e4230.

O'Dell JR et al. Therapies for active rheumatoid arthritis after methotrexate failure. **N Engl J Med** 2013 Jul 25; 369:307.

O'Dell JR et al. Validation of the methotrexate-first strategy in patients with early, poor-prognosis rheumatoid arthritis. **Arthritis Rheum** 2013 Aug; 65:1985.

Smolen JS et al. Adjustment of therapy in rheumatoid arthritis on the basis of achievement of stable low disease activity with adalimumab plus methotrexate or methotrexate alone (OPTIMA trial). **Lancet** 2013 Oct 26 (epub).

Lee EB et al. Tofacitinib versus methotrexate in rheumatoid arthritis. **N Engl J Med** 2014 Jun 19; 370:2377.

Restless Legs Syndrome

Trotti LM, Bhadriraju S, Becker LA. Iron for restless legs syndrome. **Cochrane Database of Systematic Reviews** 2012, Issue 5. Art. No.: CD007834. DOI: 10.1002/14651858.CD007834.pub2.

Scholz H, Trenkwalder C, Kohnen R, Kriston L, Riemann D, Hornyak M. Levodopa for the treatment of restless legs syndrome. **Cochrane Database of Systematic Reviews** 2011, Issue 2. Art. No.: CD005504. DOI: 10.1002/14651858.CD005504.pub2.

Scholz H, Trenkwalder C, Kohnen R, Kriston L, Riemann D, Hornyak M. Dopamine agonists for the treatment of restless legs syndrome. **Cochrane Database of Systematic Reviews** 2011, Issue 3. Art. No.: CD006009. DOI: 10.1002/14651858. CD006009.pub2.

Allen RP et al. Comparison of pregabalin with pramipexole for restless legs syndrome. **N Engl J Med** 2014 Feb 13; 370:621.

Eeden VD et al. . Risk of Cardiovascular Disease Associated with a Restless Legs Syndrome Diagnosis. **Sleep** 2015 Jul 1;38(7):1009-15. doi: 10.5665/sleep.4800.

Sciatica

Cohen SP et al. Epidural steroids, etanercept, or saline in subacute sciatica. **Ann Intern Med** 2012 Apr 17; 156:551.

Moreland LW et al. A randomized comparative effectiveness study of oral triple therapy versus etanercept plus methotrexate in early aggressive rheumatoid arthritis. **Arthritis Rheum** 2012 Sept; 64:2824.

Pinto RZ et al. Epidural corticosteroid injections in the management of sciatica: Meta-analysis. **Ann Intern Med** 2012 Nov 13 (epub).

El Barzouhi A et al. Magnetic resonance imaging in follow-up assessment of sciatica. **N Engl J Med** 2013 Mar 14; 368:999.

Goldberg H et al. Oral steroids for acute radiculopathy due to a herniated lumbar disc. **JAMA** 2015 May 19; 313:1915.

Chou R et al. Epidural corticosteroid injections for radiculopathy and spinal stenosis: a meta-analysis. **Ann Intern Med** 2015 Aug 25; (online).

Sexual Dysfunction

Hyde Z et al. Prevalence of sexual activity and associated factors in men aged 75 to 95 years. **Ann Intern Med** 2010 Dec 7; 153:693.

Aldemit M et al. Pistachio diet improves erectile dysfunction parameters and serum lipid profiles in patients with erectile dysfunction. **Int J Impot Res**. 2011; 23:32.

Lorenz TA et al. Acute Exercise Improves Physical Sexual Arousal in Women Taking Antidepressants. **Ann Behav Med**. 2012 Jun; 43(3): 352–361.

Spitzer M et al. Effect of testosterone replacement on response to sildenafil citrate in men with erectile dysfunction. **Ann Intern Med** 2012 Nov 20; 157:681.

Finkelstein JS et al. Gonadal steroids and body composition, strength, and sexual function in men. **N Engl J Med** 2013 Sep 12; 369:1011.

Vigen R et al. Association of testosterone therapy with mortality, myocardial infarction, and stroke in men with low testosterone levels. **JAMA** 2013 Nov 6; 310:1829.

Skeldon S, et al. Erectile dysfunction and undiagnosed diabetes, hypertension, and hypercholesterolemia. **Ann Fam Med** 2015 July/Aug; 13(4):331.

Shingles
Himal Lal, M.D., et al. Efficacy of an Adjuvanted Herpes Zoster Subunit Vaccine in Older Adults. **N Engl J Med** 2015 May 28; 372:2087

Phuc Le and Rothberg B. Cost-effectiveness of herpes zoster vaccine for persons aged 50 years. **Ann Int Med** 2015 Sept 8 (Online First).

Sinusitis
Vaidyanathan S et al. Treatment of chronic rhinosinusitis with nasal polyposis with oral steroids followed by topical steroids. **Ann Intern Med** 2011 Mar 1; 154:293.

Garbutt JM et al. Amoxicillin for acute rhinosinusitis. **JAMA** 2012 Feb 15; 307:685.

Rudmik L and Soler ZM. Medical therapies for adult chronic sinusitis: a systematic review. **JAMA** 2015 Sept 9; 314(9): 926.

Sprains, Strains, and Muscle Tears
Wise BL et al. Impact of age, sex, obesity and steroid use on quinolone-associated tendon disorders. **Am J Med** 2012 Dec; 125:1228.

Khan M et al. Arthroscopic surgery for degenerative tears of the meniscus: a systematic review and meta-analysis. **CMAJ** 2014 Aug 25; 10:1503.

Katz JN et al. Surgery versus physical therapy for a meniscal tear and osteoarthritis. **N Engl J Med** 2013 Mar 18; (epub).

Sihvonen R et al. Arthroscopic partial meniscectomy versus sham surgery for a degenerative meniscal tear. **N Engl J Med** 2013 Dec 26; 369:2515.

Dunn WR et al. Symptoms of pain do not correlate with rotator cuff severity. **J Bone Joint Surg Am** 2014 May 21; 96:793.

Rhon DI et al. One-year outcome of subacromial corticosteroid injection compared with manual physical therapy for the management of the unilateral shoulder impingement syndrome. **Ann Intern Med** 2014 Aug 5; 161:161.

Gibbons CH et al. Clinical implications of delayed orthostatic hypotension. **Neurology** 2015 Oct 20; 85:1362.

Kukkomen J et al. Treatment of nontraumatic rotator cuff tears. **J Bone Joint Surg Am** 2015 Nov 4; 97:1729.

Stroke

Ciccone A et al. Endovascular treatment for acute ischemic stroke. **N Engl J Med** 2013 Mar 7; 368:904.

Broderick JP et al. Endovascular therapy after intravenous t-PA versus t-PA alone for stroke. **N Engl J Med** 2013 Mar 7; 368:893.

Aburto NJ et al. Effect of increased potassium intake on cardiovascular risk factors and stroke. Meta-analyses. **BMJ** 2013 Apr 4; 346:f1378.

Zaidat OO et al. Effect of a balloon-expandable intracranial stent vs medical therapy on risk of stroke in patients with symptomatic intracranial stenosis. The VISSIT randomized clinical trial. **JAMA** 2015 Mar 24/31; 313:1240.

Goya, M, et al. Randomized Assessment of Rapid Endovascular Treatment of Ischemic Stroke. **N Engl J Med** 2015 March 12; 372:1019-1030

Thyroid

Turner MR et al. Levothyroxine dose and risk of fractures in older adults. **BMJ** 2011 Apr 28; 342:d2238.

Asvold BO et al. Serum TSH within the reference range as a predictor of future hypothyroidism and hyperthyroidism: 11 year follow-up of the HUNT study in Norway. **J Clin Endocrinol Metab** 2012 Jan; 97:93

Somwaru LL et al. The natural history of subclinical hypothyroidism in the elderly. **J Clin Endocrinol Metab** 2012 Jun; 97:1962.

Vita R et al. Impaired absorption of levothyroxine induced by proton pump inhibitors. **J Clin Endocrinol Metab** 2014 Dec; 99:4481.

Urinary Tract

Beerepoot MAJ et al. Lactobacilli vs. antibiotics to prevent urinary tract infections. **Arch Int Med** 2012 May 14; 172:704.

Cai T et al. The role of asymptomatic bacteriuria in young women with recurrent urinary tract infections: To treat or not to treat? **Clin Infect Dis** 2012 Sep 15; 55:771.

Wise BL et al. Impact of age, sex, obesity and steroid use on quinolone-associated tendon disorders. **Am J Med** 2012 Dec; 125:1228.

Gordon LB et al. Overtreatment of presumed urinary tract infection in older women presenting to the emergency department. **J Am Geriatr Soc** 2013 May; 61:788.

Etminan M et al. Oral flouroquinolone use and risk of peripheral neuropathy. **Neurology** 2014 Sept 30; 83:1261.

Grigoryan L et al. Diagnosis and management of urinary tract infections in the outpatient setting: A review. **JAMA** 2014 Oct 22/29; 312:1677.

Venous Insufficiency

Warson JM et al. Use of weekly, low dose, high frequency ultrasound for hard to heal venous leg ulcers. **BMJ** 2011 Mar 8; 342:d1092.

Evangelista MT et al. Simvastatin as a novel therapeutic agent for venous ulcers. **Br J Derm** 2014 May; 170(5): 1151.

Brittenden J et al. Surgical ligation, laser ablation or foam sclerotherapy for varicose veins? **N Engl J Med** 2014 Sept 25 (epub).

Venous Thrombosis

B Charlton, et al: The trouble with dabigatran, editorial. **BMJ**; July 23, 2014: 349.

Gomez-Outes A et al. Dabigatran, rivaroxaban, or apixaban versus enoxaparin for thromboprophylaxis after total hip or knee replacement: **BMJ** 2012 Jun 14; 344:e3675.

Baillargeon J et al. Concurrent use of warfarin and antibiotics and the risk of bleeding in older adults. **Am J Med** 2012 Feb; 125:183

Brighton TA et al. Low-dose aspirin for preventing recurrent venous thromboembolism. **N Engl J Med** 2012 Nov 4 (epub).

Schulman S et al. Extended use of dabigatran, warfarin, or placebo in venous thromboembolism. **N Engl J Med** 2013 Feb 21; 368:709.

Southworth MR et al. Dabigatran and postmarket reports of bleeding. **N Engl J Med** 2013 Apr 4; 368:1272.

Castellucci LA et al. Efficacy and safety outcomes of oral anticoagulants and antiplatelet drugs in the secondary prevention of venous thromboembolism: a meta-analysis. **BMJ** 2013 Aug 30; 347:f5133.

Lozano F et al. Home versus in-hospital treatment of outpatients with acute deep venous thrombosis of the lower limbs. **J Vasc Surg** 2014 May; 59:1362.

Sardar P et al. New oral anticoagulants in elderly adults. A meta-analysis. **J Am Geriatr Soc** 2014 May; 62:857.

Mismetti P et al. Effect of a retrievable inferior vena cava filter plus anticoagulation vs anticoagulation alone on risk of recurrent pulmonary emboli. **JAMA** 2015 Apr 28;313:627.

Carrier M et al. Screening for occult cancer in unprovoked venous thromboembolism. **N Engl J Med** 2015, Jun22; DOI 10.1056.

Pollack CV et al. Idarucizumab for dabigatran reversal. **N Engl J Med** 2015 Jun 22 (epub).

Cannegieter SC et al. Risk of venous and arterial thrombotic events in patients diagnosed with superficial vein thrombosis. **Blood** 2015 Jan 8; 125:229.

Eerenberg ES et al. Clinical impact and course of major bleeding with rivaroxaban and vitamin K antagonists. **J Thromb Haemost** 2014 Sep; 13:1590.

Weight Loss

Owan T et al. Favorable changes in cardiac geometry and function following gastric bypass surgery. **J Am Coll Cardiol** 2011 Feb 8; 57:732.

Gadde KM et al. Effects of low dose, controlled release, phentermine plus topiramate combination on weight and associated comorbidities in overweight and obese adults (CONQUER trial). **Lancet** 2011 Apr 16; 377:1341.

Elder CR et al. Impact of sleep, screen time, depression and stress on weight change in the intensive weight loss phase of the LIFE study. **Intnl J of Obesity** 2012 Jan. 36:86

Bhaskaran K, et al. Body-mass index and risk of 22 specific cancers: a population based cohort study of 5.24 million UK adults. **Lancet**. 14 August 2014.

Lee D-C et al. Changes in fitness and fatness on the development of cardiovascular disease risk factors: Hypertension, metabolic syndrome, and hypercholesterolemia. **J Am Coll Cardiol** 2012 Feb 14; 59:665.

Jolly K et al. Comparison of range of commercial or primary care led weight reduction programmes with minimal intervention control for weight loss in obesity. **BMJ** 2011 Nov 3; 343.

Sjostrom L et al. Bariatric surgery and long-term cardiovascular events. **JAMA** 2012 Jan 4; 307:56.

Schauer PR et al. Bariatric surgery versus intensive medical therapy in obese patients with diabetes. **N Engl J Med** 2012 Mar 26.

Ebbeling CB et al. Effects of dietary composition on energy expenditure during weight loss maintenance. **JAMA** 2012 Jun 27; 307:2627.

Adams TD et al. Health benefits of gastric bypass surgery after 6 years. **JAMA** 2012 Sept 19; 308:1122.

Hooper L et al. Effect of reducing total fat intake on body weight: Meta-analysis. **BMJ** 2012 Dec6; 345:e7666.

Flegal KM et al. Association of all cause mortality with overweight and obesity using standard body mass index categories: Meta-analysis. **JAMA** 2013 Jan 2; 309:71.

Te Morenga L et al. Dietary sugars and body weight: meta-analyses. **BMJ** 2013 Jan 15; 346:e7492.

Kullgren JT et al. Individual versus group based financial incentives for weight loss. **Ann Intern Med** 2013 Apr 2; 158:505.

Carlin AM et al. The comparative effectiveness of sleeve gastrectomy, gastric bypass, and adjustable gastric banding procedures for the treatment of morbid obesity. **Ann Surg** 2013 May; 257:791.

Block JP et al. Consumers' estimation of calorie content at fast food restaurants. **BMJ** 2013 May 23; 346:f2907.

Peterli R et al. Early results of the Swiss Multicentre Bypass or Sleeve study (SM-BOSS): comparing laparoscopic sleeve gastrectomy and Roux-en-Y gastric bypass. **Ann Surg** 2013 Nov; 258:690.

Gloy VL et al. Bariatric surgery versus non-surgical treatment for obesity. Meta-analysis. **BMJ** 2013 Oct 22; 347:f5934.

Kramer CK et al. Are metabolically healthy overweight and obesity benign conditions? A systematic review and meta-analysis of the effect of body mass index and metabolic status phenotypes on all-cause mortality and cardiovascular events. **Ann Intern Med** 2013 Dec 3; 159:758.

Courcoulas AP et al. Weight change and health outcomes at 3 years after bariatric surgery among individuals with severe obesity. **JAMA** 2013 Dec 11; 310:2416.

DuPree CE et al. Laparoscopic sleeve gastrectomy in patients with preexisting gastro-esophageal reflux disease. **JAMA Surg** 2014 Feb 5; (epub).

Krakauer NY, Krakauer JC Dynamic Association of Mortality Hazard with Body Shape. **PLoS ONE** 2015, Feb 20; 9(2): e88793.

Johnston BC et al. Comparison of weight loss among named diet programs in overweight and obese adults: A meta-analysis. **JAMA** 2014 Sep 3;312:859.

Bhaskaran K et al. Relation between excess weight and cancer incidence. **Lancet** 2–14 Aug 14 (epub).

Ikramuddin S et al. Effect of reversible intermittent intra-abdominal vagal nerve blockade on morbid obesity. **JAMA** 2014 Sep 3; 312:915.

Vinson JA et al. Retraction of study to evaluate the efficacy and safety of a green coffee bean extract in overweight subjects. **Diabetes, Metabolic Syndrome and Obesity**: Targets and therapy. 2014 Oct 3. (epub).

Arterburn D et al. Comparative effectiveness of laparoscopic gastric banding vs laparoscopic gastric bypass. **JAMA Surg** 2014 Oct 29 (epub).

Poirier SR et al. Long term effects of 4 popular diets on weight loss and cardiovascular risk factors: A meta-analysis. **Circ Cadiovasc Qual Outcomes**. 2014, November (online at American Heart Association).

Crous-Bou M et al. Mediterranean diet and telomere length in Nurse's Health Study. **BMJ** 2014 Dec 2; 349:g6674.

Zhang P et al. Visceral adiposity is negatively associated with bone density and muscle attenuation. **Amer J Nutr**. 2014 Feb; 101 (2): 337.

Gudzone K et al. Efficacy of commercial weight loss programs: An updated systematic review Efficacy of Commercial weight-loss programs. **Ann Intern Med** 2015, March; 162(7): 501.

Alison Fildes, PhD, et al. Probability of an Obese Person Attaining Normal Body Weight: Cohort Study Using Electronic Health Records. **Am J Public Health**, 2016 July 16 (epub).

Parretti HM et al. Efficacy of water preloading before main meals as strategy for weight loss in primary care patients with obesity. **Obesity** 2015 Aug 3 (Online).

Toledo E et al. Mediterranean diet and invasive breast cancer among women at high cardiovascular risk in the PREDIMED trial. **JAMA Intern Med** 2015 Sept 14 (epub).

Shuval K et al. Standing, Obesity, and Metabolic Syndrome. **Mayo Clin Proc**. 2015 Nov; 90(11): 1524.

Shakyan KR et al. Normal-weight central obesity: Implications for total and cardiovascular mortality. **Ann Int Med** 2015 Nov 10 (Online First).

Zeevi D, et al. Personalized Nutrition by Prediction of Glycemic Responses. **Cell** 2015 Nov 19. Volume 163, Issue 5, Pages 1079–1094.

Hogstrom G et al. Aerobic fitness in late adolescence and the risk of early death. **Intl J Epidemiol**. 2015 Dec 20 (online).

Wounds

Greer N et al. Advanced Wound Care Therapies for Non-Healing Diabetic, Venous, and Arterial Ulcers: A Systematic Review Washington (DC): Department of Veterans Affairs; 2012 Nov.

Cereda E et al. A nutritional formula enriched with arginine, zinc and antioxidants for the healing of pressure ulcers. **Ann Intern Med** 2015 Feb 3; 162:167.

APPENDIX

References, Referrals and Ordering

*I*MPORTANT NOTE: For updates, errata, scheduled events, interviews, and additional information, go to *www.DoctorSayWhat.com*. Also visit the author's *Facebook* page and follow him on *Twitter*.

Web References for Recommended Treatments

Low-Level Energy Laser
www.ML830.com
www.Erchonia.com
www.Theralase.com

Herbs and Supplements (Quality Assessments)
www.NaturalDataBase.com
www.ConsumerLab.com
www.USP.org (US Pharmacopeia)

Chinese Medicine (Acupuncture, Chinese Herbs)
www.NCCAOM.org
www.HealthConcerns.com
www.evherbs.com (Evergreen)
www.CraneHerb.com
www.nqa.org (QiGong/Tai Chi)

Naturopathy
www.Naturopathic.org

Homeopathy
www. nationalcenterforhomeopathy.org

Manual Therapy
Osteopathic
www.osteopathic.org/Pages/default.aspx

Chiropractic
www.acatoday.org

Alexander Technique
www.amsatonline.org
www.alexandertechnique.com

Feldenkrais Method
www.feldenkraisinstitute.com/

Rolfing
www.rolfing.org

Medical Newsletter
Berkeley Wellness
www.BerkeleyWellness.com

Medical Research Review
NEJM Journal Watch: www.JWatch.org

www.UpToDate.com

Mind-Body Techniques

Hypnosis
http://www.asch.net/
http://www.hypnosis.edu/aha/

Imagery
http://acadgi.com/

Biofeedback
www.aapb.org/providers.html

Interactive Imagery/ Active Imagination
http://www.deanschlecht.com/

Nambudripad Allergy Elimination Therapy
www.NAET.com

Nutrition
WWW.EatRight.org

Yoga
www.americanyogaassociation.org/

Important note: There are many other excellent references, but space does not allow mentioning them all. Information obtained from the above sources has been referenced throughout this book.

88406371R00372

Made in the USA
Columbia, SC
04 February 2018